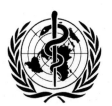

World Health Organization Classification of Tumours

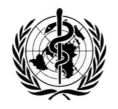

WHO   OMS

International Agency for Research on Cancer (IARC)

4th Edition

WHO Classification of Tumours of the Breast

Edited by

Sunil R. Lakhani

Ian O. Ellis

Stuart J. Schnitt

Puay Hoon Tan

Marc J. van de Vijver

International Agency for Research on Cancer

Lyon, 2012

World Health Organization Classification of Tumours

Series Editors   Fred T. Bosman, MD
Elaine S. Jaffe, MD
Sunil R. Lakhani, MD
Hiroko Ohgaki, PhD

WHO Classification of Tumours of the Breast

Editors   Sunil R. Lakhani, MD
Ian O. Ellis, MD
Stuart J. Schnitt, MD
Puay Hoon Tan, MD
Marc J. van de Vijver, MD, PhD

Technical Editors   Heidi Mattock, PhD
Rachel Purcell, PhD

Layout   Alberto Machado
Delphine Nicolas

Printed by   Participe Présent
69250 Neuville s/Saône, France

Publisher   International Agency for
Research on Cancer (IARC)
69372 Lyon Cedex 08, France

This volume was produced with support from the

MEDIC Foundation

The WHO Classification of Tumours of the Breast
presented in this book reflects the views of a Working Group
that convened for a Consensus and Editorial Meeting at the
International Agency for Research on Cancer (IARC), Lyon
September 1–3, 2011.

Members of the Working Group are indicated
in the List of Contributors on pages 196–202

Published by the International Agency for Research on Cancer (IARC),
150 cours Albert Thomas, 69372 Lyon Cedex 08, France

© International Agency for Research on Cancer, 2012

Distributed by
WHO Press, World Health Organization, 20 Avenue Appia, 1211 Geneva 27, Switzerland
(Tel: +41 22 791 3264; Fax: +41 22 791 4857; e-mail: bookorders@who.int).

Format for bibliographic citations:
Lakhani S.R., Ellis I.O., Schnitt S.J., Tan P.H., van de Vijver M.J. (Eds.):
WHO Classification of Tumours of the Breast.
IARC: Lyon 2012

IARC Library Cataloguing in Publication Data

WHO classification of tumours of the breast / edited by Sunil R Lakhani ... [et al.] – 4th edition

(World Health Organization classification of tumours)

1. Breast Neoplasms – genetics 2. Breast Neoplasms – classification
3. Breast Neoplasms – pathology I. Lakhani, Sunil R. II. Series

ISBN 978-92-832-2433-4   (NLM Classification: WI 1)

Contents

WHO classification of tumours of the breast

EPITHELIAL TUMOURS

Microinvasive carcinoma

Invasive breast carcinoma

Invasive carcinoma of no special type (NST)	8500/3
Pleomorphic carcinoma	8022/3
Carcinoma with osteoclast-like stromal	
giant cells	8035/3
Carcinoma with choriocarcinomatous	
features	
Carcinoma with melanotic features	
Invasive lobular carcinoma	8520/3
Classic lobular carcinoma	
Solid lobular carcinoma	
Alveolar lobular carcinoma	
Pleomorphic lobular carcinoma	
Tubulolobular carcinoma	
Mixed lobular carcinoma	
Tubular carcinoma	8211/3
Cribriform carcinoma	8201/3
Mucinous carcinoma	8480/3
Carcinoma with medullary features	
Medullary carcinoma	8510/3
Atypical medullary carcinoma	8513/3
Invasive carcinoma NST with medullary	
features	8500/3
Carcinoma with apocrine differentiation	
Carcinoma with signet-ring-cell differentiation	
Invasive micropapillary carcinoma	8507/3*
Metaplastic carcinoma of no special type	8575/3
Low-grade adenosquamous carcinoma	8570/3
Fibromatosis-like metaplastic carcinoma	8572/3
Squamous cell carcinoma	8070/3
Spindle cell carcinoma	8032/3
Metaplastic carcinoma with	
mesenchymal differentiation	
Chondroid differentiation	8571/3
Osseous differentiation	8571/3
Other types of mesenchymal	
differentiation	8575/3
Mixed metaplastic carcinoma	8575/3
Myoepithelial carcinoma	8982/3

Rare types	
Carcinoma with neuroendocrine features	
Neuroendocrine tumour, well-differentiated	8246/3
Neuroendocrine carcinoma, poorly	
differentiated (small cell carcinoma)	8041/3
Carcinoma with neuroendocrine	
differentiation	8574/3
Secretory carcinoma	8502/3

Invasive papillary carcinoma	8503/3
Acinic cell carcinoma	8550/3
Mucoepidermoid carcinoma	8430/3
Polymorphous carcinoma	8525/3
Oncocytic carcinoma	8290/3
Lipid-rich carcinoma	8314/3
Glycogen-rich clear cell carcinoma	8315/3
Sebaceous carcinoma	8410/3
Salivary gland/skin adnexal type tumours	
Cylindroma	8200/0
Clear cell hidradenoma	8402/0*

Epithelial–myoepithelial tumours

Pleomorphic adenoma	8940/0
Adenomyoepithelioma	8983/0
Adenomyoepithelioma with carcinoma	8983/3*
Adenoid cystic carcinoma	8200/3

Precursor lesions

Ductal carcinoma in situ	8500/2
Lobular neoplasia	
Lobular carcinoma in situ	
Classic lobular carcinoma in situ	8520/2
Pleomorphic lobular carcinoma in situ	8519/2*
Atypical lobular hyperplasia	

Intraductal proliferative lesions

Usual ductal hyperplasia
Columnar cell lesions including flat epithelial
 atypia
Atypical ductal hyperplasia

Papillary lesions

Intraductal papilloma	8503/0
Intraductal papilloma with atypical	
hyperplasia	8503/0
Intraductal papilloma with ductal	
carcinoma in situ	8503/2*
Intraductal papilloma with lobular	
carcinoma in situ	8520/2
Intraductal papillary carcinoma	8503/2
Encapsulated papillary carcinoma	8504/2
Encapsulated papillary carcinoma with	
invasion	8504/3
Solid papillary carcinoma	
In situ	8509/2
Invasive	8509/3

Benign epithelial proliferations

Sclerosing adenosis
Apocrine adenosis
Microglandular adenosis

Radial scar/complex sclerosing lesion
Adenomas
    Tubular adenoma 8211/0
    Lactating adenoma 8204/0
    Apocrine adenoma 8401/0
    Ductal adenoma 8503/0

MESENCHYMAL TUMOURS

Nodular fasciitis 8828/0*
Myofibroblastoma 8825/0
Desmoid-type fibromatosis 8821/1
Inflammatory myofibroblastic tumour 8825/1
Benign vascular lesions
    Haemangioma 9120/0
    Angiomatosis
    Atypical vascular lesions
Pseudoangiomatous stromal hyperplasia
Granular cell tumour 9580/0
Benign peripheral nerve-sheath tumours
    Neurofibroma 9540/0
    Schwannoma 9560/0
Lipoma 8850/0
    Angiolipoma 8861/0
Liposarcoma 8850/3
Angiosarcoma 9120/3
Rhabdomyosarcoma 8900/3
Osteosarcoma 9180/3
Leiomyoma 8890/0
Leiomyosarcoma 8890/3

FIBROEPITHELIAL TUMOURS

Fibroadenoma 9010/0
Phyllodes tumour 9020/1
    Benign 9020/0
    Borderline 9020/1
    Malignant 9020/3
    Periductal stromal tumour, low grade 9020/3
Hamartoma

TUMOURS OF THE NIPPLE

Nipple adenoma 8506/0
Syringomatous tumour 8407/0
Paget disease of the nipple 8540/3

MALIGNANT LYMPHOMA

Diffuse large B-cell lymphoma 9680/3
Burkitt lymphoma 9687/3
T-cell lymphoma
    Anaplastic large cell lymphoma,
      ALK-negative 9702/3
Extranodal marginal-zone B-cell lymphoma
  of MALT type 9699/3
Follicular lymphoma 9690/3

METASTATIC TUMOURS

TUMOURS OF THE MALE BREAST

Gynaecomastia
Carcinoma
    Invasive carcinoma 8500/3
    In situ carcinoma 8500/2

CLINICAL PATTERNS

Inflammatory carcinoma 8530/3
Bilateral breast carcinoma

---

[a] The morphology codes are from the International Classification of Diseases for Oncology (ICD-O) {463B}. Behaviour is coded /0 for benign tumours, /1 for unspecified, borderline or uncertain behaviour, /2 for carcinoma in situ and grade III intraepithelial neoplasia, and /3 for malignant tumours; [b] The classification is modified from the previous WHO histological classification of tumours {1413} taking into account changes in our understanding of these lesions. In the case of neuroendocrine neoplasms, the classification has been simplified to be of more practical utility in morphological classification; * These new codes were approved by the IARC/WHO Committee for ICD-O.

TNM classification of tumours of the breast

T – Primary tumour

TX	Primary tumour cannot be assessed
T0	No evidence of primary tumour
Tis	Carcinoma in situ
Tis (DCIS)	Ductal carcinoma in situ
Tis (LCIS)	Lobular carcinoma in situ
Tis (Paget)	Paget disease of the nipple not associated with invasive carcinoma and/or carcinoma in situ (DCIS and/or LCIS) in the underlying breast parenchyma.

Note: Carcinomas in the breast parenchyma associated with Paget disease are categorized based on the size and characteristics of the parenchymal disease, although the presence of Paget disease should still be noted.

T1	Tumour 2 cm or less in greatest dimension
T1mi	Microinvasion 0.1 cm or less in greatest dimension*

Note: *Microinvasion is the extension of cancer cells beyond the basement membrane into the adjacent tissues with no focus more than 0.1 cm in greatest dimension. When there are multiple foci of microinvasion, the size of only the largest focus is used to classify the microinvasion. (Do not use the sum of all individual foci.) The presence of multiple foci of microinvasion should be noted, as it is with multiple larger invasive carcinomas.

T1a	More than 0.1 cm but not more than 0.5 cm in greatest dimension
T1b	More than 0.5 cm but not more than 1 cm in greatest dimension
T1c	More than 1 cm but not more than 2 cm in greatest dimension
T2	Tumour more than 2 cm but not more than 5 cm in greatest dimension
T3	Tumour more than 5 cm in greatest dimension
T4	Tumour of any size with direct extension to chest wall and/or to skin (ulceration or skin nodules)

Note: Invasion of the dermis alone does not qualify as T4. Chest wall includes ribs, intercostal muscles, and serratus anterior muscle but not pectoral muscle.

T4a	Extension to chest wall (does not include pectoralis muscle invasion only)
T4b	Ulceration, ipsilateral satellite skin nodules, or skin oedema (including peau d'orange)
T4c	Both 4a and 4b, above
T4d	Inflammatory carcinoma

Note: Inflammatory carcinoma of the breast is characterized by diffuse, brawny induration of the skin with an erysipeloid edge, usually with no underlying mass. If the skin biopsy is negative and there is no localized measurable primary cancer, the T category is pTX when pathologically staging a clinical inflammatory carcinoma (T4d). Dimpling of the skin, nipple retraction, or other skin changes, except those in T4b and T4d, may occur in T1, T2, or T3 without affecting the classification.

N – Regional lymph nodes

NX	Regional lymph nodes cannot be assessed (e.g. previously removed)
N0	No regional lymph-node metastasis
N1	Metastasis in movable ipsilateral level I, II axillary lymph node(s)
N2	Metastasis in ipsilateral level I, II axillary lymph node(s) that are clinically fixed or matted; or in clinically detected* ipsilateral internal mammary lymph node(s) in the absence of clinically evident axillary lymph-node metastasis
N2a	Metastasis in axillary lymph node(s) fixed to one another (matted) or to other structures
N2b	Metastasis only in clinically detected* internal mammary lymph node(s) and in the absence of clinically detected axillary lymph-node metastasis
N3	Metastasis in ipsilateral infraclavicular (level III axillary) lymph node(s) with or without level I, II axillary lymph-node involvement; or in clinically detected* ipsilateral internal mammary lymph node(s) with clinically evident level I, II axillary lymph-node metastasis; or metastasis in ipsilateral supraclavicular lymph node(s) with or without axillary or internal mammary lymph node involvement
N3a	Metastasis in infraclavicular lymph node(s)
N3b	Metastasis in internal mammary and axillary lymph nodes
N3c	Metastasis in supraclavicular lymph node(s)

Note: * "Clinically detected" is defined as detected by clinical examination or by imaging studies (excluding lymphoscintigraphy) and having characteristics highly suspicious for malignancy or a presumed pathological macrometastasis based on fine-needle aspiration biopsy with cytological examination. Confirmation of clinically detected metastatic disease by fine-needle aspiration without excision biopsy is designated with an (f) suffix, e.g., cN3a(f).

Excisional biopsy of a lymph node or biopsy of a sentinel node, in the absence of assignment of a pT, is classified as a clinical N, e.g., cN1. Pathological classification (pN) is used for excision or sentinel lymph node biopsy only in conjunction with a pathological T assignment.

M – Distant metastasis

M0	No distant metastasis
M1	Distant metastasis

pN – Regional lymph nodes

The pathological classification requires the resection and examination of at least the low axillary lymph nodes (level I). Such a resection will ordinarily include six or more lymph nodes. If the lymph nodes are negative, but the number ordinarily examined is not met, classify as pN0.

pNX   Regional lymph nodes cannot be assessed e.g. previously removed, or not removed for study)

pN0   No regional lymph-node metastasis*

Note: *Isolated tumour cells (ITC) are single tumour cells or small clusters of cells not more than 0.2 mm in greatest extent that can be detected by routine H & E stains or immunohistochemistry. An additional criterion has been proposed to include a cluster of fewer than 200 cells in a single histological cross-section. Nodes containing only ITCs are excluded from the total positive node count for purposes of N classification and should be included in the total number of nodes evaluated.

pN1   Micrometastasis; or metastasis in 1–3 axillary ipsilateral lymph nodes; and/or in internal mammary nodes with metastasis detected by sentinel lymph-node biopsy but not clinically detected *

    pN1mi   Micrometastasis (larger than 0.2 mm and/or more than 200 cells, but none larger than 2.0 mm)

    pN1a   Metastasis in 1–3 axillary lymph node(s), including at least 1 larger than 2 mm in greatest dimension

    pN1b   Internal mammary lymph nodes with microscopic or macroscopic metastasis detected by sentinel lymph node biopsy but not clinically detected

    pN1c   Metastasis in 1–3 axillary lymph nodes and internal mammary lymph nodes with microscopic or macroscopic metastasis detected by sentinel lymph-node biopsy but not clinically detected

pN2   Metastasis as described below:

    pN2a   Metastasis in 4–9 axillary lymph nodes, including at least one that is larger than 2 mm

    pN2b   Metastasis in clinically detected* internal mammary lymph node(s), in the absence of axillary lymph-node metastasis

pN3   Metastasis as described below:

    pN3a   Metastasis in 10 or more axillary lymph nodes (at least one larger than 2 mm) or metastasis in

infraclavicular lymph nodes

    pN3b   Metastasis in clinically detected* internal ipsilateral mammary lymph node(s) in the presence of positive axillary lymph node(s); or metastasis in more than 3 axillary lymph nodes and in internal mammary lymph nodes with microscopic or macroscopic metastasis detected by sentinel lymph-node biopsy but not clinically detected

    pN3c   Metastasis in ipsilateral supraclavicular lymph node(s)

Note: * "Clinically detected" is defined as detected by imaging studies (excluding lymphoscintigraphy) or by clinical examination and having characteristics highly suspicious for malignancy or a presumed pathological macrometastasis based on fine-needle aspiration biopsy with cytological examination.

Not clinically detected is defined as not detected by imaging studies (excluding lymphoscintigraphy) or not detected by clinical examination.

Post-treatment ypN

- Post-treatment ypN should be evaluated as for clinical (pretreatment) N methods above. The modifier sn is used only if a sentinel-node evaluation was performed after treatment. If no subscript is attached, it is assumed the axillary nodal evaluation was by axillary-node dissection.
- The X classification will be used (ypNX) if no yp post-treatment SN or axillary dissection was performed
- N categories are the same as those used for pN.

Stage grouping

Stage 0	Tis	N0	M0
Stage IA	T1	N0	M0
Stage IB	T0, T1	N1mi	M0
Stage IIA	T0, T1	N1	M0
	T2	N0	M0
Stage IIB	T2	N1	M0
	T3	N0	M0
Stage IIIA	T0, T1, T2	N2	M0
	T3	N1, N2	M0
Stage IIIB	T4	N0, N1,N2	M0
Stage IIIC	Any T	N3	M0
Stage IV	Any T	Any N	M1

A help-desk for specific questions about the TNM classification is available at http://www.uicc.org.

References

1. American Joint Committee on Cancer (AJCC) Cancer Staging Manual 7th ed. Edge SB, Byrd DR, Compton CC, Fritz AG, Greene FL, Trotti III H. eds. New York: Springer. 2009

2. International Union against Cancer (UICC): TNM classification of malignant tumors 7th ed. Sobin LH, Gospodarowicz MK, Wittekind Ch. eds. Wiley-Blackwell. Oxford. 2009

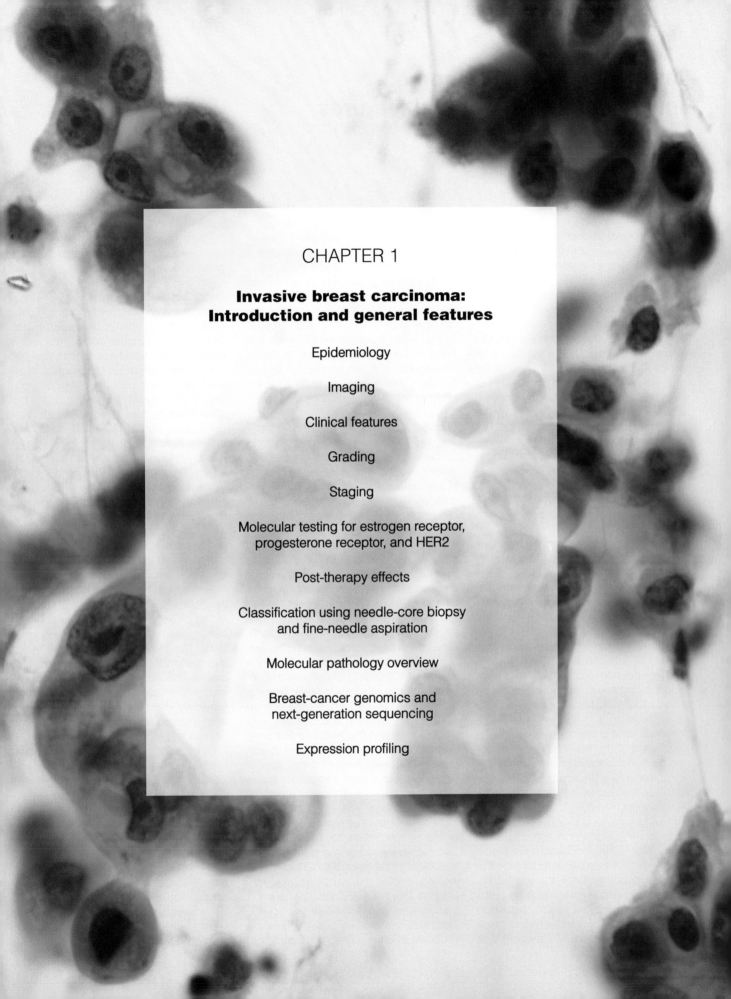

CHAPTER 1

Invasive breast carcinoma: Introduction and general features

Epidemiology

Imaging

Clinical features

Grading

Staging

Molecular testing for estrogen receptor,
progesterone receptor, and HER2

Post-therapy effects

Classification using needle-core biopsy
and fine-needle aspiration

Molecular pathology overview

Breast-cancer genomics and
next-generation sequencing

Expression profiling

Invasive breast carcinoma: Introduction and general features

Epidemiology

G. Colditz
K.S. Chia

Invasive breast cancer is the most common carcinoma in women. Accounting for 23% of all cancers in women globally and 27% in affluent countries, it is more than twice as common as cancer at any other site {432}.

As with most epithelial tumours, the incidence of breast cancer increases rapidly with age. Worldwide, the incidence of breast cancer varies 10-fold. The areas of high risk are the affluent populations of Australia, Europe and North America, where 6% of women develop invasive breast cancer before age 75 years. The risk of breast cancer is low in less developed regions of sub-Saharan Africa and in parts of southern and eastern Asia (including Japan), where the probability of developing breast cancer by age 75 years is one third that of rich countries.

Geographical variations, time trends, and studies of populations migrating from low- to high-risk areas show that the risk for migrant populations approaches that of the host country within one or two generations; this suggests an important role for environmental factors in the etiology of this disease.

The risk of developing breast cancer was increasing until the early 1980s in more and less developed countries. Rates of incidence continue to increase in less developed countries, but have been levelling off or declining in more developed countries as a result of mammographic screening. Since 2005, there has been a decrease in incidence in several countries in Europe and the USA, which is partly attributable to the decreasing use of hormone-replacement therapy.

The prognosis for patients with this disease is very good if it is detected at an early stage. While significant improvements in survival have been recorded in more developed countries since the late 1970s, advances have been dramatic in the 1990s owing to the combined effect of population screening and adjuvant hormonal treatment and chemotherapy, especially with the introduction of second- and third-generation chemotherapy agents and aromatase inhibitors. As a result, the trend towards increasing mortality observed until the 1980s has declined in several high-risk countries, e.g. Australia, Canada and the USA. During the last 10 years, mortality has been consistently decreasing in these countries, but increasing in Japan, the Republic of Korea, and Russia. Mortality rates no longer reflect trends in the underlying risk of developing the disease.

Etiology

The origin of breast cancer is multifactorial and involves diet, reproductive factors, and hormones. The etiological journey begins in utero and continues throughout life with a variety of exposures modulating risk at different times {773}. From descriptive epidemiological data it has clearly emerged that breast cancer is a disease of affluent societies that have acquired the "Western lifestyle", characterized by a high-calorie diet rich in animal fat and proteins, combined with a lack of physical exercise. Regions that have featured this lifestyle for a long time (Australia, North America, northern Europe) have reached a plateau of incidence with an annual rate of 70–90 new cases per 100 000 population, while countries that have relatively recently become industrialized and affluent show a marked increase in incidence and mortality, e.g. India, Japan and the Republic of Korea. Specific environmental exposures operative in the development of breast cancer (e.g. radiation, alcohol, exogenous hormones) have been identified, but are associated with a lower risk.

More than most other human neoplasms, breast cancer shows familial clustering. Two high-penetrance genes have been identified (*BRCA1* and *BRCA2*) that greatly increase the risk of developing breast cancer (see Chapter 16). Additional polymorphisms and genes have been recently identified, primarily via genome-wide association studies (GWAS), which are of medium or low penetrance and convey lower risks. The evidence suggests a polygenic origin for this disease.

Reproductive lifestyle

A woman's reproductive history is highly associated with the risk of breast cancer. The disease occurs more frequently among women who have an early menarche, remain nulliparous or, if parous, have few children with a late age at first delivery {981,1163}. Infertility per se appears to be a risk factor, as does lack of breast-feeding {841}. Late age at menopause also increases the risk. Most of these factors have also been found to be relevant in populations with a low risk of breast cancer, such as the Japanese and Chinese. Any delivery before the age of 30 years appears to have a protective effect {1222}.

It is believed that changes in reproductive patterns account for much of the drastic increase in risk in countries like China and Singapore. Although the data for Africa are limited, at least one study has confirmed the increased risk associated with late age at first delivery, reduced number of pregnancies and shorter breast-feeding time {794}. Controversy still surrounds the issue of abortion: some studies, but not others, have found an increased risk associated with induced abortion. Similarly, the protective effect of lactation, once considered a strong factor, has latterly been attributed less influence; its impact appears to be limited to long-term cumulative breast feeding, preferably more than 2 years {828}.

Endogenous hormones

There is overwhelming evidence from epidemiological studies that sex steroids (androgens, estrogens, progestogens) have an important role in the development of breast carcinomas. Breast-cancer incidence rates rise more steeply with age before menopause (approximately 8% per year) than after (approximately 2% per year) {279}, when ovarian synthesis of estrogen and progesterone ceases and ovarian production of androgens gradually diminishes.

Growing evidence shows a strong and consistent link between blood concentrations of estrogen and testosterone in postmenopausal women and risk of developing breast cancer. The combined prospective data show that the positive relationship between circulating hormone concentrations and breast cancer is dominant and independent of a woman's level of obesity and other risk factors {686}. In the updated analysis from the Nurses' Health Study, the risk of breast cancer increases three- to fourfold with increasing hormone concentrations from the bottom to the top quarter of the population. This increase in risk is strongest for breast tumours that are classified as positive for estrogen receptor (ER) {927}. Among premenopausal women, higher follicular concentrations of total and free estradiol are associated with an increased risk of breast cancer, as are higher concentrations of testosterone, but not progesterone or sex hormone-binding globulin (SHBG) {374}.

Higher concentrations of prolactin are associated with an increase in risk among both pre- and postmenopausal women {1380} and are more strongly related to ER-positive breast cancer {1474}. While initial studies suggested that high normal-range values for insulin-like growth factor (IGF) were associated with premenopausal but not postmenopausal breast cancer {548,1174}, further detailed analysis of common genetic variation in 18 genes in the IGF pathway showed a limited relationship between single-nucleotide polymorphisms (SNPs) and circulating concentrations of IGF and IGFBP-3 (accounting for 3.9% of variation), but no significant association with risk of breast cancer {521}.

Exogenous hormones

Oral contraceptives

It was previously believed that oral contraceptives might increase the risk of breast cancer, since they contain estrogen and progestin (a synthetic progestogen that resembles progesterone) at concentrations that may exceed those produced during a normal ovulatory cycle {122}. Combined data from more than 50 studies (53 000 cases) have provided considerable reassurance that there is little, if any, increase in risk associated with use of oral contraceptives in general, even among women who

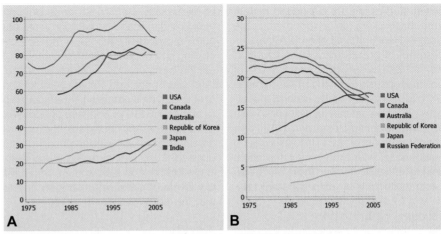

Fig. 1.01 A Incidence of breast cancer in selected countries, 1975–2005. **B** Mortality from breast cancer in selected countries, 1975–2005 {432}.

have used oral contraceptives for 10 or more years {280}. However, current users and recent users (< 10 years since last use) have a modest elevation in risk compared to never-users. The relative risk for current users compared to never-users was 1.24 (a 24% increase in risk), while the relative risks for women 1–4 years after stopping and 5–9 years after stopping were 1.16 and 1.07, respectively {280}. IARC has concluded that estrogen-progestogen oral contraceptives (combined) are a class 1 carcinogen. A more contemporary national study in the USA showed no increase in risk among current users, perhaps reflecting changes in contraceptive formulation since the earlier studies {873}.

Postmenopausal hormone-replacement therapy

The relationship between postmenopausal use of estrogens and risk of breast cancer has been investigated in many epidemiological studies over the past 30 years, with substantial advances in the past decade. Increased risk has been observed in two important subgroups – long-duration users and current users – although the magnitude of risk varies according to whether the therapy included estrogen alone, or estrogen plus progestin.

Unopposed estrogen therapy

In a large reanalysis that combined data from 51 epidemiological studies, the investigators observed a statistically significant association between current or recent use of predominantly unopposed estrogen and risk of breast cancer, with the strongest positive association among women with

the longest duration of use {281}. Among postmenopausal women who had used hormones within the previous 5 years (compared to never-users), the relative risks were 1.1 for a duration of use of 1–4 years, 1.3 for 5–9 years, 1.2 for 10–14 years, and 1.6 for 15 years or more. No significant increase in risk was noted for women who had stopped using postmenopausal hormone therapy 5 years or more previously, regardless of duration. Of note, this increase in risk was significantly higher among lean women than among obese women (who would naturally have higher levels of endogenous hormones than lean women) {281}. The Nurses' Health Study also reported that the adverse effect of postmenopausal hormones was largely limited to women with little or no adult weight gain {607}.

The randomized controlled trial within the Women's Health Initiative (WHI) among women who had had a hysterectomy showed no increase in the risk of developing invasive breast cancer over the nine years of follow-up {1371}. The mean body mass index (BMI) of these women was 27 at baseline, far greater than the level of obesity recorded in the Nurses' Health Study and in the earlier studies combined in the reanalysis {281}. Chen and colleagues showed that the risk of developing breast cancer was not elevated until after 10 years of use of unopposed estrogen, consistent with the WHI, and that after 20 years of use the risk of breast cancer was 1.42 (95% CI, 1.05–2.07) {256}. Also, the carcinomas developing were more likely to be ER-positive. Data on how recently a woman has used hormones and risk of breast cancer are sparse because many earlier studies did not distinguish current from past users. In a report from the Nurses' Health Study cohort {278}, an excess risk of breast cancer was limited to women with current or very recent use of postmenopausal hormones. Data from the UK Million Women Study confirm the excess risk of breast cancer associated with use of unopposed estrogen {117} and show the impact of timing in relationship to menopause, with greater adverse effect among leaner women and those who begin therapy within 5 years of menopause {118}.

Estrogen plus progestin
The addition of a progestin to estrogen regimens became increasingly common from the 1980s to 2000; this addition minimizes or eliminates the increased risk of endometrial hyperplasia and endometrial cancer associated with using unopposed estrogens. The impact of added progestin on the risk of breast cancer has been evaluated rigorously only in the last 15 years; overall, the results of these studies indicate that added progestin at the doses typically used in postmenopausal hormone-replacement therapy does not have a protective effect against breast cancer {281,1616}. In fact, the WHI showed a significant increase in the risk of developing breast cancer among women taking estrogen plus progestin and that this risk rose with increasing duration of use {264,1225}. Moreover, the adverse effect of combination estrogen-plus-progestin was underestimated in the WHI as some women in this randomized trial were counted in the primary analysis despite having stopped receiving the drug combination. The results of the UK Million Women Study suggested that the relative risk of breast cancer for current users of estrogen-only preparations compared to never-users was 1.30 (95% CI, 1.22–1.38), while the relative risk for current users of estrogen-plus-progestin combinations was 2.00 (95% CI, 1.91–2.09); this observed difference in the magnitudes of the associated risk was highly significant {117}. Importantly, recent data from the WHI also show that mortality from breast cancer is elevated among women who have used estrogen-plus-progestin combinations {263}.
Because widespread use of estrogen plus progestin is so recent, few data are currently available to evaluate the effect of different formulations, doses, or schedules of use of progestin on risk of breast cancer. The results from the UK Million Women

Study provide the largest range of information and indicate little variation in risk according to dose of estrogen or regimen, including oral or patch administration {117}. On the basis of a review of the evidence, IARC has concluded that the combination of estrogen plus progestin is carcinogenic to humans {618}. In addition, unopposed estrogen therapy increases the risk of breast cancer, with risk augmenting with duration of use. Furthermore, this rise in risk is greatest among lean women, who have low levels of circulating estrogen due to their low body mass.

Adiposity
The relationship between adiposity and breast cancer depends on menopausal status: in affluent industrialized populations with high rates of breast cancer, measures of body adiposity are inversely related to risk of premenopausal breast cancer, but positively related to risk of postmenopausal breast cancer.
A modest inverse relationship between adiposity (typically measured as body mass index, BMI) and incidence of premenopausal breast cancer has been consistently observed in both case–control and cohort studies {1479}. Heavier premenopausal women, even those at the upper limits of what are considered to be healthy weights, have more irregular menstrual cycles and increased rates of anovulatory infertility {1181}, suggesting that their lower risk may be due to fewer ovulatory cycles and less exposure to ovarian hormones.
In case–control and prospective studies conducted in affluent industrialized countries, the association between BMI and risk of breast cancer among postmenopausal women has been only weakly positive {602,614}. The lack of a stronger association has been surprising because plasma concentrations of endogenous estrogens are nearly twice as high in obese postmenopausal women as in lean women {547}. However, an elevated BMI in a postmenopausal woman represents two opposing risks: a protective effect due to the correlation between early weight and postmenopausal weight (those who are obese premenopausally are also obese postmenopausally), and the adverse effect of elevated plasma concentrations of endogenous estrogens attributable to adiposity after menopause. For this reason, body-weight gain between early adult life and after the menopause should be more strongly related to risk of postmenopausal

breast cancer than attained weight, and this has been consistently supported by case–control {1629} and prospective studies {278,607,765}. Another reason for failing to appreciate a greater adverse effect of excessive weight or weight gain on risk of postmenopausal breast cancer is that the use of postmenopausal hormones obscures the variation in endogenous estrogens attributable to adiposity and elevates risk of breast cancer regardless of body weight. Among women who had never used postmenopausal hormone therapy in the Nurses' Health Study, those who gained 25 kg or more after age 18 years had double the risk of breast cancer of women who maintained their weight to within 2 kg {607}. In 2002, IARC concluded that overweight and obesity cause postmenopausal breast cancer and that current levels of obesity in the USA cause approximately 10% of cases of postmenopausal breast cancer.
Weight loss in adult years and after menopause has been studied in a limited fashion, partly because few women lose weight and avoid regaining it. Recent prospective data from the Nurses' Health Study show that weight loss after menopause is associated with a reduced risk of breast cancer, particularly of ER-positive tumours {373}. Women who lose 10 kg or more and maintain this weight loss have a 40% reduction in their risk of breast cancer.

Physical activity
The relationship between physical activity and risk of breast cancer has been assessed by IARC, which concluded that higher levels of activity are associated with a reduction in risk {622,1599}. Evidence for a dose–response effect was found in most of the studies that examined the trend. Most studies have focused on postmenopausal breast cancer, although there is also some evidence for a protective effect of physical activity on premenopausal disease. Recent evidence shows that the benefit of activity is independent of race or ethnicity {123}. The strongest protection against breast cancer has been reported in women maintaining consistent high levels of activity from menarche through adult life {123,888}.

Nutrition
There is some evidence of a decrease in the risk of breast cancer in individuals with healthy dietary patterns, although a recent

meta-analysis and large cohort studies found no evidence of increased risk of breast cancer associated with "Western" unhealthy dietary patterns {27,508,671} and high intakes of fruit and vegetables are not associated with a reduced risk of breast cancer in recent studies {156}. Rapid growth and greater adult height, partly reflecting total food intake in early years, are associated with an increased risk. Similarly, a high body mass, also linked to a high total caloric intake, or intake not counterbalanced by caloric expenditure, is a risk factor for postmenopausal breast cancer. Total intake of fat, and saturated animal fat, may also increase the risk.

Consistent evidence suggests that higher consumption of meat, particularly red or fried/browned meat, is associated with a higher risk of breast cancer {671}.

Alcohol
The consumption of alcohol has been consistently associated with a moderate increase in the risk of breast cancer {1345, 1386}. According to the dose–response relationship (number of drinks per day), even a low level of consumption was associated with an increase in risk. Evidence suggests that high intake or high blood levels of folate may decrease risk {1624}.

Cigarette smoking
According to the USA Surgeon General's 2004 report on the health consequences of smoking, the evidence suggested no causal relationship between active smoking and breast cancer {1394}. Similarly, the combined data from 53 epidemiological studies showed no relationship between smoking and breast cancer among women who do not drink alcohol {538}.

However, substantial additional evidence has accumulated in the past decade, and a review conducted in 2009 by a Canadian task force concluded that active smoking is causally related to both pre- and postmenopausal breast cancer. Furthermore, this task force concluded that second-hand smoke ("passive smoking") is causally related to premenopausal breast cancer, but that the data were insufficient to allow a conclusion to be made for postmenopausal breast cancer {287}.

Single-nucleotide polymorphisms
Recent studies have included advanced methods to scan the whole genome for genetic changes (GWAS) that may convey an increased risk of breast cancer. Results to date do not show any applications for these methods to either demarcate risk or offer strategies for prevention {1101}.

Imaging

R. Wilson
P. Britton

Detection
Mammography is the baseline imaging method for the detection of breast cancer in women aged > 40 years. Invasive breast cancer is most commonly manifested on mammography as an ill-defined or spiculated mass, with or without associated calcifications, but can also present as architectural distortion, focal asymmetric density or calcifications alone. Ultrasound can be added to improve sensitivity in women with mammographically dense breasts.

Mammography is rarely helpful in younger women and its use in women aged < 40 years is confined to those with proven breast cancer. Ultrasound alone is the method of choice for imaging the breast in women aged < 40 years. Magnetic resonance imaging (MRI) is the most sensitive method for detecting breast cancer, but its use is confined to screening women at very high risk (e.g. carriers of mutations in the *BRCA1* or *BRCA2* genes) and local staging of certain breast cancers (see below).

Further assessment and staging
Imaging should always be used to assess both breasts before any treatment is implemented. Mammography and ultrasound are complementary for the pretreatment assessment of the size, extent and presence of multifocality of breast cancer. The vast majority of breast cancers should be diagnosed without the need for surgical biopsy using imaging-directed needle sampling; ultrasound-guided core biopsy is the method of choice. Ultrasound is also used routinely to assess the axilla at the time of presentation, with biopsy of any abnormal lymph nodes. MRI can be used to improve pretreatment staging of the breast where there is doubt about the extent of disease after mammography and ultrasound (e.g. in the dense breast) and routinely for invasive lobular carcinoma.

Table 1.01 Mammographic appearance of histologically malignant breast lesions

Appearance	Proportion of lesions
Stellate and circular without calcifications	64%
Stellate and circular with calcifications	17%
Calcifications only	19%

Table 1.02 Spectrum of histological diagnosis corresponding to mammographic circular/oval lesions

Histological diagnosis	Proportion of lesions
Invasive carcinoma of no special type	59%
Medullary carcinoma	8%
Mucinous carcinoma	7%
Encapsulated papillary carcinoma	5%
Tubular carcinoma	4%
Invasive lobular carcinoma	4%
Other diagnoses	13%

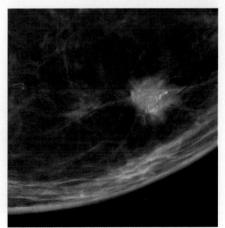

Fig. 1.02 Digital mammogram showing a typical small spiculate breast cancer with associated calcification.

Clinical features

M. Morrow
E. Rutgers

A palpable mass is the most common clinical sign of invasive breast carcinoma, although skin retraction, nipple inversion, nipple discharge – and less commonly, a change in the size or shape of the breast or a change in the colour or texture of the skin – may also be seen. Rarely, breast carcinoma will present as enlargement of the axillary lymph nodes in the absence of any abnormality in the breast. All the symptoms of breast cancer may also be caused by benign breast disease, so evaluation with imaging and histological sampling with core biopsy or fine-needle aspiration cytology are indicated to establish a definitive diagnosis.

The imaging workup of a breast mass should include diagnostic mammography with a marker placed over the lesion to ensure that it is visualized on the film. A spiculated mass is the classic appearance of cancer, but cancers may also be visualized as architectural distortion or well-circumscribed masses. About 5–15% of palpable cancers are not seen on mammogram. The majority of these will be identified with targeted ultrasound. The false-negative rate of combined mammography and ultrasound is quite low, ranging from 0% to 3% {952,1353}. Unless the presence of an unequivocally benign diagnosis such as a cyst is established based on imaging, tissue sampling is

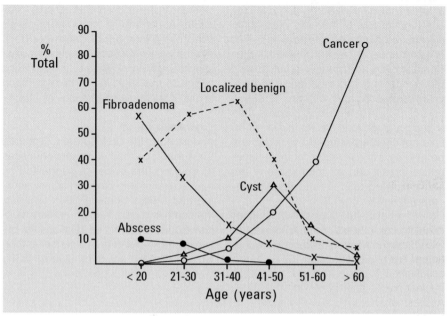

Fig. 1.03 Age distribution of benign and malignant breast lesions in patients presenting with a discrete breast lump {346}.

necessary before determining that carcinoma is not present. Magnetic resonance imaging (MRI) is not a substitute for a histological diagnosis; in one study, the negative predictive value of MRI was 85.4% (95% CI, 81.1–89.0%) {152}. When the results of the physical examination, mammography, and needle biopsy are all benign and concordant, the risk of

malignancy is extremely low. However, if any one of these modalities is non-concordant or cannot be evaluated, surgical biopsy is indicated.

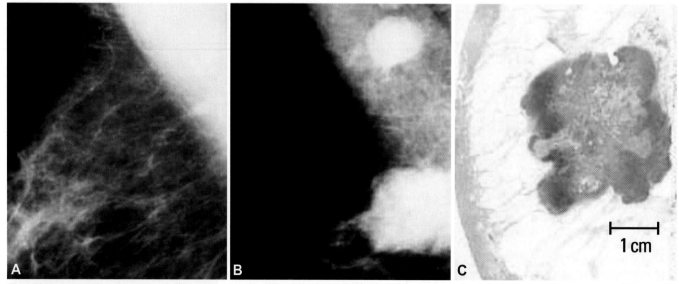

Fig. 1.04 Mammographic demonstration of the evolution of a poorly differentiated invasive carcinoma of no special type, a circular tumour mass on the mammogram. **A** Non-specific density in the axillary tail of the right breast, undetected at screening. **B** 18 months later: an ill defined, high-density lobulated tumour of > 30 mm is evident and mammographically appears to be malignant. Metastatic lymph nodes are seen in the axilla. **C** Large-section histology of the tumour.

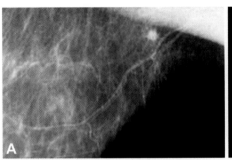
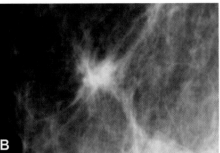
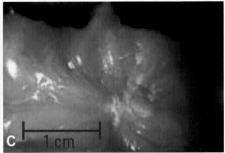

Fig. 1.05 Invasive carcinoma. **A** Mammogram of invasive carcinoma, clinically occult, < 1 cm. **B** Mammographic detail of small, non-palpable, invasive carcinoma (< 1 cm). **C** Macroscopic picture.

Grading

I.O. Ellis   J.S. Reis-Filho
J.F. Simpson   T. Decker

Invasive carcinomas of no special type (NST) and all other invasive breast carcinomas are routinely graded based on an assessment of tubule/gland formation, nuclear pleomorphism and mitotic count. Assessment of histological grade has become more objective as the original methods by Patey & Scarff {1077} and Bloom & Richardson {151} have been modified by Elston & Ellis {377}. After the adoption of these changes, many studies have demonstrated a significant association between histological grade and survival of patients with invasive breast carcinoma {1136, 1146}. Grade is a powerful prognostic factor and should be included as a component of the minimum dataset for histological reporting of breast cancer {1091} and is a key component of clinical decision-making tools such as the Nottingham Prognostic Index {146} and Adjuvant! online {1158}.

Method of grading

Three tumour characteristics are evaluated: tubule formation as an expression of glandular differentiation; nuclear pleomorphism; and mitotic counts. A numerical scoring system of 1 to 3 is used to ensure that each factor is assessed independently (Table 1.03). Glandular formation is assessed over the whole tumour and is a low-power assessment. Nuclear pleomorphism is evaluated for the area showing the worst degree of pleomorphism, and mitotic counting is performed for the area exhibiting the most proliferation.

When evaluating tubules and glandular acini, only structures exhibiting clear central lumina surrounded by polarized neoplastic cells are counted; cut-off points of 75% and 10% of glandular/tumour area are used to allocate the score.

Nuclear pleomorphism is assessed by reference to the regularity of nuclear size and shape of normal epithelial cells in adjacent breast tissue. Increasing irregularity of nuclear outlines and the number and size of nucleoli are useful additional features in allocating scores for pleomorphism. Score 1 nuclei are very similar in size (< 1.5) to those of benign pre-existing epithelial cells and show minimal pleomorphism and even chromatin pattern and nucleoli are not visible or very inconspicuous. Score 2 nuclei are larger (1.5–2× size of benign epithelial cell nuclei), with mild to moderate pleomorphism and visible but

small and inconspicuous nucleoli. Score 3 nuclei are larger in size (> 2 × size of benign epithelial cell nuclei) with vesicular chromatin, vary markedly in size and shape and often show prominent nucleoli. Evaluation of mitotic figures requires care, and relies on optimal tissue fixation and good preparation of sections. Observers

Table 1.03 Semi-quantitative method for assessing histological grade in breast tumours {377}

Feature	Score
Tubule and gland formation	
Majority of tumour (> 75%)	1
Moderate degree (10–75%)	2
Little or none (< 10%)	3
Nuclear pleomorphism	
Small, regular uniform cells	1
Moderate increase in size and variability	2
Marked variation	3
Mitotic counts	
Dependent on microscope field area	1–3 (see Table 1.04)
Final grading	
Add scores for gland formation, nuclear pleomorphism and mitotic count:	
Grade 1	Total score, 3–5
Grade 2	Total score, 6 or 7
Grade 3	Total score, 8 or 9

Table 1.04 Score thresholds for mitotic counts

Field diameter (mm)	Mitotic count (score)		
	1	2	3
0.40	≤ 4	5–9	≥ 10
0.41	≤ 4	5–9	≥ 10
0.42	≤ 5	6–10	≥ 11
0.43	≤ 5	6–10	≥ 11
0.44	≤ 5	6–11	≥ 12
0.45	≤ 5	6–11	≥ 12
0.46	≤ 6	7–12	≥ 13
0.47	≤ 6	7–12	≥ 13
0.48	≤ 6	7–13	≥ 14
0.49	≤ 6	7–13	≥ 14
0.50	≤ 7	8–14	≥ 15
0.51	≤ 7	8–14	≥ 15
0.52	≤ 7	8–15	≥ 16
0.53	≤ 8	9–16	≥ 17
0.54	≤ 8	9–16	≥ 17
0.55	≤ 8	9–17	≥ 18
0.56	≤ 8	9–17	≥ 18
0.57	≤ 9	10–18	≥ 19
0.58	≤ 9	10–19	≥ 20
0.59	≤ 9	10–19	≥ 20
0.60	≤ 10	11–20	≥ 21
0.61	≤ 10	11–21	≥ 22
0.62	≤ 11	12–22	≥ 23
0.63	≤ 11	12–22	≥ 23
0.64	≤ 11	12–23	≥ 24
0.65	≤ 12	13–24	≥ 25
0.66	≤ 12	13–24	≥ 25
0.67	≤ 12	13–25	≥ 26
0.68	≤ 13	14–26	≥ 27
0.69	≤ 13	14–27	≥ 28

must count only definite mitotic figures; hyperchromatic and pyknotic nuclei are ignored since they are more likely to represent apoptosis rather than cells in mitosis. Mitotic counts require standardization to a fixed field area. The total number of mitoses per 10 HPF is recorded. Cut-off points for scoring depend on field area. Therefore, for mitotic counting it is essential to calibrate the microscope by measuring the diameter of the HPF (40× objective; see Table 1.04). Field selection for mitotic scoring should be from the peripheral leading edge of the tumour to find the area with most mitotic activity. If there is heterogeneity, regions exhibiting a higher frequency of mitoses should be chosen. Field selection is by random meander through the chosen area. Only fields with a representative tumour-cell burden should be assessed.

The three values are added together to produce scores of 3 to 9, to which the grade is assigned as follows:

- 3–5 points: grade 1, well-differentiated
- 6–7 points: grade 2, moderately differentiated
- 8–9 points: grade 3, poorly differentiated.

For the purposes of quality assurance, it is recommended that the individual score components be reported in addition to the calculated grade.

Grading of small tissue samples such as needle-core biopsy specimens is possible, but should be recognized to have limitations particularly due to the inherent reduced ability to assess mitotic frequency accurately. This may lead to underestimation of true grade in such specimens {552}.

Molecular genetics of histological grade

Tumours of different histological grades show distinct molecular profiles at the genomic {204,970,1229}, transcriptomic {1178,1358} and immunohistochemical levels {4}. These studies suggest that most high-grade tumours are unlikely to stem from the progression of low-grade cancers and that grade 1 and 3 breast tumours are probably two different diseases that may have distinct molecular origins, pathogenesis and behaviour {970,1230,1358}. Gene-expression studies have demonstrated that histological grade reflects the molecular makeup of breast cancer better than lymph-node status or tumour size {834,1615}.

It should be noted, however, that recent meta-analyses of microarray-based expression-profiling studies have demonstrated that the prognostic impact of the signatures investigated stems from the proliferation-related genes {332,1589} and these studies are discussed in detail elsewhere in this book. Most importantly, in some studies using molecular signatures, histological grade remained an independent prognostic factor for estrogen-receptor-positive tumours even after the inclusion of gene signatures in the multivariate models {1059,1566}.

Staging

S. Lester
D. Weaver
M. Morrow

G. Cserni
S. Tuzlali

Tumour staging

The most widely used system for staging breast carcinoma is the TNM system published by the American Joint Committee on Cancer (AJCC)/Union for International Cancer Control (UICC). The most recent criteria described in the seventh edition of the TNM system are provided at the beginning of this chapter {366}. This system captures information about the extent of cancer at the primary site (tumour or T), the regional lymph nodes (nodes or N), and spread to distant metastatic sites (metastases or M). Special techniques for classification are not required and comparable information can thus be collected over time and in diverse locations.

T, N, and M are combined to create five stages (stages 0, I, II, III, and IV) that summarize information about the extent of regional disease (tumour size, skin or chest-wall invasion, and nodal involvement) and metastasis to distant sites. For individual patients, this information is important for making decisions concerning the control of local disease, as well as to determine the value of systemic therapy. Determining tumour stage is also essential for organizing groups of similar patients for comparison in clinical trials, epidemiological studies, or other types of investigations. Biological tests, such as gene-expression profiling, may complement information on stage by estimating the risk of future metastasis or recurrence or by predicting the likely response to treatment.

Both clinical staging and pathological staging are used for patients with breast cancer. Clinical stage depends on physical examination and imaging studies, with or without confirmation by fine-needle aspiration cytology. Pathological classification of T and N primarily relies on the gross and microscopic examination of surgically excised specimens. T is based on the size of the invasive carcinoma in the majority of patients. If multiple areas of invasion are present, T classification is based on the largest focus. A small cancer is sometimes best evaluated by measuring size on glass slides. Often correlation between gross, microscopic, and imaging findings is necessary to determine the best T category. Lymph nodes should be evaluated by thinly slicing and examining all nodal tissue in order to identify all macrometastases (metastases > 0.2 cm). M classification is primarily determined by the results of radiological studies, with pathological confirmation after biopsy in some cases.

An important change in the seventh edition of the TNM system is the introduction of a new stage IB for patients with T1 carcinomas (2.0 cm or less) and only micrometastases to axillary nodes (pN1mi). Although these metastases have statistical significance {515,1125,1561}, the effect on prognosis is so small that it is more appropriate to classify them separately rather than together with stage II patients having macrometastases.

The increasingly common practice of initiating therapy before definitive surgical treatment (i.e. neoadjuvant or presurgical therapy) requires a combination of information from clinical examination, imaging, and pathological examination to determine the most likely T, N, and M classifications before treatment. Post-treatment yT and yN classifications are determined after definitive surgery. Determining stage both before and after treatment provides important prognostic information {221, 650}.

Lymphatic and blood-vessel invasion

Lymph-vascular invasion (also termed lymphovascular invasion, angiolymphatic invasion, vascular invasion, or LVI) is the finding of carcinoma within small vessels outside the main tumour mass, most frequently at the periphery of an invasive carcinoma (peritumoral LVI). Although LVI is associated with lymph-node metastasis, it is also an independent prognostic factor for local and distant recurrence and is used to help in clinical decision-making (NCCN guidelines www.nccn.org/professionals/physician_gls/f_guidelines.asp) {324,505,772,1108}. The presence of both LVI and nodal metastases confers a worse prognosis than either alone. Vascular-space involvement can serve as a reservoir for tumour cells in the skin or chest wall that cannot be removed by conventional surgery. In addition, intravascular tumour may be less susceptible to treatment, as demonstrated by reported cases of residual cancer present only as LVI after neoadjuvant chemotherapy.

LVI in the dermis is a particularly poor prognostic factor owing to frequent association with local recurrence and distant metastases {10}. When extensive, LVI in the dermis often causes the skin changes characteristic of inflammatory carcinoma. LVI is frequently noted when multiple lymph-node metastases are present, although not in the unusual cases in which the observation of LVI is hindered by the biological characteristics of the carcinoma. For example, LVI is rare in lobular carcinomas, possibly because of the lack of adhesion of this tumour type to vessel walls. In other cases, extensive LVI may be difficult to diagnose if the tumour cells completely fill vascular spaces and mimic ductal carcinoma in situ (DCIS). Conversely, LVI is present in approximately 15% of patients without axillary nodal metastases and it is more important as a prognostic factor in this group of patients. Lymphatic drainage for some cancers may be to other nodal basins.

Alternatively, some subtypes of cancers are associated with a lower incidence of lymph-node metastases and may metastasize primarily via blood vessels {930,931}. For example, "triple-negative" carcinomas (negative for estrogen, progesterone, and HER2 receptors), often do not involve lymph nodes, but frequently spread to distant sites {467,1581}. In general, the involved vessels are the size of capillaries. Metastases in larger blood vessels with muscular walls are exceedingly rare.

The use of LVI as a prognostic factor has been hampered by the lack of universal consensus on how to define its presence and whether there is a need to separate lymphatics from blood vessels or measure the extent of LVI. In the majority of cases, LVI can be reliably identified on haematoxylin-and-eosin (H&E) slides by using strict histological criteria {1203}. Immunohistochemical studies can be used to distinguish lymphatics from small capillaries and, in some cases, additional subtle foci can be identified {929,930}. However, the currently available markers are not completely specific or sensitive. In daily practice, it is not necessary to distinguish the vessel type, as both have prognostic significance. It is not yet clear if the foci only seen by special studies have sufficient prognostic significance to justify their routine use or whether they will dilute the overall significance of LVI as a prognostic variable.

Lymph-node status

The status of the axillary lymph nodes is the most important single prognostic factor for all except a small subset of breast carcinomas. Nodal metastases are strongly correlated with tumour size and the number of invasive carcinomas {213,230,1451,1581}. Disease-free survival and overall survival diminish with each additional positive node {920,976,1521}. The ratio of positive to negative nodes also provides prognostic information and can adjust for differences in surgical and pathology practices that result in variable numbers of nodes evaluated {1522,1596}. Positive nodes are a marker of distant dissemination, as surgical removal of nodes does not appear to have a major effect on survival {495}.

Macrometastases, defined as being > 0.2 cm in size, have been shown in multiple studies to have prognostic significance. They can be reliably detected by thinly sectioning nodes (into slices of 0.2 cm), embedding all slices in paraffin blocks, and examining a representative H&E slide from each block. However, failure to examine all nodal tissue can result in missing macrometastases in up to 40% of positive nodes {149,1343}. Detection of smaller metastases may require additional levels into paraffin blocks and/or immunohistochemical studies.

Although these small metastases, classified as either micrometastases (> 0.02 cm, up to 0.2 cm, or > 200 cells in a single nodal cross-section) or isolated tumour-cell clusters (ITCs; no larger than 0.02 cm,

or < 200 cells in a single nodal cross-section) do have statistical significance, the actual impact on prognosis (after all macrometastases have been excluded) is < 3% at 5 and 10 years when compared with node-negative women {515,1125,1560,1561}. In addition, the presence of micrometastases or ITCs on additional deeper levels is not a discriminatory variable for predicting recurrence or survival. More than 80% of these women survive without recurrence at a median follow-up of 8 years {1561}. Thus, there is little value in performing additional levels or immunohistochemical studies that will find some but not all of these deposits {1560}.

In current practice, there is wide variation in how nodes are evaluated intraoperatively and on permanent sections {297,298,1562}. The role of molecular approaches, such as reverse-transcriptase polymerase chain reaction (RT-PCR), in routine practice is unclear since the size of the metastasis is uncertain and both false-positive and false-negative results can occur {366,839}. In selected cases in which larger metastases may be difficult to detect, such as lobular carcinomas, immunohistochemical studies may be helpful {299,1490}.

Neither palpation nor readily available imaging techniques are reliable for the exclusion of nodal metastases, as most patients present with only a few nodes involved by small metastases. Cancers drain to one or two sentinel nodes in the axilla, or rarely to other nodal basins, which can be identified intraoperatively by either dye or radioactive tracer. If cancer is not detected in the sentinel node(s), < 10% of patients will have other nodes involved. Intramammary nodes are rarely sentinel nodes; however, when involved by cancer, they are included with axillary nodes for staging {366,1126}. Sentinel-node biopsy has proven to be a useful technique to separate node-positive from node-negative patients with reduced morbidity {74,682,839}. A completion axillary dissection is not required for patients with negative sentinel nodes and may not be necessary for selected patients with only limited nodal involvement {495,721}.

In the setting of presurgical or neoadjuvant therapy, small nodal metastases are indicative of an incomplete response to systemic therapy and have the same significance as larger metastases {699}. A complete response in known lymph-node metastases is more predictive of ultimate outcome than is the response in the primary carcinoma {350,1226}. Thus to obtain the most information, it is preferable to document positive nodes before therapy by fine-needle aspiration or needle-core biopsy, rather than surgical removal. Sentinel-node biopsy can be employed after treatment, although the false-negative rate is slightly higher {198,1050}.

Although negative nodes are a very favourable prognostic factor, 10–30% of patients will eventually develop distant metastases. In some cases, the cancers will have spread to other nodal groups that are not routinely evaluated, such as internal mammary nodes {641}. There is also a small group of cancers that appear to metastasize haematogenously without

the involvement of nodes. For example, although basal-like carcinomas are a poor prognostic group, this is the molecular subtype least likely to exhibit extensive nodal involvement {1581}. For these patients, other prognostic markers will be more important than nodal staging.

Molecular testing for estrogen receptor, progesterone receptor, and HER2

C. Allred
K. Miller
G. Viale

E. Brogi
J. Isola

Introduction
Three molecular biomarkers are used in the routine clinical management of patients with invasive breast cancer: estrogen receptor (ER), progesterone receptor (PR), and HER2. Since all are targets and/ or indicators of highly effective therapies against invasive breast cancer in various clinical settings, accurate assessment is essential and mandatory {33,242, 360}. It is the responsibility of every pathology laboratory evaluating these biomarkers to provide accurate and reproducible results.

ER
ER is a nuclear transcription factor that, when activated by the hormone estrogen,

stimulates the growth of normal breast epithelial cells {272}. Proliferation may also be activated in the cells of invasive breast cancers expressing ER which, of course, is detrimental {1274}. ER expression has been measured in invasive breast cancers by various methods for almost 40 years. Today nearly all testing is performed by immunohistochemistry, a sensitive, specific, easy and inexpensive technique that can be performed on routinely prepared histological samples, primarily formalin-fixed paraffin-embedded (FFPE) tissue sections. Stained slides are evaluated microscopically to determine the proportions and intensity of positive cells. By immunohistochemistry, about 80% of invasive breast

cancers express nuclear ER, in a proportion ranging from < 1% to 100% positive cells {558}.

Many clinical studies, including large randomized clinical trials, have demonstrated that ER is a strong predictive factor for response to hormonal therapies such as tamoxifen {360,1274}; this is the main reason for routine evaluation. Tamoxifen binds ER and blocks estrogen-stimulated growth, resulting in significantly longer disease-free and overall survival in patients with ER-positive invasive breast cancers, compared with those that are ER-negative. The clinical response to newer types of hormonal therapies, such as the aromatase inhibitors (that suppress the production of

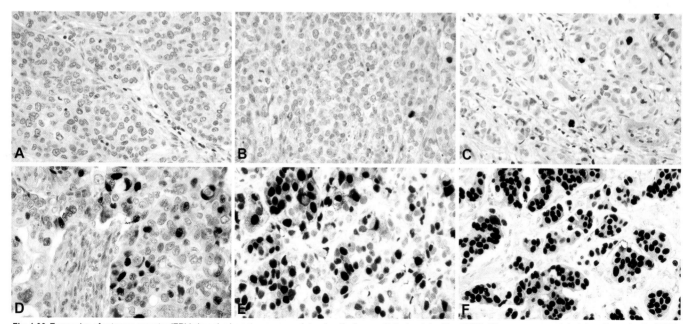

Fig. 1.06 Expression of estrogen receptor (ER) in invasive breast cancers, as determined by immunohistochemistry. About 80% of these cancers and ductal carcinoma in situ (DCIS) express ER in tumour-cell nuclei with a range of < 1% to 100 % (**A** 0% ; **B** Approx. 1%; **C** Approx. 10%; **D** Approx. 30%; **E** Approx. 60%; **F** Approx. 100%). Approx. 65% express progesterone receptor (PR), with a similar broad range. The remaining tumours are entirely negative (0% of cells; **A**). A clinically positive test for both receptors is defined as nuclear staining in ≥ 1% of tumour cells, and a negative result as < 1%.

estrogen) is also dependent on ER status; only tumours that are positive for ER respond {33,1274}. There is a direct correlation between the likelihood of response to hormonal therapies and the level of expression, although even tumours expressing very low levels of ER show a significant benefit far above that of entirely negative tumours, which are essentially unresponsive {558}. The results of many immunohistochemistry studies provide strong support for defining "ER-positive" clinically as ≥ 1% positive-staining tumour cells {541}; this has also been endorsed by a committee of international experts in recently published guidelines {541}. These guidelines make many other recommendations intended to promote accurate reproducible results, such as mandatory confirmation of unlikely negative results (e.g. ER-negative tubular carcinomas, tumours of low histological grade), and the implementation of comprehensive quality assurance programmes.

PR

PR is also routinely assessed by immunohistochemistry in invasive breast cancers {33,1274}. ER regulates the expression of PR, so the presence of PR usually indicates that the estrogen–ER pathway is intact and functional {272}. Once expressed, PR is activated by the hormone progesterone, which also stimulates the growth of tumour cells {46, 242,1274}. Very like ER, PR is expressed in the nuclei of 60–70% of invasive breast cancers, with expression that varies on a continuum ranging from 0% to 100% positive cells. There is a direct correlation between levels of expression and response to hormonal therapies, and even tumours with very low levels (≥ 1% positive cells) have a significant chance of responding {932, 1274}. Although the expression of PR is highly correlated with that of ER, the correlation is imperfect, resulting in four possible phenotypes of combined expression. Each combination is associated with significantly different rates of response to hormonal therapy, which would not be apparent if measuring ER or PR only {103}. The phenotype ER-positive/PR-positive is most frequent (70%), and is associated with the best rate of response (60%). ER-negative/PR-negative is the next most common combination (25%) and these tumours are essentially unresponsive (0%). The remaining two discordant phenotypes are associated with intermediate response

rates, although there is debate as to whether ER-negative/PR-positive tumours actually exist.
Several new molecular methods for determining the status of hormone receptors, as well as other important biomarkers, which may be more powerful than immunohistochemistry in predicting response to hormonal therapy and prognosis, are being developed {840, 843,1024,1059,1359}.

HER2 oncogene and oncoprotein

The *HER2* gene (standard nomenclature, *ERBB2*), located on chromosome 17, encodes a growth factor receptor on the surface of normal breast epithelial cells {383}. HER2 expression has been evaluated in invasive breast cancers for about 25 years. Studies demonstrate that the gene is amplified in approximately 15% of tumours in patients with primary breast cancer, and that amplification is highly correlated with elevated protein expression {33,242,383}. The reported frequency of HER2-positive invasive breast cancers was higher in the past, before widespread screening mammography; later detection may have allowed more time for genetic alterations to accumulate as tumours evolved {713}.
HER2 status is primarily determined by immunohistochemistry and/or fluorescence in situ hybridization (FISH) on FFPE samples, providing results that are essentially equivalent, and occasionally complementary, in terms of clinical efficacy {383,1591}. Other chromogenic methods of in situ hybridization that can accurately determine gene copy number using routine bright-field microscopy are becoming popular {1087A}. As with hormone receptors, guidelines have been developed to

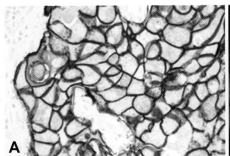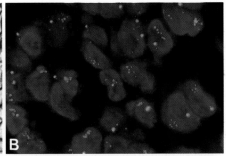

Fig. 1.07 HER2 testing in invasive breast cancers. Immunohistochemistry (IHC) and fluorescence in situ hybridization (FISH) are the most comprehensively validated assays for use in routine clinical practice. A clinically positive IHC test is defined as strong circumferential membrane staining in > 30% of tumour cells (**A**), while a negative result is defined as weak or entirely absent staining. A positive FISH result is defined as a *HER* gene : chromosome 17 ratio of > 2.2 (**B**), while a negative result is defined as < 1.8. Both assays may return equivocal results, and HER status in these tumours must be confirmed by testing using the alternative method (i.e. FISH by IHC, and IHC by FISH).

promote accurate testing for HER2, and it is prudent for laboratories to follow the principles established {1591}.
The relationship between HER2 status and clinical outcome is complex and varies with setting {242,1591}. Recent studies demonstrate that HER2-positive invasive breast cancers respond favourably to therapies that specifically target the HER2 protein (e.g. trastuzumab and lapatinib) {112,383}. The main reason for assessing HER2 status today is to identify candidates for this type of targeted therapy. HER2-positive tumours are defined as those tumours that show strong circumferential staining (referred to as 3+ staining) in > 30% of cells by immunohistochemistry, and/or *HER2*-gene amplification detected by in situ hybridization; or tumours that show moderately strong circumferential membrane staining (referred to as 2+ staining) and *HER2*-gene amplification detected by in situ hybridization {542, 1591}. These HER2-positive tumours show the best response to HER2-targeted therapy in any clinical setting {112,326}. Tumours that show little or no protein expression by immunohistochemistry (referred to as 0 or 1+ staining) almost always have the normal number of copies of the *HER2* gene as assessed by in situ hybridization and are reported as HER2-negative.

Post-therapy effects

F. Symmans
S. Lester
S.E. Pinder
J. Kulka

Definition

In the widest sense, post-therapy effects include morphological and biological alterations in cancers and normal tissue after any treatment. However, the term is most commonly used to describe changes seen after neoadjuvant therapy (also termed "primary systemic therapy" or "presurgical therapy"), in which treatment (chemotherapy, endocrine therapy, and/or targeted therapy) is administered before surgical excision. Observed alterations in cancers are used to evaluate the response in vivo.

Morphological characteristics of carcinomas after treatment

Based on the results of imaging and needle-core biopsy findings (grade, histological type, necrosis, proliferation rate, hormone-receptor status, and HER2 status), any patient who is eligible for systemic therapy can be treated with neoadjuvant therapy. Although neoadjuvant therapy does not provide survival benefit, response to treatment is a strong prognostic factor and is useful for individual patient care, and also represents a short-term end-point for clinical trials {162,441, 599,727,849,1105}. In addition, some patients with large cancers may consequently become eligible for breast conservation {163,175}.

Post-therapy specimens

The residual carcinoma or tumour bed must be found in order to evaluate response to therapy, and this is facilitated by the placement of clips before treatment. In large specimens, lack of such markers may lead to difficulty identifying the tumour bed, which may render a statement about pathological complete response (pCR) problematic. In cases of pCR, the tumour bed can often be identified macroscopically as a fibrous, rubbery area. However, gross changes may be subtle, making pretreatment clip placement valuable. Residual cancers typically become softer and more difficult to palpate, except in cases of absent or minimal response. The macroscopic size of identifiable residual tumour or multiple tumour foci, as well as distances from the resection margins, should be recorded. Changes in the residual tumour cells, if present, are very variable in degree. In therapy-resistant cancers, no morphological alteration may be detected. More commonly, carcinomas become less cellular and are often present as scattered small nests across the tumour bed. The size and cellularity of foci of the overall residual cancer should be recorded, since the extent of residual invasive carcinoma, together with lymph-node status, is a powerful predictor of long-term survival {221}. In a few cases, the remaining cancer cells become bizarre, possessing large and irregular nuclei. The cytoplasm of the residual tumour cells may become vacuolated in about 40% of cases {939}. In some cases, the only residual cancer is in lymphatic spaces and this finding has been associated with recurrence after neoadjuvant therapy {250A}. The mitotic count is often lower in the residual carcinoma. Nevertheless, histological grade remains a prognostic factor after neoadjuvant therapy and should be reported {179}. After a complete response, only a loose, oedematous, vascularized fibroelastotic area of connective tissue with chronic inflammatory cells and macrophages may mark the tumour bed. When only small foci of atypical cells are present, immunohistochemical studies may be helpful to distinguish cancer cells from

Table 1.05 Comparison of systems for evaluating response to neoadjuvant therapy for breast cancer: pathological evaluation

Name of system	Reference	Factors evaluated in the breast	pCR in the breast	Lymph nodes included	No. of categories of partial response
B-18	{449}	Any treatment effect on invasive carcinoma	No invasive carcinoma	Yes,[a] size of largest metastasis	1
Chevallier	{262}	Presence of invasive carcinoma with sclerosis or fibrosis	No invasive or in situ carcinoma	Yes	1
Sataloff	{1266}	Presence of invasive carcinoma Presence of treatment effect	Total or near total therapeutic effect	Yes, ± treatment effect	2
Miller-Payne	{1023}	Presence of invasive carcinoma Cellularity	No invasive carcinoma	No	3
RCB (residual cancer burden)	{1390}	Size of tumour bed in two dimensions Cellularity of residual invasive carcinoma	No invasive carcinoma	Yes, number and size of largest deposit	2 (with individual scores calculated for each case)
AJCC (y)	{221}	Size of invasive carcinoma	No invasive carcinoma	Yes, number	Up to 4 (dependent on the initial AJCC T and N categories)
MNPI (Modified Nottingham Prognostic Index)	{11}	Size of invasive carcinoma Tumour grade	No invasive carcinoma	Yes, number	3
Pinder	{1109}	% of tumour remaining in breast	No invasive carcinoma	Yes, presence of evidence of response	Breast: 3 Lymph nodes: 1

AJCC, American Joint Committee on Cancer; ER, estrogen receptor; N, node; pCR, pathological complete response; T, tumour.

[a] Survival according to lymph-node status was analysed separately from response in the breast.

benign histiocytic cells and invasive carcinoma from carcinoma in situ.

Primary endocrine therapy may be used, but rarely results in pCR. The treated cancers may have a central area of fibrous scarring {1432}.

Ductal carcinoma in situ (DCIS) may be present in the absence of residual invasive carcinoma. This finding does not exclude classification as a pCR and these patients have a good prognosis {162,449, 727}.

Lymph nodes

To obtain the maximum amount of information from neoadjuvant therapy, the lymph nodes should be evaluated before treatment. Enlarged nodes, or those identifiable by ultrasound, may be sampled by fine-needle aspiration or needle-core biopsy. If no metastatic carcinoma is seen, a sentinel node can be biopsied. In lymph nodes removed following neoadjuvant therapy, areas of fibrosis (sometimes wedge-shaped) or large collections of macrophages, can be seen and are interpreted as representing response of metastatic disease to the neoadjuvant therapy. As in the breast tissue, immunohistochemistry for keratins can be helpful in the identification of small-volume residual metastatic carcinoma. However, metastases can completely resolve without leaving histological evidence of prior nodal involvement. Without pretreatment evaluation, the distinction between negative nodes before treatment and a nodal pCR cannot be made with certainty. The response in the nodes has more prognostic importance than does response in the breast {726}. Small metastases after treatment, including isolated tumour cells, are representative of an incomplete pathological response. In the setting of neoadjuvant therapy, the presence of isolated tumour cells seen by H&E should be interpreted with caution, and as node-positive disease.

Classification of response

In most studies, 10–30% of patients have a pCR, 10–15% of patients have no or little response, and the majority has a partial response to therapy. The extent of this response is associated with outcome. More than eight systems have been proposed to classify the degree of tumour response to therapy. Some systems compare carcinomas pre- and post-therapy (e.g. Miller-Payne, Pinder) {1023,1109}, whereas

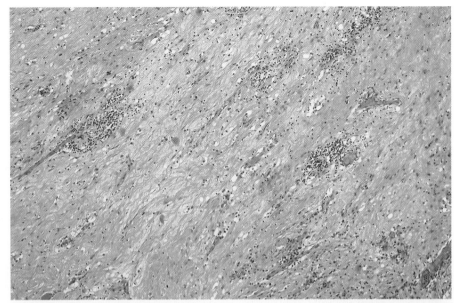

Fig. 1.08 Pathological complete response following neoadjuvant therapy; poorly cellular oedematous connective tissue and chronic inflammatory cell infiltrates are present.

others quantify the amount of residual carcinoma (e.g. AJCC; and RCB, residual cancer burden) {221,1390}. Identifying AJCC stage before and after treatment is important and provides additional prognostic information {650}.

Morphological changes in normal tissues after treatment

Normal breast epithelial structures may show atypia, in the form of enlarged and occasional pleomorphic nuclei, after neoadjuvant therapy. These may be present at some distance from the site of the invasive tumour and can be present throughout the specimen rather than in the vicinity of the tumour bed; care should be taken not to over-diagnose these as in situ disease.

Radiation can cause the stroma to be dense and hypocellular. The epithelial cells of ducts and lobules may show slightly irregular and hyperchromatic nuclei, and lobules may become sclerotic. Radiation fibroblasts may be seen and bizarre stromal cells may also be present.

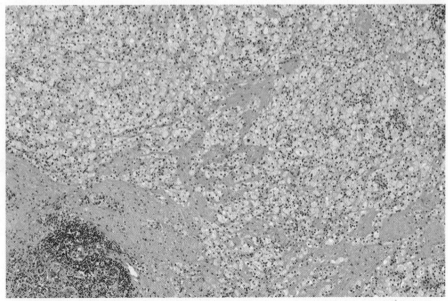

Fig. 1.09 Pathological complete response following neoadjuvant therapy; foamy histiocytes mark the tumour bed.

It is important that these changes are not reported as signs of sui generis atypia or recurrent malignancy {1283}. Atypical vascular proliferations can occur in the skin, and sarcomas, particularly angiosarcoma, may arise in the radiated skin and/or breast years after radiotherapy.

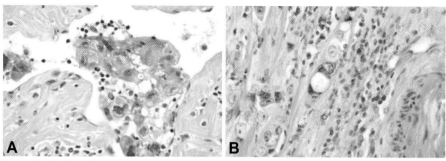

Fig. 1.10 A Residual (intravascular) tumour cells showing marked pleomorphism following neoadjuvant therapy. **B** The residual bizarre tumour cell in the middle of the field bears a large intracytoplasmic vacuole.

Classification using needle-core biopsy and fine-needle aspiration

F. Schmitt
N. Sneige
A. Lee

Fine-needle aspiration (FNA) and needle-core biopsy (NCB) have been extensively used for years in the diagnosis of breast lesions and have good sensitivity for the diagnosis of malignancy in palpable lesions {704,966}. There is evidence that NCB is more sensitive for the detection of impalpable lesions and is recommended for the evaluation of microcalcifications and FNA findings that are suspicious {187}. It is essential that these techniques are used in combination with clinical and radiological assessment, the "triple approach" {186}.

It is not possible to distinguish between in situ and invasive carcinoma using FNA. False-positive diagnosis of adenocarcinoma is uncommon with FNA (< 1%). By NCB, a false-positive diagnosis of invasive carcinoma or ductal carcinoma in situ (DCIS) is rare {1139}. Furthermore, in patients with microcalcifications detected at mammography, about 20% of diagnoses of DCIS made by NCB are upgraded to invasive carcinoma on excision. Preoperative diagnosis using FNA or NCB can allow definitive decisions regarding treatment to be made before surgery and may affect surgical outcome {1578,1580}. In other instances, such information can help avoid unnecessary surgery in patients with benign lesions. The rate at which malignancies are missed with NCB is rare, with a low impact on patient management {1143}.

Classification using FNA
A definitive diagnosis of carcinoma is made when the aspirates display high cellularity, a monomorphic cell population, conspicuous loss of cell cohesion with numerous isolated single epithelial cells, and aniso-nucleosis. Some carcinomas, such as lobular, tubular, papillary invasive carcinomas or invasive carcinomas of low nuclear grade may be difficult to recognize on FNA and should be confirmed by NCB {966}. The distinction of metastases to the breast from primary cancers elsewhere may be possible using NCB or FNA if there are distinctive features and/or pertinent clinical history {1000}.

Classification using NCB
Experience to date has indicated that there is excellent correlation between the findings of NCB with those of open biopsy {805, 1593}. Furthermore, the level of diagnostic agreement among pathologists in the interpretation of NCB specimens is extremely high {285}. The use of strict diagnostic criteria, coupled with immunohistochemistry, is useful to avoid a misdiagnosis. However, a definitive diagnosis is not always possible and a classification that includes borderline categories such as "suspicious," "equivocal" or "uncertain malignant potential" is useful in patient management {1142}. The

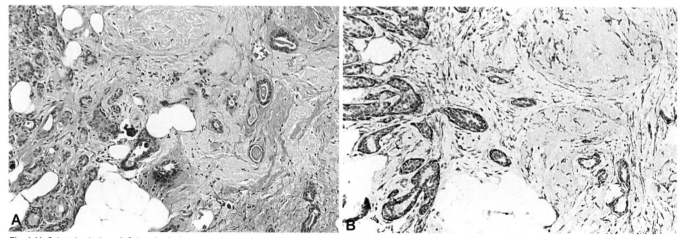

Fig. 1.11 Sclerosing lesion. **A** Sclerosing lesion on needle-core biopsy, thought to be suspicious for invasive carcinoma. **B** Immunostaining for smooth-muscle actin highlights an intact layer of myoepithelial cells surrounding the tubular structures, supporting the diagnosis of non-invasive carcinoma.

finding of atypical ductal hyperplasia (ADH), papilloma, lobular neoplasia, radial scar or mucocele-like lesion on NCB has been associated with variable rates of missed carcinoma in the subsequent surgical excision {140,178,654,988}. As a result, the appropriate management of such lesions after diagnosis by NCB has been controversial. It must be noted however that the frequency of missed carcinoma is influenced by the type of biopsy device used, the number of cores obtained, the gauge of the needle used, and the percentage of the lesion removed {594,824}. Excision is often recommended after NCB diagnosis of these lesions; however, for some individuals, in whom careful correlation of imaging and histological findings is concordant {988}, or breast magnetic resonance imaging (MRI) is normal, follow-up without surgical excision may be appropriate {1325}.

Prognostic and predictive markers

Histological grade can be assessed on NCB with about 70% of agreement with the grade determined in the surgical specimen {552,944}. Both FNA and NCB can give an indication of histological type, but neither is definitive because of the existence of tumours with mixed types. Estrogen receptor status and HER2 status can be reliably assessed on NCB, with agreements of about 98–99% {70,586}. The analysis of prognostic and predictive factors using FNA should be limited to cases of distant metastasis and cases with no available tissue material {704}. Ultrasound-guided NCB or FNA of axillary lymph nodes can be helpful in the management of invasive carcinoma, for the preoperative diagnosis of metastases {309}.

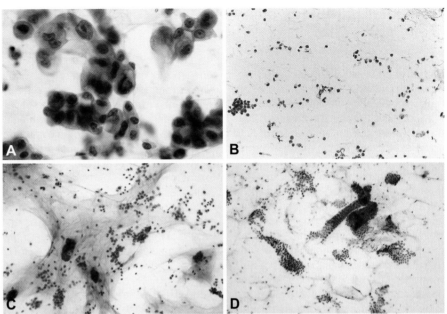

Fig. 1.12 Morphological aspects on fine-needle aspiration (Papanicolaou staining). **A** Invasive carcinoma of no special type. **B** Invasive lobular carcinoma, classical type. **C** Invasive mucinous carcinoma. **D** Tubular carcinoma.

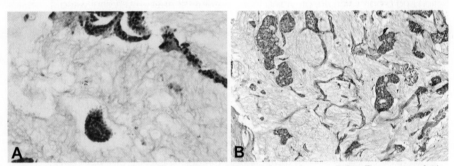

Fig. 1.13 A Mucocele-like lesion on needle-core biopsy, misinterpreted as mucinous carcinoma. The presence of strips of bland epithelium which represent the lining of a ruptured cystic space, and the absence of thin blood vessels crossing the mucinous lakes should be the key to the diagnosis. Contrast this image with that of mucinous carcinoma (**B**).

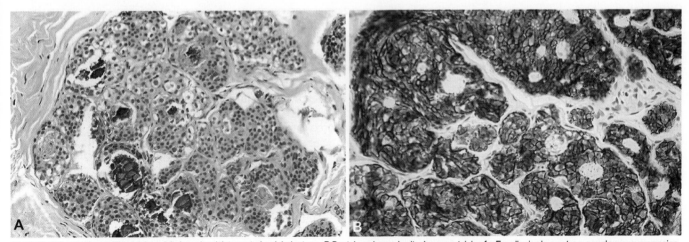

Fig. 1.14 A Carcinoma in situ involving a lobular unit, misinterpreted as lobular type. **B** Ductal carcinoma in situ. Immunostaining for E-cadherin shows strong membranous expression, establishing the presence of ductal differentiation.

Molecular pathology overview

S.R. Lakhani
J.S. Reis-Filho
M.J. van de Vijver

Breast cancer is a heterogeneous disease with multiple subtypes, variable size, grade, metastatic potential and with varying prognosis. Hence, the choice of therapy for patients with breast cancer is to some extent defined by information provided by the pathological assessment. The examination of the standard haematoxylin and eosin (H&E)-stained section is still an efficient, cost-effective and powerful mode of providing information to inform classification and hence clinical management {1146}. The pathological subtype (e.g. tubular versus metaplastic), grade (1 versus 3), size, vascular permeation and nodal status will provide informative data to define the likeliest outcome for patients with breast cancer and the need for adjuvant systemic therapies. Nonetheless, developments in our understanding of the molecular and cellular basis of cancer initiation and progression are providing tools for refining the taxonomy of breast cancer and opening up new avenues for the classification and treatment of breast cancer {941,1090}

The use of immunohistochemistry for differentiating benign from in situ and invasive malignancy using a variety of cell- and tissue-specific molecules, such as keratins (keratins 5/6, 14), p63 and basement-membrane markers (collagen IV, laminin) has had a significant impact on clinical management. This is particularly important in breast-screening practice, where small amounts of tissue removed using core biopsies have to be evaluated subsequent to the detection of an abnormality on radiological examination. Sclerosing lesions pose particular diagnostic difficulties.

Staining for estrogen receptor (ER), progesterone receptor (PR) and HER2 is becoming standard practice and increasingly, gene-amplification studies for *HER2* (*ERBB2*) have also been incorporated into testing. Guidelines for the assessment of hormone receptors have been published by the American Society of Clinical Oncology (ASCO) and thresholds for positivity have been established {541, 1591}. The use of tamoxifen or an aromatase inhibitor and the addition of chemotherapy with or without trastuzumab are dictated by the results of these studies; it is important that the information derived from the analysis is robust with good quality controls in the pre-analytical, analytical and post-analytical stages. Quality assurance programmes exist to help standardize protocols and it is recommended that laboratories engaged in the analysis should participate {107}. These simple molecular tests already help us to stratify breast cancers into meaningful groups for determining prognosis and treatment.

Recently, genomic and expression microarray technology, enabling us to simultaneously examine changes in thousands of genes, has been used to subclassify breast cancer and establish "signatures" for the prediction of "good versus bad" and "responsive versus non-responsive" cancers {1486} Proteomic methods are also available and a number are suitable for use with paraffin-embedded material. Proposals for identifying and substratifying patients using more clinically useful grading systems (i.e. stratifying intermediate grade into low-risk/grade 1 and high-risk/grade 3 {1358} and those with tumours that are likely to recur (recurrence scores) {1409} have been suggested. Much remains to be done in terms of standardization of platforms, use of appropriate quality controls, statistical methods for analysis and cut-offs used to separate cancers into different groups. Nevertheless, the technology holds much promise for adding to and extending the current classification of breast cancer to help optimize patient management.

Breast-cancer genomics and next-generation sequencing

J.S. Reis-Filho
S.R. Lakhani
P. Devilee

Comparative genomic hybridization and microarray-based comparative genomic hybridization have demonstrated that breast cancers are remarkably heterogeneous at the genomic level {15B,262C, 262D,463,574,664,970A}, and that there is a correlation between the patterns of gene copy-number aberrations and histological grade and estrogen receptor (ER) expression in both ductal carcinomas in situ (DCIS) and invasive carcinomas of no special type (NST) {15B,204,205,273B, 574,664,970A,970B,1520}. Grade 1 invasive carcinomas NST are usually diploid or near-diploid, and have been shown to harbour recurrent deletions of 16q (> 85%), gains of 1q (60%) and gains of 16p (40%), which may result from an unbalanced chromosomal translocation involving chromosomes 1 and 16 in up to 40% of cases {451,831,970,1466A}. Grade 3 cancers, on the other hand, are remarkably heterogeneous, and often frankly aneuploid. Despite the greater number and complexity of copy-number aberrations found in grade 3 carcinomas, deletions of 16q are found in only approximately 30% of cases, and are almost restricted to ER-negative lesions {970}. In fact, approximately 50% of grade 3 ER-positive cancers harbour the typical pattern of gene copy-number aberrations found in grade 1 tumours (i.e. deletion of 16 and gain of 1q) {831,970}. This information has led to the hypothesis that progression from low- to high-grade breast cancer is an uncommon biological phenomenon, which may be restricted to tumours of ER-positive phenotype {970,970A}. Intermediate-grade DCIS and grade 2 invasive carcinoma NST harbour more complex genomes than grade 1 lesions; however, deletions of 16q and gains of 1q are found in a substantial number of cases. These observations suggest that these lesions are the result of progression of grade 1 DCIS and invasive carcinomas.

In a way akin to low-grade DCIS and invasive carcinomas NST, lobular carcinomas also harbour deletions of 16q, gains of 1q and 16p {26A,258,520A,827,1173}. There is evidence to suggest that the differences between low-grade ductal and lobular proliferations is the target gene of 16q deletions; while in low-grade ductal proliferations the target gene of 16q deletions remains to be identified {613A,730A, 1135A,1495A}, the target gene in lobular lesions has been shown to be *CDH1* {128, 129,273A,1528}. This gene encodes E-cadherin, an adhesion molecule that mediates homophylic and homotypic adhesions in epithelial cells; loss of E-cadherin expression has been shown to lead to the characteristic discohesiveness and patterns of invasion and metastasis of lobular carcinomas {331B,1568}.

In addition to the *CDH1* loss of function and lobular phenotype, additional genotypic-phenotypic correlations have been recorded in breast cancers. For instance, secretory carcinomas {1442} and adenoid cystic carcinomas {1092,1577A} have been shown to harbour recurrent chromosomal translocations, namely t(12;15) and t(6;9), respectively. These translocations lead to the formation of the chimaeric fusion genes *ETV6-NTRK3* {1442} and *MYB-NFIB* {1092,1577A}. Furthermore, micropapillary {875, 876} and mucinous {739} carcinomas have been shown to harbour distinct patterns of gene copy-number aberrations when compared to grade- and ER-matched invasive carcinomas NST.

Despite the associations between the phenotypical characteristics of DCIS and invasive carcinomas NST and the patterns of gene copy-number aberrations in breast cancer, there is still a great degree of heterogeneity in grade 2 and grade 3 lesions. Furthermore, although the "intrinsic" subtypes as defined by gene-expression array analysis have distinctive patterns of gene copy-number aberrations, each subtype comprises a rather heterogeneous group of tumours in terms of the patterns of genetic aberrations observed {15B,118A,262C,262D,463,574, 664,970A,1242A}.

With the advent of next-generation sequencing, it has become possible to characterize the entire genome, transcriptome and epigenome of a tumour {63A}. Complete genomic sequencing studies of breast cancers have demonstrated that breast cancers are incredibly heterogeneous in terms of the mutations, structural variations and copy-number aberrations they harbour {343A,676A,970C,1297A, 1375}. In fact, few mutations have been shown to be highly recurrent (e.g. *TP53*, *PIK3CA* and *PTEN*) in invasive carcinomas NST {519A, 676A,1374,1374A}. With the clinically defined subgroup of breast cancers (i.e. ER-positive/HER2-negative, HER2-positive and ER-negative/HER2-negative), a great degree of heterogeneity in terms of the patterns and types of gene copy-number aberrations, mutations and somatic rearrangements has been documented. Next-generation sequencing has also revealed the existence of a "mutator" phenotype {1375}, which is characterized by the presence of multiple tandem duplications and is reported to be found more frequently in ER-negative/HER2-negative breast cancers. In addition, complete sequencing of matched primary and metastatic breast cancers have demonstrated that tumours are likely to be composed of mosaics of subclones of cancer cells that harbour genetic aberrations in addition to the founder genetic events, and that breast-cancer metastasis may stem from genetically distinct subclones from the primary tumour {343A,1297A}. With the combined efforts of The Cancer Genome Atlas (TCGA), the International Cancer Genome Consortium (ICGC) and numerous individual academic projects, > 25 000 cancer genomes will be sequenced in the next 5 years {703B}. These data will undoubtedly unravel the complete landscape of mutations in different types of breast cancer and lead to the identification of novel "drivers" of the disease, which can be exploited therapeutically.

Expression profiling

M.J. van de Vijver
C.M. Perou
J.S. Reis-Filho

D. Hayes
C. Sotiriou

Introduction

There is a large body of literature on the association of gene alterations or changes in gene/protein expression of one or of a limited number of genes with prognosis and response to therapy in breast cancer {1146,1223}. Although many statistically significant associations have been identified, the overwhelming majority are not strong enough to be clinically useful. This is not entirely surprising because many of these genes already correlate with known biomarkers (estrogen receptor, ER; HER2; Ki67), and the behaviour of cells or tumours is determined by the coordinated expression of many genes, making it unlikely that the analysis of one or a few genes can accurately predict clinical behaviour beyond what is already known. Genome-wide analysis of gene expression using DNA microarrays is used in translational research to identify novel prognostic and predictive factors, and a number of diagnostic tests based on the assessment of patterns of gene expression in tumours are commercially available. The use of microarray analysis makes it possible to assess the level of expression of all genes in the human genome. Tumour-cell behaviour is determined by the coordinate expression pattern of genes involved in the regulation of cell growth and other important aspects of cell behaviour. Therefore, the analysis of global gene-expression patterns may facilitate the prediction of tumour behaviour, including the risk of developing distant metastases and response to specific therapies.

In most studies, gene expression has been analysed using RNA isolated from frozen tumour material, without attempting to enrich for tumour cells. The expression pattern of a tumour is also determined by gene expression in the many other cell types that are present in the clinical tumour mass (e.g. fibroblasts, endothelial cells, and inflammatory cells) and thus these non-tumour cells may also contribute to tumour behaviour.

Technical principles of microarray analysis

A microarray is an ordered arrangement of known DNA molecules of predetermined sequence (the "probes") attached to a solid support. One array may contain many thousands of probes and can be obtained by a number of different manufacturing methods. The probes attached to the solid support can be complementary DNAs (cDNAs), oligonucleotides of varying length, or genomic sequences (i.e. bacterial artificial chromosomes, BACs). The array may be formatted by applying the DNA (cDNA, oligonucleotides) to the array by pins or inkjet technology, by in situ photolithographic synthesis of oligonucleotides, or by bead-based methods. The target sequence hybridized to the probes on the array may be radioactively or fluorescently labelled. The isolation of RNA, which is then converted to cDNA, followed by high-throughput sequencing of all cDNAs, can now also be used for the analysis of gene-expression patterns.

The result of each of the techniques used to assay gene-expression profiles is that the expression level of each gene on the array is measured quantitatively for each tumour sample.

Bioinformatics techniques

The combination of clinical and microarray studies produces a database of gene-expression data and clinical/pathological data; each patient or sample is represented by thousands of data-points that then have to be analysed. Of the many analytical techniques that can be used to correlate gene-expression data with clinical and pathological parameters, unsupervised hierarchical cluster analysis is very important, as are supervised classification methods, and the use of existing gene-expression signatures.

Unsupervised hierarchical cluster analysis

When an unsupervised approach is used to analyse gene-expression data for a series of tumours, the clinical or pathology information available for the tumour samples is not used. For the analysis of microarray data, the most frequently used method has been hierarchical cluster analysis. This is a mathematical algorithm that can be used to order gene-expression data. Thus gene-expression analysis can be used in selected circumstances to subclassify tumours on the basis of hierarchical cluster analysis into specific subgroups {416,1090,1356}.

Supervised classification

To find gene-expression patterns that can predict the clinical behaviour of tumours, it is more appropriate to use a supervised method that specifically searches for genes that correlate with a given clinical parameter, such as survival or response to therapy. Fundamental to this approach is the identification of the patterns of expression of a combination of genes that can predict tumour behaviour (e.g. risk of

development of distant metastases, responsiveness to specific forms of chemotherapy).

An essential step is to validate a predictive gene-expression pattern in an independent series of tumours/patients. It is obvious that the robustness of the predictive gene-expression profiles will improve with increasing sample size.

Existing gene-expression signatures

A major advantage of microarray analysis is that specific properties of cells can be recognized by the expression level of a large set of genes. This has been operationally defined as "expression signatures" or "multigene predictors". A gene-expression signature can be defined by the cell type in which its component genes are expressed (e.g. "T-cell signature") or by the biological process in which its component genes are known to function (e.g. "proliferation signature" or "wound signature").

Studies of gene expression in clinical samples of breast cancer

For the clinical use of gene-expression profiling, the main aim is to identify profiles associated with specific clinical endpoints and to implement gene-expression profiling in the diagnostic process for patients with breast cancer. The first step towards this goal is to obtain tumour tissue that is suitable for use in gene-expression profiling. At present, studies of gene-expression profiling mainly employ RNA isolated from frozen tissue. To this end, tumour samples from a representative part of the surgical specimen must be processed within 30–60 minutes after surgery. The tumour sample is most commonly snap-frozen in liquid nitrogen and stored at –70 °C or in liquid nitrogen, but commercial reagents are also available in which tissue can be stored for up to 7 days, preserving the quality of the RNA. The tissue composition of the frozen sample, including the percentage of tumour cells, should be assessed under the microscope. The source of RNA is usually surgical-excision specimens, but RNA isolated from fine-needle aspirates and needle-core biopsies can also be used for microarray analysis. It is also possible to perform gene-expression studies using RNA from formalin-fixed, paraffin-embedded (FFPE) tissue sections; however, the methods involved require painstaking design and testing of individual gene-expression probes, thus precluding the use of the

global microarray-type format for FFPE material.

Subgroups of breast cancer as defined by gene-expression profiles

When unsupervised hierarchical cluster analysis is used to analyse series of breast carcinomas, a striking division of the tumours into ER-positive and ER-negative categories is observed {1090,1496}. The ER-positive group is characterized by the expression of many genes specific to breast luminal cells, whereas most of the ER-negative tumours express genes characteristic of myoepithelial cells.

Based on the subgroups that are observed using hierarchical cluster analysis, several subgroups of breast carcinomas can be categorized with distinct clinical outcomes: basal-like type tumours (ER-negative tumours expressing myoepithelial/"basal" genes such as keratin 5, 14, and 17); HER2-like tumours (ER-negative tumours that overexpress the *HER2* gene); luminal A and luminal B (both ER-positive tumours clustering together) {1090}. Other dominant subgroups that can be recognized are normal epithelial-like tumours and claudin-low tumours, the latter of which show features of stem cells {1122}.

Gene-expression profile-defined signatures predicting clinical outcome

The supervised approach of classifying tumours has identified a 70-gene and a 76-gene prognosis signature {1090,1486, 1549}. "Activated" and "quiescent" subgroups of tumours can be recognized on the basis of a wound-like signature {241}; while "genomic high grade" and a "genomic low grade" groups of tumours can be recognized on the basis of a histological grade-related signature {1358}. In addition, a reverse transcription polymerase chain reaction (RT-PCR) 21-gene expression profile for prognosis in patients with tamoxifen-treated node-negative breast cancer has been identified {1059}. Probably the most promising and clinically useful area for the application of microarray analysis is the prediction of response to treatment, including chemotherapy {629}, hormonal therapy {846}, and radiation; there are fewer of these predictive signatures, but many are under development. The prognostic gene-expression profiles that can be used in clinical practice are listed below.

70-gene signature

A 70-gene prognosis signature has been developed as a microarray-based test that can be used to determine the prognosis of patients with stage 1 or 2, node-negative invasive breast cancer of tumour size < 5.0 cm. It requires fresh or frozen samples with a tumour-cell content of > 30%. This dichotomous test classifies tumours into "good" or "poor" prognosis, which is an independent predictor of distant metastasis {1486,1496}. The prognostic value of the 70-gene prognosis signature is supported by level II evidence {211A,703A,944A,1486}. Consistent with the notion that the prognostic information provided by the 70-gene signature largely stems from the expression levels of ER-related and proliferation-related genes {1173A,1177A,1589}, the prognostic information provided for ER-negative cancers is limited or non-existent.

Genomic grade index (GGI)

GGI is a prognostic signature that was developed based on the evidence that histological grade is a strong prognostic factor in ER-positive disease and that reproducibility of tumour grade by histological analysis is suboptimal. A microarray-based gene signature that could classify invasive breast cancers into GGI grades I and III was derived {1358}. This signature not only accurately classified histological grade 1 and 3 tumours into GGI grade I and III, respectively, but was also shown to substratify histological grade 2 cancers into grade I-like, which have a low frequency of distant relapses, and grade III-like, which have a clinical behaviour similar to that of histological grade 3 cancers {1358}. GGI was initially developed as a microarray-based test that required fresh or frozen samples {1358}; a quantitative real-time RT-PCR (qRT-PCR) version of this signature has been recently developed

and validated {1452A}. There is level III evidence to demonstrate that GGI is a prognostic factor for ER-positive breast cancers {331A}. In a way akin to histological grade and the 70-gene prognosis signature, the prognostic information provided by GGI primarily stems from the expression levels of proliferation-related genes.

"Intrinsic" subtypes

Hierarchical cluster analysis of genes that vary more between tumours than between repeated samples of the same tumour (i.e. "intrinsic genes") revealed the existence of at least five molecular subtypes of breast cancer, namely luminal A, luminal B, HER2-enriched, basal-like and normal breast-like. Importantly, the most stable separation was shown to be between basal-like tumours and tumours classified as of another "intrinsic" subtype {1126A,1569A}.

Different lists of "intrinsic genes" and single-sample predictors to classify breast cancers into the "intrinsic" subtypes have been described; however, it has been demonstrated that different methods may assign the same patients into different "intrinsic" subtypes and only the basal-like cancers can be reproducibly identified regardless of the analysis methods employed {356A,838A,849A,1089A,1355A, 1569A}. The lack of standardization and reproducibility was in part addressed by the development of PAM50 {1073A}, a 50-gene set that classifies invasive breast cancers into luminal A, luminal B, HER2-enriched and basal-like subtypes. A prognostic test based on the expression levels of these 50 genes assessed by qRT-PCR has been developed and is applicable to FFPE archival samples. Level II evidence for its prognostic impact has been demonstrated in retrospective analyses of prospective clinical trials {376A,997A}.

It must be emphasized that the classification

of tumours into luminal A, luminal B, HER2-enriched and basal-like types by PAM50 and the classification of breast cancers on the basis of immunohistochemical analysis of ER, PR and HER2 is not equivalent. When the results of PAM50 and immunohistochemical analysis of ER, PR and HER2 are discrepant, patients should be managed according to the current immunohistochemical markers.

Additional molecular subtypes of tumours that are preferentially ER-negative have been proposed, including the molecular apocrine {346A,422} and claudin-low {1122} tumours. The biological and clinical relevance of these novel subtypes remains to be determined.

21-gene recurrence score

The 21-gene recurrence score is a qRT-PCR-based signature based on the expression of 21 genes (16 cancer-related and 5 reference genes) that can be applied to RNA extracted from FFPE tissue samples {1059}. The 21-gene recurrence score is a mathematical function developed to predict the risk of distant relapse at 10 years for patients with ER-positive, lymph node-negative breast cancers {1059}. It is a continuous variable (ranging from 0 to 100) that is associated with the risk of distant relapse within 10 years, and an independent prognostic factor for ER-positive, node-negative patients with breast cancer treated with adjuvant endocrine therapy (i.e. tamoxifen and aromatase inhibitors) {353A,1059,1609A}. On the basis of the 21-gene recurrence score, patients can be classified into three categories, including low risk (recurrence score [RS] < 18), intermediate risk (RS 18–31) and high risk (RS ≥ 31), which equate with 10-year relapse rates of 7%, 14% and 30%, respectively. The 21-gene recurrence score also correlates with benefit from chemotherapy in ER-positive breast cancers {1059A}.

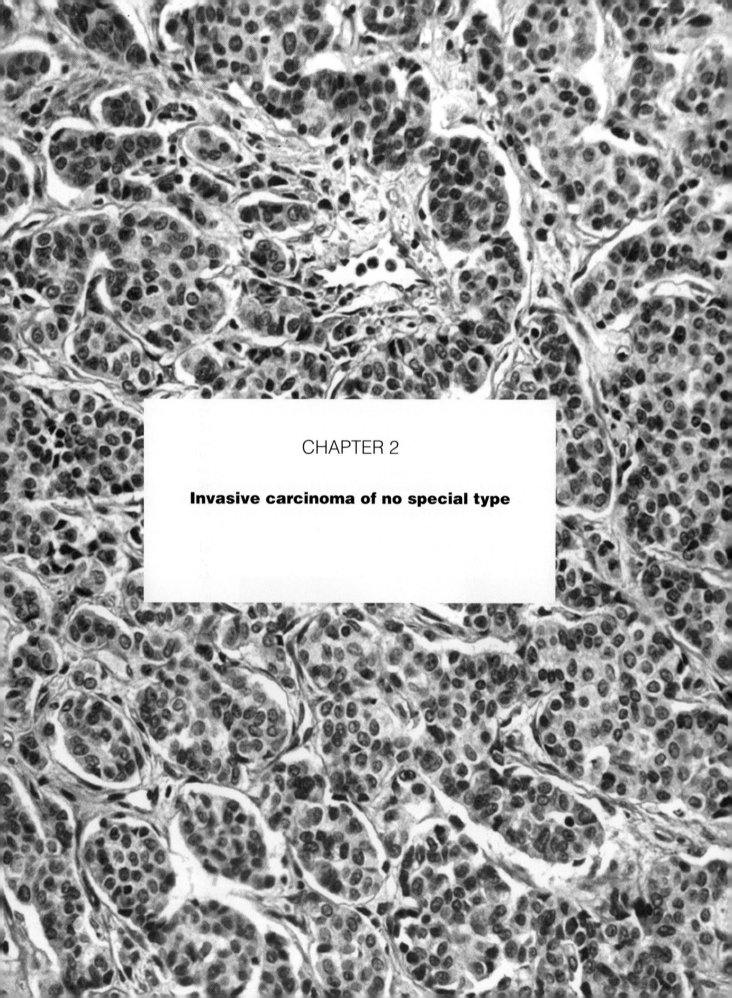

CHAPTER 2

Invasive carcinoma of no special type

Invasive carcinoma of no special type

I.O. Ellis
L. Collins
S. Ichihara
G. MacGrogan

Definition

Invasive breast carcinoma of no special type (NST), commonly known as ductal carcinoma NST, comprises the largest group of invasive breast cancers. It is not an easily defined entity as it represents the heterogeneous group of tumours that fail to exhibit sufficient characteristics to achieve classification as a specific histological type, such as lobular or tubular carcinoma.

ICD-O code   8500/3

Synonyms and historical annotation

Invasive carcinoma of no specific type (ductal NST); invasive carcinoma, not otherwise specified (ductal NOS); infiltrating ductal carcinoma. Many other names have been used historically for this form of breast carcinoma, including scirrhous carcinoma, carcinoma simplex and spheroidal cell carcinoma. "Infiltrating ductal carcinoma" has been used in the past, but was revised in the last edition of the WHO Classification of Tumours {1413} to recognize the non-specific nature of this term. Use of the term "ductal" perpetuates the traditional but incorrect concept that these tumours are derived exclusively from mammary ductal epithelium in distinction from lobular carcinomas, which were deemed to have arisen from within lobules, for which there is also no evidence. In addition it has been shown that the terminal-duct lobular unit (TDLU) should be regarded as a single entity from the point of view of the site of origin of most breast carcinomas {84, 1573}. Some groups {445} have retained the term "ductal" but added the phrase "not otherwise specified", while others {1052} prefer to use "no special type" to emphasize the distinction from specific-type tumours. "Carcinoma of no special type" is increasingly accepted internationally and preferred, but since "ductal" is still widely used, the terms "ductal NST," "ductal NOS," or "invasive ductal carcinoma" are alternative terminology options.

Epidemiology

Invasive carcinoma NST forms a large proportion of mammary carcinomas and its epidemiological characteristics are similar to those of the group as a whole (see Chapter 1: *Epidemiology*). It is the most common "type" of invasive carcinoma of the breast, comprising between 40% and 75% of cases in published series. This wide range is largely attributable to the lack of application of strict criteria for inclusion in the special types and also the fact that tumours with a combination of invasive carcinoma NST and special-type patterns are not universally recognized as a separate mixed category, but may be included with tumours of "no special type". Invasive carcinoma NST, like all forms of breast cancer, is rare below the age of 40 years, but the proportion of tumours classified as such in young women with breast cancer is in general similar to that in older women {708}.

There are no well-recognized differences between the known risk factors

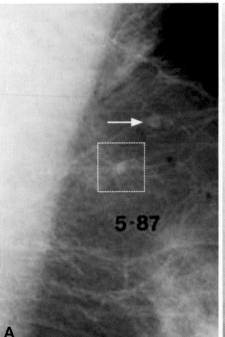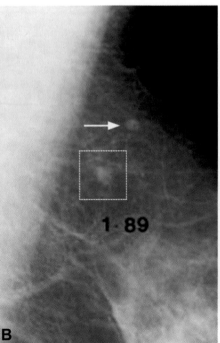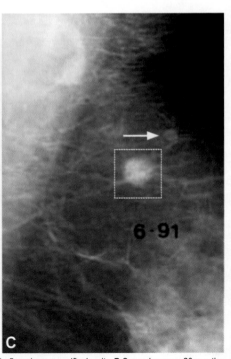

Fig. 2.01 Invasive carcinoma of no special type, grade 1. **A** First screen: Intramammary lymph node (arrow) and small (< 5 mm) non-specific density. **B** Second screen, 20 months later: the density has grown a little. **C** Third screen, after another 29 months: the 10 mm tumour is more obvious but still not palpable.

(e.g. geography, cultural/lifestyle factors, reproductive variables) for breast cancer in general and ductal NST cancers in particular. Among the tumours developing subsequent to the diagnosis of conditions conferring an increased risk of breast cancer, such as atypical ductal hyperplasia and lobular neoplasia, invasive carcinoma NST is less frequent than tumours of special type, namely tubular and classical lobular carcinoma {1055,1056}.

Macroscopy

These tumours have no specific macroscopic features. There is a marked variation in size from < 10 mm to > 100 mm. They can have an irregular, stellate outline or nodular configuration. The tumour edge is usually moderately or ill-defined and lacks sharp circumscription. Classically, invasive carcinoma NST is firm or even hard on palpation, and may have a "gritty" feel when cut with a knife. The cut surface is usually grey-white with yellow streaks.

Histopathology

Designation as this histological type of breast cancer is essentially through a process of exclusion of recognized special types. As a consequence, morphological features vary considerably from case to case. All types of tumour margins can be observed, from highly infiltrative,

permeating the lobular stroma and disrupting the normal lobular units, to continuous pushing margins. Architecturally, the tumour cells may be arranged in cords, clusters and trabeculae, whilst some tumours are characterized by a predominantly solid or syncytial infiltrative pattern with little associated stroma. In a proportion of cases, glandular differentiation may be apparent as tubular structures with central lumina in tumour-cell groups. Occasionally, areas with single-file infiltration or targetoid features are seen, but these lack the cytomorphological characteristics of invasive lobular carcinoma. The carcinoma cells also have a variable appearance. The cytoplasm may be abundant and eosinophilic. Nuclei may be regular and uniform or highly pleomorphic with prominent, often multiple, nucleoli. Mitotic activity may be virtually absent or extensive. In up to 80% of cases, foci of associated ductal carcinoma in situ (DCIS) will be present. Any associated DCIS is usually of same nuclear grade as the invasive carcinoma.

Some histopathologists recognize a subtype of invasive carcinoma NST, "infiltrating ductal carcinoma with extensive in situ component." The stromal component is extremely variable. There may be a highly cellular fibroblastic proliferation, a scanty element of connective tissue or marked

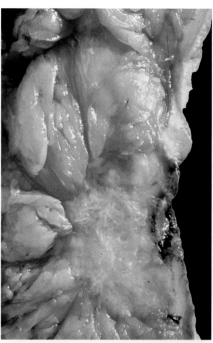

Fig. 2.02 Invasive carcinoma of no special type. A mastectomy specimen from a patient aged 84 years.

hyalinization. Foci of elastosis may also be present in a periductal or perivenous distribution. Focal necrosis may be present and this is occasionally extensive with secondary formation of cysts. In a minority of cases, a distinct lymphoplasmacytoid infiltrate can be identified.

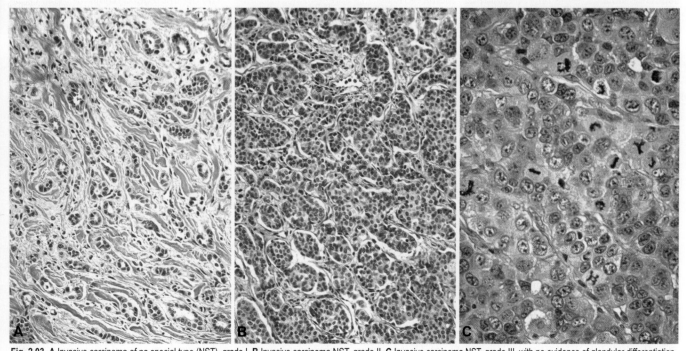

Fig. 2.03 A Invasive carcinoma of no special type (NST), grade I. **B** Invasive carcinoma NST, grade II. **C** Invasive carcinoma NST, grade III, with no evidence of glandular differentiation. Note the presence of numerous cells in mitosis, with some abnormal mitotic figures present.

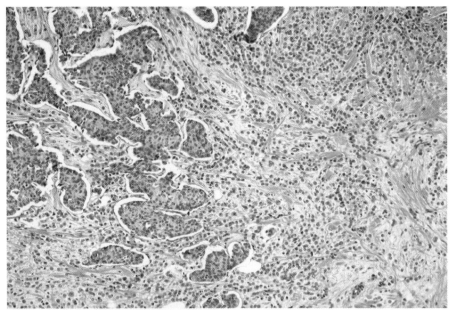

Fig. 2.04 Invasive carcinoma of no special type and invasive lobular carcinoma. Two distinct morphological patterns are seen in this tumour, no special type on the left and lobular on the right.

Lympho-vascular tumour emboli can be observed throughout the tumour, but only those localized outside the tumour carry a prognostic effect.

Carcinoma of mixed type

For a tumour to be typed as invasive carcinoma NST, it must have a non-specialized pattern in > 50% of its mass as judged by thorough examination of representative sections. If the non-specialized pattern comprises between 10% and 49% of the tumour, the rest being of a recognized special type, then it will fall into one of the mixed groups: mixed invasive NST and special type or mixed invasive NST and lobular carcinoma. Apart from

these considerations, there are very few lesions that should be confused with invasive carcinoma NST.

Rare morphological variants of invasive carcinoma NST

These morphological forms of breast cancer are not currently recognized as distinct special types of invasive breast cancer but as variants of invasive carcinoma NST.

Pleomorphic carcinoma

ICD-O code   8022/3

Pleomorphic carcinoma is a rare variant of high-grade invasive carcinoma NST, which is characterized by a proliferation

of pleomorphic and bizarre, sometimes multinucleated, tumour giant cells comprising > 50% of the tumour cells in a background of adenocarcinoma or adenocarcinoma with metaplastic spindle and squamous differentiation {1321}. In the original series described, the patients ranged in age from 28 to 96 years with a median of 51 years. Most patients present with a large palpable mass (mean size, 5.4 cm); in 12% of cases, metastatic tumour is the first manifestation of disease.

The tumour giant cells in pleomorphic carcinoma account for > 75% of tumour cells in most cases. The tumours are typically of grade 3 with a high mitotic frequency and central necrosis. There may be associated high-grade DCIS and lymphovascular invasion. Hormone-receptor expression is usually negative, but a proportion of cases overexpress HER2 protein {1626}. Axillary lymph-node metastases are present in 50% of patients, with involvement of three or more lymph nodes in most of these. Many patients present with advanced disease. One recent study found that poor outcome in these tumours is associated with presence of a spindle-cell metaplastic component {989}.

Carcinoma with osteoclast-like stromal giant cells

ICD-O code   8035/3

The common denominator of these carcinomas is the presence of osteoclastic giant cells (OGCs) in the stroma {571}. The giant cells are generally associated with an inflammatory, fibroblastic, hypervascular stroma, with extravasated erythrocytes, lymphocytes and monocytes

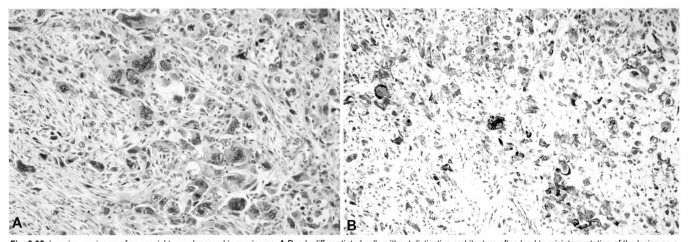

Fig. 2.05 Invasive carcinoma of no special type: pleomorphic carcinoma. **A** Poorly differentiated cells without distinctive architecture often lead to misinterpretation of the lesion as a sarcoma. **B** Immunostaining for keratin (AE1/AE3) confirms the epithelial nature of the process.

along with mononucleated and binucleated histiocytes, some containing haemosiderin. The giant cells vary in size and have a variable number of nuclei. They appear to embrace the epithelial component or are found within lumina formed by the cancer cells. The giant cells contain a variable number of non-atypical bland nuclei. The giant cells and hypervascular reactive stroma can be observed in lymph-node metastases and in recurrences {1454}. The carcinomatous part of the lesion is most frequently a well- to moderately differentiated invasive carcinoma NST but all the other histological types have been observed particularly invasive cribriform carcinoma {986,1103}, and also tubular, mucinous, papillary {1552}, lobular {986,1103}, squamous and other metaplastic patterns {571,1323} and pleomorphic carcinoma {735}.

The giant cells show uniform expression of CD68 {571} and are negative for S100 protein and actin, and negative for keratin, epithelial membrane antigen (EMA), estrogen and progesterone receptors (ER and PR) {1414}. The giant cells are strongly positive for acid phosphatase, non-specific esterase and lysozyme, but negative for alkaline phosphatase, which is indicative of morphological similarity to histiocytic cells and osteoclasts {1207, 1414,1454}. Ultrastructural and immuno-histochemical studies have confirmed the histiocytic nature of the osteoclastic cells present in these unusual carcinomas {1454,1513}. OGCs appear in relation to inflammatory hypervascular stroma around breast carcinoma regardless of histology. Cytokines that promote macrophage migration and angiogenesis, such as VEGF

and MMP12, are secreted from both tumoural and non-tumoural cells. It is likely that the OGCs are generated by syncytial fusion of macrophages, but not by mitosis without cell division. The phenotypic resemblance of OGCs to osteoclasts in the bone has been confirmed by the observation of expression of MMP9, TRAP, and cathepsin K {1255,1314}.

About one third of the reported cases had lymph-node metastases. The 5-year survival rate is around 70%, which is similar to, or better than, patients with ordinary invasive carcinomas {1552}. Prognosis is related to the characteristics of the associated carcinoma and does not appear to be influenced by the presence of stromal giant cells.

Carcinoma with choriocarcinomatous features

Patients with invasive carcinoma NST may have elevated levels of serum human chorionic gonadotrophin (HCG) {1303} and as many as 60% of invasive carcinomas NST have been found to contain HCG-positive cells {596}. Histological evidence of choriocarcinomatous differentiation, however, is exceptionally rare with only a few cases reported {487,518,1250}. All were in women aged between 50 and 70 years.

Carcinoma with melanotic features

A few case reports have described exceptional tumours of the mammary parenchyma that appear to represent combinations of invasive carcinoma NST and malignant melanoma {1005,1051, 1237} and in some of these cases, there appeared to be a transition from one cell type to the other. A genetic analysis of one

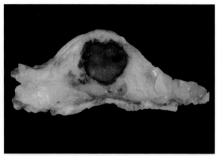

Fig. 2.06 Invasive carcinomas with stromal osteoclastic giant cells often have vascular stromal tissue with accumulation of haemosiderin pigment, giving them a brown macroscopic appearance.

such case showed loss of heterozygosity at the same chromosomal loci in all the components of the tumour, suggesting an origin from the same neoplastic clone {1005}. The mere presence of melanin in breast cancer cells should not be construed as evidence of melanocytic differentiation, since pigmentation of carcinoma cells with melanin can occur when breast cancers invade the skin and involve the dermoepidermal junction {85}. In one study, focal expression of melan A was found in 18% of breast cancers. The presence and extent of melan A expression was statistically significantly associated with a reduction in tumour-cell differentiation, but not tumour type, size, lymph-node metastasis, hormone-receptor status or HER2 expression. Expression of melanocytic markers in breast tissue appears to be related to lineage infidelity {87}. In addition, care must be taken to distinguish tumours showing melanocytic differentiation from breast carcinomas with prominent cytoplasmic deposition of lipofuscin {1309}.

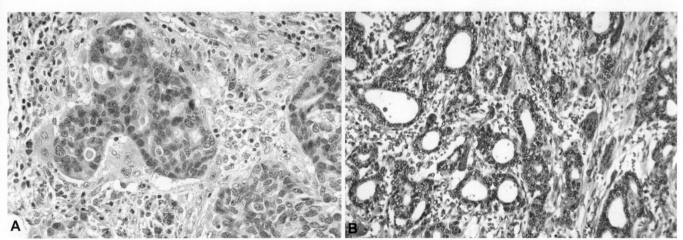

Fig. 2.07 A Invasive carcinoma of no special type (NST) with stromal osteoclastic giant cells and haemosiderin-laden macrophages. **B** The invasive carcinoma NST is of low grade. Multinucleated giant cells are evident in the stroma.

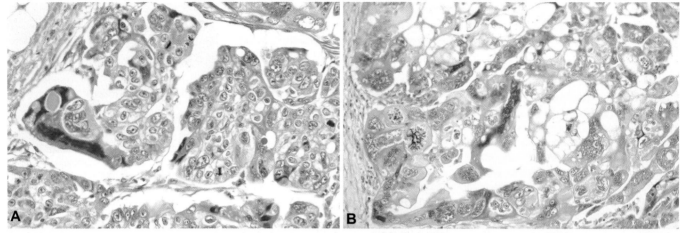

Fig. 2.08 Invasive carcinoma of no special type: carcinoma with choriocarcinomatous features. **A, B** Multinucleated tumour cells with smudged nuclei extend their irregular, elongated cytoplasmic processes around clusters of monocytic tumour cells, mimicking the biphasic growth pattern of choriocarcinoma. **B** Note the abnormal mitotic figures in this high-grade carcinoma.

Most melanotic tumours of the breast represent metastases from malignant melanomas originating in extra-mammary sites {1323}. Primary melanomas may arise anywhere in the skin of the breast, but an origin in the nipple–areola complex is extremely rare {1070}. The differential diagnosis of malignant melanoma arising in the nipple-areolar region must include Paget disease, the cells of which may occasionally contain melanin pigment {1267} (see Chapter 12).

Genetics

Cases of familial breast cancer associated with mutations in *BRCA1* are commonly of invasive carcinoma NST type but have medullary carcinoma-like features, exhibiting higher mitotic counts, a greater proportion of the tumour with a continuous pushing margin, and more lymphocytic infiltration than sporadic cancers {747}. Cancers associated with mutations in *BRCA2* are also often of invasive carcinoma NST type, but exhibit a high score for tubule formation (fewer tubules), a higher proportion of the tumour perimeter with a continuous pushing margin and a lower mitotic count than sporadic cancers {747}.

The genetic variation seen in breast cancer as a whole is apparent in invasive carcinoma NST. Recent observations associating specific genetic lesions or regions of alteration with a particular histological type or grade imply that the group of breast cancers of invasive carcinoma NST type includes a number of different types of tumour that have developed via unrelated genetic evolutionary pathways {204}, and that show fundamental differences to some tumours of special type, including lobular {528} and tubular carcinoma {1230}. Furthermore, cDNA microarray analysis has clearly demonstrated that invasive carcinoma NST can be classified into subtypes on the basis of gene-expression patterns {1090, 1356} and that many of the special types of breast cancer have characteristic alterations (see Chapter 1: *Expression profiling* and *Breast-cancer genomics and next-generation sequencing*).

Prognosis and predictive factors

Invasive carcinoma NST forms the bulk (50–80%) of cases of breast cancer and its prognostic characteristics and management are similar or slightly worse with a 35–50% 10-year survival {376} compared to breast cancer as a whole with around a 55% 10-year survival. Prognosis is influenced profoundly by the classical variables of histological grade, tumour size, lymph-node status and vascular invasion (see Chapter 1: *Grading* and *Staging*) and by predictors of therapeutic response, such as ER and HER2 status (see Chapter 1: *Molecular testing for estrogen receptor, progesterone receptor and HER2*). Approximately 70–80% of invasive breast carcinomas NST are ER-positive and approximately 15% of cases are HER2-positive. The management of invasive carcinoma NST is also influenced by these prognostic and predictive characteristics.

CHAPTER 3

Special subtypes

Invasive lobular carcinoma

Tubular carcinoma and cribriform carcinoma

Carcinoma with medullary features

Metaplastic carcinoma

Carcinomas with apocrine differentiation

Salivary gland/skin adnexal type tumours

Adenoid cystic carcinoma

Mucoepidermoid carcinoma

Polymorphous carcinoma

Mucinous carcinoma and carcinomas
with signet-ring-cell differentiation

Carcinomas with neuroendocrine features

Invasive papillary carcinoma

Invasive micropapillary carcinoma

Inflammatory carcinoma

Bilateral breast carcinoma
and non-synchronous breast carcinoma

Exceptionally rare types and variants

Invasive lobular carcinoma

S.R. Lakhani
E. Rakha
P.T. Simpson

Definition

An invasive carcinoma composed of non-cohesive cells individually dispersed or arranged in a single-file linear pattern in a fibrous stroma. It is usually associated with lobular carcinoma in situ (LCIS).

ICD-O code   8520/3

Epidemiology

Invasive lobular carcinoma (ILC) represents 5–15% of invasive breast tumours {376,789,795,1264,1444,1587}.
Since the 1980s, the incidence of ILC has increased relative to that of invasive carcinoma of no special type (invasive carcinoma NST) {789,790}. This might be attributable to the increased use of hormone-replacement therapy {168,308,789,796, 1016,1162} or increased consumption of alcohol {791,793}. The mean age of patients with ILC is 57–65 years, slightly higher than that of patients with invasive carcinoma NST {73,795,1138,1264,1444}.

Clinical features

Most women present with an ill-defined palpable mass involving any part of the breast, although centrally located tumours were found to be slightly more common in patients with ILC than with invasive carcinoma NST in one study {1587}. Radiologically, the most common mammographic findings are a spiculated mass or architectural distortion. Calcification is infrequent. Compared with invasive carcinoma NST, mammography has a reduced sensitivity for detecting ILC (57–89%) with high false-negative rates of up to 19% {577,723,764}. Ultrasound is more sensitive (78–95%), although the size of the tumour can be underestimated {211,237, 243,409,1189,1295,1556}. Magnetic resonance imaging (MRI) is more helpful in diagnosing ILC, particularly multifocal lesions, although this technique can lead to false positives and overestimation of tumour size {342,1273}.
A high rate of multicentric tumours has been reported in some studies {341,785} but this has not been found in other series based on clinical {1264} or radiological

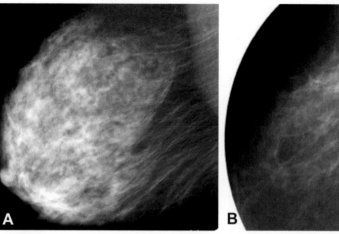

Fig. 3.01 Mammography of invasive lobular carcinoma. **A** Architectural distortion in the axillary tail, corresponding to a palpable area of thickening. **B** Magnified view of the architectural axillary distortion.

{764} analysis. An incidence of contralateral tumours, particularly synchronous tumours, of 5–19% has also been reported (see *Bilateral breast carcinoma*), which is higher than for invasive carcinoma NST {73,190,257,341, 426,1094,1326}.

Macroscopy

ILCs frequently present as irregular and poorly delimited tumours that can be difficult to define macroscopically because of the diffuse growth pattern of the cell infiltrate {1326}. The size of the ILC is also difficult to determine, although it has been reported to be slightly larger than that of invasive carcinoma NST in some series {1264,1326,1587}.

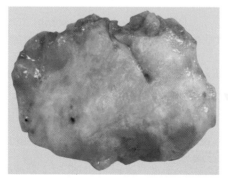

Fig. 3.02 Macroscopy of an invasive lobular carcinoma displays an ill-defined lesion.

Histopathology

The classic pattern of ILC {455,885,1555} is characterized by a proliferation of small cells, which lack cohesion and appear individually dispersed through a fibrous connective tissue or arranged in single-file linear cords that invade the stroma. These infiltrating cords frequently present a concentric pattern around normal ducts. There is often little host reaction or disturbance of the background architecture. The neoplastic cells have round or notched ovoid nuclei and a thin rim of cytoplasm with an occasional intracytoplasmic lumen {1128}, often harbouring a central mucoid inclusion. Mitoses are typically infrequent. These classic cytological features are the same as those seen in lobular neoplasia, which is associated with ILC in 58–98% of cases {6,341,345,984}.

Histological variants

A number of variants of ILC have been described that share either the cytological or growth pattern of classic ILC, but all lack cell-to-cell cohesion.
The *solid type* is characterized by the typical non-cohesive and small cells of lobular morphology but these cells grow in sheets, are often more pleomorphic and have a higher frequency of mitoses than the classic type {427}.

Cells of the *alveolar variant* are mainly arranged in globular aggregates of at least 20 cells {1316}.

Pleomorphic lobular carcinoma (PLC) retains the distinctive growth pattern of lobular carcinoma but exhibits a greater degree of cellular atypia and pleomorphism and a higher mitotic rate than classic ILC {396,922,1565}. This variant is frequently associated with LCIS composed of the same pleomorphic cytological features. PLC may show apocrine {396} or histiocytoid {1541} differentiation and may be composed of signet ring cells.

The *tubulolobular variant* is composed of the admixture of a tubular growth pattern and small uniform cells arranged in a linear pattern {446}. LCIS is observed in about one third of tubulo-lobular carcinomas.

A *mixed group* is composed of cases showing an admixture of the classic type with one or more of these variant patterns {345}. The classic ILC type and mixed variants contribute to the majority of lobular tumours, comprising up to 75% of all cases {1043,1137}. In addition, both invasive carcinoma NST and lobular features of differentiation are present in about 5% of invasive breast cancers {795,885} (see *Mixed-type carcinoma*).

Histological grading

The relevance of the three-tiered Nottingham histological grading system for ILC has been a matter for debate due to the characteristic absence of tubule formation (except in the tubulo-lobular variant), the uniformity of neoplastic cells and the low mitotic count. Some studies report the limited prognostic value of grading ILC {1332,1395}, while several studies suggest that grade is an independent predictor of patient outcome {98,937,1089, 1137}. Most (approximately 76%) classic ILCs are grade 2, whereas ILC of grade 3 are mostly of non-classic type {1043,

1395}. Of the three components of tumour grading, the mitotic index is the most useful predictor of outcome; a high mitotic count is associated with a worse prognosis {1137}.

Immunoprofile

Although the literature suggests that 80–95% of ILCs are positive for estrogen receptor (ER), in current practice, classic ILCs are almost invariably ER-positive. In comparison, 70–80% of invasive carcinomas NST are ER-positive. Progesterone receptor (PR) positivity is found in 60–70% of both tumour types {73,1138, 1264,1617}. ER was found to be expressed in the classic form and in variants, but the rate of positivity was highest (100%) in the alveolar variant {1316} and lowest (10%) in PLC {1130}. HER2 amplification and overexpression are rare in ILC {73,1117,1138,1231,1354}, although evident in some PLCs {922,1329}. The expression of p53, basal markers (keratin 14, keratin 5/6, EGFR) and myoepithelial markers (smooth-muscle actin and p63) is rare in ILC {348,413,1138}. The proliferation rate, measured by MIB1/Ki67 labelling, is generally low in ILC, although higher in the variants {1004,1043}. One of the most consistent molecular alterations in ILC and its variants is the loss of expression of the cell–cell adhesion molecule E-cadherin, which contributes to the characteristic discohesive nature of lobular cells {322,469,938,1032,1060,1144, 1155,1329}. Most ILCs also show altered integrity of E-cadherin complex molecules, with loss of alpha-, beta- and gamma-catenins, and the mislocalization of p120 catenin from the cell membrane to the cytoplasm {304,1144,1262}.

Analysis of expression of E-cadherin and p120 may help to differentiate between lobular and low-grade invasive carcinoma NST that are difficult to classify on the

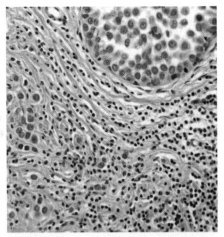

Fig. 3.03 In situ and invasive lobular carcinoma. The larger cells on the left and lower part of the field are invasive tumour cells.

basis of morphological criteria; however, about 15% of ILCs do express E-cadherin and so positive staining should not be used to re-classify a lobular lesion as invasive carcinoma NST {14, 303,1144}.

Genetics

Using flow cytometry, ILCs were found to be near diploid in about 50% of cases {451}. ILCs have fewer and different patterns of genomic alterations than invasive carcinoma NST {451,827,1004,1329}. The most frequently identified alterations in DNA copy number are loss of chromosomal arm 16q and gain of material on 1q and 16p {389, 617,827,1004,1173}. Other alterations are more heterogeneous, although recurrent gains (8q), amplifications (1q32, 8p12–p11.2, 11q13) and losses (8p23–p21, 11q14.1–q25, 13q) are identified.

PLCs exhibit similar alterations but in addition contain amplifications at loci such as 8q24, 17q12 and 20q13, which are characteristic of high-grade invasive carcinoma NST {1329}.

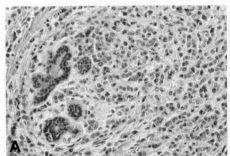
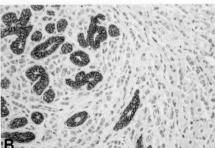
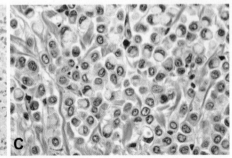

Fig. 3.04 A Invasive lobular carcinoma. **B** Loss of E-cadherin expression is typical of lobular carcinoma cells. Note immunoreactivity of entrapped normal ductules. **C** There is a large number of signet ring cells and intracytoplasmic lumina (targetoid secretion).

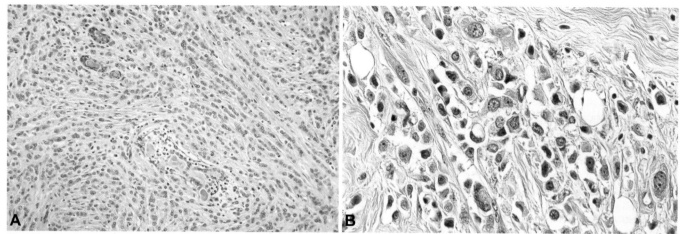

Fig. 3.05 A Classic invasive lobular carcinoma with uniform, single-cell files compared with (B). **B** Invasive pleomorphic lobular carcinoma with characteristic pleomorphic, atypical nuclei.

Inactivation of E-cadherin is the most commonly identified genetic alteration in ILC and occurs as an early event in oncogenesis {1528}. Somatic, truncating mutations within the E-cadherin gene (*CDH1*, mapping to 16q22.1), together with loss of heterozygosity and promoter methylation contribute to this loss of expression {128,354,678,1528}.

Gene-expression profiling studies have demonstrated that ILCs are most frequently classified as luminal A type molecular tumours, but they can also be classified as luminal B, HER2, normal-like or basal-like {1569}. In support of genomic data, gene-expression data indicate that ILCs differ from grade- and ER-matched invasive carcinoma NST and tubular carcinomas in the expression of genes associated with cell adhesion, cell-to-cell signalling and actin cytoskeletal signalling {717,1469,1568,1625}.

Prognosis and predictive factors

Despite the favourable prognostic features of ILC (low grade, ER-positive, HER2-negative, low proliferative index),

there remains controversy as to whether the outcome differs for patients with ILC or invasive carcinoma NST. Several studies have reported a more favourable outcome for ILC than invasive carcinoma NST {345,355,376,1326,1444}, whereas others found no significant differences {73,716,940,1084,1138,1514,1526} or a worse prognosis for ILC {75,1094,1138}. In large series, ILCs were more likely to be of larger size (> 5 cm), more advanced tumour stage (stage III/IV) and with more lymph-node positivity than invasive carcinoma NST {73,795}. An important observation made in two series shows that patients with ILC have a better or similar outcome than patients with invasive carcinoma NST in the first 10 years after diagnosis; however, the long-term outcome associated with ILC is worse than for invasive carcinoma NST {1094,1138}. The higher incidences of distant metastases, recurrences and mortality in ILC are long-term events following diagnosis.

When the histological subtypes of ILC were analysed separately, a more favourable outcome was reported for the classic type

than for the variants, namely pleomorphic and solid {203,341,345,355,396,1043, 1565}. However, tubulo-lobular carcinoma and alveolar ILC have been considered to be low-grade tumours {519,1316}.

A lower frequency of axillary nodal metastasis in ILC than in invasive carcinoma NST has been reported in some series, the difference ranging from 3% to 10% {636, 757,1264,1326,1444}.

The metastatic pattern of ILC differs from that of invasive carcinoma NST. A higher frequency of tumour extension to bone, gastrointestinal tract, uterus, meninges, ovary and diffuse serosal involvement is observed in ILC, while extension to the lung is more frequent in invasive carcinoma NST {73,170,433,554,636,757,1264, 1326,1444}.

Immunohistochemistry using antibodies to GCDFP-15, keratin 7, ER, PR and E-cadherin may help to establish an intra-abdominal tumour as a metastatic ILC.

Tubular carcinoma and cribriform carcinoma

E. Rakha
S.E. Pinder
S.J. Shin
H. Tsuda

Tubular carcinoma

Definition
A special type of breast carcinoma with a particularly favourable prognosis, tubular carcinoma (TC) is composed of well-differentiated tubular structures with open lumina lined by a single layer of cells.

ICD-O code   8211/3

Epidemiology
Pure TC accounts for approximately 2% of invasive breast cancers in most series. Higher frequencies are found among small breast cancers of stage T1 and in mammographic screening programmes {672,820,832,1141}.

Clinical features
There is no specific clinical feature that distinguishes TC from the more common invasive carcinomas of no special type (NST) or other types. When compared with low-grade invasive carcinoma NST, TC is more likely to be smaller, less frequently shows lympho-vascular invasion and nodal involvement and a better patient outcome is typical {340,428,672,780, 1071,1141}. Approximately 10–20% of TCs have been reported to be multifocal {519,928}.
Mammographically, 22–57% of TCs do not show a mass lesion, but others are frequently spiculated and calcifications are variably present {526,1307,1621}. On ultrasound, a hypoechoic mass with ill-defined

margins and posterior acoustic shadowing are seen {526,1302,1307,1621}.

Macroscopy
TC often presents as an ill-defined grey to white, firm or hard mass measuring between 0.2 cm and 2 cm in diameter; most are 1.5 cm or less {340,428,1021,1141}.

Histopathology
The characteristic feature of TC is the predominance of open tubules composed of a single layer of epithelial cells enclosing a clear lumen. These should compose > 90% of the tumour. The tubules are generally an admixture of oval or rounded and angulated shapes and are arranged haphazardly. The cells are small to moderate in size, regular with little nuclear pleomorphism, inconspicuous nucleoli and scanty mitotic figures. Multilayering of nuclei, marked nuclear pleomorphism or high mitotic activity are contraindications for a diagnosis of TC. Apical snouts are seen in up to a third of cases, but are not pathognomonic. Myoepithelial cells are absent around the tubules, but some may have an incomplete surrounding layer of basement membrane.
A secondary, but important feature is the cellular desmoplastic stroma, commonly accompanying the tubular structures. TC occurs in association with flat epithelial atypia, low-grade ductal carcinoma in situ (DCIS) and, less commonly, lobular neoplasia {435, 506,1141}. These epithelial proliferations typically share nuclear grade,

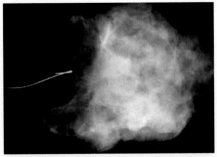
Fig. 3.06 Tubular carcinoma. Specimen X-ray.

immunophenotype and genotypical features {7,79,1141}. An association with radial scar has also been proposed {1340}. There is a lack of consensus concerning the proportion of tubular structures necessary for a diagnosis of TC, with the requirement being set at between 75% and 100% {227,428,672,780,898,1096,1383, 1621} but pragmatically, 90% purity offers a practical solution and is recommended {1141,1413}. Tumours exhibiting between 50% and 90% tubules admixed with another morphology should be regarded as being of mixed type.
TC is nearly always positive for estrogen and progesterone receptors, has a low growth fraction, and is typically negative for HER2, EGFR, P-cadherin, p53 and high-molecular-weight keratins {1071,1141}.

Differential diagnosis
Sclerosing adenosis can be distinguished from TC by its lobular architecture and the compression and distortion of glandular structures. Myoepithelial cells are always present in sclerosing adenosis and can be highlighted with immunostaining. Similarly, a fully retained basement membrane can be shown by immunostaining for collagen IV and laminin in sclerosing adenosis. Complex sclerosing lesions/radial scars have central fibrosis and elastosis containing a few small, often distorted, tubular structures around which myoepithelial cells are present. In a minority of cases of radial scar, attenuated or focally absent staining of myoepithelial cells is seen, particularly in areas of marked sclerosis. The peripheral glandular structures

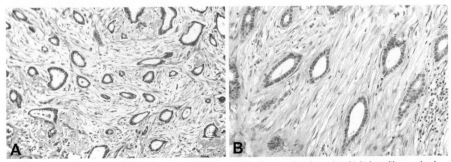
Fig. 3.07 Tubular carcinoma. **A** There is a haphazard distribution of rounded and angulated tubules with open lumina, lined by only a single layer of epithelial cells separated by abundant reactive, fibroblastic stroma. **B** The neoplastic cells lining the tear-drop-shaped tubules lack significant atypia.

in a radial scar show varying degrees of dilatation and ductal epithelial hyperplasia. Microglandular adenosis can be more difficult to differentiate, because of the rather haphazard, diffuse, infiltrative pattern of the tubules and lack of myoepithelial cells around the tubules, in contrast to the localized growth found in TC. Importantly, the tubules of microglandular adenosis are more rounded and regular and often contain colloid-like secretory material compared to the often angulated tubules of TC.

TC should be distinguished from low-grade invasive carcinomas NST and tubulo-lobular carcinomas. The presence of single-layered angulated tubules in > 90% of the lesion, along with an absence of marked pleomorphism and mitoses distinguishes TC from the former. The tubular structures in tubulo-lobular carcinoma are different from those in TC, being small and round rather than angulated in shape, and are admixed with a classic lobular component.

Genetics

TCs of the breast have a low frequency of genetic alterations. Using loss-of-heterozygosity (LOH) and comparative genomic hybridization (CGH) techniques, alterations are seen most frequently at chromosomes 16q (loss) (78–86%), followed by 1q (gain) (50–62%), and they usually occur concomitantly. Other alterations include 16p gain and loss of 8p, 3p (FHIT

gene locus) and 11q (ATM gene locus) {79,865,1186,1540}. Although these chromosomal alterations are common among other low-grade breast cancers, i.e. low-grade invasive carcinoma NST, and lobular carcinomas, small yet important differences at the transcriptome level have been demonstrated {831,1186}. Chromosomal alterations found commonly in invasive carcinoma NST, such as 17p loss, are infrequent in TC. Profiling studies of global gene expression have demonstrated that TC belongs to the "luminal A" molecular class of breast cancer {1569}.

Prognosis and predictive factors

Women with TC have an excellent long-term outcome {227,645,898,1021,1096, 1525}, which in some series is similar to that of age-matched women without breast cancer {340,428,1141,1383}. Recurrence after complete excision is rare. Following breast conservation, whilst taking into account multifocality and associated in situ disease, the risk of local recurrence is so low that some centres consider that adjuvant radiotherapy is unnecessary. Ten-year disease-free survival and overall survival rates after mastectomy or partial resection have been reported to be 93.1–99.1% and 99–100%, respectively {645,820,1141}. Axillary-node metastases occur infrequently (average, 10%; range, 0–22%) and rarely involve more than one axillary lymph node. Even when patients have axillary metastases

from TC, the prognosis is very good and the use of systemic adjuvant therapy and axillary-node dissection are considered unnecessary by some groups {340,428, 672,780,1071}.

Cribriform carcinoma

Definition

An invasive carcinoma with an excellent prognosis that grows in a pattern similar to that seen in intraductal cribriform carcinoma; a 50% component of tubular carcinoma may be admixed.

ICD-O code   8201/3

Epidemiology

Invasive cribriform carcinoma (ICC) accounts for 0.3–0.8% of breast carcinomas {795,832,889,1136}; however, a frequency of up to 4% has been reported in some series {1053,1508}. Mean patient age is 53–58 years {1053,1317,1508}.

Clinical features

The tumour may present as a mass, which may be radiologically occult. However, on mammography, ICCs typically form a spiculate mass, frequently containing microcalcifications {1003,1317, 1379}. Multifocality is observed in 10–20% of cases {889,1053}.

ICC is positive for estrogen receptor in all cases and positive for progesterone receptor in 69% of cases {1508}.

Macroscopy

There is no specific macroscopic feature that distinguishes cribriform carcinoma from invasive carcinoma NST or mixed types. Mean tumour size is 3.1 cm {1053}.

Histopathology

Pure ICC consists of an invasive cribriform pattern in > 90% of the lesion. The tumour is arranged as invasive, often angulated, islands, in which well-defined cribriform spaces are formed by arches of cells (sieve-like pattern). Apical snouts are common. Mucin-positive secretion bearing microcalcifications can be present within lumina {1053,1317,1574}. The tumour cells are small to moderate in size, with a mild or moderate degree of pleomorphism. Mitoses are rare. A prominent fibroblastic stroma is common; in occasional cases, osteoclast-like giant cells of histiocytic origin are found {588,986,

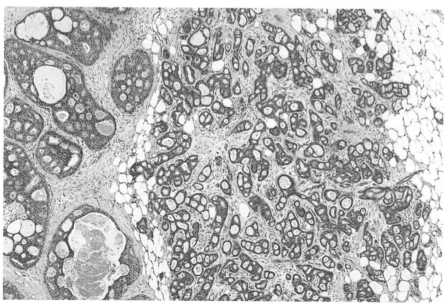

Fig. 3.08 Invasive cribriform carcinoma. The haphazard distribution of irregularly shaped and angulated invasive areas contrasts with the rounded configuration of the ducts with cribriform ductal carcinoma in situ on the left-hand side.

1257}. DCIS, generally of cribriform architecture, is frequent (80% of cases) {1053}. Axillary lymph-node metastases occur in 14.3% of cases {1053}, typically with retention of the cribriform pattern. Invasive carcinoma with a cribriform arrangement but associated with a component (< 50%) of TC is also included in the category of ICC {1053}. Cases with a 10–49% component of another morphological type (other than TC) are regarded as being of mixed type {1053,1508}.

Differential diagnosis
ICC should be differentiated from well-differentiated neuroendocrine tumour and adenoid cystic carcinoma. The former has intracytoplasmic argyrophilic granules, while the latter has a second population of cells as well as intracystic secretory and basement membrane-like (e.g. laminin-positive) material {1574}. ICC is distinguished from cribriform DCIS by the lack of a myoepithelial-cell layer around its invasive islands, its haphazard distribution and irregular configuration. Carcinomas rich in osteoclast-like giant cells are mostly seen in ICC, but such giant cells may be seen in other types of invasive mammary carcinoma and are not diagnostic for ICC.

Genetics
Both ICC and TC have similar genomic and transcriptomic features (both belong to molecular class "luminal A") and immunophenotype (e.g. consistent expression of hormone receptors and lack of HER2 overexpression) and are associated with the same family of low-grade precursor lesions {1569}.

Prognosis and predictive factors
As for TC, the outcome for patients with ICC is favourable {376,1053,1508}; 10-year overall survival is between 90% {376} and 100% {832,1053}. The outcome for patients with mixed ICC is less favourable than for patients with the pure form, but better than for invasive carcinoma NST {1053}. The biological behaviour of ICC is similar to that of TC {376}; however, many tumours have no tubular component and the definition of ICC as a distinct clinico-pathological entity appears to be justified.

Carcinomas with medullary features

J. Jacquemier
J.S. Reis-Filho
S.R. Lakhani
E. Rakha

Definition

Carcinomas with medullary features include medullary carcinomas (MC), atypical MC, and a subset of invasive carcinomas of no special type (NST). These tumours demonstrate all or some of the following features: a circumscribed or pushing border, a syncytial growth pattern, cells with high-grade nuclei, and prominent lymphoid infiltration.

ICD-O code

Medullary carcinoma	8510/3
Atypical medullary carcinoma	8513/3
Invasive carcinoma NST with medullary features	8500/3

Epidemiology

Classic MC is rare, representing < 1% of all breast carcinomas, although higher rates have been reported, depending on the stringency of the diagnostic criteria used. Studies with higher prevalence likely include examples of atypical MC and/or invasive carcinomas NST with medullary features. The average age at diagnosis reported for patients with these tumours ranges from 45 to 52 years, but 26% are diagnosed at < 35 years {48,239,884,1534}

Clinical features

These tumours are often well-defined clinically and on imaging studies.

Macroscopy

Tumours in this group are often well-circumscribed, soft to moderately firm. Foci of necrosis or haemorrhage are frequent, leading in some cases to cystic degeneration. Median diameter varies from 2 to 2.9 cm.

Histopathology

Classically, the following criteria were used to define MC {1082,1184}: syncytial architecture in > 75% of the tumour mass, histological circumscription or pushing margins, lack of tubular differentiation, a prominent and diffuse lymphoplasmacytic stroma infiltrate, and round tumour cells with abundant cytoplasm and pleomorphic high-grade vesicular nuclei containing one or several nucleoli. Mitoses are

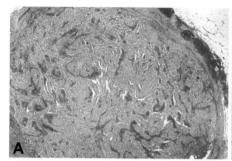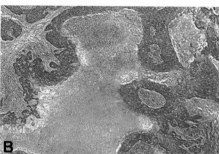

Fig. 3.09 Medullary carcinoma **A** Typical medullary carcinoma, > 75% well-circumscribed. **B** Typical medullary carcinoma with > 75% syncytium. Note the necrotic area and the prominent lymphocytic infiltrates.

numerous and atypical giant cells may be observed. The terms "atypical medullary carcinoma" and "carcinoma with medullary features" have been proposed for tumours that do not fulfil all these criteria. These diagnostic criteria are difficult to apply, resulting in poor inter-observer reproducibility. Therefore, we recommend that classic MC, atypical MC and invasive carcinoma NST with medullary features be grouped within the category of carcinomas with medullary features.

Immunoprofile

Tumours in this group are most often negative for estrogen and progesterone receptors (ER and PR) and HER2 ("triple-negative") and variably express keratins 5/6 and 14, smooth-muscle actin, EGFR, P-cadherin, p53, and caveolin-1.
Immunophenotyping suggests that the lymphoid infiltrates show a predominance of CD3+ T-lymphocytes and increased levels of CD8+ cytotoxic T-lymphocytes {530,734,1041}.

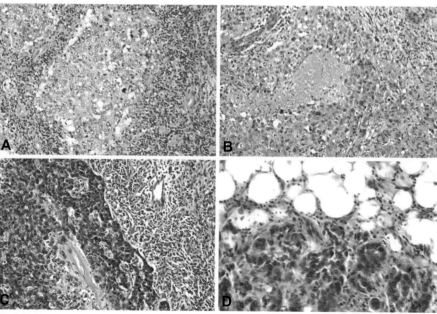

Fig. 3.10 Medullary carcinoma. **A** Typical medullary carcinoma comprising high-grade malignant tumour cells and admixed lymphoplasmacytic infiltrates. **B** Histological necrosis. **C** Syncytial tumour nests accompanied by abundant lymphocytes and plasma cells. **D** Grade 3 invasive carcinoma of no special type without lymphoid stroma shows similar high-grade tumour cells.

Differential diagnosis

Although Epstein-Barr virus (EBV)-associated lymphoepithelial-like carcinomas in the breast share some morphological features with tumours in this group, only a few cases have been found to be associated with EBV, in contrast to the 31–51% rate of EBV-positivity found among common invasive carcinoma NST {166}.

Genetics

A large proportion of tumours in this group are now recognized as basal-like. Genomic instability is a common feature of these lesions {126}. Most tumours in patients with germline mutations in *BRCA1* have medullary features {368, 369,1500}. However, only about 13% of patients with carcinomas harbouring medullary features were confirmed to have *BRCA1* germline mutations in a key consortium study {746}. Somatic mutations and *BRCA1* promoter hypermethylation have been observed in these tumours, suggesting a possible role for this gene in the development of these tumours {1044}. The most frequent somatic alteration detected is mutation of *TP53* {329,1519}.

Prognosis and predictive factors

MC was traditionally considered to be associated with a relatively favourable prognosis compared with grade-matched invasive carcinoma NST. In a cohort of 1444 breast carcinomas, 46 cases of MC were diagnosed in a double-reading examination {1534}; the distant relapse-free survival rate of 10 years was significantly better for MC than for the control group of invasive carcinoma NST (94.9% versus 77.5%; $p = 0.028$). However, the low level of reproducibility of a diagnosis of MC has resulted in an increase in the use of the concept of "medullary-like features" {1194} and to the practice of treating MC, like basal-like triple-negative carcinomas, with aggressive therapy.

In a series of invasive carcinomas NST of grade 3, it was demonstrated that the presence of a prominent lympho-plasmacytic infiltrate is associated with good prognosis {1135,1147}. Independent gene-expression profiling studies have demonstrated that the expression levels of immune response genes, in particular a B-cell/plasma-cell metagene, are independent predictors of outcome in ER-negative and ER-positive highly proliferative breast cancers {1195}. Consistent with these observations, a MC signature was shown to identify prognostic subgroups of triple-negative/basal-like carcinomas {1247}. These results suggest that the relatively good outcome of carcinomas with medullary features may be related to the prominent lymphoplasmacytic infiltrate.

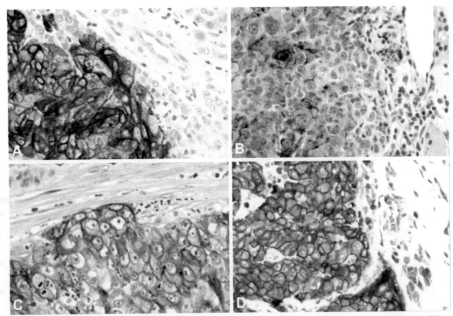

Fig. 3.11 Medullary carcinoma. Markers of the basal-like features in a typical medullary carcinoma. **A** Keratin 5/6. **B** Keratin 14. **C** EGFR. **D** P-cadherin.

Table 3.01 Comparative immunohistochemical profiles (% of cells expressing the given marker)

Immunohistochemical markers	Typical medullary breast cancer {634}	Invasive carcinoma with medullary features {1194}	Invasive carcinoma, grade 3 {1135}
Nielsen Basal profile (ER-negative/HER2-negative and keratin 5/6-positive and/or EGFR-positive)	Not evaluated for this signature	62.9%	18.9%
ER-negative	89.5%	94.3%	38.5%
PR-negative	48.7%	77.1%	34%
HER2-negative	97.7%	100%	76.2%
Keratin 5/6-positive	54.8%	60%	17.9%
P-cadherin-positive	65.6%	40%	7.9%
p53-positive	69.3%	65.7%	31.6%
Ki67 > 50%	54.5%	91.2%	63.2%
Cyclin E	31.4%	65.2%	26.2%
P-cadherin-positive/Ki67 > 50% HER2-negative/p53-positive	54%	20%	0%

EGFR, epidermal growth factor receptor; ER, estrogen receptor; HER2, human epidermal growth factor receptor 2; PR, progesterone receptor.

Metaplastic carcinoma

J.S. Reis-Filho
S.R. Lakhani
H. Gobbi
N. Sneige

Definition

Metaplastic carcinoma encompasses a group of neoplasms characterized by differentiation of the neoplastic epithelium into squamous cells and/ or mesenchymal-looking elements {616A,1551A–D,1552}, including but not restricted to spindle, chondroid, osseous, and rhabdomyoid cells. These neoplasms may be either entirely composed of metaplastic elements, or a complex admixture of carcinoma and metaplastic areas.

ICD-O codes

Metaplastic carcinoma	8575/3
Low-grade adenosquamous carcinoma	8570/3
Fibromatosis-like metaplastic carcinoma	8572/3
Squamous cell carcinoma	8070/3
Spindle cell carcinoma	8032/3
Carcinoma with mesenchymal differentiation	
Chondroid differentiation	8571/3
Osseous differentiation	8571/3
Other types of mesenchymal differentiation	8575/3
Myoepithelial carcinoma	8982/3

Synonyms

Given the multiple histological appearances exhibited by metaplastic breast cancers, a plethora of terms have been coined to refer to subgroups of metaplastic breast cancers, including carcinosarcoma {537A}, sarcomatoid carcinoma {469A}, carcinoma with pseudosarcomatous metaplasia {679B}, carcinoma with pseudosarcomatous stroma {659A}, spindle cell carcinoma {485A,1551A}, spindle cell metaplastic tumour {485A,499}, matrix-producing carcinoma or matrix-producing breast cancer {353B,1551B}, adenosquamous carcinoma {1594A}, low-grade adenosquamous carcinoma {1215A}, squamous cell carcinoma {1551D}, and fibromatosis-like metaplastic carcinoma or tumour {499,1113A,1171A,1347}.

Epidemiology

Metaplastic breast carcinomas account for 0.2–5% of all invasive breast cancers {448,679A,1363A,1569C}. The prevalence varies to such an extent, given the different definitions adopted by different authors. It should be noted that if only tumours with mesenchymal metaplasia are considered, metaplastic breast cancers account for approximately 1% of invasive breast cancers.

Clinical features

Metaplastic carcinomas present similar clinical features and age distribution to other estrogen-receptor (ER)-negative invasive carcinomas of no special type (NST) {233,616A,679A,1019A,1552,1569C}.

Macroscopy

The gross appearance of metaplastic carcinomas is not distinctive, and these tumours can either be well-circumscribed or show an indistinct or irregular border. Cystic degenerative changes are not infrequent, particularly in metaplastic squamous cell carcinoma. In general, metaplastic carcinomas tend to be relatively large tumours, compared to invasive carcinomas NST, with a mean size of 3.9 cm (range, 1.2 to > 10 cm) {105A,233,262A, 1100A,1551A–D,1552}.

Histopathology

Metaplastic carcinomas comprise a heterogeneous group of tumours. The consensus of the Working Group was that a descriptive classification system should be adopted.

Low-grade adenosquamous carcinoma

Low-grade adenosquamous carcinomas show well-developed glandular and tubular formation intimately admixed with solid nests of squamous cells in a spindle-cell background. The carcinomatous component is characterized by small glandular structures, with rounded rather than angulated contours, and solid cords of epithelial cells, which may contain squamous cells, squamous pearls or squamous cyst formation. The invasive neoplastic component typically shows long, slender extensions at the periphery and infiltrate between normal breast structures {354A, 1215A,1493A}. Clusters of lymphocytes are often observed at the periphery, sometimes in a "cannon ball" pattern. The association between these tumours and adenomyoepithelioma {459A} and sclerosing proliferative lesions {331,499A} has been reported.

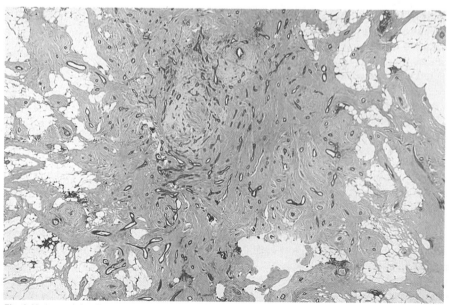

Fig. 3.12 Low-grade adenosquamous carcinoma. A highly infiltrative growth pattern is responsible for the high frequency of local recurrence associated with many lesions.

Fibromatosis-like metaplastic carcinoma

Fibromatosis-like metaplastic tumours of the breast are characterized by bland spindle cells with a pale eosinophilic cytoplasm and slender nuclei with tapered edges and finely distributed chromatin embedded in stroma with varying degrees of collagenization. Nuclear atypia is mild or absent. The spindle cells are often arranged in wavy, interlacing fascicles, or form long fascicles with finger-like extensions infiltrating the adjacent breast parenchyma. Cords and clusters of plump spindled and more epithelioid cells are often found; not uncommonly, these cells are arranged in a pattern reminiscent of a perivascular distribution {317A,499, 499A, 1113A,1347}. Focal squamous differentiation may be found. A gradual transition from plump cells to the spindle cell component is frequently observed. These tumours are almost invariably p63-positive {707,1168B,1171A}; keratins are invariably expressed in these lesions, occasionally focally and not uncommonly restricted to the plump spindle and epithelioid cells.

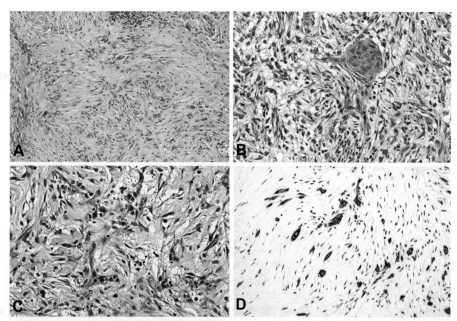

Fig. 3.13 Low-grade fibromatosis-like carcinoma, composed of deceptively bland-looking spindle cells arranged in wavy, interlacing fascicles (**A**). Focal squamous differentiation is not uncommonly found (**B**). Cords of spindle cells immersed in loose myxoid stroma can be observed (**C**), which are highlighted by immunohistochemistry with antibodies to high-molecular-weight keratins (**D**).

Squamous cell carcinoma

Squamous cell carcinomas usually present as a cystic lesion, where the cavity is lined by squamous cells with varying degrees of nuclear atypia and pleomorphism. The neoplastic cells infiltrate the adjacent stroma in the form of sheets, cords and nests, which elicit a conspicuous stromal reaction. Inflammatory infiltrate is usually prominent. The infiltrating squamous elements may vary in degrees of squamous differentiation, with spindle cells commonly observed at the invasive fronts of the tumour {659A,1551D}. The acantholytic variant of squamous cell carcinoma, characterized by the formation of irregular spaces lined by atypical squamous cells leading to a pseudoglandular or pseudoangiosarcomatous appearance, should be considered as a potential differential diagnosis with angiosarcoma {398A}. Metaplastic squamous cell carcinoma may be pure or mixed with coexisting invasive carcinoma NST {448,659A, 1551D}. It should be noted that squamous differentiation can also be found in carcinomas with medullary-like features (see *Medullary carcinoma*). For a diagnosis of primary squamous cell carcinoma of the breast to be rendered, a primary squamous cell carcinoma from other sites, especially skin, must be ruled out {1551D}.

Spindle cell carcinoma

Spindle cell carcinomas are characterized by atypical spindle cells, arranged in a multitude of architectural patterns ranging from long fascicles in herringbone or interwoven patterns to short fascicles in a storiform ("cartwheel") patterns {233,485A, 1551A}. Most often, a mixture of different patterns is observed. The cytoplasm ranges from elongated to plump spindle. Nuclear pleomorphism is usually moderate to high. Inflammatory infiltrate is often found in a proportion of cases, often with lymphocytes and dendritic cells percolating

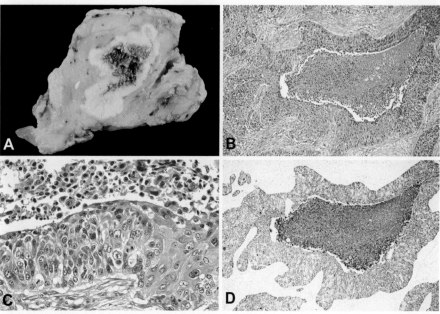

Fig. 3.14 Squamous cell carcinoma. **A** Macroscopically, there are often central cystic areas. **B** Variously shaped spaces lined by squamous epithelium are characteristic. **C** Higher magnification showing a range of squamous-cell differentiation with most differentiated at the right. **D** Immunostaining for keratins 5/6 is positive as expected for squamous epithelium.

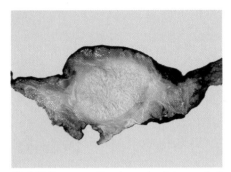

Fig. 3.15 Squamous cell carcinoma. A well-circumscribed mass shows numerous irregularly shaped depressions on cut surface.

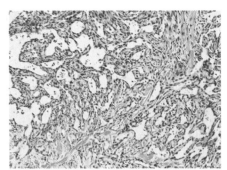

Fig. 3.16 Squamous cell carcinoma, acantholytic variant, which is often mistaken for angiosarcoma.

the tumour bulk. Areas where the neoplastic cells form small clusters, with more epithelioid morphology or squamous differentiation can be found. It should be noted that this group of tumours includes lesions that are likely to constitute the end of the spectrum of spindle squamous cell carcinomas on one hand, and malignant myoepithelioma/myoepithelial carcinoma on the other {613}. At present, there are no definitive criteria to differentiate these two lesions, nor are there data to suggest that these lesions display distinct clinical behaviour. Metaplastic spindle cell carcinoma should always be considered as a main differential diagnosis of atypical spindle cell proliferations of the breast. A diagnosis of metaplastic spindle cell carcinoma can be rendered based on the presence of any evidence of epithelial differentiation by histopathological and/or immunohistochemical analysis (see below). In addition, the presence of ductal carcinoma in situ (DCIS) at the periphery or

admixed with the lesion should prompt a diagnosis of spindle cell metaplastic carcinoma.

Metaplastic carcinoma with mesenchymal differentiation

Metaplastic breast carcinomas with mesenchymal elements are often composed of an admixture of mesenchymal components, including chondroid, osseous, rhabdomyoid and even neuroglial differentiation, with carcinomatous areas, which can be in the form of glandular tubules, solid clusters and/ or foci of squamous differentiation {233,353B,1019A,1551B, 1551C}. The mesenchymal components can either appear differentiated with minimal atypia to exhibiting frankly malignant features that to some extent recapitulate the patterns found in true sarcomas of the soft tissues. Historically, the term "matrix-producing carcinomas" was applied to a subgroup of metaplastic carcinomas with mesenchymal elements where an abrupt

transition from epithelial to the mesenchymal components without the presence of intervening spindle cells was found {353B,1551B}. In such tumours, true chondroid differentiation or chondroid matrix is often found. It should be noted that although in the vast majority of cases areas of epithelial differentiation can be readily found, in some cases, extensive sampling is required for the carcinomatous areas to be documented. Importantly, immunohistochemical analysis also reveals the expression of epithelial markers, usually high-molecular-weight keratins.

Mixed metaplastic carcinomas

It should be noted that upon extensive sampling, a large proportion of metaplastic breast cancers display a mixture of different elements. These cases should be reported as metaplastic carcinomas and the distinct elements recorded in the final report.

Different types of metaplastic carcinomas have been described arising in association with complex sclerosing lesions and papillomas {331,499A}.

Immunohistochemistry

Immunohistochemical analysis of metaplastic carcinomas has revealed that > 90% of these cancers are negative for ER, progesterone receptor (PR) and HER2, and express keratins 5/6 and 14, and EGFR {354A,568A,568C,1169A,1170A,1347, 1464A}. The identification of epithelial differentiation in metaplastic breast carcinomas requires the use of more than one

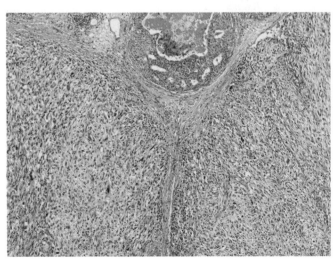

Fig. 3.17 Spindle cell carcinoma. Although the tumour is entirely composed of neoplastic spindle cells, the presence of ductal carcinoma in situ at the periphery and admixed with the lesion should prompt a diagnosis of spindle cell carcinoma.

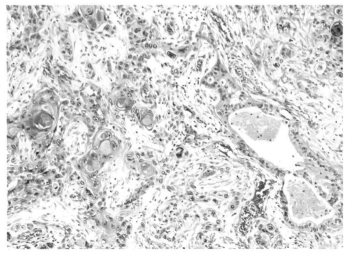

Fig. 3.18 Metaplastic carcinoma with squamous elements. Both glandular and squamous differentiation coexist in this carcinoma.

immunohistochemical marker. Usual markers are high-molecular-weight keratins, in particular 34betaE12, keratins 5/6 and 14, and AE1/AE3; low-molecular-weight keratins are commonly negative {15A,356}. It should be noted that the expression of keratins is often variable, and not uncommonly focal. P63, which is expressed in > 90% of metaplastic breast carcinomas, has proven to be a useful marker for the identification of these tumours and for their differentiation with other spindle and mesenchymal malignancies {233,707, 1169A,1171A}. Markers useful for differentiating metaplastic breast cancers from phyllodes tumours with sarcomatous overgrowth include keratins, p63, CD34 and BCL2: keratins and p63 are negative in phyllodes tumours and positive in metaplastic breast cancers, and CD34 and BCL2 show the opposite distribution {356,770}.

In a pure spindle cell lesion, unequivocal expression of high-molecular-weight keratins and/ or p63 in any proportion of cells should prompt a diagnosis of metaplastic carcinoma. Adequate sampling of the lesion is strongly advised.

Genetics

Microarray-based gene-expression profiling has demonstrated that metaplastic breast tumours are preferentially classified as of basal-like subtype {1569, 1569B}. Independent studies, however, have suggested that a subgroup of these cancers, in particular those with spindle cell metaplasia, display transcriptomic features consistent with those of cells undergoing epithelial-to-mesenchymal transition (i.e. down-regulation of genes usually found in epithelial cells and overexpression of genes usually found in fibro-

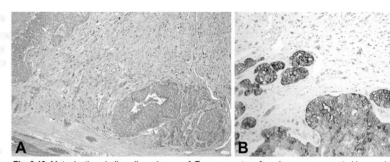

Fig. 3.19 Metaplastic spindle cell carcinoma. **A** Two aggregates of carcinoma are separated by neoplastic spindle cells. **B** Immunostaining shows absence of reactivity with a pan-keratin antibody cocktail in the mesenchymal component, while the epithelial cells are positive.

blasts) {568B,806A,1122,1569B}, and can be classified into a recently described molecular subtype named claudin-low. Claudin-low tumours are reported to be enriched in cells with epithelial-to-mesenchymal features and in the so-called cancer stem cells {1122}.

Genetic analysis of metaplastic breast cancers has been performed in a limited number of samples and only in part substratified according to histological type. These tumours, as a group, have complex genomes, characterized by complex patterns of gene copy-number gains and losses, similar to those found in other types of triple-negative and basal-like breast cancers {485B,485C,568B, 1170A}. Mutations of the tumour suppressor gene *TP53* are found in the vast majority of these cancers {806B}. Loss of *CDKN2A* (*p16*) and *PTEN* are found in subgroups of the disease {568B,951A}. Recurrent mutations of *PIK3CA* {568B, 951A} and of genes pertaining to the Wnt pathway {559A} have been reported in metaplastic breast cancers. Importantly, the high prevalence of *CTNNB1* mutations reported in one study (i.e. 26% of cases)

{559A} was not validated in subsequent independent analyses {568B,738}. Amplification and high polysomy of the *EGFR* gene have been reported in 10–25% of metaplastic breast cancers {489A,168A, 1170A}, and are more prevalent in tumours with squamous and/ or spindle cell elements {1169A}.

Genomic characterization of the different elements from metaplastic breast cancers performed to date has revealed that the histologically distinct components are clonally related in the vast majority of cases {485C,1436A}; however, specific genetic aberrations may be restricted to specific components within a cancer.

Prognosis and predictive factors

Lymph-node metastases are significantly less frequently found in metaplastic breast cancers than in invasive carcinomas NST of similar size and grade {233,317A,499A, 568A,616A,1019A,1111A,1551A–D,1552. In a way akin to other triple-negative breast cancers, distant metastases can be found in the absence of lymph-node metastases, and preferentially affect brain and lungs. At present, there are no validated

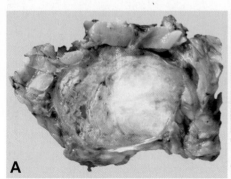
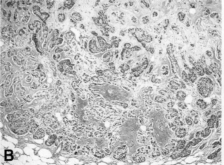
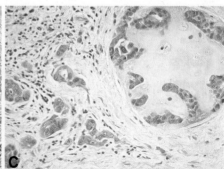

Fig. 3.20 A Metaplastic carcinoma with mesenchymal differentiation (matrix-producing carcinoma), mastectomy from a patient aged 77 years. **B** Carcinoma with mesenchymal (benign osseous and chondroid) differentiation. Typically, these carcinomas have a well-delineated pushing margin. Areas of osseous and/or chondroid differentiation are variably scattered in an otherwise typical invasive carcinoma of no special type (NST). **C** The adenocarcinoma is admixed, in part, with chondroid matrix containing lacunar spaces and rare chondrocytes.

prognostic markers for metaplastic carcinomas. Although specific subtypes have been associated with a better or worse prognosis, the retrospective design of the studies, the consultation nature of the samples included, and differences in definitions of the lesions studied do not lead to definitive conclusions with regard to the prognostic information that can be derived from the presence of specific metaplastic elements. Importantly, there is evidence to suggest that, as a group, metaplastic breast cancers have lower response rates to conventional adjuvant chemotherapy and a worse clinical outcome than those of other forms of triple-negative breast cancers {568A–C,670A, 836A}. It should be noted, however, that there is evidence from independent studies to suggest that low-grade fibromatosis-like tumours/carcinomas and low-grade adenosquamous carcinomas may have a better clinical outcome than other types of metaplastic breast cancer {499,1113A, 1215A,1493A}. The prognostic value of histological grading of metaplastic breast carcinomas is uncertain.

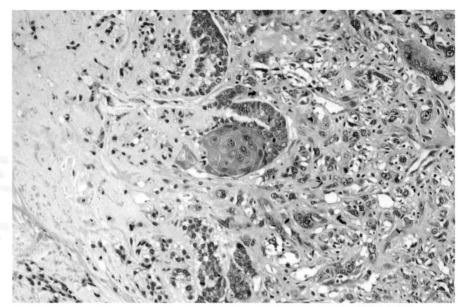

Fig. 3.21 Mixed metaplastic carcinoma with spindle, mesenchymal (chondroid) and squamous differentiation.

Carcinomas with apocrine differentiation

F. O'Malley
V. Eusebi
S.R. Lakhani

Definition
Any invasive carcinoma in which the cells show the cytological features of apocrine cells.

ICD-O code
These tumours are coded according to the primary invasive type.

Epidemiology
Focal apocrine differentiation is a common feature in invasive carcinomas of no special type (NST) as well as some special types. However, extensive apocrine differentiation is seen in approximately 4% of invasive breast carcinomas {398,1214}.

Clinical features
Carcinomas with apocrine differentiation are indistinguishable clinically and radiologically from those without apocrine features.

Macroscopy
These tumours can present as a mass of any size and at any site in the breast.

Histopathology
Apocrine differentiation is seen in invasive carcinomas NST and in special-type carcinomas (including tubular, lobular, micropapillary and medullary) {3,396,398}. Apocrine differentiation is also seen in lobular carcinoma in situ and ductal carcinoma in situ {258,292,390,768}. The constituent cells have enlarged nuclei with prominent nucleoli and either abundant granular, eosinophilic cytoplasm that shows diastase-resistant periodic-acid–Schiff (PAS) positivity (type A cells), or abundant foamy cytoplasm (type B cells), or a combination of both. Intracytoplasmic lipid has also been demonstrated in tumours with apocrine differentiation {398, 947}.

Immunoprofile
Areas of the tumour with apocrine differentiation are typically BCL2-negative and GCDFP-15–positive, although GCDFP-15 expression may be lost in advanced-stage tumours {519A}. Staining for estrogen and progesterone receptors (ER and PR) is usually negative, but a novel isoform of ER (ER-alpha36) has recently been shown to be frequently overexpressed {1532}. Tumours that show androgen receptor positivity, in combination with ER and PR negativity and HER2 positivity overwhelmingly demonstrate apocrine features histologically {132,998,1387}. It is likely that this immunophenotype identifies tumours that have the distinct "apocrine molecular signature," as discussed below.

Differential diagnosis
Tumours composed entirely of type A cells may be confused with a granular cell tumour and those in which type B cells predominate may resemble an inflammatory reaction or a histiocytic proliferation {395}; antibodies to keratin can aid diagnosis in such cases {1416}.

Genetics
Comparative genomic hybridization (CGH) has revealed copy-number changes in carcinomas with apocrine differentiation, with chromosomal gains of 1p, 1q and 2q and losses of 1p, 12q, 16q, 17q and 22q {657A}. These are common regions of alterations for breast carcinomas in general. An "apocrine molecular signature," identified by gene-expression array analysis, is characterized by increased androgen signalling and significant overlap with the "HER2 group," as defined by microarray studies {422, 1090,1356,1357}. It should be noted that the molecular apocrine subtype as defined by gene-expression array analysis is not equivalent to apocrine differentiation in breast cancer. Approximately half of carcinomas with apocrine differentiation show this molecular signature, including most pleomorphic lobular carcinomas with apocrine features {396}. However, overall, carcinomas with apocrine differentiation

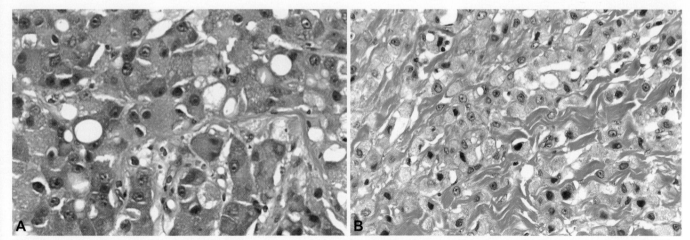

Fig. 3.22 Carcinoma with apocrine differentiation. **A** Note the abundant, granular, intensely eosinophilic cytoplasm and the enlarged nuclei with prominent nucleoli (type A cells). **B** This example shows cells with abundant, foamy cytoplasm (type B cells).

do not form a distinct cluster and are composed of "apocrine" and "luminal" molecular subtypes {1569}. Hence the data suggest that apocrine differentiation is a common feature of many subtypes of breast cancer, and that "apocrine carcinomas" do not represent a distinct entity.

Prognosis and predictive factors

Some studies have shown that carcinomas with apocrine differentiation have the same clinical outcome as invasive carcinomas NST, when matched for grade and stage {3,301}, although one preliminary study suggests better prognosis {642}. An in silico analysis using microarray-derived readings of two sets of prognostic genes, showed that carcinomas with apocrine differentiation clustering with the "molecular apocrine signature" had a high 21-gene recurrence score and a poor 70-gene prognosis signature, suggesting worse prognosis {1569}. The androgen signalling associated with these tumours may lead to the development of new therapeutic modalities for these tumours in the future.

Salivary gland/skin adnexal type tumours

A. Sapino
N. Sneige
V. Eusebi
M. Michal

Definition
Cylindroma and clear cell hidradenoma (CCH) of the breast show features similar to cutaneous homonymous neoplasms of the adnexa.

ICD-O code
Cylindroma   8200/0
Clear cell hidradenoma   8402/0

Synonyms
CCH is also known as nodular hidradenoma or eccrine acrospiroma.

Epidemiology
Primary breast cylindroma {26,502,1547} and CCHs are extremely rare {351,438, 681,1025}. Both occur in adult to elderly women.

Clinical features
Breast cylindromas may be associated with lobular and invasive carcinoma NST {26} and occasionally occur in patients with Brooke-Spiegler syndrome {1011, 1547}. CCHs are circumscribed tumours often found in the subareolar area, without connection to the overlying skin.

Macroscopy
Cylindromas are well-circumscribed, non-encapsulated tumours (usually < 2 cm). CCHs are sharply demarcated from the surrounding areas and show an indistinct lobulated architecture protruding into cystic spaces filled by clear mucous substance without haemorrhage {351,438,681,1025}.

Histopathology
Cylindromas are composed of multiple variously shaped and sized epithelial lobules arranged in a jigsaw puzzle simulating a pseudoinfiltrative pattern. Occasional sebaceous-cell differentiation may be found {26}. Homogeneous eosinophilic hyaline periodic-acid-Schiff (PAS)-positive extracellular matrix surrounds most of the lobules and round masses of similar material are present within the lobules. The neoplastic lobules are composed of two cell types: small basal cells with scanty cytoplasm and hyperchromatic nuclei mostly located at the periphery, and larger cells with pale cytoplasm and oval vesicular nuclei usually situated in the centre. Occasional ductal structures may contain secretory material. Mitoses, necrosis and haemorrhage are absent. The peripheral cells of the lobules display alpha-smooth-muscle actin and p63, as may the outer cells in the ductal structures. The luminal cells stain with antibodies to epithelial membrane antigen. Reactive Langerhans cells may be abundant and these are strongly positive for S100 and CD1a. The tumours are negative for estrogen and progesterone receptors and GCDFP-15. CCH nodules are composed of cuboidal monomorphous cells and larger clear cells, which often predominate (hence the term "clear cell" hidradenoma). Large mucinous cells with granular cytoplasm may be found. Occasional secondary lumina rimmed by one layer of basophilic cells are filled by PAS- and mucicarmine-positive mucin. The intervening stroma may be hyalinized. Columnar cell hyperplasia may be found in the vicinity of CCH {681}. Tumour cells are always negative for S100 and there is no evidence of myoepithelial-cell differentiation.

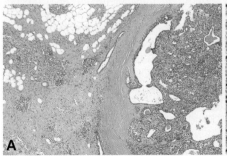
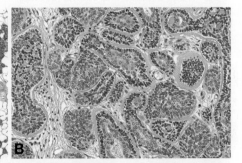

Fig. 3.23 Cylindroma. **A** Multiple variously shaped and sized epithelial lobules into the adipose tissue simulating a pseudoinfiltrative pattern. **B** The tumour is composed of two cell types: small basal cells with scanty cytoplasm and hyperchromatic nuclei, and larger cells with pale cytoplasm and oval vesicular nuclei in the centre of neoplastic nodules.

Genetics
Germline *CYLD* mutation (at 16q12–13) may be etiologically implicated in patients with Brooke-Spiegler syndrome, who may occasionally develop cylindromas {1011,1547}. The *MYB-NFIB* fusion gene, also found in adenoid cystic carcinomas, has been reported in up to 60% of cylindromas {429}. In one CCH case, a 120-bp *CRTC1-MAML2* fusion transcript was identified {681}. This t(11;19) translocation is present in approximately 50% of cutaneous CCHs {1588}.

Prognosis and predictive factors
In none of the reported patients did the cylindroma of the breast recur or metastasize {26,502,1547}. CCH is invariably a benign tumour.

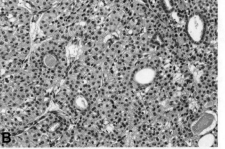

Fig. 3.24 Clear cell hidradenoma. **A** Indistinct lobulated architecture protruding into cystic spaces. **B** The neoplastic nodules composed of cuboidal monomorphous cells and larger clear cells. Occasional lumina rimmed by one layer of basophilic cells are filled by mucin.

Adenoid cystic carcinoma

A. Sapino
N. Sneige
V. Eusebi

Definition
A carcinoma of low malignant potential, histologically similar to its counterpart in the salivary gland.

ICD-O code   8200/3

Synonyms
Carcinoma adenoides cysticum; adeno-cystic basal cell carcinoma; cylindroma-tous carcinoma

Epidemiology
Adenoid cystic carcinoma (ACC) is rare, comprising < 0.1% of breast carcinomas {486}. The mean age at diagnosis is 64 years {486,1384}. The incidence ratio for black women is 39% lower than for white women {486}.

Clinical features
About 50% of cases are found in the sub-areolar region {486}. They may be painful {897}. The mammographic and sono-graphic appearances are non-specific {496}.

Macroscopy
ACC are usually circumscribed tumours ranging from 0.5 to 12 cm in size (aver-age, 3 cm). Occasionally, pink, tan or grey microcysts are evident {1416}.

Histopathology
ACC of the breast is very similar to that of the salivary gland, lung and skin {83,459, 496} and is formed by epithelial and my-oepithelial cell types arranged into clas-sic tubular or cribriform architecture. A solid variant with striking basaloid fea-tures may be encountered {466,1310}. In situ lesions are occasionally observed but can be difficult to distinguish from the in-vasive component.

Neoplastic cells are polarized around two types of structures: true glandular spaces and pseudolumina. True glandular spaces, surrounded by luminal cells, are small, difficult to see and contain neutral peri-odic acid-Schiff (PAS)-positive mucin. Pseudolumina, which result from intralu-minal invaginations of the stroma (stromal space) are surrounded by basal–myoepi-thelial cells {758,1416}. These pseudolu-mina are of varying shape, mostly round, and contain a myxoid acidic stromal sub-stance that stains with Alcian blue {892} or straps of collagen with small capillar-ies {1416}. With immunohistochemistry, a rim of laminin and collagen IV-positive material outlines these stromal spaces. Sometimes the pseudolumina are filled by small spherules or cylinders of hyaline ma-terial, which has been shown ultrastruc-turally and immunohistochemically to be basal lamina {261}.

Ultrastructurally, the basaloid cells have myoepithelial features {1619} and are im-munohistochemically positive for smooth-muscle actin, p63, and calponin {82,459, 892} as well as for high-molecular-weight keratins (keratins 14, 5/6), while being negative for CD10 {979}. Nevertheless, most basaloid cells are nondescript ele-ments showing few filaments and or-ganelles without specific features on electron microscopy {1416}.

The luminal cells are positive for keratins 7 and 8/18 {82}. CD117 positivity, which is well-known in salivary ACC, is also rec-ognized in breast ACC {82,892}. In con-trast to ACC of the salivary gland, squamous metaplasia of luminal cells may be relatively frequent {758}. ACC has been seen in association with adenomyo-epithelioma {1491} and low-grade syringo-matous (adenosquamous) carcinoma {1200}, which suggests a close relation-ship between these combined epithelial and myoepithelial tumours.

A third type of cells that have sebaceous differentiation can be rarely identified {1418}, but these elements can occasion-ally be numerous {1416}.

ACC is generally negative for estrogen and progesterone receptors (ER and PR) and HER2 {82,293,1261,1569}. Recently, a novel 36 kDa isoform of the full-length ER (ER-alpha36) has been detected in ACC {1533}. Overexpression of EGFR has been shown in 65% of cases {1531}.

Differential diagnosis
ACC must be distinguished from collage-nous spherulosis {273} and from invasive cribriform carcinoma {892} that shows

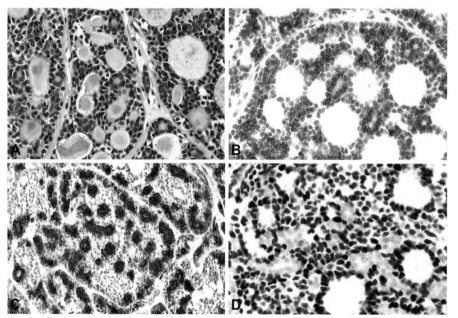

Fig. 3.25 Adenoid cystic carcinoma. **A** With a cribriform pattern. Cells around glandular lumina are positive for CD117 (**B**) and keratin 5/6 (**C**), while the majority of the cells around spherules of basement membrane material are positive for p63 (**D**).

roundish spaces lined by a single cell type that is ER-positive {1416}. A solid variant of ACC with basaloid features is distinguished from small cell carcinoma, solid papillary carcinoma or metaplastic carcinoma on basis of the presence of intercalated ducts and immunohistochemistry {1310}.

Genetics

Like salivary-gland ACCs, breast ACCs display the recurrent chromosomal translocation t(6;9)(q22–23;p23–24), which generates fusion transcripts involving the genes *MYB* and *NFIB* {1092} in > 90% of cases. Somatic mutations of *PIK3CA* and *PTEN* have been shown in one primary ACC and in its renal metastasis {1530}.

Prognosis and predictive factors

ACC is a low-grade malignant tumour that is generally cured by simple mastectomy. Ro et al. {1190} performed tumour grading according to the criteria accepted for salivary-gland ACC and suggested that cases classified as grade 3 (solid growth pattern) may have a higher rate of metastasis and recurrence. This result has not been confirmed by other studies {700, 758}. Like its analogue in the salivary gland, breast ACC rarely spreads via the

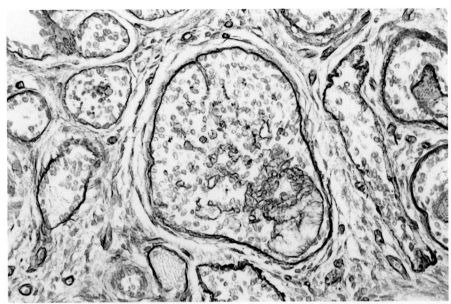

Fig. 3.26 Adenoid cystic carcinoma. Immunostaining for laminin decorates the basement membranes.

lymphatic system and rarely involves regional lymph nodes and most cases are associated with excellent survival {486}. The solid variant of ACC with basaloid features may have a greater propensity for axillary metastasis than conventional ACC {1310}.

Local recurrence is related to incomplete excision, but patients have been reported to survive 16 years after the excision of the recurrent tumour {1095}. The reported 5-year and 10-year survival rates for patients with breast ACC are > 95% and 90%, respectively {877}.

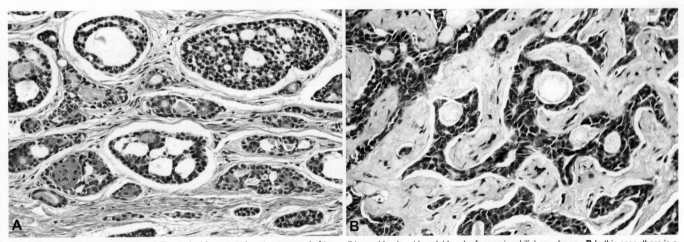

Fig. 3.27 Adenoid cystic carcinoma. **A** The typical fenestrated nests composed of two cell types (dominant basaloid and a few eosinophilic) are shown. **B** In this case, there is a predominant tubular architecture.

Mucoepidermoid carcinoma

A. Sapino
N. Sneige
V. Eusebi

Definition
A primary breast carcinoma that is histologically similar to its counterpart in the salivary gland, and that concomitantly shows basaloid, intermediate, epidermoid and mucinous cells.

ICD-O code   8430/3

Epidemiology
Mucoepidermoid carcinomas (MEC) are very rare tumours of the breast. The estimated incidence is approximately 0.3% of all breast cancers {448}.

Clinical features
Clinically, MECs are similar to invasive carcinomas of no special type (NST). Nipple discharge can be the first symptom of MEC located in the retro-areolar region {338}.

Macroscopy
Tumour size ranges from 0.5 to 15 cm. Low-grade MECs are well-circumscribed, sometimes containing mucoid cysts.

Histopathology
MECs of the breast are comparable to those of the salivary gland. Central nests of "epidermoid or mucus-secreting" cells and cysts that are positive for keratin 7 and 18 are lined by "basaloid" cells that are positive for keratin 14 and "intermediate" cells that are positive for keratin 5/6 and p63 {338,1104}. Intermediate cells may express EGFR {598}. Most MECs in the breast are of low grade with a prevalence of mucus cells {218}. High-grade MECs are rare, generally solid, and contain

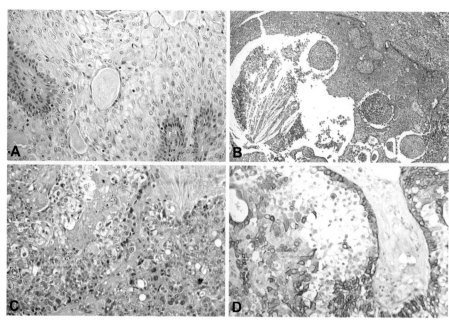

Fig. 3.28 Mucoepidermoid carcinoma (MEC). **A** Low-grade MEC. **B** Cystic low-grade MEC. **C** High-grade MEC. **D** Immunostaining for keratin 14 indicates basaloid cells.

predominantly intermediate and squamous cells {549,559,719,783}. An intraductal component may be present {218,338}. Hormone-receptor status was negative in the three cases studied {559,598}.

Differential diagnosis
MEC must be differentiated from invasive carcinoma NST with squamous-cell differentiation. True keratinization with formation of squamous pearls should exclude MEC and favour the diagnosis of metaplastic carcinoma with squamous differentiation {459}.

Genetics
In one case of breast MEC, partial deletion of 11q21 (*MAML2*) has been described {218}.

Prognosis and predictive factors
Accurate grading is important for prognosis {338}. All reported patients with low-grade MEC have been disease-free in the follow-up period, whereas high-grade MECs show usually aggressive behaviour with metastasis to axillary nodes and distant organs {338}.

Polymorphous carcinoma

A. Sapino
N. Sneige
V. Eusebi

Definition
Tumour with histological features similar to those referred to as "polymorphous low-grade carcinoma" in salivary glands {407,408}.

ICD-O code　　　　8525/3

Epidemiology
The true incidence of polymorphous carcinoma is not known as it has been recognized very recently and studies on large series are lacking. Only three cases have been reported to date {76}.

Clinical features
Patients' age ranges from 37 to 74 years {76}.

Macroscopy
Polymorphous carcinoma in the breast produces nodules ranging in size from 1.5 to 4 cm.

Histopathology
In analogy to polymorphous carcinoma of minor salivary glands {1104}, polymorphous carcinoma of the breast displays solid nests, surrounded at the periphery by alveolar, cribriform and trabecular as well as single-file patterns, which simulate an invasive lobular carcinoma. In contrast to adenoid cystic carcinomas, polymorphous carcinoma is constituted by a single cell-type, which shows round to ovoid nuclei and numerous mitoses. The neoplastic cells stain strongly for BCL2 and are faintly immunoreactive for keratin 7

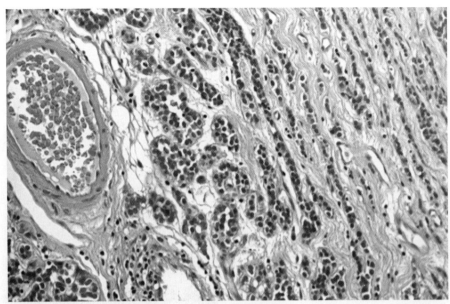

Fig. 3.29 Polymorphous carcinoma with alveolar and single-cell pattern.

and E-cadherin. Staining for epithelial membrane antigen, estrogen receptor, progesterone receptor, keratin 14, actin, HER2 and CD117 is consistently negative {758}.

Genetics
There are no available data on the genetic features of these lesions.

Prognosis and predictive factors
One case out of the three described in the literature showed aggressive behaviour, with the patient dying of widespread disease 3 years after diagnosis. All cases were of grade 2 and large size at the moment of diagnosis. It thus seems that the biological behaviour and morphological features of polymorphous carcinoma are those of a high-grade carcinoma and the term "low grade" as used for polymorphous carcinoma of salivary glands does not seem to be appropriate to tumours seen in the breast. Six cases of polymorphous carcinoma of the skin with aggressive behaviour were reported {1385} as "polymorphous sweat gland carcinoma", a name that was adopted for polymorphous carcinoma of the breast for the same reason {76}.

Mucinous carcinoma and carcinomas with signet-ring-cell differentiation

G. Bussolati
A. Sapino

Mucinous carcinoma

Definition
Mucinous carcinoma is characterized by clusters of generally small and uniform cells floating in large amounts of extracellular mucin.

ICD-O code   8480/3

Synonyms
Colloid carcinoma; mucoid carcinoma; gelatinous carcinoma; mucinous adenocarcinoma.

Epidemiology
Pure mucinous carcinoma accounts for about 2% of all breast carcinomas {337, 1157,1290}. It often occurs in patients aged > 55 years {104}.

Clinical features
Mammography of mucinous carcinoma simulates a benign process; magnetic resonance imaging (MRI) shows a typical dynamic enhancement pattern {1609}. Sonographically, almost all tumours are hypoechoic {821}.

Macroscopy
Gross examination shows a glistening gelatinous lesion with pushing margins and a soft consistency that is readily recognizable. The tumours range in size from < 1 cm to > 20 cm {104}.

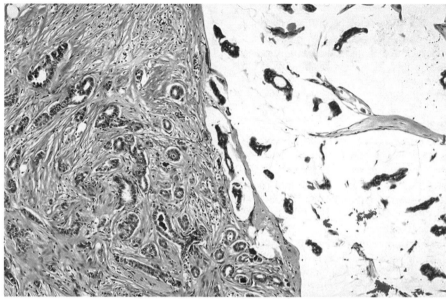

Fig. 3.30 Combined mucinous and invasive carcinoma of no special type (NST). The favourable prognosis associated with pure mucinous carcinoma is no longer expected when it is admixed with regular invasive carcinoma NST.

Histopathology
Mucinous carcinoma is characterized by nests of cells floating in lakes of mucin partitioned by delicate fibrous septae containing capillary blood vessels. The cell clusters are variable in size and shape; sometimes with a tubular arrangement. Nuclear atypia is generally low in classic mucinous carcinoma, but in rare cases atypia and mitoses may prevail {1407}. A micropapillary or cribriform intraepithelial component is rarely seen {1407}. Mucinous carcinoma presenting with large cell clusters, reported by Capella {219} as hypercellular or type B mucinous carcinoma, shows frequent neuroendocrine differentiation, as demonstrated by expression of chromogranin and synaptophysin {1187,1259}. Type A mucinous carcinoma with larger quantities of extracellular mucin represents the "classic" non-endocrine variety. Pure and mixed variants have been described {712,1407, 1443}. The most common admixture is with invasive carcinoma of no special type (NST). A pure tumour must be composed of > 90% mucinous carcinoma {1407}.

Differential diagnosis
The main challenge on core biopsy is the differential diagnosis of mucinous carcinoma with mucocoele-like-lesion (MLL) with extravasated mucin {113}. The presence of ducts distended by mucinous material and of myoepithelial cells adhering to the strips of cells floating in the lakes of mucin serve as important clues to differentiate benign MLL {1407} from mucinous carcinoma. However, several studies have described MLL associated

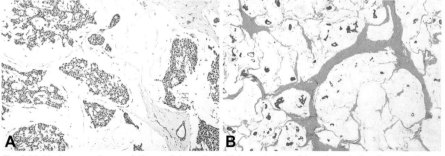

Fig. 3.31 Mucinous carcinoma. **A** Hypercellular variant with large clusters of densely packed malignant cells. **B** Hypocellular variant. Lakes of mucus are separated by fibrous septae. A few isolated or clusters of carcinoma cells are floating in the mucus lakes.

with atypical ductal hyperplasia or ductal carcinoma in situ (DCIS) {539, 1564}, suggesting that MLL and mucinous carcinoma may represent two ends of the pathological spectrum of mucinous lesions of the breast {113}.

Immunoprofile

Typically, mucinous carcinoma is positive for estrogen and progesterone receptors (ER and PR) {104}, while androgen receptors are expressed at a low level {1073} and HER2 is not amplified {739}. Pure and mixed mucinous carcinomas are reported to express WT1 {349}.

Genetics

Transcriptomic studies have demonstrated that mucinous tumours are of luminal A molecular subtype {1569}, and transcriptionally distinct from grade- and molecular subtype-matched invasive carcinomas NST {1567}. The transcriptomic features of mucinous A are distinct from those of mucinous B tumours, the latter showing a pattern of gene expression that is similar to that of neuroendocrine carcinomas {1567}. The Lacroix-Triki group {739} has shown that pure mucinous carcinomas harbour a low level of genetic instability and rare recurrent amplifications, and that the genomic profiles of the different tumour components of mixed mucinous tumours are remarkably similar to those of pure mucinous cancers.

Prognosis and predictive factors

Pure mucinous carcinomas are generally associated with low rates of local and distant recurrence and excellent 5-year disease-free survival rates {104,337,340, 832}. The 10-year overall survival ranges from 80% {712} to 100% {431}. Mixed mucinous carcinomas have a far worse prognosis and higher incidence of lymph-node metastases than do pure mucinous carcinomas {712,1012}. Late distant metastases may occur in pure mucinous carcinoma {1157,1443}.

Carcinomas with signet-ring-cell differentiation

Definition

Carcinomas with signet-ring-cell differentiation are characterized by abundant intracellular mucin that pushes the nucleus to one side, creating the characteristic signet-ring-cell morphology.

ICD-O code

These tumours are coded according to the primary invasive type.

Epidemiology

Primary breast carcinomas composed predominantly or exclusively of signet ring cells are rare; focal signet-ring-cell differentiation is seen more commonly.

Clinical features

No specific clinical features have been described.

Macroscopy

There are no specific macroscopic features.

Histopathology

Prominent signet-ring-cell differentiation is most common in invasive lobular carcinomas but may also be seen in invasive carcinoma NST and other special-type cancers. As such, carcinomas with signet-ring-cell differentiation do not represent a distinct entity. Two cytological types of carcinomas with signet-ring-cell differentiation have been described in the breast. One type is characterized by large intracytoplasmic vacuoles, with a "target" appearance owing to the presence of large intracytoplasmic lumina containing a periodic acid-Schiff (PAS)/Alcian blue and HMFG2-positive central globule {679,915}. This cytological pattern is observed in lobular neoplasia {412,1258}, in classic invasive lobular carcinoma and it has also been associated with the pleomorphic variant of lobular carcinoma {258}. The other cytological type is similar to the cells of diffuse gastric carcinoma, and is characterized by acidic muco-substances that diffusely fill the cytoplasm and dislodge the nucleus to one pole of the cell. This type of signet-ring cell may populate DCIS.

Primary carcinomas of the breast with signet-ring-cell differentiation have to be distinguished from metastases to the breast of signet ring cell carcinomas from other organs, particularly from the stomach. Hormone receptors (ER and PR) and GCDFP-15 are frequently expressed in breast carcinomas with signet-ring-cell differentiation; lack of staining for all three favours a primary gastric carcinoma {1014}.

Genetics

There are no available data on the genetic features of these tumours.

Prognosis and predictive factors

The prognostic significance of tumours with prominent signet-ring-cell differentiation is uncertain.

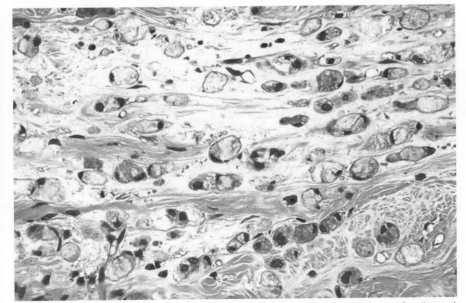

Fig. 3.32 Carcinoma with signet-ring-cell differentiation. The invasive cells assume a lobular growth pattern and contain abundant intracytoplasmic mucin, conferring a signet-ring-cell appearance to the cells.

Carcinomas with neuroendocrine features

G. Bussolati
S. Badve

Definition

Carcinomas with neuroendocrine differentiation exhibit morphological features similar to those of neuroendocrine tumours of the gastrointestinal tract and of the lung. All tumours express neuroendocrine markers to a greater or a lesser degree. Other invasive breast carcinomas of no special type (NST), and some special variants, may show neuroendocrine differentiation.

ICD-O code

Neuroendocrine tumour,
   well-differentiated   8246/3
Neuroendocrine carcinoma, poorly
   differentiated/small cell carcinoma
                         8041/3
Invasive breast carcinoma with
   neuroendocrine differentiation 8574/3

Synonyms

Endocrine carcinoma; carcinoid tumour of the breast

Epidemiology

Carcinomas with neuroendocrine differentiation represent < 1% of breast carcinomas. Most patients are in the sixth or seventh decades of life {1259}. However, since neuroendocrine markers are not routinely used on breast tumours with solid, alveolar and nested patterns of growth, the true incidence is difficult to assess.

Neuroendocrine differentiation as determined by histochemical and immunohistochemical analysis occurs more frequently (up to 30%) in invasive carcinoma NST and other special types, particularly mucinous carcinomas.

Clinical features

There are no notable or specific differences in presentation from other tumour types. Clinical syndromes related to hormone production are extremely rare. Serological tests may detect circulating neuroendocrine markers such as chromogranin A.

Macroscopy

Neuroendocrine breast carcinomas can grow as infiltrating or expansile tumours. The consistency of tumours with mucin production is soft and gelatinous.

Histopathology

Neuroendocrine tumour, well-differentiated

These tumours consist of densely cellular, solid nests and trabeculae of cells that vary from spindle to plasmacytoid and large clear cells {1260} separated by delicate fibrovascular stroma. The classic features of carcinoid tumours of the gastrointestinal tract or lung, i.e. ribbons, cords and rosettes, are not features of

neuroendocrine carcinomas of the breast. The majority are of low or intermediate grade {1259}.

Neuroendocrine carcinoma, poorly differentiated/small cell carcinoma

This carcinoma is morphologically indistinguishable from its counterpart in the lung on the basis of histological and immunohistochemical features {1308}. The tumours are composed of densely packed hyperchromatic cells with scant cytoplasm and display an infiltrative growth pattern. Large numbers of mitotic figures and focal areas of necrosis are present {1259}. An in situ component with the same cytological features may be detected. Lymphatic tumour emboli are frequently encountered.

Invasive breast carcinoma with neuroendocrine differentiation

Neuroendocrine differentiation as determined by histochemical and immunohistochemical analysis occurs more frequently (up to 30%) in invasive carcinoma NST and other special types, particularly mucinous carcinomas. Mucinous carcinomas, hypercellular variant, represent approximately one quarter of mammary carcinomas with neuroendocrine differentiation {1259}, are almost invariably of low grade {1004}. Solid papillary carcinomas

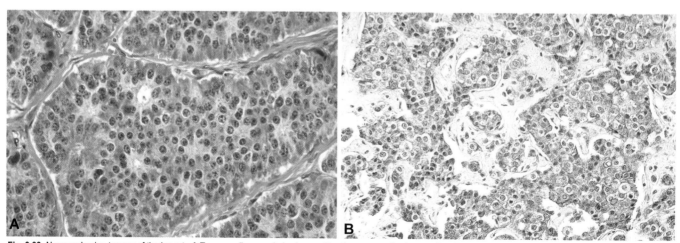

Fig. 3.33 Neuroendocrine tumour of the breast. **A** Tumour cells are polarized around lumina; some cells show eosinophilic granules (carcinoid-like pattern). **B** Immunostaining is positive for chromogranin.

(see Chapter 7) frequently show neuroendocrine differentiation in both in situ and invasive components.

Differential diagnosis
Since primary mammary carcinoma with neuroendocrine features is rare, metastatic well-differentiated neuroendocrine tumour (carcinoid) and poorly differentiated neuroendocrine carcinoma/small cell carcinoma should be excluded before making a definite diagnosis {391}. The presence of ductal carcinoma in situ (DCIS) with similar cytological features is supportive of origin in the breast.

Immunoprofile
Expression of chromogranin proteins and/or synaptophysin is the characteristic feature of carcinomas with neuroendocrine differentiation. About 50% of low- or intermediate-grade neuroendocrine tumours express chromogranin and only 16% express synaptophysin {1259}. A monoclonal antibody to neurone-specific enolase (NSE) has also been used and is expressed in 100% of poorly differentiated/small cell carcinomas of the breast {1308}, whereas chromogranin A and synaptophysin are expressed in about 50% of such cases.
Estrogen and progesterone receptors (ER and PR) are expressed in the majority of tumour cells in well-differentiated tumours and in > 50% of poorly differentiated/small cell carcinomas.

Ultrastructure
Different types of dense core granules, whose neurosecretory nature is confirmed

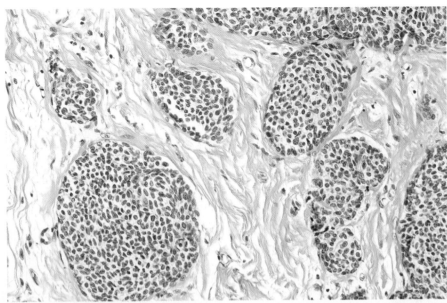

Fig. 3.34 Neuroendocrine carcinoma of the breast. Alveolar pattern with rounded solid nests of spindle cells invading a dense collagenous stroma.

by ultrastructural immunolocalization of chromogranin A have been identified by electron microscopy in carcinomas with neuroendocrine differentiation {220}. The presence of clear vesicles of presynaptic type is correlated with the expression of synaptophysin. Both dense core granules and mucin vacuoles are present in neuroendocrine mucinous carcinomas {611}.

Genetics
The only relevant gene-expression studies have used genome-wide oligonucleotide microanalysis and demonstrated that solid papillary and mucinous carcinomas exhibiting neuroendocrine differentiation of the breast fall within the luminal A subgroup. No transcriptomic differences were detected between the subtypes of these tumours {1567}.

Prognosis and predictive factors
Histological grading and staging are important prognostic parameters. However no specific guidelines exist for grading carcinomas with neuroendocrine differentiation and grading is probably not clinically significant.

Invasive papillary carcinoma

G. Tse
T. Moriya
Y. Niu

Definition

An invasive papillary carcinoma is an invasive adenocarcinoma which has a predominantly papillary morphology (> 90%) in the invasive component. Invasive non-papillary carcinoma associated with encapsulated papillary carcinoma and solid papillary carcinoma should not be classified as invasive papillary carcinoma, but categorized according to the individual invasive component. As a consequence, true invasive papillary carcinomas are rare. Papillary metastases from other primary sites should therefore be considered in the differential diagnosis.

ICD-O code   8503/3

Epidemiology

As this rare group of tumours has not been well-defined in the past, there are currently no specific epidemiological data available.

Clinical features

True invasive papillary carcinomas have no specific or known clinical characteristics.

Macroscopy

There are no specific macroscopic features.

Histopathology

As these lesions are extremely rare, histological characteristics are not well-documented. Invasive elements harbour a papillary architecture with papillae formed by malignant epithelial cells intimately related to fine fibrovascular cores. These tumours have a permeative front.

Genetics

There are no available data on the genetic features of these tumours.

Differential diagnosis

The main differential diagnosis is a papillary metastasis originating from another organ site, particularly ovary or lung. These tumours should be distinguished from invasive carcinoma arising in con-

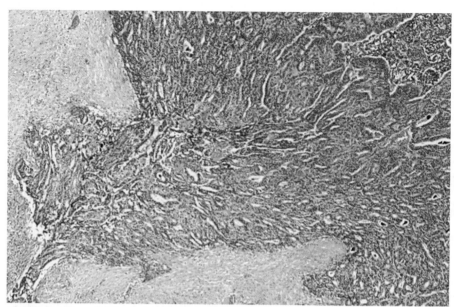

Fig. 3.35 Invasive papillary carcinoma showing crowded papillary structures lined by malignant cells. The invasive edge is broad.

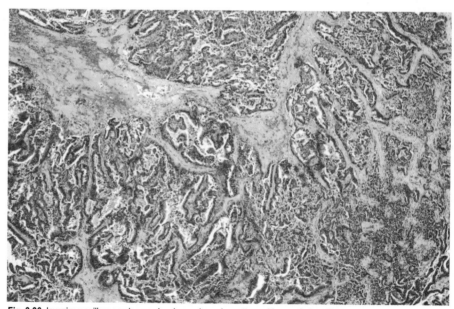

Fig. 3.36 Invasive papillary carcinoma showing an irregular pattern with crowded papillae.

junction with encapsulated and solid papillary carcinoma (see Chapter 7).

Prognosis and predictive factors

Survival data are scanty. Prognosis is related to grade and stage of the tumour.

Invasive micropapillary carcinoma

J.S.Reis-Filho
I.O. Ellis

Definition
A carcinoma composed of small, hollow or morula-like clusters of cancer cells, surrounded by clear stromal spaces. The neoplastic cells characteristically display a reverse polarity, also known as an "inside-out" growth pattern, whereby the apical pole of the cells faces the stroma and not the luminal surface.

ICD-O code   8507/3

Synonyms
Micropapillary carcinoma

Epidemiology
Pure micropapillary carcinomas are rare, accounting for approximately 0.9–2% of invasive breast cancers {527,1076,1335}. The presence of areas with a micropapillary pattern is found in up to 7.4% of all invasive breast cancers {529,1544,1622}. The mean age at presentation of patients with pure or mixed micropapillary carcinoma is consistent with that of patients with estrogen-receptor positive (ER-positive) invasive carcinoma of no special type (NST) {529,837,1335,1544}. Single case reports of invasive micropapillary carcinomas in men are on record {18, 384}.

Clinical features
The vast majority of micropapillary carcinomas present as a palpable mass. Mammography usually reveals a dense, irregular mass with indistinct margins and microcalcifications. By ultrasound analysis, micropapillary carcinomas are preferentially hypoechoic but occasionally isoechoic, homogeneously hypoechoic, irregular or microlobulated masses with or without posterior acoustic shadowing {18, 527,676,725}.

Macroscopy
Invasive micropapillary carcinomas appear not to have any specific features on gross analysis.

Histopathology
Micropapillary carcinomas are characterized by the presence of hollow or morula-

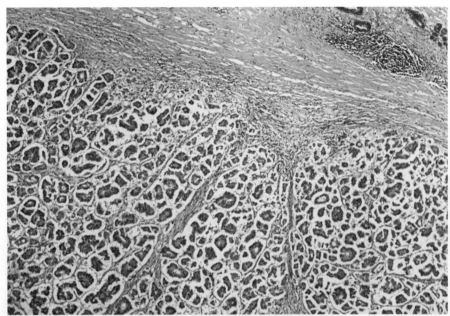

Fig. 3.37 Invasive micropapillary carcinoma. Tumour cell clusters with irregular central spaces proliferate within empty stromal spaces. Some clusters have reversed polarity with an "inside-out" morphology.

like aggregates of cuboidal-to-columnar neoplastic cells devoid of fibrovascular cores, surrounded by empty stromal spaces, which at first glance confer an appearance reminiscent of that of lymphovascular invasion. The empty stromal spaces, although resembling dilated lymphatic channels, have been shown not to be lined by endothelial cells, and may potentially constitute a fixation artefact. Cytologically, the cytoplasm is eosinophilic, and either dense or finely granular; in some cases, overt apocrine features can be identified. Nuclear pleomorphism is variable, but rarely pronounced. Mitotic activity ranges from low to moderate. Necrosis and brisk lymphocytic infiltrate are rare findings.

Characteristically, the neoplastic cells of micropapillary carcinomas display a reverse polarity (i.e. "inside-out" pattern), whereby the apical pole of neoplastic cells faces the empty stromal spaces rather than the hollowed central aspects of the tumour cell aggregates. This pattern can be easily appreciated by immunohistochemical analysis with MUC1 antibodies, and is useful for distinguishing be-

tween invasive micropapillary carcinomas and artefactual stromal retraction in an invasive carcinoma NST. Up to 75% of invasive micropapillary carcinomas are of Nottingham histological grades 2 or 3 {529,819, 837,875,876,923,1076,1099,1335,1453, 1544}.

The vast majority of micropapillary carcinomas are ER-positive (61–100%) and progesterone receptor-positive (PR-positive) (46–83%) {733,837,838,875,876, 1076,1453,1544,1603}; however, in other series a lower prevalence of hormone-receptor expression has been described (25–32% for ER, and 13–20% for PR) {923,1099}. Conflicting results on HER2 expression in micropapillary carcinomas have also been reported; while in some studies, up to 100% of micropapillary carcinomas displayed HER2 "overexpression" {923,1099,1499}, more recent studies adopting current criteria for HER2 overexpression documented HER2 positivity in < 10% to 35% of cases {733,838,875, 876,1603}. In addition, *HER2* mRNA overexpression and *HER2* gene amplification appear to be less frequent (10–30% of cases) {875,876,1569}.

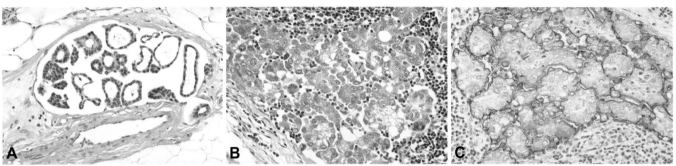

Fig. 3.38 Invasive micropapillary carcinoma. **A** Note the prominent vascular invasion and occasional pyknotic nuclei within the central spaces. **B** Lymph-node metastasis. **C** Positive staining for epithelial membrane antigen on the peripheral cell membranes is suggestive of an "inside-out" morphology.

Genetics

Consistent with the high prevalence of ER expression, microarray gene-expression profiling of invasive micropapillary carcinomas has revealed that these tumours are classified as of luminal A or B subtype {1569}. Expression of "basal" markers is vanishingly rare {693,875,876,1569}. Microarray-based comparative genomic hybridization analyses have demonstrated that these tumours display recurrent gains of chromosome 8q, 17q and 20q and deletions of chromosomes 6q and 13q {875,1438}; in fact, pure and mixed invasive micropapillary carcinomas have been shown to be characterized by a repertoire of gene copy-number aberrations distinct from that of grade- and ER-matched invasive carcinomas NST {808, 875,876}. Interestingly, in mixed micro-papillary carcinomas, the non-micropapillary component displays genetic aberrations remarkably similar to those found in the micropapillary areas {875,876}. In a small series of invasive micro-papillary carcinomas, recurrent amplifications of *MYC*, *CCND1* and *FGFR1* were found in 33%, 8% and 17% of the tumours, respectively {876}.

Prognosis and predictive factors

Micropapillary carcinomas significantly more frequently present with lympho-vascular invasion and lymph-node metastasis at diagnosis than do invasive carcinomas NST {693,802,967,1614}.

It remains to be determined whether the micropapillary phenotype is an independent prognostic factor.

Inflammatory carcinoma

E. Charafe-Jauffret
H. Tsuda
E. Rutgers

Definition

Inflammatory carcinoma is a rare but very aggressive form of breast carcinoma with distinct clinical and/or pathological criteria {836}. The clinical inflammatory symptoms are due to the presence of numerous dermal lymphatic emboli, that alone define "occult" inflammatory breast carcinoma {167,1253}.

ICD-O code   8530/3

Epidemiology

The incidence rate is about 2.5 per 100 000 women-years and is increasing. There are considerable racial disparities since incidence is highest in African-American women and lowest in Asians and Pacific Islanders {545,1192}. The reported frequency of inflammatory breast carcinoma varies between 1% and 10%, according to the diagnostic criteria used to define this disease {375,545}. Inflammatory breast carcinoma shows a prominent geographic pattern (more common in north Africa, including Egypt and Tunisia) {177,245,

1349}. At present, there are few established risk factors for inflammatory breast carcinoma, but a high body-mass index, and a younger age at disease onset have been suggested in African-Americans {1192}.

Clinical features

The clinical inflammatory symptoms are rapid breast enlargement and changes in the overlying skin (redness, oedema, "orange-peel" skin) often without a discrete palpable mass {1192}. Diffuse firmness of the breast is common.They involve more than one third of the breast. Palpable, firm ipsilateral, axillary nodes are common findings. Inflammatory carcinoma is recognized as T4d carcinoma of the breast for staging purposes.

Macroscopy

Usually there is no clinically discrete mass; biopsies of the tumour are facilitated by diagnostic imaging. When a generalized increase in breast density is the only imaging finding, random needle

biopsies are often diagnostic. Nipple involvement is not a diagnostically defining clinical feature, but flattening, retraction and crusting may be frequent.

Histopathology

The pathognomonic feature is the presence of numerous dermal lymphatic emboli in the skin overlying the breast. The emboli may not always be found in small punch biopsies, so the absence of dermal lymphatic invasion does not exclude the diagnosis. The emboli cause dermal lymphatic obstruction and subsequent oedema, but are not associated with any significant degree of inflammatory cell infiltration. The underlying invasive carcinoma is often of no special type (NST), and grade 3. Inflammatory breast carcinomas are highly angiogenic, lymph-angiogenic and vasculogenic {37,896, 1512}.

Immunoprofile

The immunoprofile reflects the aggressive nature of these tumours: inflammatory

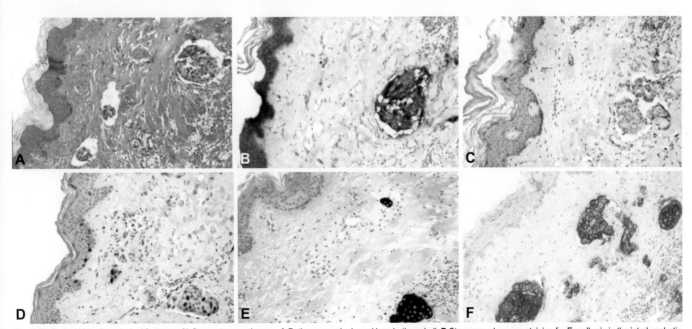

Fig. 3.39 Typical histophenotypical features of inflammatory carcinoma. **A** Pathognomonic dermal lymphatic emboli. **B** Strong membranous staining for E-cadherin in the intralymphatic tumour cells. **C** Absence of estrogen-receptor expression in tumour cells. **D** High proliferation index in tumoral nuclei (Ki67 staining). **E** Intense and diffuse MUC1 staining in cytoplasm of tumour cells. **F** Strong and crisp membranous staining for HER2.

breast carcinoma often lacks hormone receptors (up to 50% of cases), overexpresses HER2 (about 40%) and, less frequently, EGFR {523,1487} and highly expresses p53 and sialomucin MUC1 {414,1487}. E-cadherin overexpression is a hallmark of inflammatory breast carcinoma and sustains the cohesion of tumoral clumps forming emboli {37,701}.

Differential diagnosis

Clinical features can be confused with infection (mastitis or abscess), other tumours with skin changes, and locally advanced breast cancers, which can all be excluded on the basis of morphological and immunohistochemical findings {246,523,1494}.

Genetics

There is no genetic hallmark of inflammatory breast carcinoma, but HER2 amplification and TP53 mutations are common {523,1472,1494}. Molecular subtyping often classifies this carcinoma within the HER2 or basal subtype {1494}.

Most genetic studies have described overexpression of RhoC GTPase (90%) and a loss of Wnt-inducible signalling protein 3 (WISP3/CCN6) {703,1492,1493, 1494}. Microarray technology has suggested a role for other specific pathways, such as NFkappaB, IGF-1 signalling activation or angiogenic pathways {702,1494, 1489}. Recent studies have demonstrated a high level of the translation initiation factor eIF4GI, which regulates p120-catenin that anchors E-cadherin {1322}.

Very recent data have suggested that there is a highly specific and unknown alteration in activation of the anaplastic lymphoma kinase (ALK) pathway related to ALK gene amplification at the 2p23 locus in inflammatory breast cancer. If ongoing studies confirm ALK amplification, patients with inflammatory breast cancer might be eligible for specific targeted therapies {1192A}.

Prognosis and predictive factors

The use of neoadjuvant therapy has improved survival rates from 25% to 50%, but survival outcomes for patients with inflammatory breast carcinoma are still worse than those for patients with non-inflammatory locally advanced breast cancers {294,295,318,1266}. Pathologically complete response to chemotherapy is a very strong prognostic factor for overall and disease-free survival {1266}.

Classic prognostic factors in breast cancer do not have a real prognostic value in inflammatory carcinoma, with the exception of expression of ER and BCL2 {244, 1351}. The cancer stem-cell population contains the tumorigenic and metastatic fraction {244,1351,1602} and ALDH1, a marker for cancer stem cells, is an independent prognostic indicator for inflammatory breast carcinoma {244}.

Bilateral breast carcinoma and non-synchronous breast carcinoma

G. MacGrogan
T. Tot
E. Rakha
M. Morrow

Definition

Breast carcinoma is designated as bilateral when a primary carcinoma develops in each breast.

Although reported time intervals vary, bilateral breast carcinoma (BBC) is generally considered to be synchronous when a contralateral breast carcinoma (CBC) is diagnosed within 3 months, and metachronous when CBC is diagnosed more than 3 months after diagnosis of the first tumour {555}; however, 12 months would seem more appropriate from an epidemiological point of view {615}.

Before establishing the diagnosis of BBC, metastatic cancer in the contralateral breast must be excluded. Patients with evidence of local, regional or distant metastasis are at a higher risk of having metastatic disease in the contralateral breast than of having a primary cancer. Conversely, the presence of carcinoma in situ or differences in histological type and grade between the two tumours is evidence for BBC {248}. Several studies, using different molecular methods, have shown that BBCs are most likely to be genetically non-identical {620,1164,1304}.

Epidemiology

BBC accounts for between 2% and 6% of all breast cancers {555}. The incidence of BBC ranges from 3.8 to 9.3 per 1000 person-years in patients with a first primary breast cancer {257}. Women who already have breast cancer have a two- to sixfold risk of developing CBC compared with the risk of developing a first primary breast cancer among other women, and the risk is inversely correlated with age at initial diagnosis {15,257,546,593}. Median time between diagnosis of the first breast cancer and metachronous CBC varies from 3.9 to 7.7 years {15,555,593}.

In a Swedish nationwide population-based study covering three decades, BBC was reported in 5.3% of patients with primary breast carcinoma; of these, 1.5% were synchronous tumours and 3.8% were metachronous. Between 1970 and 2000, an increase in the incidence of synchronous BBC was observed, consistent with the introduction of bilateral mammography, while a decrease of one third was observed in the incidence of metachronous BBC, owing to the introduction of systemic adjuvant therapy {555}.

Women who have hormone receptor-positive primary breast cancers have a more than twofold risk of developing a contralateral tumour, and women who have hormone receptor-negative breast cancers have nearly a fourfold risk, compared with the general population, after adjusting for age, race, and year. Those with hormone receptor-negative first tumours are much more likely to develop hormone receptor-negative second tumours, especially when the first diagnosis is made before age 30 years {732}.

Although exposure to radiotherapy does not affect risk of BBC in the general population, young patients (< 45 years) with breast cancer treated by postlumpectomy radiotherapy using tangential fields experience an increased risk of CBC, especially women with a family history of breast cancer {157,271,471,593,1378}. The risk is highest for cancers of the medial part of the contralateral breast that is exposed to the highest dose of radiation {593}. Women having undergone mantle radiation in their youth for the treatment of Hodgkin disease also have an increased risk (range, 9–29%) of developing BBC {110,134}.

It is recognized that adjuvant systemic hormone therapy reduces the incidence of CBC by 39–55%, depending on menopausal status and disease status {360}; this benefit seems to last for up to 5 years after the first diagnosis {125}. Adjuvant chemotherapy is also associated with a reduction (–20%) in the incidence of CBC in women aged < 50 years, but not in women aged 50 years and older {360}. One study in women aged < 55

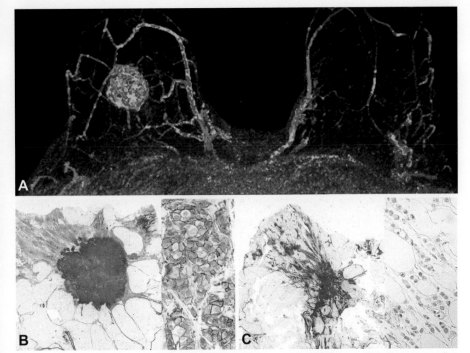

Fig. 3.40 Bilateral breast carcinoma (BBC). **A** Magnetic resonance imaging of synchronous BBC. The corresponding histological sections and HER2 immunohistochemistry are shown. **B** Invasive carcinoma of no special type, grade 3, with strong overexpression of HER2. **C** Invasive lobular carcinoma grade 2 and negative HER2 immunohistochemistry.

years with primary breast cancer has found that chemotherapy was associated with a lower risk of CBC (relative risk, 0.57; 95% CI, 0.42–0.75) than no chemotherapy {125}. For patients aged < 50 years, the duration of the protective effect of adjuvant chemotherapy varies from 5 to 10 years {125,593} and seems to be stronger among women who become postmenopausal within 1 year after the diagnosis of primary cancer {125}.

Clinical features
There are no specific clinical features.

Macroscopy
There are no specific macroscopic features.

Histopathology
Synchronous BBC tends to be more often of lobular histological type, lower histological grade and hormone-receptor positive than unilateral breast cancer {257, 623,1114,1272}. One large epidemiological study found that the estrogen-receptor (ER) status of two bilateral tumours was highly concordant (odds ratio, 7.64; 95% CI, 7.00–8.35). The strength of the association in ER status between the two

tumours appeared to decrease as the time between initial diagnoses of the two tumours increased, levelling off after 12 months, although it was still highly significant, even for two tumours separated by 10 years {615}. Similar but weaker trends were observed for progesterone-receptor (PR) status, tumour type and tumour grade. These results indicate that there is no biological cut-off point for synchronous breast cancer and that the biological closeness of two tumours is a function of time {615}. The similarities between the two bilateral tumours can be explained by the fact that they develop in the same genetic background and in the same hormonal and environmental milieux.
However, despite the statistical similarities, substantial differences may exist in hormone-receptor and HER2 status between the tumours in BBC in individual cases, therefore separate assessment of these parameters is recommended in routine practice.

Genetics
Women with a first-degree relative with breast cancer experience a 50% higher relative risk of BBC than those without a family history {556}.

Compared with non-carriers, women with BRCA1 and BRCA2 mutations have 4.5-fold and 3.4-fold risks of BBC, respectively {862}. The relative risk of CBC for carriers of BRCA1 mutations increases as age at first diagnosis decreases {862}. The risk also approximately doubles in carriers of rare low-penetrance inactivating variants of CHEK2, ATM, BRIP1, and PALB2 {555}. Conversely, carriers of common variants of the ATM gene have a reduction in risk of CBC {288}.

Prognosis and predictive factors
Assessment of prognosis in BBC is difficult as the outcome cannot be attributed unequivocally to the first or second cancer. Survival of patients with synchronous BBC seems to be dependent on the tumour with the worst pathological features {625}. Women aged > 50 years with synchronous BBC or who develop CBC within 5 years have respectively a twofold and a fourfold risk of dying of cancer compared with women with unilateral cancer. Women with BBC diagnosed > 10 years after the first cancer have a prognosis similar to that women with unilateral breast cancer {555}.

Exceptionally rare types and variants

V. Eusebi
S. Ichihara
A. Vincent-Salomon
N. Sneige
A. Sapino

Secretory carcinoma

Definition
A rare, low-grade, translocation-associated invasive carcinoma with a solid, microcystic and tubular architecture composed of cells that produce intracellular and extracellular secretory material.

ICD-O code   8502/3

Synonyms
Juvenile breast carcinoma {899}

Epidemiology
Secretory carcinomas account for < 0.15% of all breast cancers {171}. These tumours have been reported in both sexes {66}. The median age of presentation is 25 years (range, 3–87 years) {1019,1213,1416}.

Clinical features
Secretory carcinomas are well-circumscribed mobile masses located near the areola, especially in men and children.

Macroscopy
The tumours measure an average of 3 cm (range, 0.5–12 cm). The cut surface varies from grey-white to yellow-tan in colour.

Histopathology
Secretory carcinomas show pushing borders, but areas of frank invasion are frequent. Three patterns are seen in various combinations: microcystic, solid and tubular. The microcystic pattern is composed of small cysts mimicking thyroid follicles that can merge into solid islands. The tubular pattern shows lumina containing secretions. Most tumours contain all three patterns. Sclerotic tissue in the centre of the lesion may be observed. Cells are polygonal with granular eosinophilic to foamy cytoplasm. Nuclei are regular with inconspicuous nucleoli. Mitotic activity is minimal.
The presence of intracellular and extracellular secretory material that is positive on staining with periodic acid-Schiff (PAS) or Alcian blue is a consistent finding.

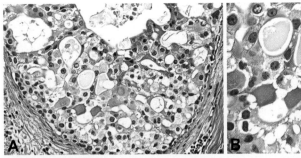

Fig. 3.41 Secretory carcinoma. **A** The tumour cells have abundant pink eosinophilic cytoplasm. **B** Abundant intracellular and extracellular secretory material is evident.

In situ carcinoma, when present, displays similar secretory features, occasionally with necrosis, or can be of low-grade type {740}.

Immunoprofile
Epithelial membrane antigen (EMA), alpha lactoalbumin and S100 protein are frequently expressed. Estrogen receptor (ER), progesterone receptor (PR), HER2 and p63 are negative, while E-cadherin, keratins 8 and 18, CD117, and alpha-smooth-muscle actin can be expressed {572,740}.

Ultrastructure
The variably sized intracytoplasmic lumina contain secretory material. The cells are attached to one another by desmosomes and surround extracellular spaces filled with secretory material {1417}.

Genetics
Tognon et al. {1442} have shown that secretory carcinoma is associated with a characteristic balanced translocation, t(12;15), that creates a *ETV6-NTRK3* gene fusion.
Paradoxically, secretory carcinoma harbours a translocation known to be oncogenic in two other tumour types (including mesenchymal tumours), while also demonstrating true epithelial differentiation with secretory activity. Alteration of the *ETV6*

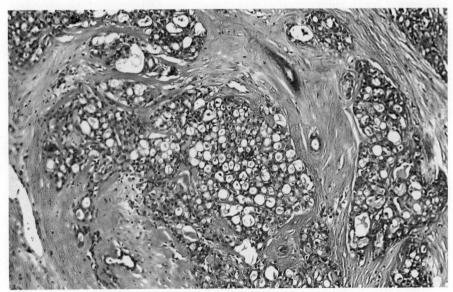

Fig. 3.42 Secretory carcinoma. The tumour cells show a honeycombed growth pattern composed of microcystic glands.

gene is present in both the in situ and invasive components when analysed by fluorescence in situ hybridization (FISH) {740}.

The differential diagnosis with acinic carcinoma is based on the absence of the *ETV6-NTRK3* translocation in acinic carcinomas {1170}.

Prognosis and predictive factors

Secretory carcinoma has a low-grade clinical course and is associated with a favourable prognosis {997}, especially in children and young adults aged < 20 years {1416}. However, in older patients, a more aggressive course is manifested with late recurrences arising after up to 20 years {722,859}.

Axillary lymph-node metastases rarely involve more than three lymph nodes. Distant metastases are extremely rare {66, 572}.

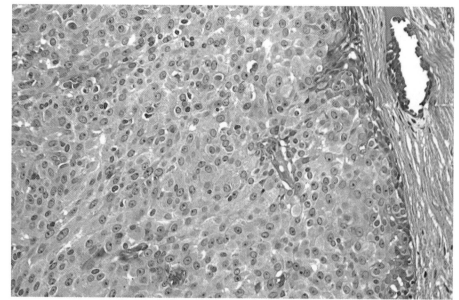

Fig. 3.43 Oncocytic carcinoma. Note the well-circumscribed nodule and cells with abundant eosinophilic cytoplasm.

Oncocytic carcinoma

Definition

A breast carcinoma composed of > 70% of cells showing oncocytic characteristics. Oncocytes are defined as cells with eosinophilic cytoplasm due to high numbers of mitochondria.

ICD-O code   8290/3

Epidemiology

The mean age at presentation is 66 years. Cases occur rarely in men.

Although generally regarded as a very rare form of breast carcinoma in its pure form, in one series, mitochondrion-rich features, defined as strong positive mitochondrial immunocytochemical staining of > 50% of the tumour cells, represented 19.7% out of 76 invasive carcinomas of the breast {1131}.

Clinical features

Clinical features are not distinctive from those of invasive carcinoma of no special type (NST). Lymph-node metastases are present at diagnosis in 44% of patients.

Macroscopy

The mean tumour size is 3 cm.

Histopathology

Oncocyte (a Greek-derived word) means "swollen cell", which in this case is attributable to an accumulation of mitochondria.

The term "oncocyte" is used when diffusely dispersed mitochondria occupy not less than 60% of the cytoplasm.

Three cases were originally reported by Damiani et al. {312} who, using immunohistochemistry for mitochondria, found that 70–90% of cells were packed with immunoreactive granules. Ragazzi et al. {1131} classified cases as oncocytic carcinoma if at least 70% of the tumour cells showed strong immunopositivity (3+) for mitochondria.

Oncocytic carcinoma shows a solid pattern of growth with pushing margins. The cells are characterized by abundant, granular, strongly eosinophilic cytoplasm and well-defined borders, while nuclei vary from monotonous to pleomorphic with prominent nucleoli.

Immunoprofile

In addition to immunoreactivity for mitochondria, EMA was present in all 32 cases described in one series. Keratin 7 was present in 27 (84%), GCDFP-15 in 11 (34%), ER in 25 (78%), PR in 20 (62.5%) of cases and HER2 was strongly expressed in 8 (25%) cases, respectively {1131}.

Oncocytic carcinomas can be distinguished from apocrine and neuroendocrine carcinomas by their immunophenotype.

Ultrastructure

Numerous mitochondria are scattered throughout the cytoplasm, without evidence of polar condensation. No secretory granules are observed.

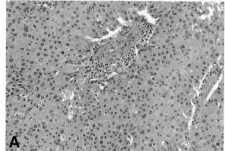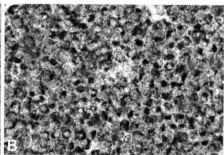

Fig. 3.44 Oncocytic carcinoma. **A** Cells with abundant eosinophilic granular cytoplasm and irregular nuclei. **B** Immunostaining with an antibody to mitochondria highlights coarse cytoplasmic granules.

Genetics

Breast oncocytic carcinomas often display chromosomal gains of 11q13.1–q13.2 and 19p13, similar to oncocytic tumours of the kidney and thyroid, respectively.

Prognosis and predictive factors

Overall survival is similar to that for invasive carcinoma NST when matched for grade and stage.

Sebaceous carcinoma

Definition

A breast carcinoma with prominent sebaceous differentiation in no less than 50% of cells. There should be no evidence of origin from cutaneous adnexal sebaceous glands.

ICD-O code   8410/3

Epidemiology

Only nine examples of this rare mammary tumour have been reported (age range, 45–85 years) {582,894,956,1124,1150,1414, 1497}. One case manifested in a man.

Clinical features

Patients usually present with a palpable mass.

Macroscopy

Tumour size ranges from 2 to 20 cm. The tumour has sharply delineated margins and shows a bright yellow cut surface.

Histopathology

The tumour has a nested structure. Sebaceous cells with abundant finely vacuolated Oil Red O-positive cytoplasm are intermingled with smaller ovoid to spindle cells showing eosinophilic cytoplasm without any vacuolization. The nuclei of both cell types are globoid with up to two nucleoli. Mitotic figures can be numerous. Squamous morules may be present focally.
In the three cases examined ultrastructurally, the cytoplasm of all cells was filled with numerous non-membrane-bound lipid droplets {956,1414,1497}.
The tumour cells stain for keratins, and ER, PR, androgen receptor and HER2 can be expressed {582,956, 1150,1497}.

Differential diagnosis

Carcinoma with apocrine differentiation, lipid-rich carcinoma and liposarcoma enter the differential diagnosis {1416}. Squamous morules are characteristic of

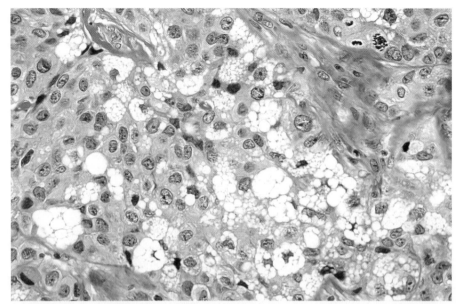

Fig. 3.45 Sebaceous carcinoma. Cells with moderate amounts of eosinophilic or abundant microvacuolated cytoplasm and variably compressed nuclei resembling lipoblasts are admixed.

sebaceous carcinoma. Sebaceous differentiation is also seen in adenoid cystic carcinomas {1416}. The extent of the sebaceous differentiation varies in different cases, and the term "sebaceous carcinoma" applies only where sebaceous differentiation is evident in no fewer than 50% of the neoplastic cells {894,1124,1414}.

Genetics

There are no available data on the genetic features of these tumours.

Prognosis and predictive factors

Not much is known about the behaviour of these tumours. A tumour of 7.5 cm in diameter was treated by radical mastectomy, but none of the 20 axillary lymph nodes was positive for metastases. Two cases were reported to be associated with metastases to axillary nodes {582, 956}, and one patient had distant metastases 10 years after surgery {1497}.

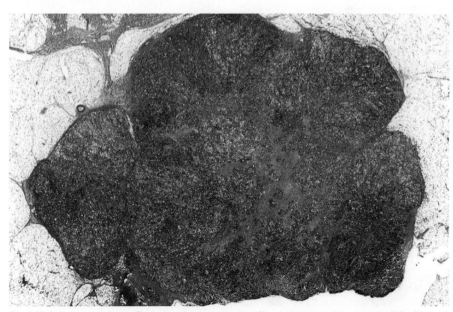

Fig. 3.46 Sebaceous carcinoma. The tumour shows neat borders. Clear (sebaceous cells) represent > 50% of the total neoplastic proliferation.

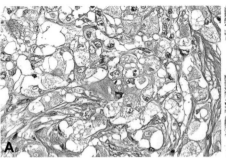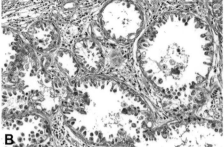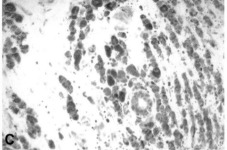

Fig. 3.47 Lipid-rich carcinoma. **A** Cells have abundant eosinophilic or microvacuolated cytoplasm with pleomorphic nuclei. **B** In situ neoplasm showing hobnail features. **C** Oil red O staining shows abundant intracytoplasmic lipids within every cell.

Lipid-rich carcinoma

Definition
An invasive breast carcinoma in which no fewer than 90% of the cells contain abundant cytoplasmic neutral lipids.

ICD-O code   8314/3

Synonyms
Lipid-secreting carcinoma

Epidemiology
If morphological features and histochemical confirmation are used to identify lipid-rich carcinoma, the incidence is < 1–1.6% {8,1152,1485}. Age at presentation ranges from 33 to 81 years {1485,1600}. An association with neuroleptic drugs has been reported {1465}.

Clinical features
One case presented as Paget disease {8}. A metastatic lipid-rich carcinoma producing pancreatic-type isoamylase has been reported {1572}.

Macroscopy
Tumour size varies from 1.2 to 15 cm {1485,1600}.

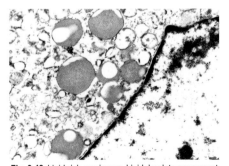

Fig. 3.48 Lipid-rich carcinoma. Lipid droplets are present in the cytoplasm.

Histopathology
Two thirds to three quarters of breast carcinomas contain cytoplasmic lipid droplets to some extent {8,444}. Lipid-rich carcinoma is characterized by cytoplasmic vacuoles containing lipids in no fewer than 90% of the tumour cells. In most cases, lipid-rich carcinoma is classified as histological grade 3.

Apocrine histiocytoid carcinoma closely mimics lipid-rich carcinoma, suggesting a kinship between the two entities {947, 1416}. Chondroid metaplasia may be seen {1498}. The associated DCIS may show cells with hobnail or lactational features {1465,1485}.

Immunoprofile
Tumour cells stain positively for alpha-lactoalbumin {21,1465,1572,1600}, lactoferrin {1572,1600}, CEA {1572}, EMA {21, 234,1498} and adipophylin and are negative for ER and PR {21,731,809,894, 1166,1465,1498,1600}. HER2 and basal-type keratin were both negative in one case {1166}.

Ultrastructure
Well-developed Golgi apparatus and lipid droplets of different sizes are recognized in the cytoplasm {1152,1510}, as well as intramitochondrial needle-like crystals {809, 1152}.

Differential diagnosis
Lipid-rich carcinoma has to be distinguished from glycogen-rich, histiocytoid, secretory, signet-ring, myoepithelial {228}, metastatic renal cell carcinomas {343} and breast carcinomas modified by hormonal therapy and chemotherapy {22, 683}. Fat necrosis and xanthogranulomatous mastitis may simulate lipid-rich carcinoma {714}.

Genetics
There are no available data on the genetic features of these tumours.

Prognosis and predictive factors
Of 37 female patients who underwent axillary dissection, 19 (51.4%) showed lymph-node metastases at presentation {21,234,731,894,1152,1166,1465,1485, 1498,1600}. In patients with follow-up longer than 2 years, 12 out of 21 (57.1%) developed distant metastases {234,760, 809,1166,1510,1600}. In the largest series published so far, a first-year mortality rate of 38.5% was reported {1152}.

Glycogen-rich clear cell carcinoma

Definition
A carcinoma in which > 90% of the neoplastic cells have abundant clear cytoplasm containing glycogen.

ICD-O code   8315/3

Synonyms
Clear cell carcinoma   8310/3
Glycogen-rich carcinoma   8315/3

Epidemiology
The incidence is between 1% and 3% of breast carcinomas, with an age range of 41–78 years (median, 57 years).

Clinical features
The features of these tumours at presentation are similar to those of invasive carcinoma NST.

Macroscopy
The tumour ranges from 1 to 8 cm in size.

Histopathology
A strict definition for glycogen-rich clear cell carcinoma is necessary for two reasons.

Firstly, carcinomas that have a clear-cell appearance are uncommon in the breast and can be an artefact of the extraction of intracytoplasmic substances during tissue processing. The substances that are extracted differ, as does their biological significance {343}. Secondly, intracytoplasmic glycogen has been observed without a significant clear-cell appearance in 60% of breast carcinomas.

The lesions have the structural features of intraductal and invasive carcinoma NST and rarely those of lobular, medullary or tubular types {1416}. Glycogen-rich clear cell carcinoma may have either circumscribed or infiltrative borders.

The in situ component, either in the pure form or in association with most invasive cases, has a compact solid, comedo or papillary growth pattern.

The tumour cells tend to have sharply defined borders and polygonal contours. The clear or finely granular cytoplasm contains PAS-positive diastase-labile glycogen. The nuclei are hyperchromatic, with clumped chromatin and prominent nucleoli.

Immunoprofile

ER is positive in 50% of cases, while PR is negative {1215}. Cases that are positive for HER2 and negative for ER and PR have been seen {1416}. Staining for smooth-muscle actin, GCDFP-15 or CD10 is consistently negative.

Differential diagnosis

Glycogen-rich clear cell carcinoma must be differentiated from lipid-rich carcinoma, histiocytoid apocrine carcinoma, adenomyoepithelioma, clear cell hidradenoma, metastatic renal cell carcinoma and tumours comprised of perivascular epithelioid cells (PEComa) {1416}.

Genetics

There are no available data on the genetic features of these tumours.

Prognosis and predictive factors

Although most reports suggest that glycogen-rich clear cell carcinoma is more aggressive than invasive carcinoma NST, Hayes et al. {562} contend that prognosis is no different once glycogen-rich clear cell carcinoma and conventional mammary carcinomas are matched by tumour size, grade, and lymph-node status.

Acinic cell carcinoma

Definition

A breast carcinoma similar to the acinic cell carcinoma of the parotid gland that shows (serous) differentiation with zymogen-type cytoplasmic granules.

ICD-O code   8550/3

Epidemiology

Acinic cell carcinoma (ACCA) of the breast is a rare tumour but its true incidence is not known as studies on large series are lacking. First reported in 1996 by Roncaroli et al. {1198} as the counterpart of similar tumours of the salivary gland, no more than 20 additional cases have been reported since {314,1276}. Carcinomas showing serous secretion, and probably related to ACCA, have also been described {621,705}. ACCA affects women aged between 35 and 80 years (mean, 56 years) {314}.

Clinical features

ACCA may present as a palpable nodule ranging from 1 to 5 cm in size {1416}.

Macroscopy

The tumour shows infiltrating growth.

Histopathology

ACCA varies from well-differentiated and easily recognizable to structurally solid (dedifferentiated) {1416}. Some show microcystic and microglandular areas, or solid nests with comedo-like necrosis and a rim of microglandular structures at the periphery {1198}. The cells have irregular round to ovoid nuclei, evident single nucleoli and abundant cytoplasm, which is usually granular, amphophilic to eosinophilic. Granules can be large and coarse,

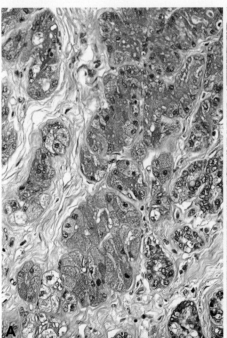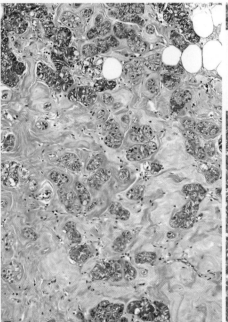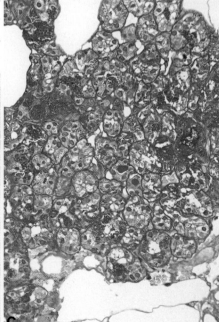

Fig. 3.49 Three examples (A, B, C) of acinic cell carcinoma with a microglandular-like infiltrative pattern and cells with abundant clear cytoplasm containing eosinophilic granules.

bright red in colour, reminiscent of those seen in Paneth cells and ultrastructurally similar to zymogen-like granules {314, 1198,1276}. Cells with clear "hypernephroid" cytoplasm are a feature and may predominate. Mitoses can number up to 15 per 10 high-power fields {314}. In almost all tumours, cells express a high level of alpha-1-antichymotrypsin, salivary-gland amylase, lysozyme, EMA and S100 protein {314}. The mucoapocrine marker GCDFP-15 can be focally positive. ACCAs are consistently negative for ER, PR, androgen receptors {1083} and HER2 {459}.

Kahan et al. {673} reported a case of ACCA that merged with microglandular adenosis and suggested a close relationship between the two lesions. One of the typical features of ACCA is the presence at the edge or within the bulk of the tumour of small carcinomatous tubules {1198, 1416}. These tubules have been interpreted as the malignant transformation of microglandular adenosis {637,705,1177, 1311} and the term "microglandular carcinoma" has been used to describe some cases. Nevertheless, some of the morphological, immunohistochemical and ultrastructural features of these lesions are different {1416} such that at the moment a histogenetic link remains to be proven.

Differential diagnosis
ACCA has to be differentiated from secretory carcinoma {580}, which lacks hypernephroid features and all the proteins of the salivary-gland counterpart of ACCA.

Genetics
From a molecular point of view, ACCA does not show the t(12:15)*ETV6-NTRK3* rearrangement typical of secretory carcinoma {1170,1336}.

Prognosis and predictive factors
None of the patients reported have died as a consequence of this tumour, although follow-up is limited to a maximum of 10 years (mean, 3.3 years) {1416}. Axillary lymph-node metastases may be observed.

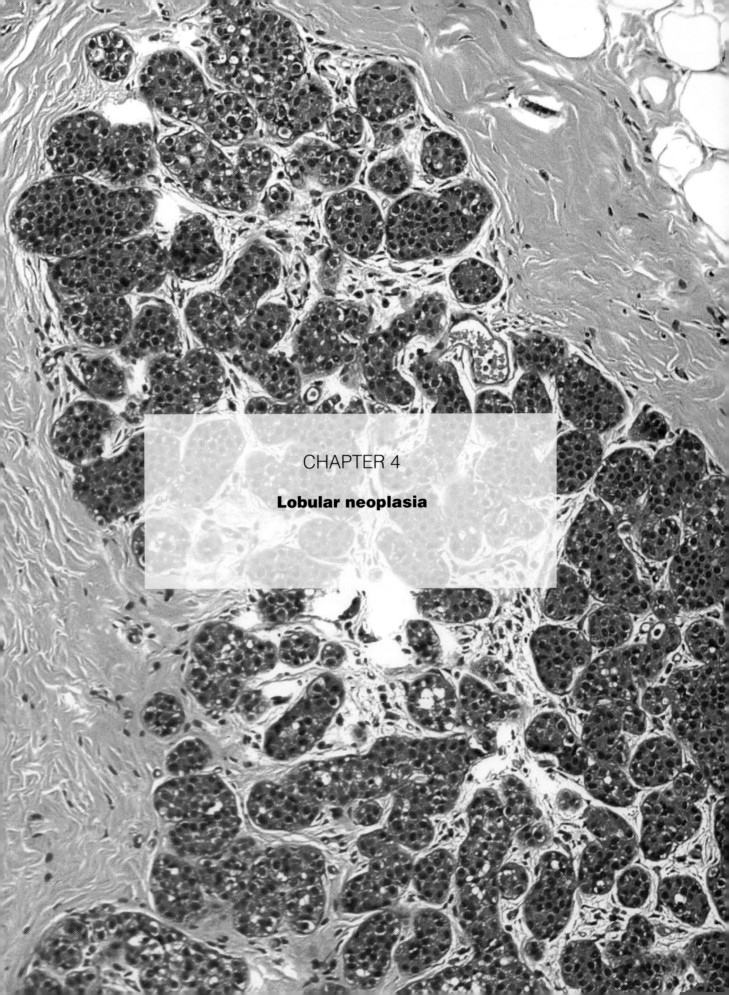

CHAPTER 4

Lobular neoplasia

Lobular neoplasia

S.R. Lakhani
S.J. Schnitt
F. O'Malley
M.J. van de Vijver
P.T. Simpson
J. Palacios

Definition

Lobular neoplasia (LN) refers to the entire spectrum of atypical epithelial lesions originating in the terminal-duct lobular unit (TDLU) and characterized by a proliferation of generally small, non-cohesive cells, with or without pagetoid involvement of terminal ducts. The designations atypical lobular hyperplasia (ALH) and lobular carcinoma in situ (LCIS) are widely used to describe the variable extent of proliferation of the lesion. The distinction between atypical lobular hyperplasia and classic lobular carcinoma in situ is based on the extent of involvement of individual lobular units {1055,1056,1058}.

ICD-O codes

Lobular carcinoma in situ	8520/2
Pleomorphic lobular carcinoma in situ	8519/2

Epidemiology

LN is found in 0.5–4% of otherwise benign breast biopsies. LN has been diagnosed in women of all ages, but is predominantly found in premenopausal women with an average age of 49 years {130,464,533}. Analysis of the Surveillance, Epidemiology and End Results (SEER) database show that the age-adjusted incidence rates for LN increased between 1978 and 1998 {788,792}.

Clinical features

There are no specific clinical features for LN.

Macroscopy

LN is not associated with any grossly recognizable features.

Histopathology

LN is a proliferation within the TDLU {1573} and may have pagetoid involvement of the terminal ducts. The lesion is multicentric in as many as 85% of patients and bilateral in 30–67% {130,532,984, 1221,1414}. On low-power examination, while lobular architecture is maintained, the acini are expanded to varying degrees by a monomorphic proliferation of dyshesive cells, with uniform round nuclei,

indistinct nucleoli, uniform chromatin and scant cytoplasm. Intracytoplasmic lumina are often present but are not specific to LN {45}. These lumina can be large enough to produce signet-ring cell types. In addition to the usual setting within a lobular unit, LN may also involve a variety of lesions, including sclerosing adenosis, radial scars, papillary lesions, fibroadenomas and may be associated with collagenous spherulosis.

Classic LCIS is diagnosed when more than half of the acini of a lobular unit are distended and distorted by a dyshesive proliferation of cells with small, uniform nuclei. Lesser involvement by the characteristic cells is diagnosed as atypical lobular hyperplasia. Pagetoid spread along the terminal duct is a common feature.

Examples of LCIS with mild to moderate degree of nuclear variability are best categorized as classic LCIS. The two forms of LCIS have previously been termed types A and B, a distinction which is of no known significance {533}.

More recently, several variants of LCIS have been recognized with increasing frequency because of the presence of microcalcifications detected on screening mammography. These mammographically-detected lesions include: (1) lesions in which the LCIS cells show the cytological features of classic LCIS (type A or B) but in which there is marked distention of involved spaces with areas of comedo necrosis; and (2) lesions that show marked nuclear pleomorphism (equivalent to that seen in high-grade ductal carcinoma in situ (DCIS), with or without apocrine features and comedo necrosis (pleomorphic LCIS). All lesions in these groups typically lack E-cadherin expression and display genomic alterations by array-based comparative genomic hybridization (CGH) typical of lobular lesions (16q losses and 1q gains) {258, 1346}. While anecdotal data suggest that these variants may have a different clinical course than classical LCIS, the clinical significance and appropriate management of these LCIS variants is at this time uncertain.

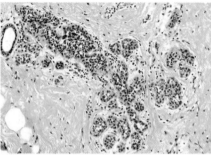

Fig. 4.01 Atypical lobular hyperplasia. Uniform cells are present without distorting the involved acini.

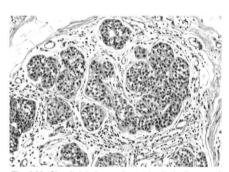

Fig. 4.02 Classic lobular carcinoma in situ is diagnosed because the characteristic cells distend and distort the acini.

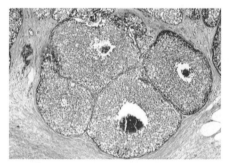

Fig. 4.03 Pleomorphic lobular carcinoma in situ. Solid growth of neoplastic cells with central necrosis and calcification.

Immunoprofile

The classical variety of LN has an immunoprofile similar to that of its invasive counterpart, invasive lobular carcinoma, and to low-grade DCIS. Lesions are frequently (up to 90%) positive for estrogen receptor (ER) and progesterone receptor (PR) and rarely overexpress HER2 or p53 protein {25,209,494,1066, 1148,1234}. Pleomorphic LCIS is more likely to be negative for ER, particularly in the apocrine variant {258}, positive for HER2 and p53 and to have a higher Ki67 proliferative index {116,258,922,1172,1346}. In pleomorphic LCIS, apocrine differentiation has been described, and the cells also express GCDFP-15 (gross cystic disease fluid protein-15). Intracytoplasmic immunoreactivity for casein has also been reported {977,1054}. Some authors have reported that positive staining of LN for keratin 34betaE12 is useful in distinguishing LN from solid DCIS (which is typically negative for keratin 34betaE12), but this finding has not been reproducible and may be related to methodological details of the immunostaining procedure {180, 936}.

In contrast to the majority of ductal lesions, classic and pleomorphic types of LN and invasive lobular carcinoma are negative for E-cadherin in about 80–90% of cases {469,1062}. Approximately 10–16% of cases will express E-cadherin, although this is usually aberrant and this pattern should not be used to make a diagnosis of ductal carcinoma {303,1144}. Beta-catenin, alpha-catenin and p120-catenin, proteins found to complex with E-cadherin, respond differently to functional loss of E-cadherin. Whereas beta-catenin and alpha-catenin are also lost together with E-cadherin, p120 is aberrantly located in the cytoplasm and, in some instances, in the nuclei of cells of LN {304, 891,938,1155,1262}.

Differential diagnosis

Distinction of LN from a solid DCIS of low nuclear grade can be difficult on morphological grounds alone, particularly when DCIS remains confined to the lobule without unfolding it (so-called lobular cancerization). The presence of secondary lumina or a rosette-like arrangement of cells indicates a DCIS. Pleomorphic LCIS can also sometimes be difficult to differentiate from high-grade DCIS. The absence of E-cadherin may be useful to help differentiate DCIS and LCIS or to classify indeterminate lesions {304,633, 1382}. However careful analysis of staining and morphology should be used to make the diagnosis since LN can sometimes be positive for E-cadherin {303, 1144}. In some cases, apparent positivity for E-cadherin might be due to admixture in the same TDLU of E-cadherin-negative neoplastic cells with residual E-cadherin-positive normal epithelial cells. In addition, some mutations in the E-cadherin gene might produce non-functional E-cadherin protein that can be immunohistochemically detected with aberrant (cytoplasmic) or normal membrane staining. If after careful assessment of morphological and immunohistochemical features, a case cannot be definitively classified as DCIS or LCIS, then a designation of "carcinoma in situ with mixed ductal and lobular features" should be rendered. In addition, LN can often be found to co-exist with low-grade DCIS within the same ductal-lobular unit and so cases of mixed ductal and lobular lesions or mixed E-cadherin staining should be recorded.

When LN involves sclerosing lesions, it can be confused with an invasive carcinoma. The presence of a myoepithelial cell layer around the neoplastic cell clusters excludes the possibility of an invasive carcinoma; immunostaining for smooth-muscle actin, p63, keratin 14 or keratin 5/6 can reveal myoepithelial cells, thus facilitating the distinction. The presence of isolated cells invading the stroma around a focus of LN can cause diagnostic problems. The absence of myoepithelial cells around the individual cells and their haphazard distribution accentuated by any of the epithelial markers (optimally with double immunostaining techniques) can help establish the presence of stromal invasion by individual or small clusters of neoplastic cells. Poor tissue preservation may give a false impression of loosely cohesive cells leading to over-diagnosis of LN.

Genetics

Molecular analysis has demonstrated that LN is a clonal neoplastic proliferation and a precursor for invasive cancer. Loss of heterozygosity (LOH) at loci frequently observed in invasive carcinoma, such as 11q13, 16q, 17p and 17q, has been reported {744,971}. Loss of chromosomal material from 16p, 16q, 17p and 22q and gain of material to 6q was also identified in equal frequency by CGH in 14 ALH and 31 LCIS lesions {835}, and by array-based CGH {890} suggesting that both are "neoplastic" and at a similar stage of genetic evolution. Array-based CGH demonstrated that LN and pleomorphic LCIS share recurrent genomic alterations, such as frequent gains on chromosome 1q and losses of 16q and complex, high-level amplifications of 11q13 encompassing the *CCND1* locus. Pleomorphic LCIS harbours greater genomic instability with increased copy-number alterations, including at 8p, 16p, 17q and amplifications at loci including 8q24 and 17q12 {160,258,1172}. These alterations are more common in high-grade ductal carcinomas and reflect the more aggressive features of pleomorphic LCIS compared with LN.

Analysis of synchronous LN and invasive lobular carcinoma and of synchronous pleomorphic LCIS and pleomorphic lobular carcinoma demonstrated concordant genomic profiles providing strong evidence for LN and pleomorphic LCIS being non-obligate precursor lesions for classic invasive lobular carcinoma and pleomorphic lobular carcinoma respectively {617,1172}. In LN and pleomorphic LCIS, the deletion

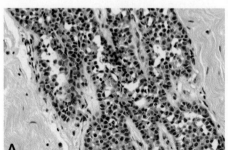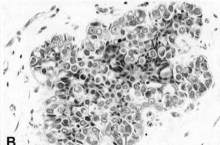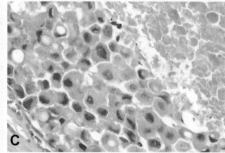

Fig. 4.04 Cytological features of lobular carcinoma in situ (LCIS). **A** Classic LCIS shows small uniform nuclei. **B** This tumour shows mild degrees of nuclear enlargement, but is appropriately diagnosed as classic LCIS. **C** Pleomorphic lobular carcinoma in situ: nuclear enlargement, variability, and prominent nucleoli are associated with abundant cytoplasm.

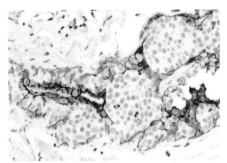

Fig. 4.05 Pleomorphic lobular carcinoma in situ lacks expression of E-cadherin.

on chromosomal 16q is accompanied by other mutational events (e.g. gene mutation and promoter methylation) to inactivate the E-cadherin gene, *CDH1*, which is found at 16q22.1 {127,128,354,1630}. In one study {129}, 27 of 48 (56%) invasive lobular carcinomas had a mutation in *CDH1*, while none of 50 breast cancers of other types showed any alteration. It was subsequently demonstrated that truncating mutations identified in invasive lobular carcinoma were also present in the adjacent LN, supporting the concept that LN is a precursor lesion {1528}.

Prognosis and predictive factors

While ALH and classic LCIS represent a morphological and biological continuum, the diagnostic separation is useful from an epidemiological and clinical point of view, because the risk of subsequent invasive cancer development associated with ALH is half that of LCIS.

The relative risk for subsequent development of invasive carcinoma among patients with LN ranges from 4 to about 12 times that expected in women without LN {47,533}. The variation in reported subsequent cancer incidence is related to differences in lengths of follow-up, which LN lesions were included (ALH alone, LCIS alone or both) and lack of complete pathological review. Early studies suggested that both breasts were at equal risk for later cancer development {53A}; however, recent carefully conducted cohort studies show that approximately two thirds of subsequent carcinomas occur in the ipsilateral breast {881,1058}.

There is controversy regarding the time-course for developing invasive carcinoma after a diagnosis of LN. Some studies find continued risk, while others show a decrease after menopause.

The type of invasive cancer that may arise following LN can be either lobular or ductal. Although all types of invasive carcinoma have been observed after a diagnosis of LN, invasive lobular carcinoma or special-type carcinomas are seen with higher frequency than in the general breast-cancer population {6,268,447, 1056}.

Features useful for identifying which patients diagnosed with LCIS will eventually develop an invasive carcinoma have not been elucidated through clinical or pathological features {1056,1219}.

The current consensus is that LN constitutes both a risk factor and a non-obligate precursor for subsequent development of invasive carcinoma in either breast, of either ductal or lobular type, but only in a minority of women after long-term follow-up. As defined in large epidemiological follow-up studies, ALH and classic LCIS are generally incidental findings. For this reason, when ALH or classic LCIS is diagnosed on needle-core biopsy, careful radiology/pathology correlation should be performed to determine the need for surgical excision. Studies that have shown a substantial rate of upgrades generally show a selection bias.

The management of patients with ALH and classical LCIS when diagnosed on needle-core biopsy is controversial. Reported rates of upgrade to a worse lesion on excision vary widely due to variations in study design {1018}. There is consensus that excision should be performed if there is another lesion which by itself would warrant excision or if there is pathological-mammographic discordance. In cases where ALH or LCIS on core biopsy is a completely incidental finding, radiological–pathological correlation is recommended for determining further management. In contrast, excision should be performed for cases of classical LCIS with comedo necrosis, bulky mass-forming LCIS lesions and cases of pleomorphic LCIS identified on needle-core biopsy.

Information on the natural history of pleomorphic LCIS is extremely limited. Although the nuclear pleomorphism and necrosis suggest a more "aggressive" lesion, it remains unproven that the lesion is associated with a higher risk of subsequent breast cancer than that associated with classic LCIS. Obtaining natural history data will be difficult because these lesions are often treated as DCIS (complete excision with or without radiation therapy). More than 180 cases originally diagnosed as DCIS in clinical trial NSABP-B-17 were later categorized as LCIS. These lesions probably represented pleomorphic LCIS based on their presentation and were associated with ipsilateral recurrence in 14% of cases. In the absence of better information on the natural history of pleomorphic LCIS, caution should be exercised in recommending more aggressive management strategies, such as excision to negative margins or mastectomy as a routine practice after a diagnostic surgical biopsy reveals pleomorphic LCIS. Decisions regarding the need for excision to negative margins should be considered after a careful review of the pathological criteria used for the diagnosis of pleomorphic LCIS, the extent of surgery required for complete excision, as well as the patient's suitability for, and acceptance of, non-surgical risk-management strategies.

Histological features, including degree of pleomorphism, bulk of disease, solid-duct involvement and presence of comedo necrosis are being used to distinguish potentially more aggressive and established forms of LCIS that would appear from the limited existing evidence to merit consideration for complete excision. The definition of what constitutes bulky disease or "florid" LCIS remains debatable, but would generally incorporate involvement of several contiguous lobules by LCIS often with accompanying mass formation. Importantly for cases of classic LCIS, there is no indication that excision to negative margins is useful, and we do not recommend reporting margin status for classic LCIS. Likewise, we do not advocate the need to report presence of classic LCIS at margins when areas of pleomorphic LCIS in the same case have already been completely excised. Classic LCIS with comedo necrosis at margins can be problematic, and will require careful pathological review as stated above, as well as close discussion with the clinical managing team.

CHAPTER 5

Intraductal proliferative lesions

Intraductal proliferative lesions: Introduction and overview

S.J. Schnitt
I.O. Ellis
M.J. van de Vijver
D. Sgroi

S.R. Lakhani
J. Simpson
C. Allred
A. Vincent-Salomon

Definition

Intraductal proliferative lesions are a group of cytologically and architecturally diverse proliferations, typically originating in the terminal-duct lobular unit (TDLU) and confined to the mammary ductal-lobular system. They are associated with an increased risk, albeit of different magnitudes, for the subsequent development of invasive carcinoma. Some of these lesions are best considered as risk indicators whereas others are recognized as true precursors of invasive breast cancer.

Clinical features

The age range of women with intraductal proliferative lesions is wide, spanning seven to eight decades post-adolescence. All these lesions are extremely rare before puberty; when they do occur among infants and children, they are generally a reflection of exogenous or abnormal endogenous hormonal stimulation. The mean age at which ductal carcinoma in situ (DCIS) is diagnosed is between 50 and 59 years. Although most often unilateral, about 22% of women with DCIS in one breast develop either in situ or invasive carcinoma in the contralateral breast {1551}.

Macroscopy

A vast majority of intraductal proliferative lesions, particularly those detected mammographically, are not evident on macroscopic inspection of the specimen. In a small proportion of cases, high-grade DCIS may be sufficiently extensive and exhibit such an abundance of intraluminal necrosis or associated stromal reaction that it presents as multiple areas of round, pale comedo necrosis or a firm, gritty mass. Specimen radiography is an important component in the pathological evaluation of mammographically detected lesions.

Localization

The vast majority of intraductal proliferative lesions originate in the TDLU {1573}. A substantially smaller proportion originates in larger and lactiferous ducts.

DCIS is a segmental disease, originating in the TDLU and progressing within the duct system toward the nipple and into adjacent branches of a given segment of the duct system. The rare lesions that develop within the lactiferous ducts may progress toward the nipple, resulting in Paget disease {1027,1028,1031}.

Terminology

Intraductal proliferative lesions of the breast have traditionally been divided into three categories: usual ductal hyperplasia (UDH), atypical ductal hyperplasia (ADH) and DCIS. It should be noted, however, that the term "DCIS" encompasses a highly heterogeneous group of lesions that differ with regard to their mode of presentation, histopathological features, biological markers, genetic and molecular abnormalities, and risk of progression to invasive cancer. Heterogeneity may exist even within a given DCIS lesion {36}. In most cases, the histopathological distinction between different types of intraductal proliferation can be made on morphological grounds alone, particularly with standardization of histopathological criteria. However, even then, the distinction between some of the lesions (particularly between ADH and some small, low-grade forms of DCIS) remains problematic. In addition, population-based mammographic screening has resulted in increased detection of lesions that show low grade cytological atypia with or without intraluminal proliferation that do not fulfil the combined cytological and architectural criteria for the diagnosis of ADH or DCIS. Those lesions lacking appreciable proliferation have been described in the past as "clinging carcinoma (monomorphic type)", "atypical cystic lobules", and "atypical columnar cell change", among other terms, and are currently categorized as "flat epithelial atypia".

Progression to invasive breast cancer

Clinical follow-up studies have indicated that intraductal proliferative lesions are associated with different levels of risk for subsequent development of invasive breast cancer, that range from approximately 1.5 times that of the reference population for UDH, to 3–5-fold for ADH, and 8–10-fold for DCIS {450}. Recent immunophenotypical and molecular-genetic studies have provided new insights into these lesions and have indicated that the long-held notion of a linear progression from normal epithelium through UDH, ADH and carcinoma in situ to invasive cancer is overly simplistic; the inter-relationship between these various intraductal proliferative lesions and invasive breast cancer is far more complex. In brief, these data have shown that: (1) UDH shares few similarities with most ADH, DCIS or invasive cancer; (2) ADH shares many similarities with low-grade DCIS; (3) low-grade DCIS and high-grade DCIS appear in most cases to represent genetically distinct disorders leading to distinct forms of invasive breast carcinoma; and (4) flat epithelial atypia represents a clonal, neoplastic lesion that shares morphological, immunohistochemical and molecular features with ADH and low-grade DCIS. These data support the notion that flat epithelial atypia, ADH and all forms of DCIS represent "intraepithelial neoplasias." UDH is not a significant risk factor and in most cases is unlikely to represent a precursor lesion. However, there are some genomic data to suggest that a small proportion of UDH can harbour clonal populations of cells, which indicates that clonal lesions such as ADH may occasionally arise in this setting {507,751}.

Classification and grading

These emerging genetic data and the increasingly frequent detection of ADH and low-grade DCIS by mammography have raised important questions about the manner in which intraductal proliferative lesions are currently classified. Although used by pathology laboratories worldwide, the traditional classification system suffers from inter-observer variability, in particular, in distinguishing between ADH and some small, low-grade DCIS. Over the last decade, it has been proposed that the traditional terminology be replaced by the ductal intraepithelial neoplasia (DIN) system, reserving the term "carcinoma" for invasive tumours. The DIN terminology has not gained widespread acceptance, in part because no new diagnostic criteria are used and the change in terminology would therefore not help with improving inter-observer variability. Molecular analysis has started to refine and should help to improve upon the traditional classification {36,1520}. Hence, the classification of intraductal proliferative lesions should be viewed as an evolving concept that may be modified as additional molecular and genetic data become available.

Diagnostic reproducibility

Multiple studies have assessed reproducibility in diagnosing the range of intraductal proliferative lesions, some with emphasis on the borderline lesions {153, 1064,1065,1199,1284,1338,1339}. These studies have clearly indicated that inter-observer agreement is poor when no standardized criteria are used {1199}. Diagnostic reproducibility is improved with the use of standardized criteria {1284}. However, discrepancies in diagnosis persist in some cases, particularly in the distinction between ADH and limited forms of low-grade DCIS since much of this distinction is based on quantitative rather than qualitative features. In one study, consistency in diagnosis and classification did not change significantly when interpretation was confined to specific images as compared with assessment of the entire tissue section on a slide, reflecting inconsistencies secondary to differences in morphological interpretation {379}. While clinical follow-up studies have generally demonstrated increasing levels of risk of breast cancer associated with UDH, ADH and DCIS respectively, concerns about diagnostic reproducibility have led some to question the practice of using these risk estimates at the individual level {153}.

Etiology

In general, the factors that are associated with the development of invasive breast carcinoma are also associated with increased risk for the development of intraductal proliferative lesions {684,736} (see Chapter 1: *Epidemiology*).

Genetics of precursor lesions

The morphological similarities between invasive and in situ carcinomas of similar grade and their intimate association within the breast suggest that these proliferations are biologically related. The relationships between in situ and invasive lesions have been investigated using a variety of methods, including immunohistochemistry, loss of heterozygosity (LOH) assays, comparative genomic hybridization (CGH) and gene-expression profiling. These data show close relationships between DCIS and invasive carcinoma {205, 206,745,835,844,1015}. The distinct molecular features found in different grades of invasive carcinomas are also mirrored in pre-invasive lesions of comparable morphology {844}. The other pre-invasive lesions are more difficult to position along the multistep pathways. UDH has traditionally been postulated as a precursor of ADH and DCIS. However, at the molecular level, relatively few and random chromosomal changes have been detected in UDH {78,658,751}. There is evidence that a minority of cases of UDH may harbour genomic alterations also observed in ADH and hence could be precursors of ADH; however, currently, the vast majority of these lesions are not thought to progress and more likely represent "dead-end" proliferations {155}. Recent data suggest that a more likely precursor to ADH and low-grade DCIS are columnar cell lesions (CCLs)/flat epithelial atypia {1281,1327}. The hallmark genetic feature of "low-grade" lesions, loss of 16q, is the most frequently detected recurrent change in CCLs/flat epithelial atypia and there is a degree of overlap in the molecular profile of CCLs/flat epithelial atypia and associated more advanced lesions {935,1327}. Genetic alterations have also been identified in normal breast tissues near to and distant from invasive carcinoma {330,743}. The genetic alterations have been seen independently in luminal and myoepithelial cell compartments {743}, suggesting that changes may have occurred very early during the development of the breast carcinoma. Genetic and transcriptomic alterations in the mammary stroma of patients with malignancy have also been described and there is currently considerable interest in understanding the relationship between the stroma and epithelial cells in breast tumorigenesis and progression {842,934}. The significance of alterations in normal breast tissues in individual patients is unclear at present but is likely to shed light on cancer development and potential preventive strategies in the future.

Usual ductal hyperplasia

L. Collins
D. Visscher
J. Simpson
S.J. Schnitt

Definition

This lesion is characterized by a solid or fenestrated proliferation of epithelial cells that often show streaming growth, particularly in the centre of involved spaces. Usual ductal hyperplasia (UDH) is not considered to be a precursor lesion in most cases. However, long-term follow-up of patients with UDH suggests that they have a slightly elevated risk for the subsequent development of invasive carcinoma.

Synonyms

Intraductal hyperplasia; hyperplasia of the usual type; epitheliosis; ordinary intraductal hyperplasia; hyperplasia without atypia.

Epidemiology

The incidence of UDH is not easily determined since it is rarely the targeted lesion in a breast biopsy. In cohorts of women who have had biopsies for lesions that proved to be benign, proliferative lesions without atypia (which includes UDH as well as other non-atypical proliferations such as sclerosing adenosis and papillomas, often admixed) represents approximately 30% of diagnoses rendered. The average age at the time of diagnosis is 53 years, which is about 5 years younger than women presenting with atypical ductal hyperplasia (ADH) {557}.

Clinical features

UDH does not present as a mass or a mammographic lesion, except in occasional instances when it may present with associated microcalcifications.

Histopathology

UDH is characterized by a cohesive proliferation of benign epithelial cells that display a haphazard orientation with respect to one another. The presence of secondary lumina or fenestrations is characteristic of this lesion. The lumina are often peripherally located and tend to be slit-like, as opposed to the very rounded, punched-out lumina seen in ADH and

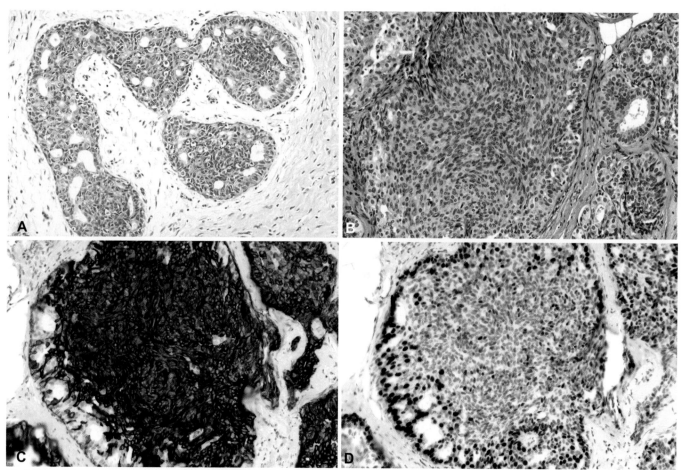

Fig. 5.01 Usual ductal hyperplasia (UDH). **A** The peripheral distribution of irregularly sized spaces is a characteristic of UDH and is readily apparent at low magnification. **B** High magnification showing a predominantly solid intraductal proliferation with pronounced cellular streaming. **C** Immunostaining for keratin 5/6 shows many positively stained cells and a few negative cells. **D** Immunostaining for estrogen receptor shows scattered positively stained nuclei.

low-grade ductal carcinoma in situ (DCIS). In some cases, the proliferation has a solid pattern and no secondary lumina are present {1054}. Occasionally, a micropapillary architecture may be present similar to that seen in gynaecomastia. The cells of UDH are irregularly placed, with indistinct borders and the nuclei are variably sized, often with grooves and intranuclear inclusions. The cells often have a streaming or syncytial pattern which is particularly evident in the centre of the proliferation. In contrast to the rigid bridges seen in low-grade atypical proliferations, epithelial bridges in UDH are thin and stretched with unevenly distributed nuclei. Micropapillations, when present, have a broad base and a narrow or pinched tip with hyperchromatic, almost pyknotic appearing nuclei. The nuclei of the cells surrounding the secondary lumina tend to run parallel rather than perpendicular to the spaces. An admixture of epithelial, myoepithelial, and even apocrine metaplastic epithelial cells can be seen within a proliferation of UDH. Foamy histiocytes, calcifications and rarely foci of necrosis may also be seen. The presence of a rare mitotic figure does not preclude the diagnosis of UDH.

The cellular population exhibits a mixed phenotype and as such stains for keratins of low and high molecular weight (keratin 5/6 or 34betaE12), the latter in a heterogeneous or mosaic pattern {154}. Staining for estrogen receptor (ER) is also heterogeneous in UDH, in contrast to the strong, diffuse staining seen in ADH and low-grade DCIS.

Genetics

Most studies have found no consistent genetic alterations associated with UDH {154,1167}. Furthermore, the characteristic alterations seen in ADH and low-grade DCIS are not found in UDH, leading to the view that these lesions are markers of, but not direct precursors of, breast cancer.

Prognosis and predictive factors

Long term follow-up of women with UDH indicates a slight increase in subsequent breast cancer risk, of the order of 1.5–2-fold. This risk is conferred on either breast and appears to be slightly higher among those with a strong family history of breast cancer {283,357,450,1279}. At present, there are no prognostic factors that can determine with any reliability which patients may develop invasive breast cancer following a diagnosis of UDH. The magnitude of breast cancer risk associated with UDH is similar to that associated with certain reproductive factors, such as early menarche and late menopause and should not alter the frequency of mammographic screening.

Columnar cell lesions

Columnar cell change and hyperplasia

A.M. Hanby
I.O. Ellis
S.J. Schnitt

Definition
Columnar cell change and columnar cell hyperplasia are lesions of the terminal-duct lobular unit (TDLU) that are characterized by enlarged, variably dilated acini lined by columnar epithelial cells.

Synonyms
Blunt duct adenosis; columnar alteration of lobules; columnar metaplasia; hyperplastic unfolded lobules; hyperplastic enlarged lobular units; enlarged lobular units with columnar alteration.

Epidemiology
There are no specific epidemiological features.

Clinical features
In current clinical practice, these lesions are being detected increasingly because of the presence of microcalcifications seen on screening mammography. They may also be revealed as incidental histological findings.

Macroscopy
Columnar cell change and hyperplasia are of microscopic size and cannot be identified on macroscopic examination.

Histopathology
Columnar cell change and hyperplasia are characterized by TDLUs with variably enlarged and dilated acini lined by columnar epithelial cells that frequently have apical cytoplasmic snouts. The involved acini usually have irregular contours. The nuclei are typically ovoid, regularly oriented perpendicular to the basement membrane, and have evenly dispersed chromatin and inconspicuous nucleoli. Luminal secretions and/or microcalcifications are commonly present. The myoepithelial cell layer may be prominent and the specialized stroma can be cellular. Lesions in which the epithelial-cell lining is only one or two cell layers thick are categorized as columnar cell change; those with cellular stratification or tufting more than two cell-layers thick are designated columnar cell hyperplasia {1110,1285}. Cytological atypia is not a feature of these lesions.

Columnar cell change and hyperplasia are often seen in association with other benign changes, such as cysts and epithelial proliferative lesions. There is a strong association between these lesions and the presence of lobular neoplasia (lobular carcinoma in situ and atypical lobular hyperplasia) {193,222,779}. Columnar cell change and hyperplasia show strong and diffuse expression of estrogen receptors and lack HER2 overexpression.

Genetics
See the Genetics section for flat epithelial atypia (FEA).

Prognosis and predictive factors
Recent follow-up studies have shown that columnar cell change and hyperplasia are associated with a very low risk for the subsequent development of breast cancer (relative risk, approximately 1.5) {72,176}. Moreover, the risk associated with these lesions is not clearly independent of the risk associated with concomitant proliferative lesions.

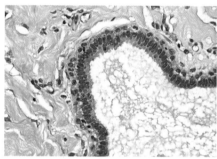

Fig. 5.02 Columnar cell change. A dilated acinus is lined by a monolayer of columnar cells exhibiting apical snouting.

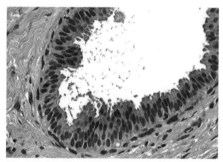

Fig. 5.03 Columnar cell hyperplasia. This space is lined by stratified layers of columnar cells with apical snouts.

Flat epithelial atypia

S.J. Schnitt
L. Collins
S.R. Lakhani

P.T. Simpson
V. Eusebi

Definition
A neoplastic alteration of the terminal-duct lobular units (TDLUs) characterized by replacement of the native epithelial cells by one to several layers of a single epithelial cell type showing low-grade (monomorphic) cytological atypia.

Synonyms
Columnar cell change with atypia, columnar cell hyperplasia with atypia

Clinical features
In current clinical practice these lesions are being detected increasingly because of the presence of microcalcifications seen on screening mammography. They may also be identified as incidental histological findings.

Macroscopy
Flat epithelial atypia (FEA) is of microscopic size and cannot be identified on macroscopic examination.

Histopathology
FEA is characterized by replacement of the native epithelial cells of the TDLUs by one to several layers of cells that lack polarity. The nuclei are round and uniform and have inconspicuous nucleoli, similar in appearance to the nuclei that characterize low-grade ductal carcinoma in situ (DCIS) {933,1280}. The cells may be cuboidal to columnar, often with apical cytoplasmic snouts. Occasional cellular tufts or mounds may be seen, but well-developed arcades, bridges and micropapillary formations are absent (hence their designation as "flat"). The acini of involved TDLUs are variably distended, usually have smooth contours, and may contain secretory or floccular material that often contains microcalcifications. Stromal lymphocytic infiltrates may be seen in some cases.
There is a strong association between these lesions and the co-existence of lobular neoplasia (lobular carcinoma in situ and atypical lobular hyperplasia [ALH]), atypical ductal hyperplasia (ADH), low-grade DCIS and low-grade invasive carcinomas including tubular carcinoma {193,222,779}. The cells of FEA are strongly and diffusely positive for estrogen receptor and do not overexpress HER2.
While lesions of this type were named by Azzopardi as "clinging carcinoma, monomorphic type," in current practice only "flat" proliferations with high-grade nuclei should be regarded as DCIS.

Genetics
Data on genetic alterations in FEA and the closely related non-atypical columnar cell lesions (i.e. columnar cell change and hyperplasia) are limited. Current evidence suggests that columnar cell lesions and FEA are the likely precursors of ADH {7,1280,1327}. Columnar cell lesions and FEA show an immunoprofile that is similar to that of ADH/low-grade DCIS {7,1280}. The degree of proliferation, architectural and cytological atypia in these lesions are mirrored at the genetic level, with a stepwise increase in the number and complexity of chromosomal copy-number changes as defined by comparative genomic hybridization (CGH) {6,1327}. The characteristic genetic alteration of "low-grade" lesions, loss of 16q, is the most frequently detected recurrent change in columnar cell lesions and FEA. It has also been demonstrated that there is a degree of overlap in the molecular genetic profiles of columnar cell lesions and FEA and those of associated, more advanced lesions, implying a precursor–product relationship {935,1327}.

Prognosis and predictive factors
FEA is of greater scientific interest as an early lesion in the low-grade breast neoplasia pathway than it is of clinical importance as a breast-cancer precursor or risk indicator. Limited available data from a few, small, retrospective studies suggest that some cases of FEA may progress to invasive breast cancer, although the risk of progression appears to be very low {138,394}. These data suggest that the risk of breast cancer associated with these lesions appears to be substantially lower than the risk associated with established forms of atypical hyperplasia (ADH and ALH). Therefore, despite the presence of "atypia" in the name, FEA should not be regarded as equivalent to ADH or ALH with regard to cancer-risk assessment or patient management.
Results from small retrospective studies have indicated that up to 30% of patients with FEA on needle-core biopsy have a worse lesion on excision. However, given the limitations of study design and the wide variation in the reported upgrade rate, the need for routine surgical excision following a diagnosis of FEA on needle-core biopsy is uncertain. Radiological-pathological correlation is recommended for determining further management.

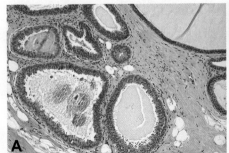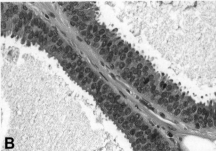

Fig. 5.04 Flat epithelial atypia. **A** A low-power view shows a portion of a terminal-duct lobular unit with variably dilated acini containing secretory material and calcifications. Apical snouts can be seen on many of the cells. **B** At high power, the spaces are seen to be lined by several layers of columnar epithelial cells with monomorphic nuclei.

Atypical ductal hyperplasia

J.F. Simpson
S.J. Schnitt
D. Visscher
M.J. van de Vijver
I.O. Ellis

Definition

Atypical ductal hyperplasia (ADH) is a proliferation of monomorphic, evenly placed epithelial cells involving terminal-duct lobular units (TDLUs). The term "ADH" identifies a group of lesions with a combination of specifically defined architectural and cytological features that predict an increased risk of subsequent breast cancer.

Synonyms

Atypical intraductal hyperplasia

Epidemiology and clinical significance

The initial long-term follow-up studies of ADH were conducted before mammography and hence the diagnosis of ADH was rare (about 4% of benign breast biopsies) {357}. In mammographic series, ADH is encountered in at least 10% of benign biopsies {1233}.

Based on the findings from several large epidemiological studies using the same histological criteria {359,557,825}, the Cancer Committee of the College of American Pathologists supports ADH being associated with a moderately increased risk for subsequent development of invasive breast cancer (relative risk, 3.0–5.0) {450}.

Histopathology

ADH is defined in terms of its resemblance to low-grade ductal carcinoma in situ

(DCIS). In fact, a diagnosis of ADH should not be made unless a diagnosis of low grade DCIS is being seriously considered. Florid examples of usual ductal hyperplasia (UDH) should not be categorized as ADH. ADH is characterized by a proliferation within TDLUs of a monomorphic population of epithelial cells that are evenly placed and lack the streaming, swirling, and overlapping of the cells that define UDH. The cell borders are distinct. The proliferation may be solid with or without subtle microacini, cribriform with round, "punched out" spaces surrounded by polarized epithelial cells, or micropapillary with epithelial projections that are typically narrower at the base than the apex. The cellular monotony and architectural patterns are similar to those seen in low-grade DCIS; however, the proliferation in ADH is either admixed with a second population of non-uniform cells in the TDLU spaces or it completely involves a limited number of those spaces. Hence, quantitative criteria play an integral role in the distinction of ADH from low-grade DCIS.

The most common quantitative criteria used to render a diagnosis of low-grade DCIS (as opposed to ADH) are the presence of homogeneous involvement of at least two membrane-bound spaces or comprising a size that is > 2 mm {359, 557,825,1419}. The two-space criterion

was used in the largest epidemiological cohort studies that evaluated the risk of breast cancer associated with ADH {359, 557,825}. The WHO Working Group did not consider that it was possible to recommend one approach rather than another, and many experts use combinations of both in their clinical practice. It should be noted that quantitative thresholds are meant to be pragmatic guidelines that are useful in preventing the categorization of very small, low-grade lesions as DCIS and, in turn, in avoiding overtreatment of patients with these minimal or equivocal lesions.

A conservative approach should particularly be used in needle-core biopsy specimens in which the differential diagnosis includes ADH and low-grade DCIS of limited extent. Categorization of such lesions as either ADH or as "atypical intraductal proliferative lesion" should be sufficient to prompt a surgical excision, and definitive categorization of such lesions should be based on evaluation of the subsequent surgical excision specimen. If no further lesion is found on the subsequent excision, the patient should be managed as for patients with ADH.

Immunoprofile

There have been attempts to refine the estimated risk of breast cancer associated

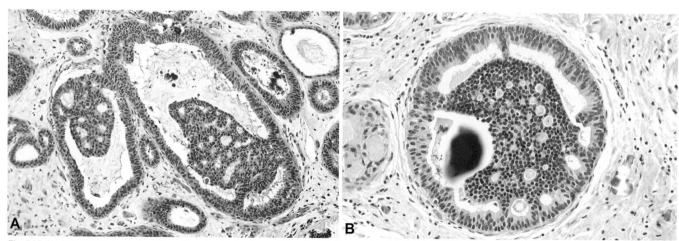

Fig. 5.05 Atypical ductal hyperplasia. **A** Two adjacent ducts showing partial involvement by a proliferation of uniform cells forming cribriform structures. **B** The central portion of this duct contains an evenly placed population of uniform cells that forms microacinar structures. Note the different cell population at the periphery, and the associated calcification.

with ADH by analysing a variety of bio-markers {1256,1524}, but at this time none of these has been validated for routine clinical use. The cells comprising the monomorphic population in ADH are typically negative for high-molecular-weight keratins (such as keratin 5/6) and diffusely positive for estrogen receptors (ER) {1046}. In contrast, the cells of UDH show variable positivity for high-molecular-weight keratins (often in a mosaic pattern) and variable positivity for ER. Immunostaining for these markers is similar in ADH and low-grade DCIS and thus cannot be used to distinguish these lesions.

Differential diagnosis
The important differential diagnoses for ADH are UDH and low-grade DCIS. Collagenous spherulosis has crisp, round spaces that may be mistaken for the "punched out" spaces in some forms of ADH; however, unlike ADH, the spaces in collagenous spherulosis represent pseudolumina that contain eosinophilic basement membrane material or basophilic myxoid material. Furthermore, these spaces are surrounded by myoepithelial cells rather than a polarized layer of epithelial cells.

Genetics
Studies using loss of heterozygosity (LOH) and comparative genomic hybridization assays have shown common patterns of genetic alteration in ADH, low-grade in situ and invasive carcinomas in the same breast, suggesting that ADH may be a non-obligate precursor lesion {742}. Frequent sites of LOH in ADH and

Table 5.01 Morphological characteristics useful in distinguishing ADH from UDH and from low-grade DCIS

Characteristic	UDH	ADH	DCIS (low grade)
Architecture	Cellular swirling and streaming; stretched or twisted epithelial bridges; peripheral, irregular, and slit-like fenestrations.	Rigid cellular bars; bulbous micropapillae; round, punched out spaces.	Rigid cellular bars; bulbous micropapillae; round, punched out spaces.
Cytology	Multiple cell types; uneven distribution and overlapping of cells and nuclei; indistinct cell borders.	Cellular uniformity; even cell placement; distinct cell borders; residual normally polarized cells.	Cellular uniformity; even cell placement; distinct cell borders; no residual normally polarized cells.
Extent	Variable, ranging from one to multiple TDLUs.	Partial involvement of multiple spaces; complete involvement of < 2 spaces or ≤ 2 mm in extent (see text).	Complete involvement of ≥ 2 spaces or > 2 mm in extent (see text).
Risk of developing breast cancer; laterality of risk	Slight risk; generalized bilateral risk.	Moderate risk; generalized bilateral risk.	High risk; regional ipsilateral risk.

ADH, atypical ductal hyperplasia; DCIS, ductal carcinoma in situ; TDLU, terminal-duct lobular unit; UDH, usual ductal hyperplasia.

invasive carcinoma include chromosomes 16q, 17p, and 11q13 {745,1015} with losses at 16q being particularly frequent {161,595, 830}. It is, however, important to remember that many of the reports of such molecular commonalities have been from studies of cases of ADH that also have established cancer, both invasive and in situ. Few studies of ADH as the most advanced lesion exist, and no studies have then established the significance of these changes through large, clinically validated patient cohorts.

Prognosis and predictive factors
ADH is associated with a relative risk of subsequent development of cancer that is three to five times that of women without ADH, and the risk applies to either breast. At present, molecular studies provide interesting insights into the biological nature of proliferative lesions, but their value in routine clinical practice remains to be determined.

Ductal carcinoma in situ

S.J. Schnitt
C. Allred
P. Britton
I.O. Ellis
S.R. Lakhani
M. Morrow

J. Palazzo
C. Reynolds
E. Rutgers
J. Simpson
M.J. van de Vijver
A. Vincent-Salomon

Definition

A neoplastic proliferation of epithelial cells confined to the mammary ductal-lobular system and characterized by subtle to marked cytological atypia and an inherent but not necessarily obligate tendency for progression to invasive breast cancer.

ICD-O code

The code 8500/2 covers all grades of ductal carcinoma in situ (DCIS).

Synonyms

Intraductal carcinoma; ductal intraepithelial neoplasia

Epidemiology

DCIS was infrequent prior to mammographic screening programmes, accounting for 2–3% of palpable breast cancers, but now accounts for 20–25% of newly diagnosed breast cancers in the USA {646}. Between 1983 and 2006, the incidence of DCIS among women aged < 50 years increased by 29% and continues to rise {38}. In women aged 50 years and older, a 500% increase in DCIS was observed between 1983 and 2003, but incidence has since decreased. Overall, the incidence of DCIS increased from 1.87 per 100 000 in 1973–1975 to 32.5 per 100 000 in 2005, with an incidence of 1.3 per 1000 screening examinations in women aged 70–84 years compared with 0.6 per 1000 screening examinations in women aged 40–49

years {386}. Family history, nulliparity, late age at first birth, late menopause, and elevated body mass index (BMI) after menopause have all been associated with an increased risk of DCIS {472}. High mammographic breast density is also associated with an increased risk of DCIS {850}.

Breast cancer-specific mortality among women with DCIS is extremely low, with 1.0–2.6% dying from invasive breast cancer 8–10 years after a diagnosis of DCIS {387}. Breast-cancer deaths after an initial diagnosis of DCIS are due to the presence of invasive carcinoma that was not detected or not recognized at the time of the initial diagnosis, or invasive recurrence after treatment, since DCIS itself does not result in mortality.

Clinical presentation

Clinical presentations of DCIS include a palpable mass, pathological discharge from the nipple with or without a mass, and Paget disease of the nipple. However, approximately 80–85% of cases of DCIS are detected mammographically in the absence of clinical findings, with an additional 5% identified as an incidental finding in a breast biopsy performed for other indications.

Calcifications are the most common mammographic presentation of DCIS and may be amorphous or pleomorphic, with a linear or segmental distribution. Classically, pleomorphic, linear calcifications

are associated with high-grade DCIS, while granular, segmental calcifications are seen with low- to intermediate-grade lesions. On magnetic resonance imaging (MRI), DCIS is typically seen as non-mass-like enhancement with delayed peak enhancement profiles {728}.

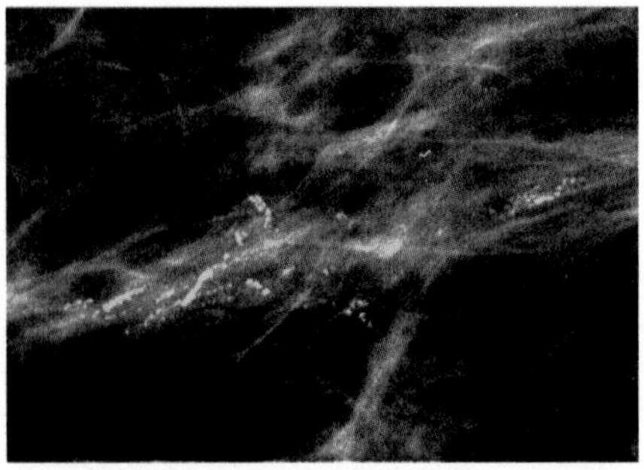

Imaging findings

The detection of DCIS has substantially increased with the widespread introduction of population screening programmes over the last 20 years {1078}. The vast majority of cases of DCIS are diagnosed following the demonstration of clustered microcalcification on screening mammograms. Approximately 20–25% of screen-detected cancers will be in situ disease {990}. Clustered microcalcification is a common finding on screening mammograms and is seen in approximately 3% of patients of screening age. Although the appearance of some clustered microcalcifications (linear branching or so-called "casting") is highly suggestive of a diagnosis of DCIS, most are indeterminate in appearance and cannot be distinguished from the myriad of benign causes. As a consequence, the majority of patients with clustered microcalcifications require a needle biopsy for a diagnosis to be reached {1542}. Such biopsies are most often performed using 11-gauge or 8-gauge vacuum-assisted biopsy using stereotactic (X-ray) guidance {630}. If adequate amounts of calcification are identified on the specimen radiograph taken of the biopsy cores, the diagnostic reliability of whether a benign or malignant process is present is extremely high {685}. Despite dramatic technological improvements, ultrasound helps infrequently with the diagnosis of DCIS. Although breast MRI is highly sensitive for the detection of invasive breast cancer, the rate of false-negatives is higher for DCIS. The utility of MRI is therefore disputed and it is not routinely required in local staging.

Classification and grading

There is currently no universal agreement on a classification system for DCIS {782}.

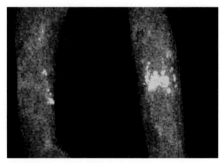

Fig. 5.06 Screening mammogram showing a cluster of microcalcification in a linear/branching pattern, highly suspicious of malignancy. Final histology revealed the presence of high-grade ductal carcinoma in situ.

Fig. 5.07 Specimen radiograph of an 11-gauge vacuum-assisted biopsy specimen showing microcalcification.

Over the past two decades, there has been a move away from the traditional architectural classification of DCIS as comedo, solid, cribriform, micropapillary and papillary types. Most modern systems use nuclear grade alone or in combination with necrosis and/or cell polarization. Several international consensus conferences have endorsed this change and recommended that, until more data emerge on clinical outcome related to pathology variables, grading of DCIS should be based primarily on nuclear features {1431}. DCIS is generally divided into three grades: low, intermediate and high. It is not uncommon to find some degree of heterogeneity of nuclear grade within the same biopsy or even within the same ductal space, although cells with low and high nuclear grade are not usually found together. When more than one grade of DCIS is present, this should be noted in the diagnosis. It is important to recognize that a three-tiered grading system does not imply progression from low-grade to intermediate- to high-grade lesions. In fact, recent molecular and genetic evidence suggests that, while progression from low- to high-grade lesions may occur in some cases {36}, low-grade and high-grade DCIS are best considered as distinct disorders {205, 830, 845, 1297}.

In their reports on DCIS, pathologists are encouraged to include, in addition to nuclear grade, comments on the presence and type of necrosis (punctate, comedo), architectural pattern(s), cell polarization, size/extent of the lesion, location of calcifications (i.e. in DCIS alone, in benign tissue alone, or both), and status of the surgical margins {1431}.

Histopathology
DCIS of low nuclear grade
DCIS of low nuclear grade is composed of small, monomorphic cells, growing in arcades, micropapillae, cribriform or solid patterns. The solid pattern may show microacini in which cells are polarized around small extra-cellular lumina in a rosette-type arrangement. The nuclei are of uniform size and have a regular chrom-atin pattern with inconspicuous nucleoli; mitotic figures are rare. Microcalcifications are often of the psammomatous type. While necrosis is uncommon, foci of either punctate or comedo-type necrosis do not preclude the diagnosis of low-grade DCIS if the neoplastic cells have the appropriate

cytological features. DCIS with a purely micropapillary pattern may be associated with a more extensive distribution, involving multiple quadrants of the breast, than that of other variants {1288}.

DCIS of intermediate nuclear grade
DCIS of intermediate nuclear grade is composed of cells that show mild to moderate variability in size, shape and placement, variably coarse chromatin, and variably prominent nucleoli. Cell polarization is not as well-developed as in low-nuclear-grade DCIS. Mitoses may be present. Punctate or comedo necrosis may be present. The distribution of amorphous or laminated microcalcifications is generally similar to that of low-nuclear-grade DCIS or may show patterns of microcalcification associated with both low-grade and high-grade DCIS.

DCIS of high nuclear grade
DCIS of high nuclear grade is composed of highly atypical cells most often proliferating in solid, cribriform or micropapillary patterns. Nuclei are pleomorphic, poorly polarized, with irregular contours and distribution, coarse, clumped chromatin and prominent nucleoli. Mitotic figures are usually common, but their presence is not required. Comedo necrosis, with abundant necrotic debris in duct lumina surrounded by a generally solid proliferation of large pleomorphic tumour cells, is frequently present. However, comedo necrosis is not obligatory. Even a single layer of highly atypical cells lining the duct in a clinging fashion is sufficient for the diagnosis of high-nuclear-grade DCIS. Amorphous microcalcifications are common and are usually associated with necrotic intraluminal debris. DCIS of high nuclear grade is usually > 5 mm in size, but even

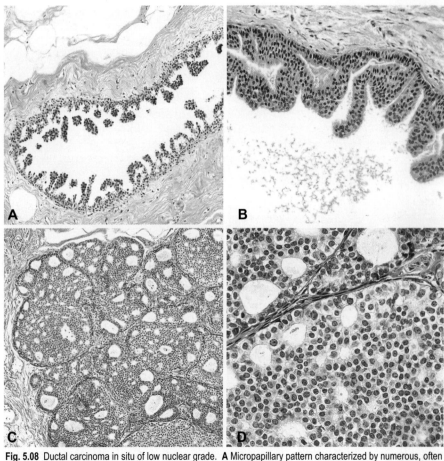

Fig. 5.08 Ductal carcinoma in situ of low nuclear grade. **A** Micropapillary pattern characterized by numerous, often bulbous epithelial projections into the duct lumen. **B** Micropapillary pattern. The micropapillae lack fibrovascular cores and are composed of uniform cells with rounded, monomorphic nuclei. **C** Cribriform pattern. Multiple adjacent ducts are distended by a sieve-like proliferation of monotonous uniform cells. The multiple spaces within the proliferation are rounded and distributed in an organized fashion. **D** Cribriform pattern. A highly uniform population of cells with round nuclei distributed equidistant from one another and polarized around extracellular lumina.

a single space with the typical morphological features is sufficient for diagnosis.

Unusual variants

A minority of DCIS lesions is composed of apocrine, signet ring, neuroendocrine, spindled, squamous or clear cells. There is no consensus or uniform approach to the grading of these unusual variants. Some experts believe that assessment of nuclear features and necrosis can also be applied to grading of the unusual variants.

Biomarkers: estrogen receptor (ER), progesterone receptor (PR), and others

Testing for ER and PR in DCIS

Currently, ER is the only biomarker validated for routine clinical practice in DCIS {33,35,542}. However, clinical validation is far less comprehensive than with invasive breast cancer, primarily because there

have been only a few randomized clinical trials of adjuvant hormonal therapy in DCIS, and only one, NSABP-B-24, created a tumour bank to support biomarker studies {34,442}. A recently published study using this resource demonstrated that adjuvant tamoxifen significantly reduces the ipsilateral risk of DCIS recurrence and/or progression to invasive breast cancer by about 50% in patients treated with lumpectomy and radiation, and that the benefit is restricted to patients with ER-positive disease {34}. A similar reduction for any breast cancer was observed in the contralateral breast. Results for PR were generally similar, but less significant, and there is a controversy regarding whether routine PR testing in DCIS is necessary. Furthermore, recent guidelines for hormone-receptor testing disagree somewhat on its use in DCIS, one favouring mandatory {35}, and the other optional testing {542}. Nonetheless,

the potential benefit of adjuvant hormonal therapy in hormone receptor-positive DCIS is widely acknowledged, and most cases are tested for ER at the present time.

The only clinically validated methodologies for evaluating ER and PR in DCIS have used immunohistochemical assays previously developed and validated in studies of invasive breast cancer {542, 558,932}. The distribution of receptor expression in DCIS is similar to that seen in invasive breast cancer: about 75–80% show positive nuclear staining for ER (ranging from < 1% to 100% cells). The frequency of PR expression in DCIS is somewhat lower. In clinical practice, for both ER and PR a positive result is defined as ≥ 1% of cells showing nuclear staining. It is unknown whether there is an association between levels of receptor expression and response to hormonal therapy because the one available clinical study (NSABP-B-24) was too small to address this question. The association between hormone-receptor expression and response to adjuvant aromatase inhibitors in DCIS has also not been studied, although benefit is probably restricted to ER-positive disease, similar to tamoxifen.

Other biomarkers

Many biomarkers have been evaluated in DCIS. Almost all biomarkers reported to be expressed in invasive breast cancers are expressed in DCIS, although the prevalence of expression of some of these markers differs in these two groups. For example, HER2 overexpression is more common in high-grade DCIS than in invasive breast cancer. Furthermore, all of the major molecular subtypes found in invasive cancer (i.e. luminal A, luminal B, HER2, basal-like) are seen in DCIS. Again, however, the frequency of these subtypes differs in DCIS and invasive cancer {32,36,161,604,830,1115}.

Clinical course and prognosis

Data accumulated from clinical, pathological, and molecular studies have indicated that DCIS is a precursor, albeit not obligate, to invasive breast cancer. Detailed radiographic-pathological correlation studies have shown that DCIS is in most cases confined to a single segment or ductal-lobular system, although involvement of the segment may be extensive and "skipped" areas may occur, especially in lesions of low nuclear grade

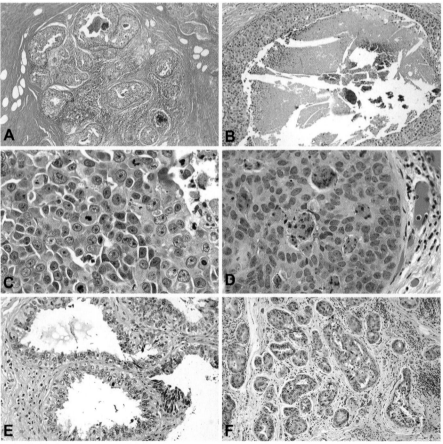

Fig. 5.09 Ductal carcinoma in situ (DCIS) of high nuclear grade. **A** Multiple spaces involved by DCIS of high nuclear grade, some with comedo necrosis and calcification. There is a chronic inflammatory cell infiltrate in surrounding stroma. **B** This space shows a rim of viable cells with high-grade nuclei. There is comedo-type necrosis and calcification. **C** Higher-power view of lesion shown in B. The cells show nuclear pleomorphism and several mitotic figures are evident. **D** Solid pattern with punctate necrosis. **E** Clinging pattern with significant nuclear pleomorphism and several mitotic figures. **F** DCIS of high nuclear grade involving lobular acini.

{587}. Several small studies from the pre-mammographic era attempted to assess the natural history of DCIS among patients in whom this lesion was identified on retrospective review of breast biopsies previously interpreted as benign. These studies showed that, among those patients in whom invasive cancer developed, most cases occurred in the same area as the original DCIS, implicating DCIS and suggesting a precursor–product relationship. The interval between DCIS and the development of invasive carcinoma is shorter for high-grade DCIS (average 5 years) {286A} than for low-grade DCIS (> 15 years) {1254A}. However, lesion size and adequacy of excision were not assessed in these studies {785A}. Additional studies have shown that approximately 50% of local recurrences after breast-conserving therapy for DCIS are invasive carcinomas and the remainder are DCIS. Rarely, tumour cells may be found in axillary lymph nodes of patients with DCIS due to unrecognized or unidentified foci of invasive carcinoma in the breast or to mechanical displacement of epithelial cells derived from the DCIS as the result of a previous biopsy procedure {149A, 228A}.

With the advent of breast-conserving therapy for invasive breast cancer and the identification of smaller DCIS lesions as a result of population-based mammographic screening, an increasing proportion of patients with DCIS choose breast-conserving therapy rather than mastectomy. There have been four randomized clinical trials comparing excision only to excision followed by radiation therapy {137,589, 600,1550}; these studies show that the addition of radiation reduces the risk of local recurrence by approximately 50%. However, radiation does not reduce the risk of metastasis or mortality from breast cancer. While these trials show the efficacy of adjuvant radiation therapy in reducing the risk of local recurrence, they do not identify patients who could safely avoid radiation. Several single-institution studies have suggested that women with small examples of DCIS treated by excision alone with adequate margins may safely forego radiation therapy {846A}. Initial results from the Eastern Cooperative Oncology Group Trial 5194 study seemed to support this approach and showed that women with low- or intermediate-grade DCIS of limited extent and clear margins had a local recurrence rate of 6% at 5

years of follow-up {609A}. However, a more recent report showed that the rate of local recurrence for these patients rose to 15.4% at 10 years, not significantly different from the rate of local recurrence for women with high-grade DCIS (15.1%) {1349A}. In one study, adjuvant tamoxifen further reduced the risk of local recurrence among patients treated with breast-conserving surgery and radiation therapy {1550}.

Prognostic and predictive factors

Prognostic and predictive factors in DCIS are used to help guide the choice of therapy. While a variety of factors such as young age, larger lesion size, high nuclear grade, comedo necrosis, and positive margin status have been associated with an increased risk of local recurrence and or progression to invasive cancer {137, 1107,1235,1324}, their relative importance and the interactions among them have not been well-defined. Algorithms

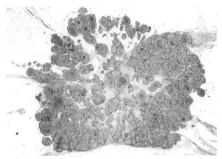

Fig. 5.10 High-grade ductal carcinoma in situ (DCIS) forming a mass.

that combine these factors to assess the risk of recurrence have been developed {1235, 1324}. In one prospective clinical trial, ER status was predictive of benefit from tamoxifen among patients with DCIS treated with lumpectomy and radiation therapy {34A}.

In the future, other systemic therapies with targeted agents may become available to reduce the risk of recurrence

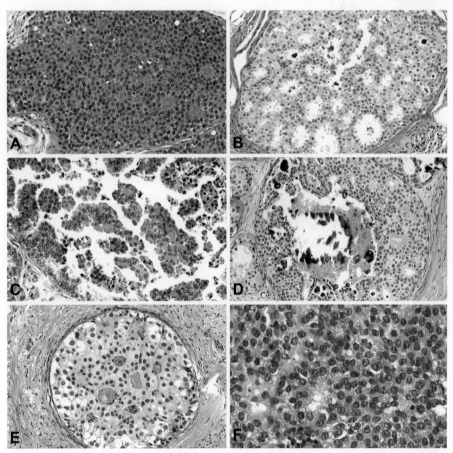

Fig. 5.11 Ductal carcinoma in situ of intermediate nuclear grade. A Solid pattern with cells polarized around a few microacini. B Cribriform pattern with scattered calcifications. C Micropapillary pattern with epithelial projections into the duct lumen that lack fibrovascular cores. D Cribriform pattern with comedo necrosis and calcifications. E Solid pattern with punctate areas of necrosis. F High-power view showing cytological detail. The cells show some variation in nuclear size and the nuclei exhibit variably prominent nucleoli.

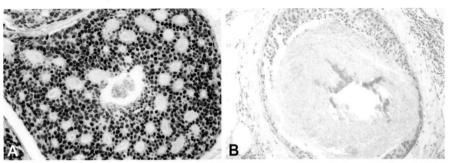

Fig. 5.12 Expression of estrogen receptor (ER) in ductal carcinoma in situ (DCIS). **A** DCIS of low nuclear grade with diffuse, strong nuclear expression of ER. **B** DCIS of high nuclear grade lacking nuclear expression of ER.

and progression to invasive cancer in patients with DCIS. Testing the pathways targeted by these agents may become an important part of evaluating DCIS, but at this time size, grade, comedo necrosis and margin status are established as critical elements in the reporting of DCIS.

Differential diagnosis

The differential diagnosis for DCIS includes usual ductal hyperplasia (UDH) and atypical ductal hyperplasia (ADH) at one end of the diagnostic spectrum, and invasive carcinoma at the other end. Intermediate-grade DCIS with a solid growth pattern can be mistaken for florid UDH. This pattern of DCIS is composed of cells with slightly spindled morphology, which can mimic the nuclear variability and streaming of UDH. Criteria to separate low-grade DCIS from ADH are presented in Table 5.01. When high-grade DCIS involves lobular units, there is often an inflammatory and fibrotic reaction that can distort the involved acini, mimicking invasion. Myoepithelial cell markers are helpful if present, but high-grade DCIS can show reduced numbers of myoepithelial cells and an altered myoepithelial immunophenotype. Finding small irregular cell clusters outside of the specialized connective tissue of the lobular unit establishes invasion. An unusual pattern of invasive carcinoma, invasive cribriform carcinoma, can be mistaken for DCIS, but recognition of an infiltrative pattern ensures the correct diagnosis. Another important differential diagnosis for DCIS of solid pattern is lobular carcinoma in situ (LCIS). Diagnostic criteria for this distinction are presented in Chapter 4.

Reproducibility

While lack of observer agreement in the diagnosis of low-grade DCIS has been publicized {1199,1268A}, when standardized diagnostic criteria are employed, the accurate diagnosis of DCIS is not difficult in most cases {1284}. In an Eastern Cooperative Oncology Group Trial of excision alone for DCIS, the agreement between the local submitting pathologist and the central reviewing pathologist was better than 90% {1326A}. For cases that are borderline between ADH and low-grade DCIS, a conservative approach is favoured, especially on needle-core biopsies. As in other areas of breast pathology, a multidisciplinary discussion including imaging findings will serve to guide a practical clinical approach.

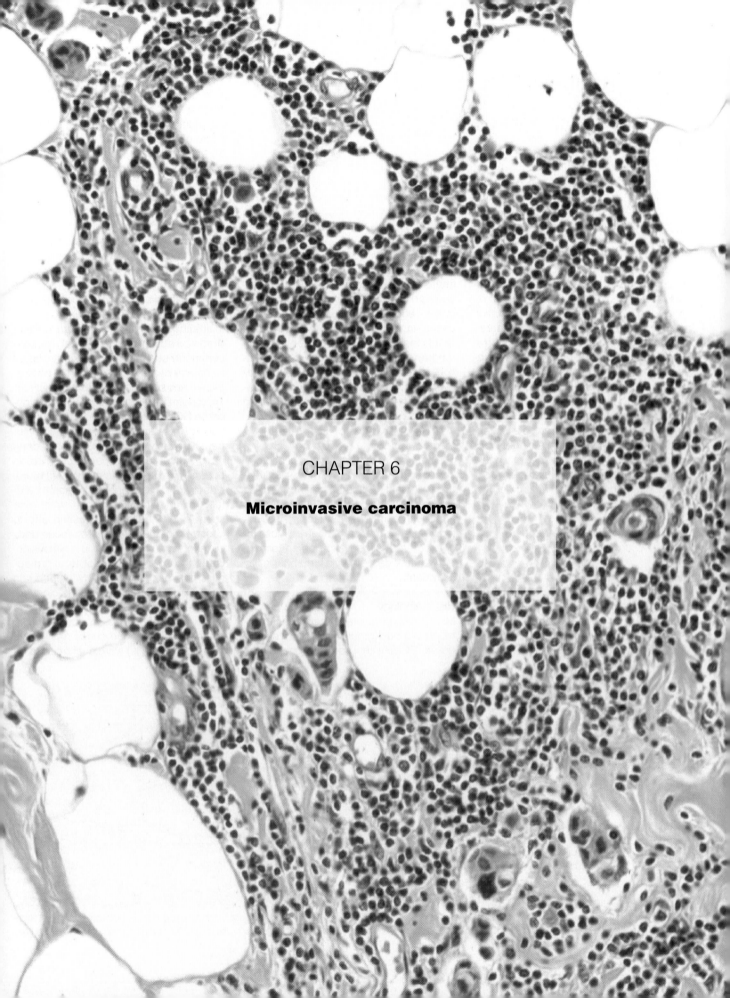

CHAPTER 6

Microinvasive carcinoma

Microinvasive carcinoma

S.E. Pinder
I.O. Ellis
S.J. Schnitt
P.H. Tan
E. Rutgers
M. Morrow

Definition

A lesion characterized by one or more clearly separate microscopic foci of infiltration of tumour cells into the mammary stroma, each less than or equal to 1 mm in size, and most commonly seen in the background of high-grade ductal carcinoma in situ (DCIS).

Historically, there has been wide variation in the definition of microinvasive carcinoma of the breast. Some authors have proposed that the definition of microinvasive carcinoma requires extension of the invasive cells beyond the specialized lobular stroma. However, it may be difficult to ascertain this, and there will be instances in which microinvasive carcinoma is diagnosed when convincing histological appearances are present, despite malignant cells or nests of cells not being clearly beyond the specialized lobular stroma.

ICD-O code

Microinvasive carcinoma does not have an ICD-O code.

Epidemiology

Microinvasive carcinoma is infrequent and is commonly over-diagnosed. It typically occurs in association with high-grade DCIS, but instances of microinvasive carcinoma accompanying lobular carcinoma in situ have been encountered and very rarely microinvasive cancer can be seen in the absence of an adjacent in situ component.

Clinical features

There are no specific clinical features associated with microinvasive carcinoma. In cases where microinvasive carcinoma arises in association with high-grade DCIS, the clinical presentation is mammographically detected microcalcifications, or less commonly a mass, asymmetry or architectural distortion. On ultrasonography, a solid hypoechoic mass has been reported in a small series {1515}.

Macroscopy

The macroscopic appearance of microinvasive carcinoma, as with the clinical features, is that of the underlying in situ lesion. Most typically, ill-defined fibrous areas with comedo-type necrosis extruding from the surface are seen on close inspection of a sliced excision specimen, but in many cases no visible abnormality is evident.

Histopathology

Microinvasion is diagnosed most commonly in a background of extensive high-grade DCIS with prominent periductal chronic inflammation. Malignant cells are seen within the stroma, most often in small angulated clusters and less frequently as single cells. There is an absence of associated myoepithelial cells. The nature of the malignant cells is typically that of invasive carcinoma of no special type (NST). When arising in association with high-grade DCIS, the appearance of the infiltrating cells is also of high nuclear grade. Additional histological features commonly seen in association with microinvasive foci are stromal oedema, desmoplasia, and chronic inflammatory cells.

Thorough sampling of large areas of high-grade DCIS should be undertaken so as not to miss foci of microinvasive (or frankly invasive) disease. Some reports have indicated that when microinvasion occurs, it is likely to be multifocal {1606}. It is therefore appropriate to search carefully for additional small foci when one such lesion has been identified and to confirm that the size of each focus does not exceed 1 mm in maximum dimension. Care should be taken not to overdiagnose this lesion, particularly in uncertain cases. Indeed, subsequent histology review frequently "downgrades" a diagnosis of microinvasion or of lesions suspicious for microinvasion; in one series, only 21 of 109 cases (19.3%) were confirmed to be

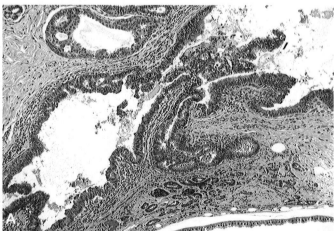
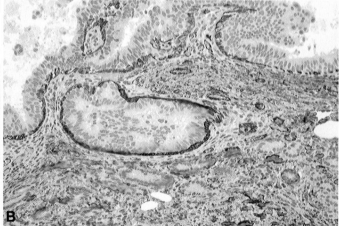

Fig. 6.01 Microinvasive carcinoma. **A** A small focus of invasive carcinoma of 0.8 mm in maximum extent is present adjacent to an aggregate of ducts displaying flat epithelial atypia (FEA) and architectural atypia. **B** Immunostaining for actin shows no evidence of a myoepithelial cell (MEC) layer around the invasive tubules, in contrast to the distinct MEC layer around the adjacent tubules with FEA.

microinvasive lesions on review {1120}, highlighting the potential for over-diagnosis of this entity.

Although microinvasive carcinoma most commonly arises in large areas of high-grade DCIS, microinvasion can arise in association with all grades of DCIS and is very rarely seen with other precursor lesions of invasive breast cancer, such as lobular carcinoma in situ {975}.

Differential diagnosis

The differential diagnosis of microinvasive carcinoma includes pure in situ disease and, conversely, frankly invasive breast carcinoma (i.e. > 1 mm in size). The size of the focus should be carefully measured with an ocular micrometer to exclude the latter. Care must also be taken to ensure that the changes do not represent DCIS involving either a terminal-duct lobular unit (TDLU) or a pre-existing benign process, such as sclerosing adenosis, radial scar or complex sclerosing lesion. Branching or distortion of ducts involved by DCIS also represents a diagnostic pitfall. Further haematoxylin and eosin (H&E) levels may be helpful in such cases.

Immunohistochemistry may also be of value in distinguishing microinvasion from its mimics. Immunostains for myoepithelial markers show that there is no myoepithelial layer surrounding microinvasive foci. Stains for keratins may be of particular value in highlighting the microinvasive foci and complement stains for myoepithelial cells. Immunostains for the basement membrane components laminin and collagen IV may be problematic since in situ lesions may show variable basement membrane loss and (micro)invasive foci may be at least partially surrounded by basement membrane. Particular difficulty in reaching a correct diagnosis may be seen when the patient has undergone previous needle biopsy (either needle-core or fine-needle aspiration) for pre-operative diagnosis, since displacement of benign epithelium (particularly from papillomas) or cells of carcinoma in situ may mimic microinvasion. The presence of granulation tissue and reparative fibrosis, adjacent fat necrosis and haemosiderin deposition, which are usually evident after

needling procedures, should be sought. When there is doubt about the diagnosis of microinvasive carcinoma or if the suspicious area is no longer seen on any further sections or immunostains, it is recommended that the case should be diagnosed as an in situ lesion with no definite evidence of established microinvasive or invasive carcinoma.

Genetics

There are no studies reporting the genetic profile of microinvasive carcinoma of the breast.

Prognosis and predictive factors

There are few data regarding prognostic or predictive significance of hormone receptor and HER2 status of microinvasive carcinoma of the breast. It seems logical to recommend assessment of these markers on this lesion; however, very commonly, the microinvasive foci are not present on the particular sections on which immunostaining is carried out, in which case the results for the associated DCIS should be reported.

The incidence of metastatic disease in axillary lymph nodes in microinvasive carcinoma of the breast is low. Review of the literature for accurate determination of the frequency of metastatic disease in sentinel lymph-node biopsy is impeded by the different definitions applied for the diagnosis of microinvasive carcinoma as well as pathological methods for handling and evaluating sentinel lymph nodes {136}. Between 0% and 20% of patients with microinvasive carcinoma are reported to have axillary metastasis (mean, 9.4%). However, caution is required in interpretation of these figures as most of these data are from very small series. For example, the highest reported frequency (20%) is reported from a series of 15 patients {291}. Nevertheless, in many centres sentinel lymph-node biopsy is undertaken in women with microinvasive carcinoma of the breast.

For the same historical reason of varying definitions of the diagnosis, robust data on the clinical behaviour of microinvasive lesions are not available. However, it appears that, if this restrictive definition is

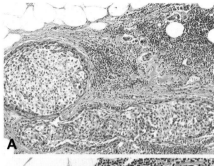
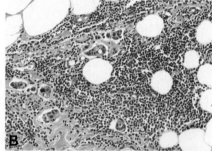
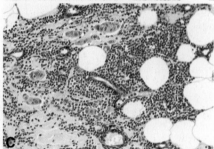

Fig. 6.02 Microinvasive carcinoma. **A** Two ducts are filled by ductal carcinoma in situ, while small clusters of carcinoma cells invade the stroma (upper right quadrant of the field) admixed with a dense lymphocytic infiltrate. **B** Higher magnification shows small invasive cell clusters within stromal spaces distributed over a 0.7 mm area and surrounded by a dense lymphocytic infiltrate. **C** Immunostaining for actin highlights the vessel walls, while absence of myoepithelial cells around the tumour cell clusters confirms their invasive nature.

applied for diagnosis, patient prognosis is excellent and not clearly different from patients with pure DCIS of equivalent size and grade. In general, this condition is managed clinically in the same way as high-grade DCIS.

No predictive factors have been identified. Microinvasive carcinoma is staged as T1mi in the TNM/AJCC classification.

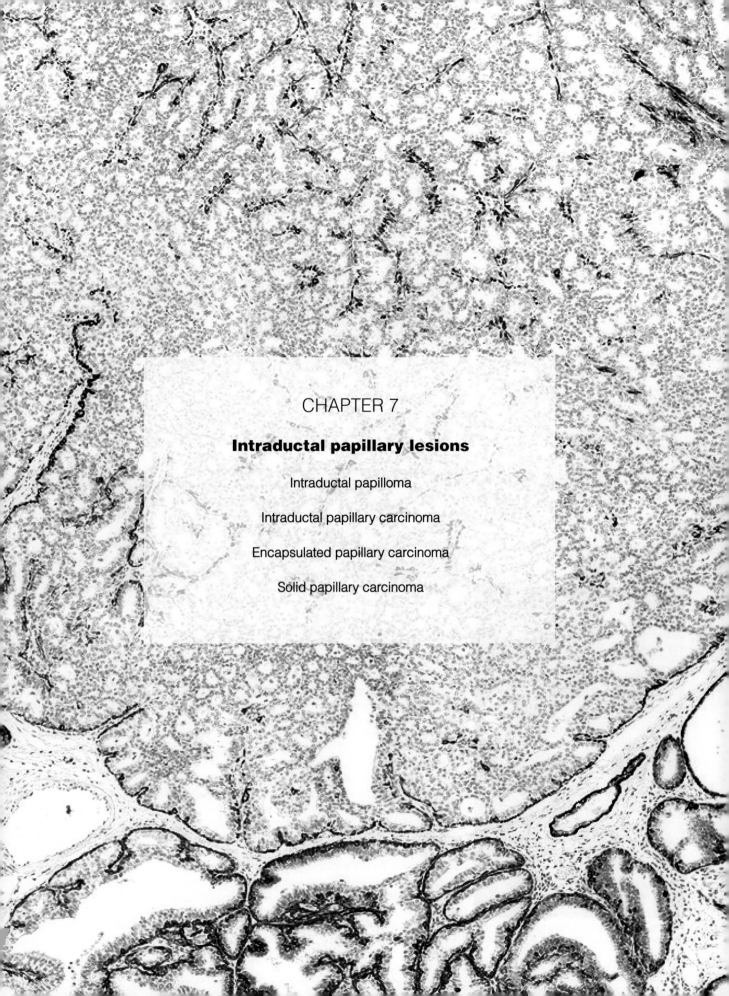

CHAPTER 7

Intraductal papillary lesions

Intraductal papilloma

Intraductal papillary carcinoma

Encapsulated papillary carcinoma

Solid papillary carcinoma

Intraductal papilloma

F. O'Malley
D. Visscher
G. MacGrogan
P.H. Tan
S. Ichihara

Definition

Intraductal papillomas are benign lesions that are characterized by finger-like fibrovascular cores covered by an epithelial and myoepithelial cell layer. They are broadly divided into two groups: central (solitary) and peripheral (multiple) {1030}. Central papillomas originate in the large ducts, usually of the subareolar region without involving the terminal-duct lobular unit (TDLU), whereas peripheral papillomas always have their roots in the TDLU, even if they extend into the ducts.

ICD-O codes

Intraductal papilloma   8503/0
Intraductal papilloma with atypical ductal
   hyperplasia   8503/0
Intraductal papilloma with ductal
   carcinoma in situ   8503/2
Intraductal papilloma with lobular
   neoplasia   8520/2

Synonyms

Central papilloma: large duct papilloma; major duct papilloma.

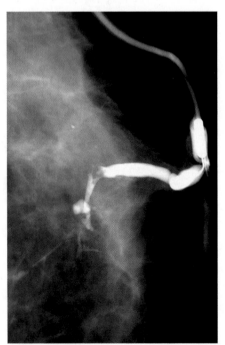

Fig. 7.03 Intraductal papilloma. Galactogram demonstrates an intraductal filling defect.

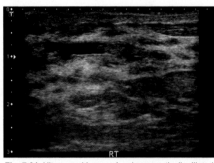

Fig. 7.01 Ultrasound image showing a cystically dilated duct containing an intraductal papilloma.

Peripheral papilloma: microscopic papilloma

Epidemiology

In a large cohort of benign breast biopsies (9108 cases), intraductal papillomas were seen in 5.3% of the cases {787}. Most papillomas are central. Patients present over a wide age range, but most cases occur between age 30 and 50 years {30,787,1282}.

Clinical features

Central papillomas present most frequently with unilateral sanguineous, or sero-sanguineous, nipple discharge. Presentation as a palpable mass is less common. Mammographic abnormalities include a circumscribed retro-areolar mass of benign appearance, a solitary retro-areolar dilated duct and, rarely, microcalcifications. Small central papillomas may be mammographically occult. Ultrasonography may show a well-defined smooth-walled, solid, hypoechoic nodule or a lobulated, smooth-walled, cystic lesion with solid components. Galactography usually shows an intraluminal filling defect or duct dilatation. Magnetic resonance imaging (MRI) may be useful in evaluating nipple discharge. Small papillomas may appear as enhancing masses with smooth margins, while larger lesions can have irregular margins {196,317}. Ductoscopy allows for direct tissue sampling and duct excision {23}.
Peripheral papillomas are often clinically

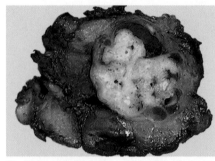

Fig. 7.02 Intraductal papilloma. A yellowish-white, broadly lobulated nodule projects into a cystically dilated duct from its attachment to the duct wall.

occult, but they can also present with nipple discharge or, less often, a mass as the result of a small cluster of papillomas. They tend to be mammographically occult, but they may manifest as peripherally located microcalcifications, nodular prominent ducts or multiple small, well-circumscribed masses. Microcalcifications may be located in the peripheral papillomas or in adjacent non-papillary intraductal proliferative lesions, such as atypical ductal hyperplasia (ADH) {30,196}.

Macroscopy

Central papillomas that are palpable may form well-circumscribed round tumours with papillary fronds attached by one or more pedicles to the wall of a dilated duct. The size of central papillomas varies from a few millimetres to > 5 cm. Focal necrosis or haemorrhage may be present, particularly in larger lesions.
In contrast, peripheral papillomas are usually grossly occult unless they are associated with other findings.

Histopathology

Both central and peripheral papillomas are characterized by a cohesive but arborescent structure composed of fibrovascular cores covered by a layer of myoepithelial cells with overlying epithelial cells. The myoepithelial layer, which is always present, may be almost inconspicuous and immunohistochemical stains for markers of myoepithelial cells such as smooth-muscle myosin heavy chain,

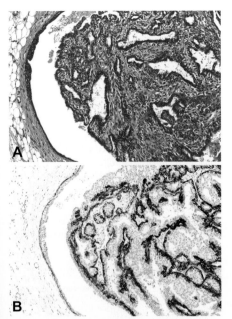

Fig. 7.04 Intraductal papilloma. **A** Note the arrangement of an epithelial layer surrounded by a myoepithelial layer. **B** Calponin immunostaining highlights the myoepithelial cells.

calponin, or p63 can be very useful in confirming their presence. In other cases the myoepithelial cells may be quite prominent and myoepithelial hyperplasia may occasionally be seen. The periphery of involved spaces is also surrounded by myoepithelial cells. The epithelial component may consist of one layer of cuboidal to columnar cells or may show foci of usual ductal hyperplasia (UDH). Apocrine change is frequently found in the epithelium of papillomas and squamous metaplasia may be seen, most often in association with areas of infarction {454}. Rarely, mucinous, clear cell and sebaceous

metaplasia may be seen {652}. Collagenous spherulosis can also involve papillomas. Epithelial cell mitoses are absent or extremely rare.

Areas of haemorrhage or infarction may occur secondary to a needling procedure or due to torsion of fibrovascular cores. Stromal fibrosis is commonly seen and can be so extensive that it obscures the underlying papillary architecture. Such lesions have been called sclerosing papillomas, a variant of which is ductal adenoma. Epithelial nests may become entrapped in the areas of fibrosis and may mimic invasive carcinoma. The epithelium, however, retains an associated myoepithelial layer, confirming its benign nature. Similarly, displacement of epithelial nests can be present in the healing biopsy site tract after fine-needle aspiration or needle-core biopsy; this may create an interpretive pitfall since such areas may be mistaken for invasive carcinoma {959}. Ducts in the region of a papilloma often show ectasia, which may be a clue to the presence of a papillary lesion in biopsy or excision specimens.

Foci of ADH or ductal carcinoma in situ (DCIS) may be seen in papillomas; these changes are more commonly associated with peripheral papillomas than central papillomas {30,1029}.

Papilloma with ADH and DCIS

Papillomas with ADH and DCIS are characterized by the presence of a focal population of monotonous cells with the cytological and architectural features of low-grade ductal neoplasia. Myoepithelial cells may be scant or absent from these foci and the atypical epithelial cells usually

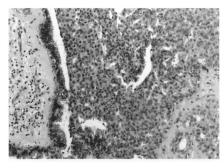

Fig. 7.05 Intraductal papilloma with usual ductal hyperplasia. The epithelial cells show crowded overlapping nuclei and are haphazardly arranged around slit-like spaces.

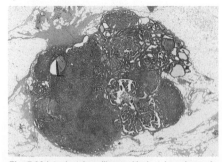

Fig. 7.06 Intraductal papilloma with ductal carcinoma in situ. Low-power magnification of an intraductal papilloma harbouring a more solid epithelial proliferation that exceeds 3 mm in size.

show lack of staining for high-molecular-weight keratins with uniform positivity for estrogen receptors {619A,955}. Extent and proportion criteria have been used to differentiate papilloma with ADH from DCIS within a papilloma. The extent cut-off according to some authorities is 3 mm; an intraductal papilloma with ADH is diagnosed when the atypical epithelial population is < 3 mm, while DCIS within a papilloma is diagnosed when this atypical

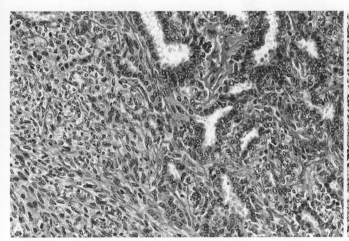

Fig. 7.07 Myoepithelial hyperplasia within an intraductal papilloma. **A** A solid proliferation of spindle cells within an intraductal papilloma. **B** Positive nuclear staining for p63 in the spindle cells indicates a myoepithelial phenotype.

population is ≥ 3 mm {1057}. While some previous authors have used a cut-off of 30% {1414}, recently revised to 90% {1477}, the WHO Working Group was of the view that size-/extent-based criteria rather than proportion criteria should be used in routine practice. It is acknowledged that this is a pragmatic guideline and that scientific evidence for this size criterion to diagnose low-grade DCIS within a papilloma is lacking {378,1282}. When epithelial proliferations with intermediate or high nuclear grade are seen, the diagnosis of DCIS within a papilloma should be made regardless of its extent. Papillomas with DCIS ought to be distinguished from papillary DCIS/intraductal papillary carcinoma. Papillary DCIS constitutes a de novo in situ malignant papillary process in which an underlying benign papilloma hosting the abnormal epithelial proliferation is not identifiable. The presence of lobular neoplasia in the context of an intraductal papilloma should be reported as such.

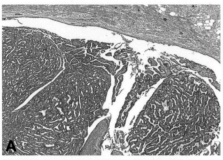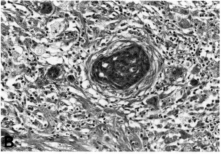

Fig. 7.08 Intraductal papilloma with epithelial displacement. **A** Low-power view shows an intraductal papilloma. **B** At higher power, epithelial nests may be seen at the periphery and can mimic invasion.

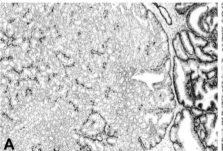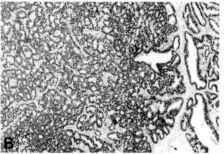

Fig. 7.09 Intraductal papilloma with ductal carcinoma in situ (DCIS). **A** Immunostaining for keratin 14 shows diminished reactivity in the abnormal cribriform epithelial population. **B** This population shows diffuse nuclear reactivity for estrogen receptor, corroborating the diagnosis of DCIS.

Genetics

Benign papillomas are monoclonal proliferations {1008}. A higher frequency of activating point mutations of *PIK3CA*, *AKT1* and *RAS* family genes was found in benign papillomas than in papillary carcinomas {1457}. Loss of heterozygosity (LOH) on chromosome 16p13 in the *TSC2/PKD1* gene region was found in benign papillary lesions as well as in papillary carcinomas, whereas LOH on chromosome 16q23 with the D16S476 marker was only found in malignant papillary lesions {336,815}.

Prognosis and predictive factors

A benign central papilloma without surrounding atypical changes is associated with a twofold increase in the risk of subsequent invasive breast carcinoma; this risk is threefold for peripheral papillomas {357,787}.

For atypical papillomas, the risk of subsequent invasive carcinoma was reported as 7.5-fold in one study and this risk was almost exclusively confined to the ipsilateral breast {1057}. Another larger study reported a relative risk of fivefold for atypical central lesions and sevenfold for atypical peripheral lesions and in this study the risk applied to both breasts {787}.

The risk of subsequent carcinoma and local recurrence associated with an atypical papilloma is obscured by the frequent concurrent presence of ADH or DCIS within the surrounding breast parenchyma. It would appear that this risk is more closely related to the presence of ADH/DCIS outside the papilloma than within it {848,1057}.

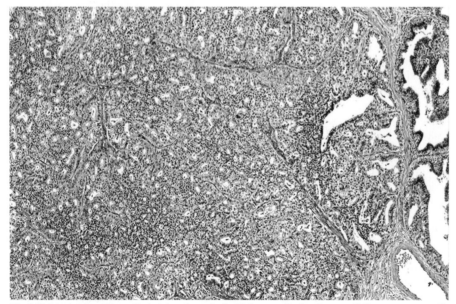

Fig. 7.10 Intraductal papilloma with ductal carcinoma in situ. Higher magnification shows a cribriform appearance with monotonous epithelial cells punctuated by well-defined rounded spaces.

Intraductal papillary carcinoma

G. MacGrogan
G. Tse
L. Collins
P.H. Tan
B. Chaiwun
J.S. Reis-Filho

Definition

Intraductal papillary carcinoma is a malignant non-invasive neoplastic epithelial proliferation with papillary architectural features occurring in the lumen of the ductal-lobular system.

ICD-O code   8503/2

Synonyms

Papillary ductal carcinoma in situ; papillary carcinoma, non-invasive

Epidemiology

Little is known about the specific epidemiology of this type of lesion owing to its rarity.

Clinical features

A clear or bloodstained nipple discharge can be the presenting symptom, whereas the more peripherally located lesions may present as a mass {706}. Otherwise, the presentation of intraductal papillary carcinoma is that of ductal carcinoma in situ (DCIS) in general, with mammographic microcalcifications being the most frequent form of presentation.

Macroscopy

There are no specific macroscopic features.

Histopathology

Microscopic examination shows ducts and/or terminal-duct lobular units (TDLU) filled with slender, branching fibrovascular stalks covered by a single cell population of neoplastic epithelial cells. The neoplastic cells can be arranged in one or several layers of columnar cells overlying the stalks in an orderly manner and with a deceptively bland appearance, also known as the stratified spindle cell pattern {1477}. The tumour cells can also form micropapillary, cribriform or solid structures obscuring the spaces between the papillary fronds. The tumour cells usually display low- or intermediate-grade nuclear features. There are no or scant myoepithelial cells interposed between the papillae and the epithelial proliferation.

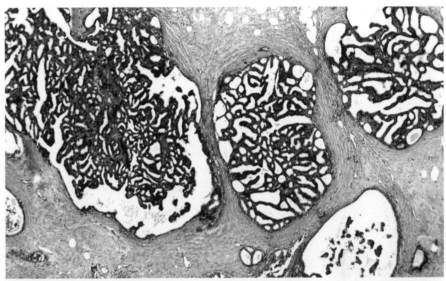

Fig. 7.11 Intraductal papillary carcinoma. The terminal-duct lobular units are filled with slender, branching fibrovascular stalks.

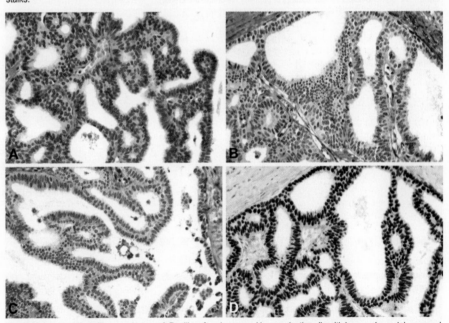

Fig. 7.12 Intraductal papillary carcinoma. **A** Papillary fronds covered by neoplastic cells with low-grade nuclei arranged in micropapillary and cribriform structures. **B** Immunostaining for p63: scant myoepithelial cells present at the periphery of the lesion. **C** Immunostaining shows that keratin 5/6 is not expressed in neoplastic epithelial cells. **D** Estrogen-receptor immunostaining shows strong and diffuse expression by neoplastic cells.

At the periphery of the ducts, the myoepithelial cell layer is present, but in a more or less attenuated form {575,1463}.

Some examples may also show a dimorphic cell population, with the presence of tumour cells with clear cytoplasm adjacent to the basement membrane {778}. These tumour cells with clear cytoplasm may be mistaken for myoepithelial cells and cause diagnostic confusion, although

Table 7.01 Histopathological characteristics of papillary lesions of the breast

	Intraductal papilloma	Papilloma with ADH or DCIS	Papillary DCIS	Encapsulated papillary carcinoma	Solid papillary carcinoma
Presentation	Single (central papilloma) or multiple lesions (peripheral papillomas)	Single (central papilloma) or multiple lesions (peripheral papillomas)	Multiple lesions	Single lesion	Single or multiple lesions
Architecture	Generally broad, blunt fronds	Generally broad, blunt fronds	Slender fronds, sometimes branching	Slender fronds, sometimes branching	Solid with inconspicuous delicate fibrovascular septa
Myoepithelial cells	Present throughout and at periphery	Mostly present throughout and at periphery May be attenuated in areas of ADH/DCIS	Absent or scant in papillae Present in attenuated form at the periphery of ducts	Usually absent throughout and at periphery	Absent within the solid papillary proliferation May be present or absent at the outer contours of the nodules
Epithelial cells	Heterogeneous non-neoplastic cell population: – Luminal cells – Myoepithelial cells – UDH – Apocrine metaplasia and hyperplasia	Focal areas of cells with architectural and cytological features of ADH or DCIS (usually low-grade) Background of heterogeneous non-neoplastic cell population	Entire lesion occupied by a cell population with architectural and cytological features of DCIS of low, intermediate or rarely high nuclear grade	Entire lesion occupied by a cell population with architectural and cytological features of DCIS of low, intermediate or rarely high nuclear grade Cribriform and solid patterns may be present	Entire lesion occupied by a cell population with architectural and cytological features appearing to be mostly of low nuclear grade Spindle cell component Neuroendocrine differentiation frequent Mucin production may be seen, which can be intracellular or extracellular

ADH, atypical ductal hyperplasia; DCIS, ductal carcinoma in situ; UDH, usual ductal hyperplasia.

Table 7.02 Immunohistochemical features of papillary lesions of the breast

	p63		Keratins of high molecular weight (K5/6, K14)	Estrogen receptor and progesterone receptor (PR)
	Papillary fronds	Periphery of lesion		
Intraductal papilloma	Positive	Positive	Positive: – Myoepithelial cells – UDH (heterogeneous positivity) Negative: – Apocrine metaplasia	Positive (patchy): – Luminal cells – UDH (heterogeneous positivity) Negative: – Apocrine metaplasia
Papilloma with ADH or DCIS	Positive in papilloma May be scant in the ADH/DCIS component	Positive	Positive: – Myoepithelial cells – UDH (heterogeneous positivity) Negative: – Apocrine metaplasia – ADH/DCIS	Positive (patchy): – Luminal cells – UDH (heterogeneous positivity) Negative: – Apocrine metaplasia Positive strong and diffuse: – ADH/DCIS
Papillary DCIS	Negative	Positive	Negative: – Neoplastic cell population	Positive strong and diffuse: – Neoplastic cell population
Encapsulated papillary carcinoma	Negative	Usually negative	Negative: – Neoplastic cell population	Positive strong and diffuse: – Neoplastic cell population
Solid papillary carcinoma	Solid-papillary areas are negative	May be negative or positive	Negative	Positive strong and diffuse

ADH, atypical ductal hyperplasia; DCIS, ductal carcinoma in situ; UDH, usual ductal hyperplasia.

negative immunohistochemical staining for myoepithelial markers will resolve the uncertainty.

The histopathological features of breast papillary lesions are summarized in Table 7.01.

Immunoprofile
Immunohistochemistry can assist in the recognition of these lesions (Table 7.02) by demonstrating the absence of expression of myoepithelial cell markers along the papillary fronds and showing positive staining for the same markers at the periphery of the involved ducts {284,1403, 1463}. Moreover, the neoplastic epithelial cell population is devoid of the expression of high-molecular-weight keratins (e.g. keratins 5/6 and 14) {1046,1403} and strongly expresses estrogen and progesterone receptors.

Histogenesis

The nature and origin of intraductal papillary carcinomas are subject to debate: some authors believe that they result from the gradual transformation and replacement of the epithelial component of pre-existing papillomas by a neoplastic cell population {847}, while others advocate that they are de novo neoplastic papillary proliferations {286}.

Genetics

A lower frequency of activating point mutations of *PIK3CA*, *AKT1* and *RAS* family genes was found in papillary carcinomas than in benign papillomas in a series with a limited number of samples {1457}. With the limitations applicable to loss of heterozygosity (LOH) studies performed on formalin-fixed paraffin-embedded tissues, LOH on chromosome 16p13 in the *TSC2/ PKD1* gene region was found in benign papillary lesions as well as in papillary carcinomas, whereas LOH on chromosome 16q23 with the D16S476 marker was only found in malignant papillary lesions {336,815}.

Prognosis and predictive factors

The prognosis and predictive factors for intraductal papillary carcinoma are the same as those for DCIS in general.

Encapsulated papillary carcinoma

L. Collins
F. O'Malley
D. Visscher
T. Moriya
S. Ichihara
J.S. Reis-Filho

Definition

This lesion is a variant of papillary carcinoma, characterized by fine fibrovascular cores covered by neoplastic epithelial cells of low or intermediate nuclear grade and surrounded by a fibrous capsule. In the majority of cases, there is no myoepithelial cell layer within the papillae or at the periphery of the lesion.

ICD-O codes

Encapsulated papillary carcinoma 8504/2
Encapsulated papillary carcinoma
 with invasion 8504/3

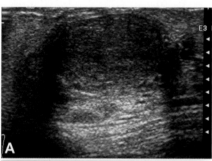

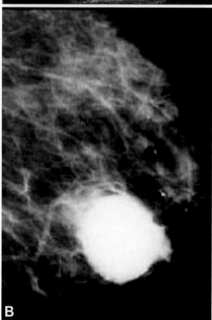

Fig. 7.13 Encapsulated papillary carcinoma. **A** Breast ultrasonography demonstrates a mass within a cystically-dilated space. **B** Left breast, medio-lateral oblique projection showing a 3 × 3 cm, solitary, high-density circular mass in the lower half of the breast.

Synonyms

Intracystic papillary carcinoma; encysted papillary carcinoma; intracystic carcinoma not otherwise specified

Epidemiology

The incidence of encapsulated papillary carcinoma is difficult to determine. Less than 2% of breast carcinomas are papillary carcinomas and only a proportion of these are encapsulated papillary carcinomas. These lesions occur in older women with an average age of 65 years (range, 34–92 years) {232,778}.

Clinical features

Encapsulated papillary carcinoma often appears as a circumscribed round mass with or without nipple discharge. These features are indistinguishable from those of benign papillary lesions.

There are no specific clinical or imaging features that distinguish encapsulated papillary carcinomas from other papillary lesions. However, encapsulated papillary carcinomas tend to be larger at presentation.

Macroscopy

On gross examination, a friable mass within a cystic cavity may be appreciated.

Histopathology

On histopathological examination, a thick fibrous capsule is evident on low-power examination. The capsule surrounds a nodule composed of delicate fibrovascular stalks, covered by a monomorphic population of neoplastic epithelial cells with low- or intermediate-grade nuclei. The epithelial cells are typically arranged in either solid or cribriform patterns. Occasionally, the cells may take on a more spindled appearance. Encapsulated papillary carcinomas typically lack myoepithelial cells both within the fibrovascular cores and at the periphery of the lesion. The observed lack of a myoepithelial cell layer, on haematoxylin-and-eosin-stained sections as well as with immunohistochemistry for a variety of myoepithelial cell markers, runs counter to our current

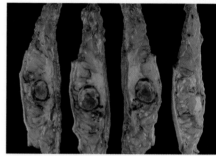

Fig. 7.14 Encapsulated papillary carcinoma. Macroscopically, the distinction between papilloma and papillary carcinoma can be difficult.

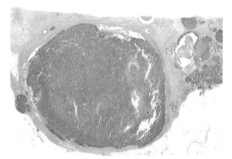

Fig. 7.15 Scanning magnification view of an encapsulated papillary carcinoma.

understanding of an in situ lesion. This is a phenomenon that has only recently been documented in the literature {284, 388,575}, but it raises the possibility that encapsulated papillary carcinomas may represent a minimally invasive, low-grade or indolent form of invasive carcinoma rather than an in situ lesion {284,575}. Others have postulated that these lesions may be a form of carcinoma "in transition" between in situ and invasive carcinoma {388,575}. A diagnosis of frank invasive carcinoma should only be rendered when neoplastic epithelial elements infiltrate beyond the fibrous capsule of encapsulated papillary carcinomas. True infiltration should also be cautiously differentiated from entrapment of neoplastic epithelial cells in the fibrous capsule and from epithelial displacement into the biopsy site, which is frequently encountered following needle-core biopsy procedures of papillary lesions (a differential that is best determined on histological examination since immunohistochemical studies for myoepithelial cells will not be helpful in this setting) {959,1612}.

Genetics

Genetic alterations involving LOH at 16q and 1q have been reported. Owing to the limited number of samples analysed, the actual prevalence of these aberrations and their significance is not yet fully characterized {336,815,1466}. A recent microarray-based comparative genomic hybridization analysis revealed that encapsulated papillary carcinoma displayed patterns of gene copy-number aberrations and prevalence of *PIK3CA* mutations similar to those of estrogen-receptor- and grade-matched invasive carcinomas of no special type {359A}.

Prognosis and predictive factors

Encapsulated papillary carcinoma of the breast in the absence of associated DCIS in the surrounding tissue or areas of infiltrating carcinoma has a very favourable prognosis with adequate local therapy alone {216,553,767,778}. In very rare instances, lymph-node metastases have been reported with the metastases revealing typical papillary features {954,1140}.

The presence of associated DCIS in the adjacent breast tissue confers a higher risk of local recurrence {231}. Complete surgical excision of encapsulated papillary carcinoma with extensive sampling of the lesion and surrounding breast tissue is essential for treatment and assessment of risk for local recurrence. Staging of encapsulated papillary carcinomas has become controversial. If there is a component of conventional invasive carcinoma associated with the encapsulated papillary carcinoma, the tumour should be staged according to the size of the invasive carcinoma. At this time there is no universal agreement on how to stage encapsulated papillary carcinomas. In the

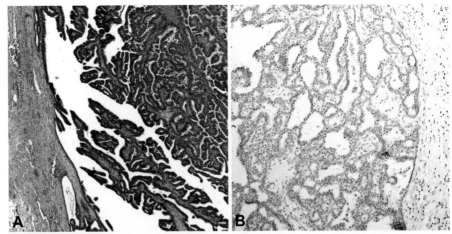

Fig. 7.16 Encapsulated papillary carcinoma. **A** Low magnification reveals the papillary fronds lined by a monotonous epithelial proliferation. **B** p63 immunostaining demonstrates the absence of myoepithelial cells both within and at the periphery of the lesion.

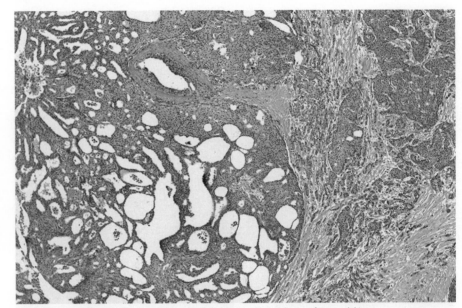

Fig. 7.17 Encapsulated papillary carcinoma with adjacent invasive carcinoma of no special type.

absence of conventional invasive carcinoma, the consensus of the WHO Working Group was that such lesions should be staged and managed as Tis disease.

Solid papillary carcinoma

D. Visscher
L. Collins
F. O'Malley
S. Badve
J.S. Reis-Filho

Definition

A distinctive form of papillary carcinoma characterized by closely apposed expansile, cellular nodules. Fibrovascular cores within the nodules are delicate and can be inconspicuous, hence the growth pattern appears solid at low magnification. Neuroendocrine differentiation is frequent. Conventional invasive growth may be present, often having mucinous and/or neuroendocrine features.

ICD-O codes

Solid papillary carcinoma in situ 8509/2
Solid papillary carcinoma
   with invasion   8509/3

Synonyms

Neuroendocrine breast carcinoma, spindle cell ductal carcinoma in situ (DCIS), neuro endocrine DCIS, endocrine DCIS

Epidemiology

This is an uncommon histological pattern accounting for < 1% of breast carcinomas {1045}. Most occur in postmenopausal women, with a mean age at presentation in the seventh decade of life {863,969}.

Clinical features

Depending on tumour size, cases may present as a mammographic abnormality or a palpable mass. Bloody nipple discharge occurs in 20–25% of cases {863}.

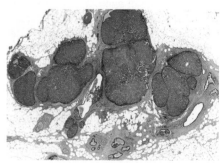

Fig. 7.18 Solid papillary carcinoma. Scanning magnification of breast tissue showing several solidified islands of epithelium.

Macroscopy

Solid papillary carcinoma may be observed as a whitish-grey or yellowish-brown, fleshy firm or soft, nodular circumscribed mass on gross examination {863}. Size may range from a few millimetres to several centimetres.

Histopathology

At low magnification, the tumour forms multiple circumscribed cellular masses comprised of closely apposed, expanded and solidified rounded duct-like structures arranged in contiguous, sometimes "geographic" patterns. These may be embedded in dense fibrous stroma. Although the cellular nests appear non-invasive because of their circumscription, they frequently lack peripheral myoepithelium as demonstrated with immunohistochemical stains {995}. Those lesions in which the nests exhibit a surrounding myoepithelial layer should be considered variants of (DCIS). However, how best to categorize lesions in which some or all of the nests lack a delimiting myoepithelial layer is controversial {286}. The precise distinction between in situ and invasive disease in solid papillary carcinoma is difficult. If there is uncertainty that there is invasion, these lesions should be regarded for staging purposes as in situ carcinoma. However, the presence of a geographic jigsaw pattern with more ragged and irregular margins, coupled with absence of myoepithelial cells, may be considered by some authors as invasive disease.

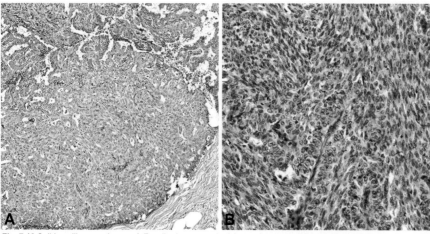

Fig. 7.19 Solid papillary carcinoma. **A** Focally, there are arborizing and anastomosing papillae with a streaming pattern of epithelial cells. Small amounts of mucin are discernible between the epithelial cells. **B** Higher magnification shows solid masses of relatively bland spindle cells with amphophilic to eosinophilic cytoplasm. Fine delicate fibrovascular septa are discovered amid the solid proliferation.

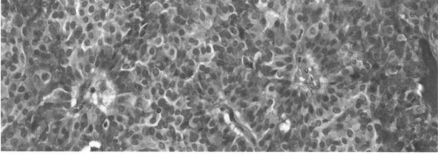

Fig. 7.20 Solid papillary carcinoma. Perivascular pseudorosettes.

The cellular proliferation in the tumour nodules of solid papillary carcinoma is homogeneous and cohesive, lacking obvious papillary or cribriform architecture, although the presence of fine, almost imperceptible vessels is a clue to its underlying papillary nature. Lesional cells often have a streaming and occasionally spindled appearance mimicking benign usual ductal hyperplasia. Extracellular mucin may be present. Fibrovascular cores can contain hyaline collagen. They are often surrounded by palisades of cells, forming perivascular pseudorosettes {863}. The neoplastic population is comprised of small, monotonous cells with hyperchromatic nuclei; the cell shape is usually polygonal, but can be spindled. Cytoplasm is moderate in amount and finely granular, though signet ring forms can be seen. Mitoses are consistently present but not numerous {424,1140,1459}.

Obvious invasive growth of the conventional infiltrative type may coexist {863, 1045, 1408} and should be classified according to its characteristics. Such invasive carcinomas frequently have mucinous and/or neuroendocrine features, although ductal, lobular or mixed histological patterns may occur {863,969,1045}.

Immunoprofile

Immunohistochemical evidence of neuroendocrine differentiation, consisting of staining for chromogranin and/or synaptophysin, is observed in at least half of cases {1045,1403A}. The tumour cell population is diffusely hormone-receptor-positive and HER2-negative, and also expresses low-molecular-weight keratins 8 and 18 {948,1129,1464,1567}.

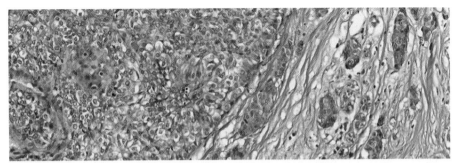

Fig. 7.21 Solid papillary carcinoma with adjacent invasive carcinoma of no special type.

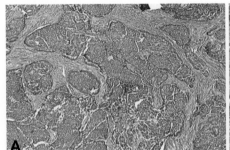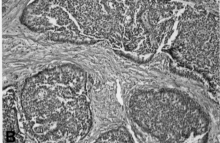

Fig. 7.22 Solid papillary carcinoma. **A** Solid cellular epithelial nodules arranged in a geographic, jigsaw-like pattern within a fibrous, focally desmoplastic background, suggesting possible invasive disease. **B** Higher magnification shows fibrovascular cores within some of the solid islands.

Differential diagnosis

The differential diagnosis includes intraductal papilloma and florid usual ductal hyperplasia. These entities lack the constellation of cellular homogeneity, mitotic activity and neuroendocrine/mucinous phenotype that characterize solid papillary carcinomas. In difficult cases, the absence of staining for high-molecular-weight keratins (e.g. keratin 5/6) in solid papillary carcinomas may have diagnostic value, this marker being positive in benign proliferative lesions {1129}.

Genetics

Gene-expression array analysis confirmed the luminal phenotype exhibited by these lesions and demonstrated a close relationship with mucinous B carcinomas at the transcriptomic level {1567,1569}.

Prognosis and predictive factors

When there is doubt about the presence of invasion, solid papillary carcinomas should be regarded for staging purposes as a form of in situ carcinoma (Tis). Metastasis may occur in patients without frankly invasive growth, but is rare {995}. Behaviour when conventional coexisting invasive carcinoma is present is consistent with its stage and grade characteristics.

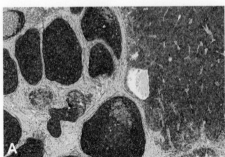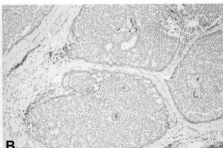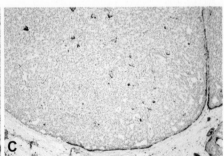

Fig. 7.23 Solid papillary carcinoma. **A** There is diffuse positivity for synaptophysin on immunohistochemistry. **B** Immunohistochemistry for smooth-muscle myosin heavy chain shows complete absence of a peripheral myoepithelial lining around the cellular nodules. Together with the geographic, jigsaw pattern of epithelial islands, this appearance may be considered invasive. **C** In these larger rounded nests, the myoepithelial cell layer is generally intact, as demonstrated by immunostaining for keratin 14, indicating an in situ process.

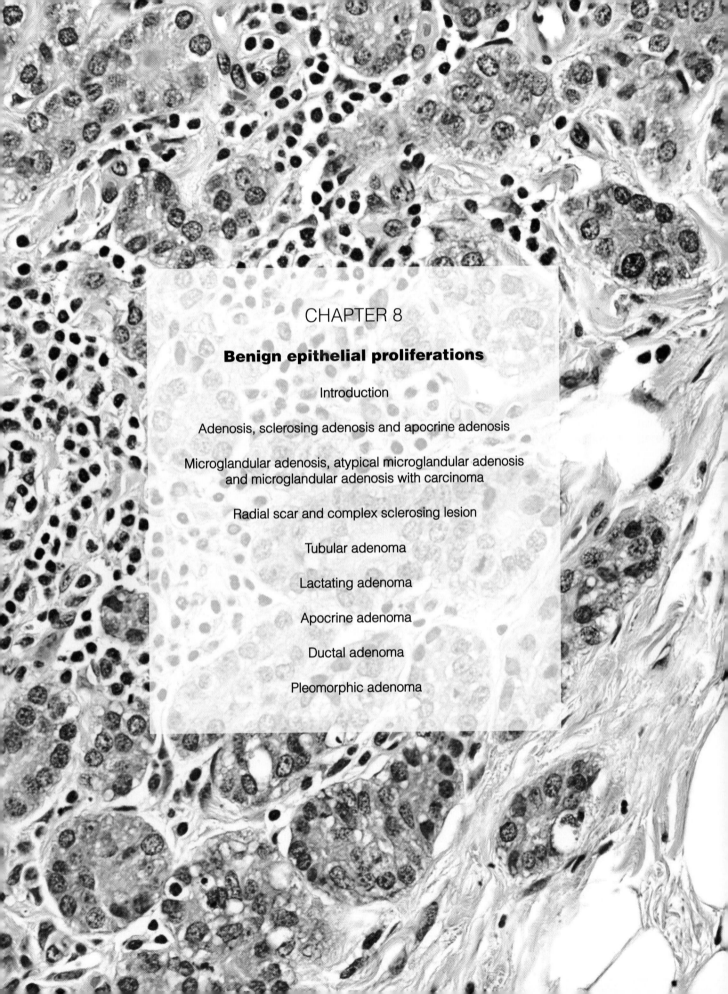

CHAPTER 8

Benign epithelial proliferations

Benign epithelial proliferations

Introduction

I.O. Ellis
J.F. Simpson

This chapter deals with benign lesions of the breast arising from the epithelial parenchyma and related structures.

Localization
With a small number of exceptions, there are no characteristic locations or laterality for most benign breast lesions. As with carcinoma, the majority arise within the terminal-duct lobular unit (TDLU). One exception is benign solitary intraductal papillomas, approximately 90% of which occur in the large subareolar ducts {870}. Other benign lesions specific to the nipple areolar complex include nipple adenoma and syringomatous tumour and are discussed in Chapter 12.

Clinical features
The predominant presenting symptoms in women attending a breast clinic have been described in detail by Haagensen {532} and Mansel {870}. The frequency of benign conditions varies considerably with the age of the patient. Fibroadenoma is most frequent in younger patients, while other localized benign lesions and cysts occur most frequently in women aged 30 to 50 years. This contrasts with carcinoma, which is rare under the age of 40 years. The mammographic appearances of benign epithelial lesions are varied, but common lesions such as cysts and fibroadenomas are typically seen as well-defined or lobulated mass lesions. Calcification is also a common feature of cysts, columnar cell change, and sclerosing adenosis. Other benign lesions such as radial scar, complex sclerosing lesion and fat necrosis can produce ill-defined or spiculated mass lesions, which are indistinguishable from some forms of breast carcinoma.

Adenosis, sclerosing adenosis and apocrine adenosis

J.F. Simpson
S.J. Shin
F. O'Malley

Definition
The term "adenosis" is used to describe a common benign proliferation of glandular structures that generally maintains normally arranged epithelial and myoepithelial components. Adenosis is a lobular-based lesion, with variably increased numbers of acinar structures. Several histological types of adenosis have been described, and their chief importance is in their occasional mimicry of an invasive carcinoma.

Epidemiology
This lesion occurs most frequently in women in the third or fourth decade of life.

Clinical features
Adenosis is most often an incidental microscopic finding, but may be detected mammographically because of associated microcalcifications.

Macroscopy
Adenosis is usually grossly inapparent. A few cases assume the appearance of a firm, rubbery grey mass (nodular adenosis or adenosis tumour). On rare occasions, associated microcalcifications may be so plentiful as to impart a gritty cut surface.

Histopathology
Adenosis in its simplest form is characterized by a lobulocentric, loosely-structured proliferation of acinar or tubular structures, composed of an epithelial and myoepithelial cell layer and surrounded by a basement membrane.
Sclerosing adenosis (SA): SA is composed of a compact proliferation of acinar structures with preservation of the luminal epithelial and the peripheral myoepithelial cell layers together with an investing basement membrane. The acini may be elongated, and often have at least a focally parallel arrangement. The normally loose intralobular connective tissue is replaced by denser fibrous connective tissue with compression and distortion of the acinar structures. Despite the expansion and alteration of the normal lobular configuration, SA retains a lobulocentric arrangement that is recognizable on low-power magnification. Psammomatous-type calcification is very commonly present within SA.

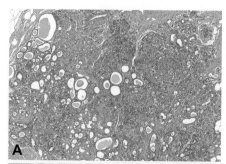

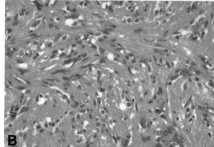

Fig. 8.01 Nodular sclerosing adenosis. **A** Note the well-delineated margins. **B** High-power view of the same lesion showing distorted and compressed tubular structures and intervening hyaline stroma. Such lesions may pose difficulties regarding the differential diagnosis with invasive lobular carcinoma.

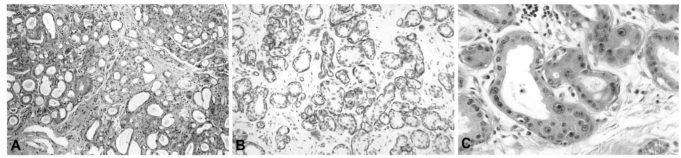

Fig. 8.02 Apocrine adenosis. **A** The small glands are lined by cells with abundant eosinophilic cytoplasm. **B** Immunostaining for actin demonstrating a myoepithelial cell layer. **C** Some degree of nuclear enlargement is acceptable.

Occasionally, atypical epithelial proliferations may populate areas of SA, specifically lobular neoplasia (atypical lobular hyperplasia (ALH), lobular carcinoma in situ (LCIS) and ductal carcinoma in situ (DCIS) {947A}. The presence of these epithelial proliferations in SA may mimic an invasive carcinoma. The recognition of SA should prompt a careful search for ALH, because breast biopsies containing SA are three times more likely to contain areas of ALH elsewhere in the specimen {648}.

In rare instances, SA may involve nerves; this feature should not be used to suggest malignancy {498}.

Apocrine adenosis: Occasionally, apocrine cells may populate areas of SA. This has been termed "apocrine adenosis," or "SA with apocrine cytology."

Differential diagnosis

The most important differential diagnostic consideration is invasive carcinoma, usually tubular carcinoma. Although compression or attenuation of the acini by surrounding fibrosis may be marked, SA always retains a lobulocentric configuration. Tubular carcinoma can be excluded because the latter has an irregular growth pattern that is not lobulocentric and often spans several lobular units, infiltrating around normal acini. If atypical lobular hyperplasia, LCIS, or DCIS populates areas of SA, the mimicry of an invasive carcinoma can be remarkable. Recognition on low power of a lobulocentric arrangement is most helpful in recognizing a non-invasive process. Immunohistochemical studies to demonstrate myoepithelial cells (sometimes attenuated), may be a useful diagnostic adjunct.

Reliable separation from microglandular adenosis can be assured by the recognition of the two-cell layer and slightly compressed acinar structures that maintain a lobular configuration in SA, whereas microglandular adenosis has an irregular pattern of proliferation of open glands with a single cell layer and a characteristic pink "secretory dot."

Genetics

There are no available data on the genetic features of these lesions.

Prognosis and predictive factors

SA is a component of proliferative breast disease, but confers only a slight increase in subsequent risk of cancer, similar to that of usual ductal hyperplasia {648}.

Apocrine adenosis is recognized as a benign process of no known clinical significance and no implications for increased risk of cancer.

Microglandular adenosis, atypical microglandular adenosis and microglandular adenosis with carcinoma

S.J. Shin
H. Gobbi

Definition

An uncommon glandular proliferation that in most cases follows an indolent clinical course but, in rare cases, gives rise to carcinoma.

Epidemiology

Microglandular adenosis (MGA) occurs over a wide age range (28–82 years), but is most common in the sixth decade of life. There are no known risk factors.

Clinical features

MGA is typically a microscopic lesion, but may present as a palpable mass.

Macroscopy

Grossly detected MGA appears as an ill-defined area of induration.

Histopathology

MGA is a non-lobulocentric, haphazard proliferation of small round glands with open lumina, composed of a single layer of flat to cuboidal epithelial cells, invested by basement membrane and lacking myoepithelium. The epithelial cells are cytologically bland with amphophilic, clear or slightly granular cytoplasm. Eosinophilic, periodic acid-Schiff (PAS)-positive luminal secretion is typically present in some glandular lumina. Oncocytic differentiation and chondroid metaplasia may be seen. In *atypical MGA*, the glandular growth pattern is retained but the epithelial cells show nuclear and architectural atypia and mitoses {1221A}.

Since MGA lacks myoepithelial cells, it is difficult to differentiate in situ from *invasive carcinoma arising in MGA*, except in those examples associated with metaplastic and adenoid cystic carcinoma {14A,686A}. However, the presence of coalescent and expanded glandular structures with solid epithelial growth and high nuclear grade is more consistent with the diagnosis of invasive carcinoma.

Differential diagnosis

MGA is most often mistaken for tubular carcinoma {272A}. In contrast to the round glands of MGA, those of tubular carcinoma are typically angulated. The cells of tubular carcinoma are positive for estrogen receptor and progesterone receptor (ER and PR) whereas those of MGA are typically negative for ER and PR. MGA glands exhibit strong expression of S100 protein and are surrounded by basement membrane, as demonstrated by laminin and collagen IV immunostains.

Genetics

MGA shows recurrent losses of chromosome 5q and gains of 8q {1311}. These genomic alterations are shared with coexistent atypical MGA and in situ and invasive carcinoma, when present, supporting a precursor–product relationship {1311}.

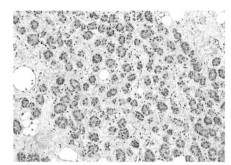

Fig. 8.03 Microglandular adenosis. A haphazard proliferation of small round glands with open lumina composed of a single layer of flat to cuboidal epithelial cells. Luminal eosinophilic secretions are typically present.

Prognosis and predictive factors

It is unclear whether MGA represents a truly benign proliferation or an indolent precursor lesion. Although atypical MGA or carcinoma may arise in the background of MGA, there are no known factors that identify which examples will likely

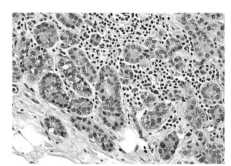

Fig. 8.04 Atypical microglandular adenosis shows more complex architecture and epithelial cells with nuclear atypia.

progress in this fashion. Subsequently, the prognosis for patients with MGA is uncertain and the requirement of complete excision is controversial. If seen in a needle-core biopsy, an excisional biopsy is recommended.

Radial scar and complex sclerosing lesion

I.O. Ellis
J.F. Simpson
S.J. Schnitt
C. Quinn

Definition

A benign lesion that on imaging, gross examination, and low-power microscopy may resemble an invasive carcinoma because the lobular architecture is distorted by a sclerosing process with associated elastosis. The term "radial scar" (RS) has been applied to small lesions, typically with a stellate configuration, while "complex sclerosing lesion" (CSL) refers to larger lesions and those with more complex features. Both may contain a variety of epithelial proliferative processes.

Synonyms

Radial scar; sclerosing papillary lesion; radial sclerosing lesion; scleroelastotic scar; stellate scar; benign sclerosing ductal proliferation; non-encapsulated sclerosing lesion; infiltrating epitheliosis.

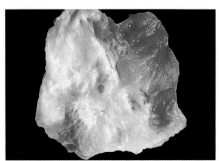

Fig. 8.05 Radial scar.

Epidemiology

The reported incidence varies depending on the mode of detection. In current practice, these lesions are most often identified by mammography. On breast imaging, the irregular stellate configuration may mimic an invasive carcinoma. Very occasionally the lesion is of sufficient size to produce a palpable mass {1340}. RS/CSL may be multiple and is frequently bilateral.

Macroscopy

These lesions may be undetected on gross examination or may be of sufficient size to produce an irregular area of firmness that can exhibit yellow streaks reflecting the elastotic stroma. The gross appearance may be indistinguishable from that of an invasive carcinoma.

Histopathology

RS is a lobulocentric proliferation that contains benign changes that may include cysts, usual ductal hyperplasia (UDH) and sclerosing adenosis. RS/CSL has a stellate outline with central dense hyalinized collagen and elastosis, which is sometimes marked. Entrapped in the central fibrous tissue are small irregular benign tubules. A two-cell layer is retained, although this may not always be visible on staining with haematoxylin and

eosin and the myoepithelial cell layer is occasionally attenuated. Around the periphery of the lesion there are various degrees of ductal dilatation, UDH, apocrine metaplasia and hyperplasia. In the larger and more complex CSLs, several of these components appear to combine and then converge with intermingling areas of sclerosing adenosis, and small, frequently sclerosing, micropapillomas and various patterns of epithelial proliferation.

Differential diagnosis

Distinction from invasive carcinoma depends on the characteristic lobulocentric architecture of RS/CSL, the presence of a myoepithelial cell layer (in most cases)

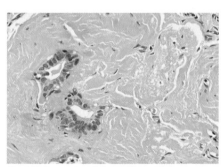

Fig. 8.06 Centre of a radial scar with two tubular structures, surrounded by hyalinized and elastotic tissue. Note the atrophic myoepithelial layer.

and basement membrane around the tubular structures, the presence of a dense hyalinized stroma with elastosis and lack of a reactive fibroblastic stroma. Demonstration of myoepithelial cells by immunohistochemistry (e.g. p63, calponin, smooth muscle myosin heavy chain) may be helpful.

Genetics

The molecular genetics of RS/CSL have not been described. The molecular characteristics of the various epithelial hyperplastic processes found within them and the forms of malignancy associated with them are described elsewhere in the relevant sections of this volume.

Prognosis and predictive factors

Despite the suggestion, especially in the radiology literature, that these lesions may be premalignant, there is no evidence to support this contention {814}. The results of two long-term follow-up studies suggest that any apparent risk is

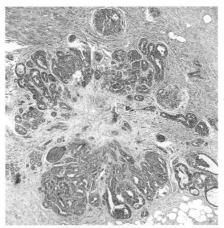

Fig. 8.07 Radial scar. A central fibrous scar is surrounded by epithelial proliferation.

related to the various patterns of associated intraductal hyperplasia {631,1254}. Recent update analysis of one of these studies has shown that RS continues to be associated with an increased risk of

breast cancer even after adjustment for histological category of benign breast disease (relative risk, 1.74), while a meta-analysis (unpublished) suggested that the magnitude of the risk was more modest (relative risk, 1.45). Atypical hyperplasia and carcinoma (both in situ and invasive) has been reported in RS/CSLs detected by mammography, particularly in lesions measuring > 0.6 cm, and in women aged > 50 years {353,1340}.

The management of RS and CSL detected by mammography remains controversial, but it has been clearly shown that lesions with associated epithelial atypia detected on needle-core biopsy sampling have a risk of associated malignancy and should be excised {372, 1142}. A rare association between CSL and metaplastic carcinoma, particularly of low-grade adenosquamous type, has been described {331}.

Tubular adenoma

M.P. Foschini
J.F. Simpson
F. O'Malley

Definition

Benign, usually round, nodules formed by a compact proliferation of tubular structures lined by epithelial and myoepithelial cells, similar to those of the normal resting breast.

ICD-O code   8211/0

Epidemiology

Tubular adenoma occurs mainly in young females {949} and is rare before menarche or after menopause {1002,1228}.

Clinical features

Tubular adenoma presents clinically as a painless, palpable, nodule. Findings on imaging studies are typically a mass with well-circumscribed borders with microcalcification rarely present {1352, 1369}.

Diagnosing tubular adenomas by fine-needle aspiration cytology may be difficult {215,1228}, and needle-core biopsy may be more reliable.

Macroscopy

Tubular adenomas are firm, well-circumscribed and homogeneous with a uniform, yellowish or tan-brown cut surface.

Histopathology

The lesions are well-circumscribed and composed entirely of small round tubules, lined by uniform epithelial cells with surrounding myoepithelial cells and separated by little intervening stroma. The latter may contain a few lymphocytes. Mitotic activity is usually low. The tubular lumina are usually empty, but may rarely contain proteinaceous material or mucin {215}.

Genetics

There are no available data on the genetic features of these lesions.

Prognosis and predictive factors

Tubular adenomas are benign lesions with no known risk of recurrence when completely excised. There is no associated risk of developing carcinoma. Rarely, carcinoma can involve a tubular adenoma {576}; this seems to be a fortuitous association.

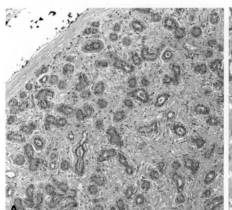
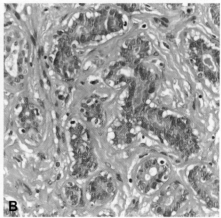

Fig.8.08 Tubular adenoma. **A** A circumscribed nodule composed of well-formed tubules. **B** At higher magnification the glands are lined by regular epithelial and myoepithelial cells.

Lactating adenoma

M.P. Foschini
J.F. Simpson
F. O'Malley

Definition
During pregnancy and lactation, the epithelial cells of a fibroadenoma or tubular adenoma may show extensive secretory changes warranting the designation of "lactating adenoma" {638,1017}. However, most lesions classified as "lactating adenoma" represent nodular areas of hyperplastic lobules with secretory or lactational changes.

ICD-O code   8204/0

Epidemiology
There are no specific epidemiological features.

Clinical features
An area of increased firmness appearing during either pregnancy or lactation. Preoperative diagnosis is based on ultrasound and magnetic resonance imaging together with fine-needle aspiration or needle-core biopsy {92,483}.

Macroscopy
Lactating adenomas vary in size, on occasion reaching large dimensions {92}.

Histopathology
The localized collections of lobules comprising the lesion show lactational changes. Infarction and haemorrhage may be present {92}.

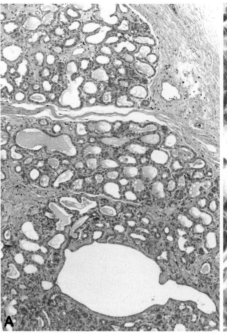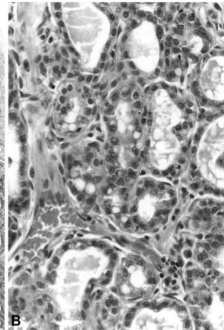

Fig. 8.09 Lactating adenoma. **A** The border of the lesion is well-circumscribed. **B** Lactating adenoma is characterized by secretory changes in the epithelial cells.

Genetics
There are no available data on the genetic features of these lesions.

Prognosis and predictive factors
Lactating adenomas are benign lesions with no known recurrences when completely excised. There is no associated risk of developing carcinoma {1248}.

Apocrine adenoma

M.P. Foschini
J.F. Simpson
F. O'Malley

Definition
A nodular collection of cysts or glands lined by apocrine metaplasia or papillary apocrine change {88,1075}.

Synonym
Nodular adenosis with apocrine metaplasia.

ICD-O code   8401/0

Epidemiology
Apocrine adenoma is a rare lesion that occurs in males and females over a wide age range.

Clinical features
A painless nodule, which mammography shows to be similar to a fibroadenoma {88,131,1075,1428}.

Macroscopy
The lesion has well-defined margins; size ranges from 3 mm to 1.7 cm {1075}.

Histopathology
Apocrine adenoma is characterized by a nodular collection of glands lined by apocrine epithelium. No cytological atypia is seen.

Genetics
There are no available data on the genetic features of these lesions.

Prognosis and predictive factors
This lesion is benign and local excision is curative.

One case has been reported in association with a breast carcinoma {131}; this is likely to be a fortuitous association since the two lesions were not spatially related.

Ductal adenoma

M.P. Foschini
J.F. Simpson
F. O'Malley

Definition
A well-circumscribed, benign glandular proliferation located, at least in part, within a duct lumen {86}.

Synonym
Sclerosing papilloma

ICD-O code   8503/0

Epidemiology
Ductal adenoma occurs over a wide age range, most frequently in women of over the age of 40 years {86,756}.

Clinical features
These lesions may present as a hard mass or, rarely, as bloody nipple discharge {756,1033}. Mammography reveals a round lesion with well-defined margins, sometimes with microcalcifications {628,1033}.

Macroscopy
Lesions may present as unilateral, single or multiple nodules {86,756}. Dimensions vary from 0.5 to 4.0 cm {86,225}. Bilateral breast involvement has been recorded in patients affected by Carney syndrome {224,225}.

Histopathology
The characteristics of these lesions are glandular structures with a typical dual cell layer of epithelial and myoepithelial cells within a central area of dense scar-like fibrosis and surrounded by a thick fibrous wall. When the myoepithelial cell proliferation is prominent, ductal adenomas can resemble adenomyoepitheliomas

{1211}. The proliferating tubules may become distorted in the sclerotic stroma, imparting a pseudoinfiltrative appearance. Apocrine metaplasia is frequent. Areas of infarction can occasionally be present {1033}.

Genetics
There are no available data on the genetic features of these lesions.

Prognosis and predictive factors
Ductal adenomas of the breast are benign lesions that do not recur if adequately excised and do not predispose to carcinoma.

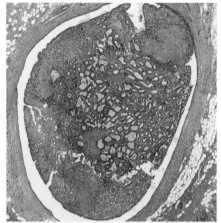

Fig. 8.10 Ductal adenoma is characterized by an intraductal glandular proliferation.

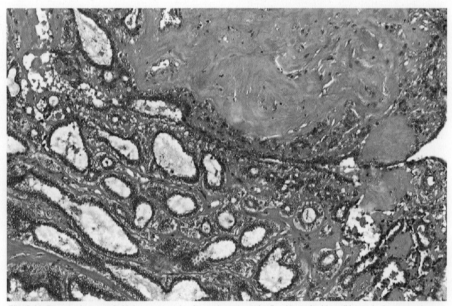

Fig. 8.11 Ductal adenoma. At higher power, glands can be seen to be lined by a double cell layer; in the present case, the myoepithelial layer is prominent.

Pleomorphic adenoma

V. Eusebi
M.P. Foschini

Definition
A tumour of the breast that is morphologically similar to pleomorphic adenoma (PA) of the salivary glands.

ICD-O code   8940/0

Epidemiology
This rare lesion occurs in women over a

wide age range {94,252} and occasionally in men {459,960}.

Clinical features
The periareolar region is usually affected.

Macroscopy
A firm nodule. Multinodular cases have been reported {252,1414}.

Histopathology
PA is composed of glands, nests and single epithelial and myoepithelial cells immersed in myxo-chondroid stroma.
Keratin 14 is present in all cells, keratin 7 is in luminal cells and p63 is observed at the edge of nests. Actin is sometimes expressed.

Differential diagnosis
PA has to be distinguished from adeno-myoepithelioma, papilloma with cartilaginous metaplasia {1220,1341,1355}, matrix-producing carcinoma and squamous cell carcinoma with myxoid stroma {459, 1416}.

Genetics
There are no available data on the genetic features of these lesions.

Prognosis and predictive factors
PA of the breast follows a benign clinical course. Recurrence can manifest as a consequence of the multinodular type of growth {653}. Malignant transformation occurs rarely {561}. Many of these lesions appear to be related to intraductal papillomas.

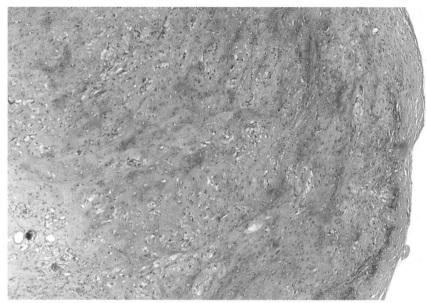

Fig. 8.12 Pleomorphic adenoma. Sparse cells immersed in myxochondroid stroma.

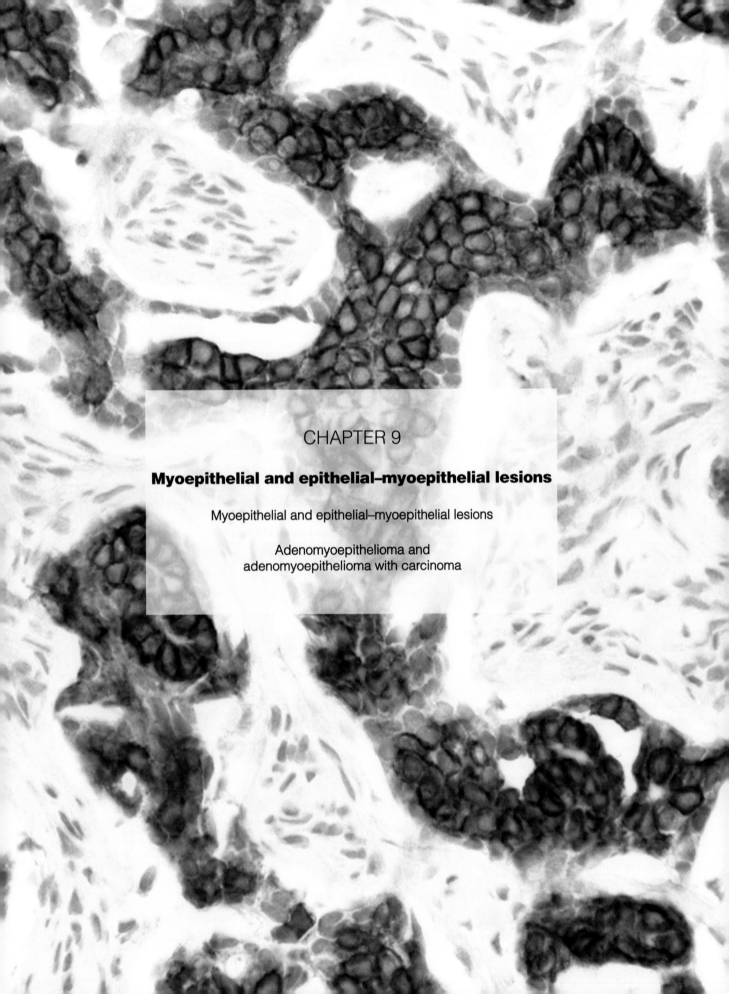

CHAPTER 9

Myoepithelial and epithelial–myoepithelial lesions

Myoepithelial and epithelial–myoepithelial lesions

Adenomyoepithelioma and
adenomyoepithelioma with carcinoma

Myoepithelial and epithelial–myoepithelial lesions

F. Schmitt
P.H. Tan
D. Dabbs
L. Jones

Definition

Myoepithelial lesions are composed of a pure or dominant population of myoepithelial cells, while epithelial–myoepithelial lesions are derived from a dual population of epithelial and myoepithelial cells. Myoepithelial lesions encompass myoepithelial hyperplasia, collagenous spherulosis and myoepithelial carcinoma (see Chapter 3: *Metaplastic carcinoma*), while epithelial–myoepithelial lesions include pleomorphic adenoma (see Chapter 8), adenomyoepithelioma, adenomyoepithelioma with carcinoma, and adenoid cystic carcinoma (see Chapter 3).

Introduction

In the normal breast and in benign lesions, myoepithelial cells are the interface between the epithelial and stromal compartments. Their function is closely reflected in their structure, since they are rich in desmosomes and hemidesmosomes by which they adhere to luminal cells and to the basement membrane, respectively, and also actin and myosin filaments, reflecting their contractile function {119,761,1242}. Lesions showing pure myoepithelial or epithelial–myoepithelial differentiation are rare and exhibit varied morphology, possibly due to the dual mesenchymal and epithelial characteristics of myoepithelial cells, leading to spindled, squamous, clear-cell or chondromyxoid appearances. While incidental microscopic changes of myoepithelial hyperplasia within lobules and ducts have been referred to by some authors as "myoepitheliosis" or "adenomyoepitheliosis" {560, 689, 1410}, we view these alterations as part of the spectrum of myoepithelial hyperplasia. Collagenous spherulosis is another incidentally discovered benign myoepithelial lesion, often seen in intraductal papillomas as well as usual ductal hyperplasia (UDH), adenosis and other breast conditions {273, 921A, 944B, 1574A,1176A}. It may sometimes be associated with microcalcifications that can be detected radiologically. Collagenous spherulosis features intraluminal eosinophilic, hyaline, acellular spherules rimmed by myoepithelial cells, histologically mimicking cribriform ductal carcinoma in situ (DCIS) or adenoid cystic carcinoma.

With the exception of myoepithelial carcinoma (malignant myoepithelioma), which merges in phenotype with metaplastic carcinoma and has a propensity for metastasis {212,458}, the prognosis for patients with myoepithelial neoplasms is generally good. It has been suggested that the infrequency and low grade of myoepithelial neoplasms is a result of the tumour-suppressive qualities of normal myoepithelial cells, which release a broad range of protease inhibitors {660, 1169, 1376} and express other recognized tumour-suppressor proteins {1328}.

Epidemiology

The spectrum of breast conditions encompassed under the rubric of myoepithelial and epithelial–myoepithelial lesions

Table 9.01 Classification of myoepithelial and epithelial–myoepithelial lesions

	Myoepithelial lesions	Epithelial–myoepithelial lesions
Benign	Myoepithelial hyperplasia	Pleomorphic adenoma
	Collagenous spherulosis	Adenomyoepithelioma
Malignant	Myoepithelial carcinoma[a]	Adenomyoepithelioma with carcinoma - Carcinoma derived from luminal epithelium - Carcinoma derived from myoepithelium - Epithelial–myoepithelial carcinoma (carcinoma derived from both luminal epithelium and myoepithelium) Adenoid cystic carcinoma

[a] Myoepithelial carcinoma (malignant myoepithelioma) is classified under metaplastic carcinoma.

Table 9.02 Antibodies for the evaluation of myoepithelial cells

Myoepithelial marker	Localization	Comments
Smooth-muscle actin	Cytoplasmic	Stains stromal myofibroblasts
Muscle-specific actin	Cytoplasmic	Stains stromal myofibroblasts
Calponin	Cytoplasmic	Stains stromal myofibroblasts
Caldesmon	Cytoplasmic	No reactivity with stromal myofibroblasts
Smooth-muscle myosin heavy chain	Cytoplasmic	May stain stromal myofibroblasts
High- molecular -weight (basal) keratins[a]	Cytoplasmic	May stain scattered epithelial/luminal cells
p63	Nuclear	May stain epithelial cells of DCIS and invasive cancer Also expressed by squamous epithelial cells and forms of metaplastic carcinoma
p75	Cytoplasmic & membranous	May stain endothelial cells, vascular adventitia, stromal cells and benign and malignant epithelial cells
CD10	Cytoplasmic	May weakly stain stromal myofibroblasts
S100	Cytoplasmic & nuclear	May stain normal, hyperplastic, and neoplastic epithelial cells
GFAP	Cytoplasmic	—
Maspin	Cytoplasmic & nuclear	May stain normal, hyperplastic and neoplastic epithelial cells
P-cadherin	Cytoplasmic & membranous	—
D2-40	Cytoplasmic	Stains endothelial cells of lymphatic vessels

DCIS, ductal carcinoma in situ; GFAP, glial fibrillary acidic protein. [a](K5, K5/6, K14, K17, 34βE12)

is relatively wide, and the age range of patients reflects this, with cases being reported in women aged 22–87 years.

Clinical features

Patients often present with radiologically detected densities or clinically palpable lumps. Collagenous spherulosis may present as radiological calcifications or be discovered incidentally on microscopy.

Immunohistochemistry

Most of the antibodies used to detect myoepithelial cells and their related neoplasms are directed against keratins and myofilaments {334}. While the appearance of myoepithelial cells in these tumours is diverse {109,1116,1410}, most are identifiable with a panel of immunostains including broad-spectrum keratins AE1/AE3, CAM5.2, and keratin 7.

Antibodies to selected high-molecular-weight keratins (keratins 5, 5/6, 14, and 17) react with most myoepithelial lesions. S100 protein is too non-specific in reactivity to be of value in the study of these lesions {489B,668A}. Antibodies to smooth-muscle actin, muscle-specific actin, calponin, and smooth-muscle myosin heavy chain all decorate normal myoepithelial cells and most tumours containing myoepithelial cells. There may however, be cross-reactivity with stromal myofibroblasts {334}. The aforementioned antibodies, both epithelial and myoepithelial, detect virtually all myoepithelial cells that are present in benign lesions, regardless of morphology {1116, 1206}. P63 is expressed in myoepithelial cells of the breast, and is also seen in tumours derived from myoepithelial cells {707,1171}. The staining pattern is strictly nuclear and is unlikely to be confused with non-specific staining of stromal elements, as may be seen with myofilament antibodies. P63 may be present in the nuclei of a variety of neoplastic cells, so its diagnostic role is largely supportive in a panel of antibodies to keratins and myofilaments.

Immunohistochemical delineation of myoepithelial cells and related lesions should thus use a panel approach, with most authors advocating a two- to three-antibody panel {334,575}. Antibodies selected for the panel depend on the type of lesion being interrogated, as some antibodies may not be as discriminatory as others in certain conditions. For example, p63 is very helpful in distinguishing in situ from invasive cancer, with myoepithelial cells being retained in the former but lost in the latter, but is not as

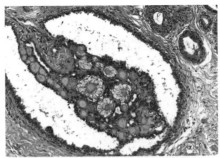

Fig. 9.01 Collagenous spherulosis in a duct, featuring round, acellular eosinophilic spherules; some appear to be rimmed by wispy radiating extensions emanating from the spherules.

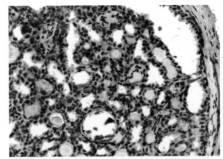

Fig. 9.02 Collagenous spherulosis: immunohistochemistry for keratin 14 shows positively stained myoepithelial cells lining the spherules.

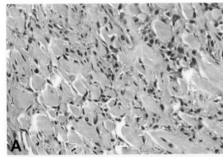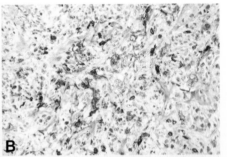

Fig. 9.03 Myoepithelial carcinoma. **A** Single strands and irregular trabeculae of plump spindled tumour cells with hyperchromatic nuclei permeating between collagen bundles. **B** Keratin AE1/AE3 decorates the spindle cells.

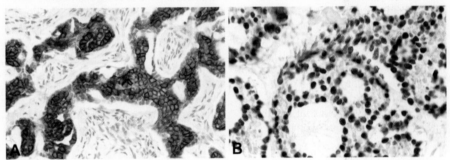

Fig. 9.04 Adenoid cystic carcinoma. **A** Membrane staining for CD117. **B** Nuclear expression of p63.

useful as high-molecular-weight keratins in corroborating UDH.

Myoepithelial cells in benign sclerosing lesions may have immunophenotypic characteristics that differ from normal myoepithelial cells {579}. Similarly, normal myoepithelial cells and those in DCIS can demonstrate different antibody sensitivities {578}. Myofilaments of myoepithelial cells in acini are not as well-developed as in those lining ducts {748}, and may show staining differences in these different locations. Additionally, there are some tumours with myoepithelial differentiation, e.g. adenoid cystic carcinoma, which incorporates luminal cells closely intermingled with myoepithelial cells, leading to a potentially varied antibody-staining pattern. Some antibodies have been used in cocktails, e.g. p63/keratin 14, to highlight myoepithelial cells.

Given their poor degree of differentiation, myoepithelial/metaplastic carcinomas are best examined with a panel that includes all antibodies to broad-spectrum keratins, all high-molecular-weight keratins, p63, as well as antibodies to myofilaments {212,233, 458,613,707,749,1145,1455}. Expression of at least one of the keratins or p63 in patchy fashion is almost universal in myoepithelial metaplastic carcinoma. EGFR expression is also common in myoepithelial carcinoma {1305}.

Benign adenomyoepithelial lesions variably express hormone receptors in the epithelial component, but myoepithelial cells remain negative. Myoepithelial carcinomas are typically completely negative for hormone receptors. Adenoid cystic carcinoma is unique in its strong membrane expression of CD117.

Adenomyoepithelioma and adenomyoepithelioma with carcinoma

S.R. Lakhani
M. Hayes
V. Eusebi

Definition

Adenomyoepithelioma (AME) is a tumour formed of a proliferation of myoepithelial cells surrounding small epithelium-lined spaces. Rarely, one or both components of AME become malignant (AME with carcinoma).

ICD-O code

Adenomyoepithelioma	8983/0
Adenomyoepithelioma with carcinoma	8983/3

Synonyms

Epithelial–myoepithelial carcinoma is a synonym for AME in which both components are malignant. Malignant AME is a synonym for AME with carcinoma.

Epidemiology

AMEs are rare tumours and most of the literature consists of individual case reports or studies of fewer than five cases {391,689,903,1206,1208,1410,1411}. AME is a tumour of adults of all ages and is rarely encountered in the male breast {1398}. AME with carcinoma is an even more infrequent tumour that usually occurs in postmenopausal women.

Clinical features

AME usually presents as a centrally located mass with or without calcifications. Patients may have nipple discharge, pain or tenderness to palpation {603,605,914, 1241}. AME with carcinoma is often preceded by a longstanding stable mass that subsequently undergoes rapid growth. On mammography, AMEs are round or lobulated, circumscribed dense masses with partially indistinct margins, with or without calcifications. Ultrasound shows either a solid or combined solid and cystic mass.

Macroscopy

AMEs are usually rounded nodules of > 1 cm {560}, with a median size of 2.5 cm. AMEs with carcinoma are large tumours that are partially well-circumscribed. Cystic degeneration, necrosis and calcifications are often seen.

Histopathology

AME is characterized by a proliferation of layers of myoepithelial cells around epithelium-lined spaces. AMEs show lobulated, papillary, tubular and mixed patterns

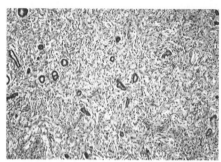

Fig. 9.05 Adenomyoepithelioma with myoepithelial carcinoma observed as a spindle cell proliferation emanating from the myoepithelial component.

on the basis of architecture. On low-power examination, most AMEs have a multilobulated architecture {903,1206, 1393,1611}. Microscopic satellite nodules may occur at the periphery of the tumour. Sclerosis and necrosis of the central area can be present. There is a relatively uniform admixture of small ducts and surrounding myoepithelial cells {81,327,1410}. The myoepithelial cells can show a range of morphology, including spindle, epithelioid, and glycogen-rich clear cells. Apocrine, squamous metaplasia, and sebaceous differentiation can be seen in the glandular elements {214,1410}.

In the spindle-cell pattern, myoepithelial cells predominate and tubules can be difficult to identify. An intraductal variant resembling leiomyoma has been described {1452}. Myoepithelial cells with abundant eosinophilic cytoplasm imparting a "myoid" appearance can also occur in all architectural variants of AME. When papillary architecture predominates, AME may be difficult to separate from intraductal papillomas with myoepithelial hyperplasia. In the tubular variant, tubular structures predominate but form a circumscribed mass. Microscopic extension into adjacent normal breast tissue may be seen, where myoepithelial prominence and hyperplasia in lobules in proximity have been described as adenomyoepitheliosis, although some authors view such microscopic lesions as part of the spectrum of myoepithelial hyperplasia {689,1151}. Mitotic activity in AME is usually low (< 2 per 10 high-power fields).

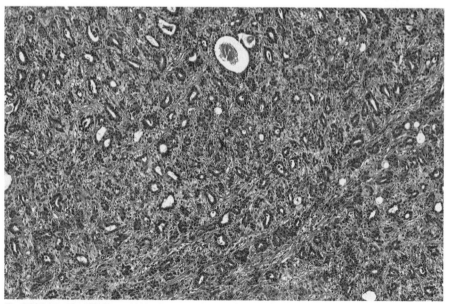

Fig. 9.06 Adenomyoepithelioma. A biphasic pattern of tubules lined by luminal epithelial cells rimmed by an outer layer of prominent pale myoepithelial cells.

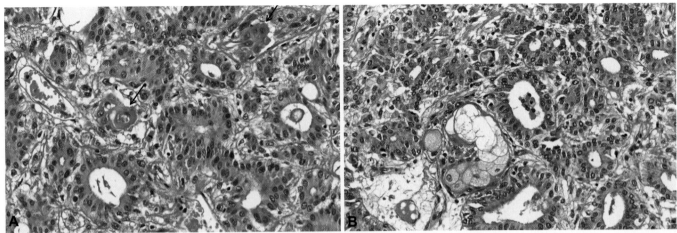

Fig. 9.07 Adenomyoepithelioma. **A** Focal squamous metaplasia (arrows) with cells acquiring more ample pink cytoplasm is noted within the tumour. **B** Focal sebaceous metaplasia with cells containing finely vacuolated cytoplasm is also observed.

Either or both cell types may undergo malignant change {20,253,417,567,696,1006, 1156}. The epithelial component of AME can give rise to invasive carcinoma of no special type (NST), undifferentiated carcinoma, or metaplastic carcinoma {459A, 921,1156}. The malignant component often shows an infiltrative growth pattern, marked cytological atypia, and a high mitotic rate. Necrosis may be present. When malignant transformation differentiates along both epithelial and myoepithelial cell lineages, the tumour can resemble poorly differentiated epithelial–myoepithelial carcinoma (EMEC) of the salivary gland {20,987}. If the high-grade malignant component shows predominantly myoepithelial differentiation, identification of a component of AME is required in order to separate it from pure/de novo malignant myoepithelioma/myoepithelial carcinoma.

The immunohistochemical features of AME and AME with carcinoma highlight their dual epithelial and myoepithelial composition {987,1399}. The presence of myoepithelial cells may be demonstrated by a variety of immunostains, including keratins 14 and 5/6, p63, actin (smooth-muscle actin, muscle-specific actin), calponin, smooth-muscle heavy-chain myosin, S100 protein, with variable positivity for H-caldesmon, but these cells are negative for desmin {101,270,579, 720,1168,1330,1399}. Immunostains for estrogen and progesterone receptors are either negative or weakly positive in a patchy pattern, while HER2 is negative {560}. Immunohistochemical identification of the luminal epithelial cell component in AME can be accomplished with antibodies to low-molecular-weight keratins.

Differential diagnosis

The tubular pattern of AME resembles tubular adenoma, although myoepithelial cells of a tubular adenoma do not assume the same degree of prominence as in an AME. Lobulated and spindle cell AME can mimic pleomorphic adenoma, but the latter usually demonstrates chondromyxoid matrix with chondroid and/or osseous metaplasia.

Genetics

Few molecular studies of AME have been reported. The gene-expression profile of an AME that exhibited reciprocal translocations between chromosomes 8 and 16 has been described {476}. Allelic imbalance and microsatellite instability have also been noted {1252}. Expression of ATM, p53, and the MRE11-Rad50-NBS1 complex has been detected in myoepithelial cells from both benign and malignant lesions, but is not specific for AME {52}. There is one case report of AME arising in association with neurofibromatosis {567}, but there are no other associated familial tumour syndromes. One case of AME with carcinoma was reported to show a mutation of the *TP53* gene {543} and the malignant areas may be aneuploid {1010}.

Prognosis and predictive factors

AMEs are cured by complete excision. Local recurrence may occur, possibly related to multinodular growth or intraductal extension of the lesion. Rare cases of AME have metastasized {829,958}.

AME with carcinoma has greater potential to recur locally and has significant metastatic potential, probably related to the grade of the transformed component {603,613} and the tumour size {20}. Metastases typically occur in patients who have high-grade malignant transformation and with tumours of ≥ 2 cm. Up to 40% of cases of AME with carcinoma reported in the literature have metastasized, but this is probably an overestimate due to selection bias. Most metastases involve the lungs {691,1455}, but may involve the liver, bone, brain and other sites {208,659}. Axillary lymph-node dissection is not indicated for these lesions unless there is clinically detected lymph-adenopathy, because metastasis to axillary nodes is unusual {1410}. There is little objective evidence to support a role for radiotherapy {419} or chemotherapy in the management of AME/AME with carcinoma.

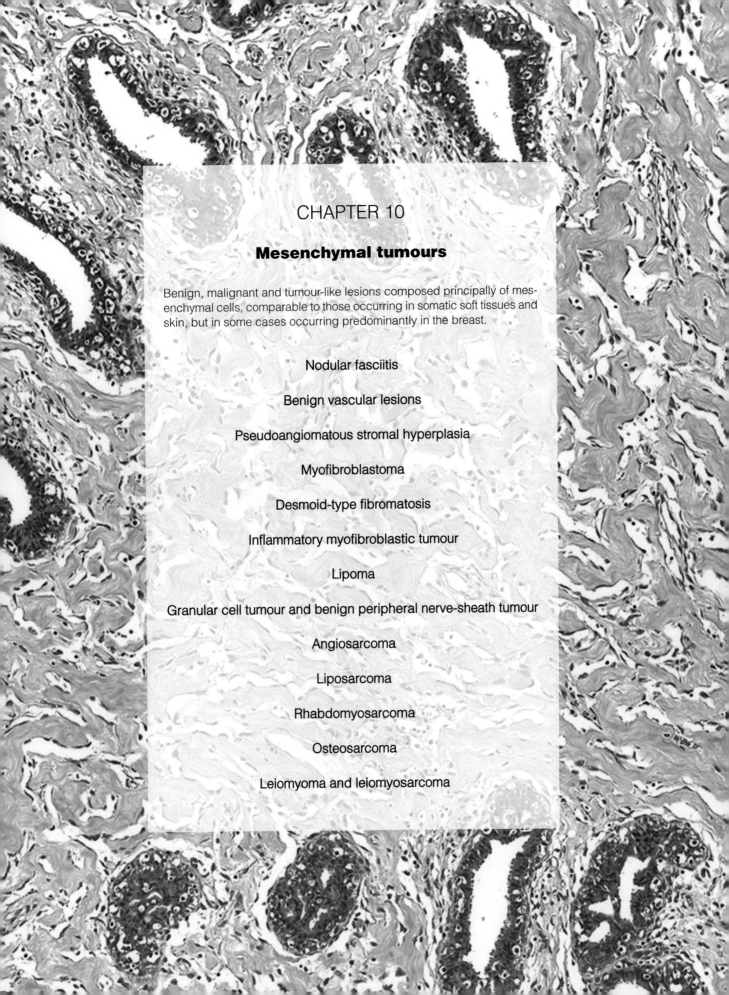

CHAPTER 10

Mesenchymal tumours

Benign, malignant and tumour-like lesions composed principally of mesenchymal cells, comparable to those occurring in somatic soft tissues and skin, but in some cases occurring predominantly in the breast.

Nodular fasciitis

Benign vascular lesions

Pseudoangiomatous stromal hyperplasia

Myofibroblastoma

Desmoid-type fibromatosis

Inflammatory myofibroblastic tumour

Lipoma

Granular cell tumour and benign peripheral nerve-sheath tumour

Angiosarcoma

Liposarcoma

Rhabdomyosarcoma

Osteosarcoma

Leiomyoma and leiomyosarcoma

Mesenchymal tumours

Nodular fasciitis

H. Gobbi
C.D.M. Fletcher

Definition
A self-limiting, mass-forming fibroblastic/ myofibroblastic proliferation that is clonal.

ICD-O code   8828/0

Synonyms
Pseudosarcomatous fasciitis

Epidemiology
Nodular fasciitis is very uncommon in the breast, but when it occurs, it most often arises in adults over a wide age range {200}. It is usually females who are affected, but rare cases occur in males {1360}.

Clinical features
Typically these lesions grow rapidly and they may be tender or painful. The usual preoperative duration is < 3–4 months and most cases measure < 5 cm in diameter. If unexcised, these lesions involute spontaneously over 1–2 months {1366}.

Macroscopy
Nodular fasciitis arises in the subcutis or, less often, in mammary parenchyma and is a well-circumscribed greyish nodule, which may show cystic change centrally.

Histopathology
Nodular fasciitis is a relatively well-circumscribed but unencapsulated lesion composed of plump fibroblastic/ myofibroblastic cells arranged in short fascicles {191,906}. The cells of the lesion have pale eosinophilic cytoplasm and plump vesicular nuclei. Mitoses may be frequent. The

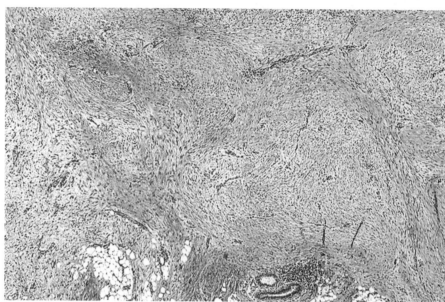

Fig. 10.01 Nodular fasciitis of the breast showing proliferation of fibroblastic/myofibroblastic cells arranged in short fascicles, more cellular at the periphery.

stroma is loose, myxoid or microcystic and contains lymphocytes, erythrocytes and thin-walled vessels. Some cases contain osteoclastic giant cells and some show keloidal hyalinization. By immunohistochemistry, the cells are consistently positive for actin but desmin positivity is rare {942}. Keratin, S100 and CD34 are typically negative {406,1571}.

Nodular fasciitis occurring in the breast should be distinguished from other benign and malignant spindle-cell lesions such as fibromatosis, low-grade spindle-cell metaplastic carcinomas, especially fibromatosis-like, and reactive spindle-cell nodules after biopsy {499,500}.

Genetics
The few cases reported have shown clonal cytogenetic aberrations {144}, in keeping with a neoplastic process. This is further confirmed by the recent identification of a consistent *MYH9–USP6* gene fusion in these lesions {384A}.

Prognosis and predictive factors
These lesions regress spontaneously. Local recurrence is very infrequent.

Benign vascular lesions

G. MacGrogan
A. Skalova
S.J. Shin

Haemangioma

Definition
A benign proliferation of mature vessels occurring in the breast.

ICD-O code
9120/0

Synonyms
Angioma

Epidemiology
Haemangiomas can be detected at any age from birth to age 80 years.

Clinical features
In most cases, haemangiomas are non-palpable and are found by breast mammography. Occasional palpable breast lesions have been described {694,1529}. Mammograms show lobular-shaped masses with circumscribed or microlobulated margins and densities equal to that of the breast parenchyma {917}. Round calcifications are seldom associated {917}. The mean size of lesions discovered on mammogram is 1.2 cm (range, 0.6–2.5 cm).

Macroscopy
Macroscopic examination reveals a circumscribed red or dark-brown spongy lesion {1217}.

Histopathology
Breast haemangiomas are characterized by the proliferation of well-differentiated vessels of varying sizes. The vascular channels can be interconnected but are most often non-anastomosing. The vessels are lined by endothelial cells showing neither nuclear atypia nor mitoses. Occasional hyperchromatic nuclei can be encountered. The vascular channels are found within the perilobular stroma, with the notable exception of perilobular angiomas where the intralobular stroma is also involved. A larger "feeding" vessel can be found within the lesion or at close proximity {1209}. Lesions are more or less well-circumscribed with isolated small vessels found in the surrounding breast tissue. Haemorrhage with disruption of the vascular channels is often encountered after needle biopsy of a mammographically detected lesion. Thrombosis,

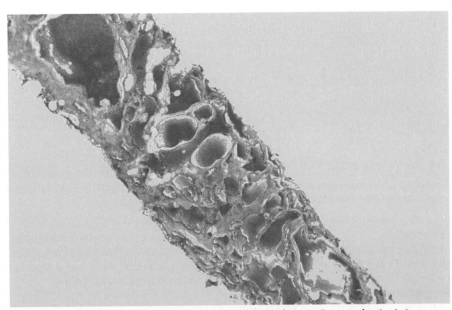

Fig. 10.02 Haemangioma, core biopsy. Despite the bland histological features, discovery of such a lesion on core biopsy should prompt surgical excision to formally exclude a well-differentiated angiosarcoma.

with secondary papillary endothelial hyperplasia can occur. Microcalcifications may be found within thrombotic channels or in surrounding fibrous stroma.

Perilobular haemangiomas/angiomas are incidental microscopic vascular lesions, measuring < 2 mm, located in the intralobular stroma or surrounding breast tissue. They are made of a more or less well-circumscribed conglomerate of small thin-walled congested capillary vessels containing erythrocytes {669}. Other types of haemangiomas (cavernous, capillary, venous {1205}) can be encountered, like elsewhere in the body.

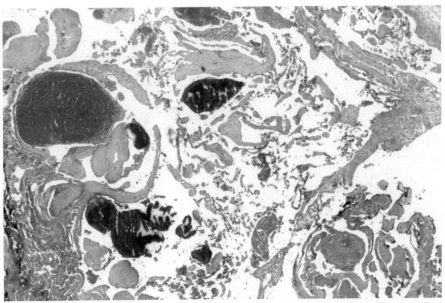

Fig. 10.03 Cavernous haemangioma. Enlarged cystic anastomosing vascular spaces are separated by fibrous septa lined by endothelial cells with non-atypical flattened nuclei. Note the presence of fractured microcalcifications.

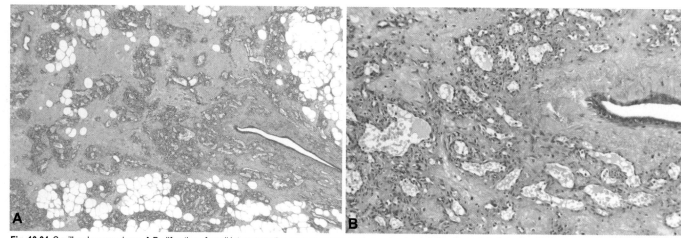

Fig. 10.04 Capillary haemangioma. **A** Proliferation of small interconnecting open or compressed vascular channels lined by endothelial cells with plump non-atypical nuclei. **B** Higher magnification showing congested capillaries arranged in congeries, adjacent to a benign duct.

Genetics

There are no available data on the genetic features of this lesion.

Prognosis and predictive factors

The discovery of a vascular lesion with features of haemangioma on a breast core biopsy should prompt surgical excision to exclude the diagnosis of well-differentiated angiosarcoma.

Angiomatosis

Definition

A diffuse proliferation of benign vessels infiltrating the breast tissue in a contiguous fashion {1154}.

Synonyms

Diffuse angioma

Epidemiology

This is a very rare vascular lesion of the breast with only a handful of case reports published in the literature. Age at

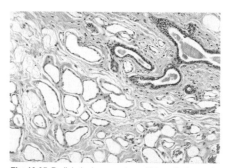

Fig. 10.05 Perilobular haemangioma. Thin-walled vessels lined by flattened endothelium are seen within the perilobular stroma.

presentation varies from birth to 60 years {188}. Most cases have been described in women, although there was a report of this lesion in a male child {1313}.

Clinical features

Lesions present as a mass in the breast with sizes varying from 9 cm to 11 cm {188}. A reticulated appearance or erythematous plaques over the breast, ulceration and tender nodules have been observed with involvement of breast skin {1604}. Massive breast enlargement during pregnancy has been documented {950}.

Macroscopy

Angiomatosis presents as red spongy lesions that can be confused with angiosarcoma.

Histopathology

Microscopically, there is a proliferation of variably-sized anastomosing vascular structures infiltrating the breast interlobular stroma displacing, but not disrupting, the lobular structures, an important feature differentiating these lesions from well-differentiated angiosarcoma {1204}. Angiomatosis can be limited to the breast stroma but can also infiltrate the underlying pectoralis muscle. The vascular channels are lined by thin walls and endothelial cells with no atypical nuclear features or mitoses. Their lumina may be filled with erythrocytes or may be empty. The vascular structures are evenly distributed throughout the lesion.

Genetics

There are no available data on the genetic features of this lesion.

Prognosis and predictive factors

Although angiomatosis is a benign lesion, local recurrences have been described and thus complete excision is commonly performed. Reduction mammoplasty and isotretinoin have been used to treat diffuse dermal angiomatosis of the breast {904, 1517}.

Atypical vascular lesions

Definition

Atypical vascular lesions of the breast are angioformative proliferations that can develop in the skin after breast conserving surgery and radiation therapy for breast cancer, and which may be precursors to angiosarcoma {188,439,867,1079,1475,1563}.

Epidemiology

Patients are women with a mean age of 61 years, who have had previous surgery and radiotherapy for breast carcinoma {1079}.

Clinical features

These atypical vascular lesions present as one or more flesh-coloured, brown or erythematous patches and papules ranging from 1 to 60 mm in size on the breast skin in the radiation field, usually occurring about 6 years after therapy {1079}.

Macroscopy

The skin shows patches, plaques and papules that are flesh-coloured, brown or erythematous.

Histopathology

Atypical vascular lesions are characterized by variably sized and dilated vessels that may anastomose and display complex branching contours, involving the superficial or deep dermis. Extension between bundles of dermal collagen may be seen. Endothelial cells lining these vessels are single-layered and often plump, with prominent nuclei {182,439, 1176}. Some authors have identified two histological types of atypical vascular lesions – lymphatic and vascular {1079}. The lymphatic type consists predominantly of thin-walled, anastomosing lymphatic channels in the superficial dermis, sometimes involving the deep dermis and subcutis. The vascular type comprises irregularly dispersed vessels that are often capillary-sized, affecting the superficial or deep dermis, accompanied by extravasated erythrocytes and haemosiderin. Endothelial atypia with nuclear and nucleolar enlargement can be observed.

Genetics
There are no available data on the genetic features of these lesions.

Prognosis and predictive factors
Reported patients have mostly followed a benign clinical course although recurrent or additional atypical vascular lesions may develop {439,1079}. A very small proportion of patients have developed subsequent angiosarcoma, but the frequency with which this occurs is not well-established {1079}. Women who have undergone surgery and radiation treatment for breast cancer should undergo careful surveillance of the skin of the irradiated breast with a low threshold for biopsy of any abnormal skin lesions {867}.

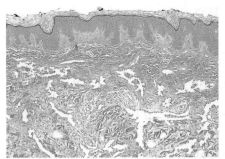
Fig. 10.06 Atypical vascular lesion. The skin shows ectatic branched thin-walled vascular channels in the superficial dermis.

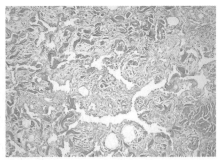
Fig. 10.07 Atypical vascular lesion. The vessels show irregular branching contours interdigitating among collagen bundles.

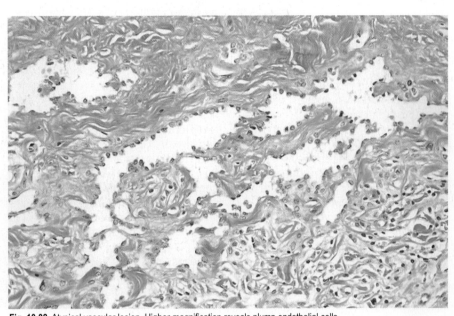
Fig. 10.08 Atypical vascular lesion. Higher magnification reveals plump endothelial cells.

Pseudoangiomatous stromal hyperplasia

M. Michal
S. Badve
S.J. Shin

Definition
A benign lesion comprising stromal myofibroblastic proliferation and having the appearance of anastomosing slit-like pseudovascular spaces lined by spindle-shaped cells {1118,1215, 1535}.

Epidemiology
Pseudoangiomatous stromal hyperplasia (PASH) most commonly occurs in premenopausal females with an average age of 37 years {1118}, but it can be observed in postmenopausal women, paediatric patients {1299} and males {89}.

Etiology
PASH is driven by hormonal imbalances in premenopausal women, and in peripubertal males in whom PASH commonly occurs in gynaecomastia. In addition, use of oral contraceptives is observed in most women with PASH. Well-developed nodular PASH in postmenopausal women is associated with use of hormone-replacement therapy {437}. It is believed that aberrant response of myofibroblasts to endogenous or exogenous hormones is an important factor in its occurrence {1118}.

Clinical features
PASH is a common incidental finding in breast tissue from men and women, mostly appearing as scattered foci in various benign and malignant breast lesions {89}. However, a palpable mass and radiologically detected lesion consisting predominantly or entirely of stromal cells (so-called nodular or tumoriform PASH) has been described rarely {1118}.
Occasionally, PASH exhibits accelerated rapid growth {919,1244,1631} and can occur as bilateral lesions {1121,1331}. In males with gynaecomastia, PASH

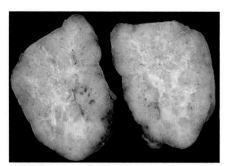

Fig. 10.09 PASH. The lesion is circumscribed with a rubbery, whitish-beige cut surface.

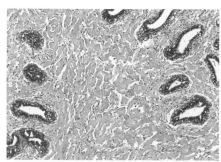

Fig. 10.10 PASH with anastomosing empty slits resembling a vascular neoplasm.

containing giant cells may herald neurofibromatosis type 1 {311, 1620}. PASH can also occur in accessory breast tissue in the axilla and vulva {668}.

Radiographically, PASH presents as a mass without calcification. Ultrasonography reveals a well-defined hypoechoic mass. Magnetic resonance imaging may feature non-mass-like contrast enhancement {661}.

Macroscopy
PASH occurs as sharply circumscribed non-encapsulated, firm to rubbery, homogeneous lobulated nodules that are tan-pink to whitish-yellow in colour on cut section and that range in size from 1 to 12 cm (mean, 6 cm) {1118}.

Histopathology
PASH is a myofibroblastic proliferation intermixed with epithelial elements. The lobular and duct structures are separated by an increased amount of hyalinized stroma. The stromal cells form a complex pattern of empty, often interanastomosing spaces in the densely collagenous stroma. Myofibroblasts with attenuated nuclei rimming the empty spaces resemble endothelial cells. Usually PASH lacks mitotic figures and atypia. There is no destruction of the normal breast tissue, no necrosis and no fat invasion.

Rarely, the myofibroblasts may accumulate in distinct bundles and fascicles in a background of conventional PASH, forming fascicular PASH. The most pronounced examples of this cellular form of PASH are reminiscent of mammary myofibroblastoma. Very rarely, PASH can be accompanied by atypia and hyperchromasia of nuclei and one genuine case of sarcoma arising in PASH is on record {968}.

Myofibroblasts of PASH react with antibodies to vimentin and reveal variable immunoreactivity with antibodies to CD34, actin, desmin, calponin and progesterone receptor. Endothelial cell markers are negative.

PASH must be histologically distinguished from true vascular lesions, in particular angiosarcoma which it mimics {1523}. Unlike PASH, angiosarcoma features anastomosing true vascular spaces lined by malignant endothelial cells.

Genetics
There are no available data on the genetic features of these lesions.

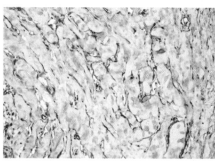

Fig. 10.11 PASH. Immunohistochemistry shows CD34-positive myofibroblasts lining the slit-like spaces.

Prognosis and predictive factors
A recurrence rate of 13–26% has been reported for PASH {520}. Although local recurrence may relate to incomplete excision of nodular PASH, it is possible that residual breast stroma remains susceptible to the same hormonal stimuli, leading to recurrence even after apparently complete removal of the tumour.

Myofibroblastoma

G. Magro
C.D.M. Fletcher
V. Eusebi

Definition
A benign tumour of the mammary stroma composed of fibroblasts and myofibroblasts.

Synonym
Benign stromal spindle cell tumour with predominant myofibroblastic differentiation.

ICD-O code   8825/0

Epidemiology
Myofibroblastoma occurs in women and men aged between 25 and 87 years {853,1416}, occasionally in association with gynaecomastia.

Clinical features
Myofibroblastoma usually presents as a solitary slowly growing nodule {853}. Imaging shows a well-circumscribed, homogeneously solid mass devoid of microcalcifications {540,670,853,1106}. Bilaterality and multicentricity have been observed rarely {540}.

Macroscopy
Myofibroblastoma is usually a well-circumscribed unencapsulated tumour ranging in size from 0.9 to 11 cm {289, 853}, with most cases not exceeding 3 cm {29}.

Histopathology
Myofibroblastoma encompasses a wide morphological spectrum, often resembling spindle cell lipoma {853, 854, 855, 1415}. It is usually composed of spindle to oval cells arranged in short, haphazardly intersecting fascicles interrupted by thick bands of brightly eosinophilic collagen {1554}. Most cases contain a variably prominent adipocytic component. Notably some cases may exhibit high cellularity, atypical cells, infiltrative margins, prominent epithelioid/deciduoid-like cells, and extensive myxoid or fibrous stromal changes {853}. Occasionally,

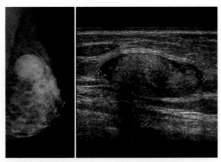

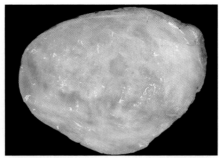

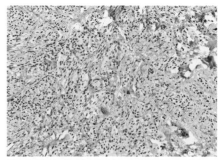

Fig. 10.12 Myofibroblastoma. Mammography (left) reveals a well-circumscribed nodule. Ultrasonography (right) also discloses a well-delineated hypoechoic mass.

Fig. 10.13 Myofibroblastoma. The gross appearance is a well-circumscribed nodule with a yellowish-white cut surface.

Fig. 10.14 Myofibroblastoma. Immunohistochemistry shows nuclear positivity for estrogen receptor, and thus potential diagnostic confusion with an invasive lobular carcinoma.

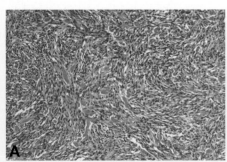

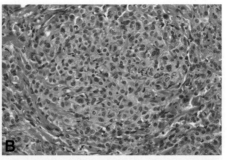

Fig. 10.15 Myofibroblastoma. **A** Classic-type myofibroblastoma showing fascicles of spindle cells, interrupted by thick bands of collagen. **B** Epithelioid cell myofibroblastoma showing plump, medium to occasionally larger cells with obvious nucleoli. Collagen bands are interspersed among neoplastic cells.

smooth-muscle, cartilaginous or osseous metaplasia may be focally evident {465, 858, 1554}. The cells have relatively abundant, pale to deeply eosinophilic cytoplasm with round to oval nuclei each containing one or two small nucleoli. Necrosis is usually absent and mitoses are only rarely observed (up to 2 mitoses per 10 high-power fields, HPF). There is usually no entrapment of mammary ducts or lobules within the tumour.

Immunohistochemistry
The neoplastic cells show variably diffuse staining for desmin and CD34.

There is also variable positivity for alpha-smooth-muscle actin, BCL2, CD99, CD10, hormone (estrogen, progesterone) and androgen receptors {854}. H-caldesmon expression is described in 2–10% of myofibroblastoma cells when there is smooth-muscle differentiation {857}.

Differential diagnosis
Myofibroblastoma should be distinguished from nodular fasciitis, fibromatosis, leiomyoma, spindle cell metaplastic carcinoma {853,906}, and the rare myofibrosarcoma {501,1368,1391}. An epithelioid

cell variant of myofibroblastoma may be confused with infiltrating lobular carcinoma, especially since both tumours express hormone receptors {854}.
Deciduoid features pose another potential diagnostic pitfall {856}. These differential diagnoses are particularly problematic on core biopsies. Myofibroblastoma is considered to be part of the same spectrum as spindle cell lipoma {855}, with which it shares the same chromosomal rearrangements affecting region 13q {858A,1081}.

Genetics
Myofibroblastoma has shown partial monosomy of chromosome 13q in two cases, one of which also showed partial monosomy of chromosome 16q; these findings are identical to those for spindle cell lipoma {1081}. The deletion of chromosome 13q14 in most cases of mammary myofibroblastoma has been confirmed recently by fluorescence in situ hybridization (FISH) {858A}.

Prognosis and predictive factors
Myofibroblastoma shows no tendency for local recurrence.

Desmoid-type fibromatosis

A. Lee
H. Gobbi

Definition
Fibromatosis (desmoid type) is a locally infiltrative lesion without metastatic potential that arises from fibroblasts or myofibroblasts. It can occur within the breast parenchyma, but frequently arises from the pectoral fascia and extends into the breast.

ICD-O code   8821/1

Synonyms
Extra-abdominal desmoid tumour; deep type fibromatosis.

Epidemiology
Mammary fibromatosis is rare, with an incidence of about 0.2% that of mammary carcinoma {356}. It occurs at a wide range of ages and is much more common

in females {1216,1553}. There is an association with previous trauma, particularly surgery, including implants {640,978}.

Clinical features
Patients typically present with a single non-tender palpable mass. Skin retraction or dimpling may be seen {978,1216,1553}. Bilateral cases are uncommon {1216}.

Mammography may show a spiculated mass suspicious for carcinoma, but can be normal {978}. Ultrasonography and magnetic resonance imaging (MRI) appear to be more sensitive for the detection of fibromatosis {978}.

Macroscopy
The typical appearance is of a poorly circumscribed mass of 0.3–15 cm in diameter with a firm white or grey cut surface {978,1216,1553}.

Histopathology
Mammary fibromatosis resembles fibromatosis arising elsewhere. It is composed of long, sweeping and intersecting fascicles of bland spindle cells. A small proportion show nuclear atypia, but this is usually mild {1216,1553}. Most show no mitoses, but a few may be seen. The cellularity may be variable and there can be very collagenous areas. The edge is infiltrative and may invade around normal structures. Lymphocytes are often present at the edge, with follicles occasionally seen. For diagnosis, fine-needle aspiration cytology is typically inadequate, but core biopsy is often possible {978}, facilitating planning of definitive surgery.

Immunohistochemistry
Nuclear expression of beta-catenin is seen in about 80% of cases {9}; however, beta-catenin can also be expressed in spindle cell carcinoma, phyllodes tumours {738} and fibrosarcoma {985}. Expression of beta-catenin appears to be negative in scar and nodular fasciitis {135,223}, although expression in a keloid has been described. In contrast to spindle cell carcinomas, keratin expression is negative {356}. Rarely, weak expression of estrogen receptor is present {333}. Expression of CD34 is absent {770}.

Differential diagnosis
A diagnosis of scar is favoured by the presence of foamy macrophages, foreign body granulomas, fat necrosis or haemosiderin-laden macrophages.
Spindle cell carcinoma, particularly the fibromatosis-like variant {499,1347}, must be excluded by looking for cohesive epithelioid foci (often squamoid), ductal carcinoma in situ and by performing immunohistochemistry using a broad panel of antibodies to keratins, including those of high molecular weight {356}. There is usually at least focal atypia in a spindle cell carcinoma.
Lipomatous myofibroblastoma may resemble fibromatosis with spindle myofibroblasts interdigitating among adipose lobules, but these are usually CD34-positive, whereas fibromatosis is negative for CD34 {356,858}.
Nodular fasciitis usually presents as a tender, rapidly enlarging subcutaneous mass and often contains myxoid stroma and haemorrhage. Occasionally the features of fibromatosis and nodular fasciitis overlap {452}.
Fibrosarcoma is more cellular than fibromatosis, with more cytological atypia and mitoses, and is very rare in the breast.
The presence of epithelial-lined clefts and CD34 expression are useful features for the diagnosis of stroma-predominant phyllodes tumour, which may mimic fibromatosis on core biopsy {356}.

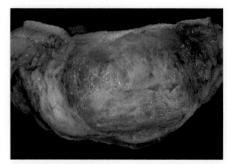

Fig. 10.16 Macroscopic specimen of mastectomy for recurrent fibromatosis, which shows a whitish whorled trabeculated appearance.

Genetics
Deep fibromatosis is clonal {800}. Mammary fibromatoses may arise in patients with familial adenomatous polyposis, but most are sporadic. Activating mutations in the beta-catenin gene are described in 45% of cases and mutations in the adenomatous polyposis coli gene or 5q loss in 33% of cases {9}.

Prognosis and predictive factors
Local recurrence is reported in 20–30% of cases. Recurrence typically occurs within 3 years of diagnosis and there is evidence that it is associated with incomplete excision {978,1216,1553}. Rarely, complete resolution without treatment is described {525}. There are no predictors of response to systemic treatment or radiation.

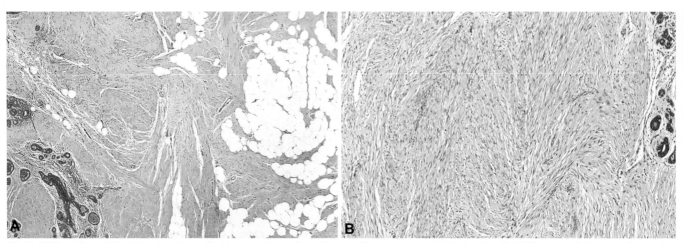

Fig. 10.17 Fibromatosis. **A** Fascicles of spindle myofibroblasts extend into adipose tissue and in between breast lobules (on the left). **B** Higher magnification shows intersecting fascicles of bland spindle cells with narrow, elongated, slightly wavy nuclei.

Inflammatory myofibroblastic tumour

C.D.M. Fletcher

Definition
A usually low-grade neoplasm composed of myofibroblastic spindle cells with prominent admixed inflammatory cells, usually plasma cells.

ICD-O code   8825/1

Synonyms
Inflammatory pseudotumour; plasma cell granuloma

Epidemiology
Inflammatory myofibroblastic tumour (IMT) is principally a tumour of the visceral or soft tissue in children and young adults, although older adults are occasionally affected {277,497}. IMT arising in the breast is very rare and fewer than 20 cases have been reported {534,687}.

Clinical features
IMT in the breast presents as a painless, circumscribed firm mass, usually < 5 cm in diameter. Reported patient age has ranged from 13 to 86 years (median, 46 years) {687}.

Macroscopy
Most cases have been described as a well-circumscribed, firm, white to yellow or grey mass.

Histopathology
These lesions are composed of fascicles of myofibroblasts with pale eosinophilic cytoplasm and ovoid or more tapering nuclei. Atypia is most often minimal. The diagnostic hallmark is the prominent admixed inflammatory infiltrate, most often dominated by plasma cells but occasionally consisting of lymphocytes or neutrophils. By immunohistochemistry, the tumour cells are positive for smooth muscle actin and occasionally for desmin and/or keratin. About 50% of cases are positive for anaplastic lymphoma kinase (ALK), mostly those in young patients.

Genetics
Approximately 50% of cases, mostly those in children and young adults, show rearrangement of the *ALK* (anaplastic lymphoma receptor tyrosine kinase) gene on chromosome 2p23, creating a variety of different fusion genes, most commonly *TPM3-ALK*, and resulting in activation of the ALK receptor tyrosine kinase {497}.

Prognosis and predictive factors
The prognosis for patients with IMT cannot be predicted reliably on morphological grounds, but the majority of lesions are benign with a local recurrence rate of 10–25%, depending on anatomical location. Fewer than 5% of cases of IMT arising at any site metastasize, metastasis being apparently more common in ALK-negative lesions {276}; metastasis from IMT arising in the breast has not yet been reported.

Lipoma

H. Gobbi
P.H. Tan

Definition
A benign tumour composed of mature adipocytes without atypia.

ICD-O code
Lipoma   8850/0
Angiolipoma   8861/0

Epidemiology
Lipomas occur in patients of all ages, most cases being in adults aged 40–60 years {698}.

Clinical features
Lipomas of the breast usually present as asymptomatic, solitary tumours, but multiple lesions may be encountered. They occur as soft, mobile masses, often located in the subcutaneous tissue overlying the breast rather than being deeply seated in the mammary parenchyma {1210,1415}.

Macroscopy
Lipomas are well-circumscribed nodules, with an average diameter of 2.5 cm, but some may exceed 10 cm {328, 1179, 1275}.

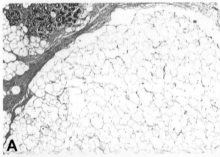
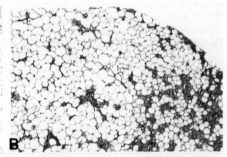

Fig. 10.18 A Histology of a lipoma shows mature adipocytes with a fairly well-circumscribed border separating it from an adjacent breast lobule. **B** Angiolipoma shows well-circumscribed mature adipose tissue incorporating congeries of small capillaries.

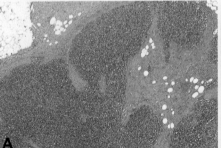
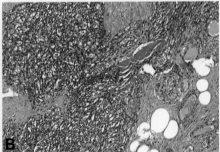

Fig. 10.19 Angiolipoma. **A** Well-circumscribed, partially encapsulated lesion composed of lobular conglomerates of cellular, densely packed congested capillaries, interspersed with broad bands of fibrous stroma. **B** Fibrin thrombi are noted in a few capillary lumina.

Histopathology

Lipomas are composed of mature adipose tissue surrounded by a thin capsule; they are difficult to distinguish from normal breast adipose tissue if a capsule is not detected {759}. Variants include angiolipomas, which are usually painless (unlike the painful angiolipomas of other sites) nodules of mature fat incorporating small vessels containing fibrin thrombi {724,1613}. A rare example of angiomyolipoma has been reported in the breast {310}. Although adenolipoma can microscopically resemble a lipoma, particularly when its fatty component predominates, it is usually classified as a hamartoma. Other variants, such as fibrolipoma, spindle cell lipoma, hibernoma and chondrolipoma, have also been described in the breast {99A,233A,240,855,1050A, 1081,1342,1357A}.

Genetics

Deletion of a limited region within 13q14, distal to the *RB1* locus, is of importance in the development of a subset of lipomatous tumours of soft tissue {305}. Chromosomal rearrangements of 13q and 16q have been reported in spindle cell lipomas {1081}.

Prognosis and predictive factors

Lipomas are essentially benign, and excisional biopsy is adequate treatment.

Granular cell tumour and benign peripheral nerve-sheath tumours

S.B. Fox
A. Lee

Granular cell tumour

Definition

A tumour with eosinophilic granular cytoplasm derived from Schwann cells of peripheral nerves.

ICD-O code   9580/0

Epidemiology

Up to 8.5% of all granular cell tumours arise in the breast {17,197,737}. Granular cell tumours of the breast occur more frequently in females and over a wide age range (17–75 years). Although they can present with coincidental carcinoma, these tumours are almost always benign (> 99%) {737}. Granular-cell changes have been found in association with mastectomy scars {1224}.

Clinical features

Granular cell tumours are usually single, but may be multiple (up to 18%) within the breast or elsewhere {17}. They can appear malignant clinically (irregular and firm mass), radiologically (ill-defined or spiculated lesions without microcalcifications) and pathologically. Granular cell tumours can cause skin retraction, nipple inversion or involve pectoralis fascia.

Macroscopy

These tumours are homogeneous, white or tan in colour, usually well-circumscribed and up to 5 cm in diameter {17, 489}.

Histopathology

Granular cell tumours have an infiltrative growth pattern, being composed of sheets, clusters or cords of round to polygonal cells that have distinct to inconspicuous cell borders, uniform round to oval nuclei, discernible nucleoli and copious, often periodic acid-Schiff (PAS)/diastase-resistant granular cytoplasm. Mitoses are generally scant {197}. Occasionally the collagenous stroma is prominent and granular cells are sparse, which can hinder diagnosis via core biopsy.

Immunoprofile

Granular cell tumours stain strongly and diffusely for S100 protein, and CD68 (lysosomal), with strong expression of PGP 9.5 and focal expression of carcinoembryonic antigen (CEA) and vimentin. Staining for myoglobin, GFAP, lysozyme, and keratins is negative and the Ki67 proliferation index is typically low (< 20%) {197,207,763, 1134}.

Cytopathology

In fine-needle aspiration samples, the granular cytoplasm and bland nuclei are useful features {370,489}, but carcinoma, particularly apocrine, and histiocytic processes must be considered.

Genetics

There are limited data available on the genetic features of granular cell tumours. These tumours have been observed in patients with Bannayan-Ruvalcaba-Riley syndrome {874}, neurofibromatosis type 1 (NF-1) {882}, LEOPARD syndrome {1285A}

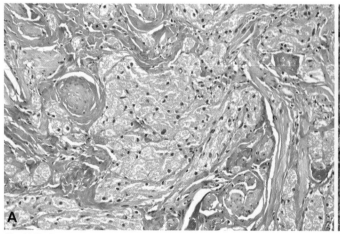
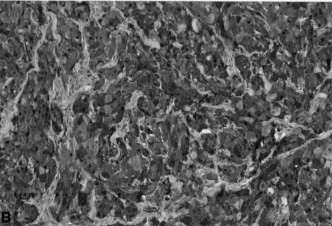

Fig. 10.20 Granular cell tumour. **A** The tumour consists of groups of cells with abundant granular, pale pink cytoplasm and inconspicuous cytoplasmic borders. Nuclei are small and bland. **B** Immunohistochemistry shows diffuse reactivity for S100 protein.

or Noonan syndrome {1149,1319}. Comparative genomic hybridization analysis of granular cell tumours of the central nervous system has shown a variety of genetic changes {1183}; one malignant granular cell tumour showed gains of chromosome 10 and loss of the *CDKNA* (p16) gene {1069}.

Prognosis and predictive factors
Treatment is by wide local excision {197}. The tumour may recur if incompletely excised. Features suggestive of malignancy include large tumour size (> 5 cm), cellular and nuclear pleomorphism, prominent nucleoli, increased mitotic activity, presence of necrosis, and local recurrence {737}.

Benign peripheral nerve-sheath tumours

Definition
A tumour derived from the sheath of peripheral nerves or showing nerve-sheath differentiation.

ICD-O code
Schwannoma	9560/0
Neurofibroma	9540/0

Epidemiology
Peripheral nerve-sheath tumours are common in the skin, including that of breast, but rarely present within the breast parenchyma. They can be benign or malignant and comprise a number of variants, but in the breast are generally neurofibroma or schwannoma (neurilemmoma) {114,812}; there are no reports of perineuroma. Malignant peripheral nerve-sheath tumours have rarely been described {335,420,907,1429,1546}.

Clinical features
Schwannoma and neurofibroma usually present as painless lumps and are more common in females (3 : 1), with an age range of 15–80 years {114,651,812, 957,1546}. Clinically, schwannomas may resemble fibroadenomas {114} and although benign, may mimic malignancy {774}. On imaging, the lesions are usually circumscribed {114}.

Macroscopy
Size ranges from several millimetres to 11 cm {114}.

Histopathology
Histologically, cytologically {1363} and phenotypically, these lesions share the characteristics (including features of malignancy) of benign and malignant nerve-sheath tumours elsewhere in the body.

Genetics
When multiple, schwannomas and neurofibromas are associated with NF-1. The lesions associated with NF-1 are also more likely to undergo malignant change. Periareolar lesions that resemble an accessory nipple in patients with NF-1 are invariably neurofibromas {463A}.

Prognosis and predictive factors
Excision is curative.

Angiosarcoma

C.D.M. Fletcher
G. MacGrogan
S.B. Fox

Definition
A malignant tumour showing endothelial differentiation.

ICD-O code
9120/3

Synonyms
Haemangiosarcoma; lymphangiosarcoma; malignant haemangioendothelioma

Epidemiology
Mammary angiosarcoma can be subdivided into: (i) primary, which arises in the breast parenchyma; and (ii) secondary, which develops in the skin, chest wall or breast parenchyma subsequent to surgery and postoperative radiation for breast cancer.
Primary angiosarcoma is rare, but is the second most common mesenchymal malignancy in the breast, after high-grade/malignant phyllodes tumour, with an incidence of about 0.05% of all primary malignancies of the breast {16}.
Secondary angiosarcoma of the breast

has been diagnosed with notably increasing frequency since the late 1980s, reflecting the trend for breast-conserving surgery with more frequent use of radiation {425,916}. At this anatomical site, angiosarcoma is the commonest type of radiation-associated sarcoma {1607}.

Clinical features
Patients with primary (de novo) angiosarcoma of breast parenchyma are almost exclusively female and aged between 15 and 75 years (median, 40 years) {964, 1218}, with exceptional cases reported in men {517,871}. These tumours are located deep within the breast tissue and present as a painless mass. Approximately 12% of patients present with diffuse breast enlargement. When the tumour involves the overlying skin, a bluish-red discoloration may ensue. Imaging is generally non-distinctive. Occasional cases are bilateral, but this is likely to represent loco-regional metastasis.
Secondary angiosarcoma of the breast

can manifest after radiation therapy in two settings. Firstly, in the chest wall subsequent to radiotherapy following mastectomy for invasive breast carcinoma, with a latent interval of 30–156 months (mean, 84–120 months). These patients are usually older than those with de novo angiosarcoma (range, 60–80 years). In such cases, the neoplastic endothelial

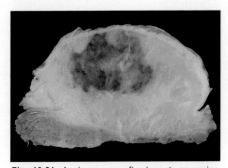

Fig. 10.21 Angiosarcoma after breast-conserving treatment. The spongy, haemorrhagic mass contains occasional solid areas. In this case, the neoplasm involves both the breast parenchyma and the skin.

proliferation is most often located in the skin. Secondly, angiosarcoma can develop in the breast after lumpectomy and radiotherapy for breast carcinoma {139, 182}. The patient age range is broad and, while the median latent interval after radiation is 5–6 years, some cases occur within as little as 2 years. This type of angiosarcoma usually involves the skin only, but occasional cases occur in mammary parenchyma or involve both tissue planes. Many of these lesions are multifocal and may be associated with preceding or synchronous atypical post-radiation vascular proliferation in the breast skin.

Macroscopy
Angiosarcomas vary in size from 1 to 25 cm (average, 5 cm) and often have a spongy haemorrhagic appearance with ill-defined borders. Poorly differentiated tumours may have more solid fibrous-appearing areas.

Histopathology
Morphologically well-differentiated angiosarcomas consist of anastomosing vascular channels that dissect through adipose tissue and lobular stroma. The neoplastic vessels have variably dilated or angulated lumina. The nuclei of the endothelium lining the neoplastic vessels are prominent and hyperchromatic, but mitoses are infrequent and there is usually no endothelial multilayering. Poorly differentiated angiosarcomas are more easily recognized as malignant since anastomosing vascular channels are intermingled with solidly cellular areas with spindled or epithelioid morphology, often with blood lakes, necrotic foci and numerous mitoses. Lesions intermediate between these two groups show endothelial multilayering or papillae, as well as readily identified

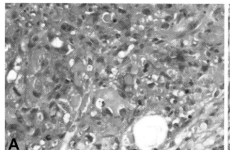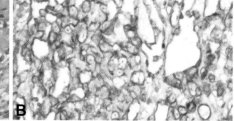

Fig. 10.22 Angiosarcoma after breast-conserving treatment. **A** As in the majority of cases, this is a poorly differentiated angiosarcoma in which vascular channels are difficult to discern. **B** Immunostaining for the endothelial marker CD31 clearly demonstrates the solid areas of endothelial cells with occasional vascular channels.

mitoses, but they lack the solidly cellular areas. Immunohistochemical staining for CD31, CD34 or sometimes podoplanin (D2-40) may be helpful for the diagnosis of poorly differentiated tumours.

The macroscopic and histological features of secondary angiosarcoma are not significantly different from those of primary de novo angiosarcoma, except for the more frequent cutaneous involvement and a somewhat higher proportion of epithelioid and poorly differentiated tumours.

Differential diagnosis
Histological differential diagnoses for well-differentiated angiosarcoma include pseudoangiomatous stromal hyperplasia (PASH), angiolipoma, benign vascular lesions and papillary endothelial hyperplasia. Epithelioid and poorly differentiated angiosarcoma may mimic spindle cell carcinoma and other sarcomas. Adjunctive immunohistochemistry using a panel approach can help to delineate these lesions. It is important to note that keratin may be expressed focally in some angiosarcomas, so this observation should be interpreted in conjunction with information on other markers.

Genetics
Activating mutations in the receptor tyrosine kinase gene *KDR* have been detected in a subset of mammary angiosarcomas, both sporadic and radiation-associated types {53}. Radiation-associated angiosarcomas also show a high level of *MYC* amplification {869}.

Prognosis and predictive factors
Although histological grading in the past was thought to be prognostically important, more recent data with more complete follow-up have shown that, in line with angiosarcomas at other locations, grade has no prognostic value {964} and even morphologically low-grade lesions often metastasize. Metastases occur mainly in the lungs, skin, bone and liver. The axillary lymph nodes are only rarely involved. Median recurrence-free survival is < 3 years and median overall survival is < 6 years.

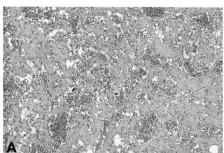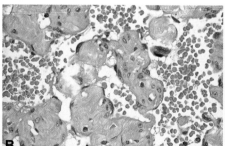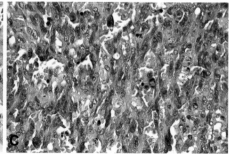

Fig. 10.23 Primary (de novo) angiosarcoma. **A** Morphologically well-differentiated angiosarcoma is composed of complex anastomosing and dissecting vascular channels. The endothelial cells have atypical hyperchromatic nuclei but endothelial multilayering and mitoses are often absent. **B** Higher magnification shows plump endothelial cells with hyperchromatic nuclei lining anastomosing spaces that contain erythrocytes. **C** Poorly differentiated angiosarcoma has a more solid, cellular growth pattern, typically with spindled morphology and more limited formation of vascular channels. There is marked nuclear pleomorphism of malignant endothelial cells with karyorrhexis and mitoses.

Liposarcoma

C.D.M. Fletcher
V. Eusebi

Definition
A malignant soft-tissue tumour showing pure adipocytic differentiation.

ICD-O code   8850/3

Epidemiology
Primary liposarcoma arising in the breast is very rare. Heterologous liposarcomatous differentiation in a malignant phyllodes tumour is a more frequent occurrence. The reported incidence of liposarcoma among sarcomas of the breast varies between 5% and 10% {147, 1427}. This tumour occurs only rarely in the male breast. Liposarcoma developing after radiation therapy for breast carcinoma has been reported {64}.

Clinical features
These tumours occur predominantly in women aged 19–76 years (median, 47 years) {80}. Rarely the tumour is bilateral. Patients present most often with a slowly enlarging, sometimes painful mass.

Macroscopy
Liposarcomas in the breast are often well-circumscribed, but about one third have an infiltrative margin. The mean size for pure liposarcoma was 8 cm (range, 3–19 cm) in the largest reported series {80}.

Histopathology
The histopathology and immunophenotype of liposarcoma of the breast is identical to that of liposarcoma at other sites. Practically every variant of soft-tissue liposarcoma has been reported in the breast. It appears that well-differentiated liposarcoma/atypical lipomatous tumour is most frequent in the primary group, while in malignant phyllodes tumours, heterologous fatty components may be either pleomorphic or well-differentiated {1119}.

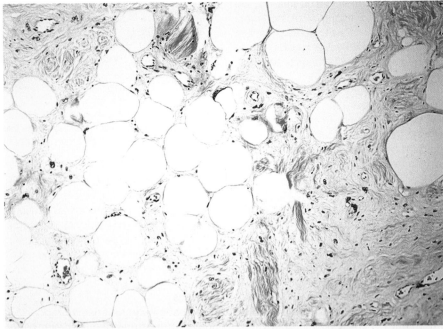

Fig. 10.24 Well-differentiated liposarcoma/atypical lipomatous tumour. Note the variation in adipocyte size and the atypical hyperchromatic nuclei in stromal cells and adipocytes.

If myxoid liposarcoma is detected in the breast, statistical probability would favour this being a soft-tissue metastasis at this site rather than a primary lesion.

Genetics
As at other locations, well-differentiated liposarcoma/atypical lipomatous tumour, and also dedifferentiated liposarcoma, contain supernumerary ring or giant marker chromosomes derived from the long arm of chromosome 12 and characterized by amplification of genes in the 12q14–15 region, principally *MDM2*, *CDK4* and *HMGA2*. Most cases of myxoid liposarcoma have t(12;16)(q13;p11), resulting in *DDIT3-FUS* gene fusion. Rare cases have a t(12;22)(q13;q12). Pleomorphic liposarcoma has a non-specific complex karyotype {1232}.

Prognosis and predictive factors
Well-differentiated liposarcoma of the breast/atypical lipomatous tumour, as at other sites, is generally cured by wide excision with clear margins. Marginal or incomplete excision is associated with a local recurrence rate of 20–30%. In any recurrence, there is a small risk of dedifferentiation and hence acquisition of metastatic potential {913,1416}. Pleomorphic liposarcoma, as at other sites, has a 30–50% risk of distant metastasis, most often to the lung {597}. The behaviour of (exceedingly rare) myxoid liposarcoma arising in the breast is dependent upon cellularity, which determines the grade. Heterologous liposarcomatous differentiation in malignant phyllodes tumours has no evident impact on prognosis or treatment of the phyllodes tumour.

Rhabdomyosarcoma

C.D.M. Fletcher
V. Eusebi

Definition
A malignant tumour composed of cells showing varying degrees of skeletal-muscle differentiation.

ICD-O code
Rhabdomyosarcoma	8900/3
Embryonal type	8910/3
Alveolar type	8920/3
Pleomorphic type	8901/3

Epidemiology
Pure primary rhabdomyosarcoma of the breast is exceedingly rare and occurs mainly in children {563}. Heterologous rhabdomyoblastic differentiation in malignant phyllodes

tumour or metaplastic carcinoma is more frequent and observed in older women, but is still very uncommon {105,457}. Metastatic rhabdomyosarcoma to the breast (most commonly from the limbs, nasopharynx/paranasal sinuses or the trunk) is also more frequent and is usually of alveolar type, affecting children or young adults {563}

Clinical features
The clinical features of this tumour depend on the context, with mass lesions that can be single or multiple, the latter often in the setting of metastasis.

Macroscopy
There are no specific macroscopic features.

Histopathology
True primary rhabdomyosarcoma of the breast is most often of alveolar type {563}. Embryonal rhabdomyosarcoma arising in the breast is exceptionally rare. On occasion, alveolar rhabdomyosarcoma in the breast, whether primary or metastatic, may need to be distinguished from invasive

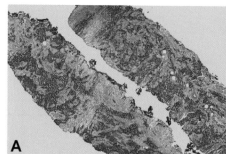
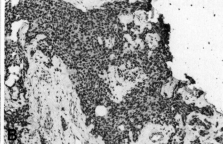

Fig. 10.25 Metastatic rhabdomyosarcoma to the breast. **A** Breast core biopsy showing groups of rhabdomyosarcoma cells with hyperchromatic nuclei and scant cytoplasm. The primary site was in the nasopharynx. **B** Immunohistochemistry shows positive nuclear staining of the tumour cells for MYOD1, reflecting myogenic differentiation.

lobular carcinoma or lymphoma. Heterologous rhabdomyoblastic differentiation in a phyllodes tumour is rare, usually resembling pleomorphic rhabdomyosarcoma {105} and has no particular prognostic significance apart from its presence defining a malignant grade.

Genetics
There have been no specific reports for primary breast rhabdomyosarcoma, but the *PAX3-FOXO1* fusion gene, resulting from a stable reciprocal translocation involving chromosomes 2 and 13, is characteristic of alveolar rhabdomyosarcoma; while embryonal rhabdomyosarcoma features loss of heterozygosity of chromosome 11p {468,811}.

Prognosis and predictive factors
Breast involvement by metastatic rhabdomyosarcoma is usually a sign of widely disseminated disease, with a very poor prognosis {302,601}.

Osteosarcoma

C.D.M. Fletcher
V. Eusebi

Definition
A malignant tumour of soft tissue elaborating osteoid or bone in the absence of any other line of differentiation (e.g. epithelial, fibroepithelial or nerve sheath).

ICD-O code   9180/3

Epidemiology
Accounting for about 12% of all mammary sarcomas, pure osteosarcomas must be distinguished from heterologous osteosarcomatous differentiation in malignant phyllodes tumour or metaplastic carcinoma. In some cases, osteosarcomatous differentiation may involve > 75% of the stroma of a phyllodes tumour and extensive sampling is necessary to establish the correct diagnosis {1416}. Less frequently, the same situation is seen for metaplastic carcinoma, where carcinomatous cells can constitute a very minute component of the whole tumour {392}. Primary osteosarcoma of breast occurs almost exclusively in women with a median age of 64.5 years (range, 27–89 years) {1320}. Occasional cases are related to

prior radiation and, very rarely, skeletal osteosarcoma may metastasize to the breast.

Clinical features
The tumour presents as an enlarging, solitary mass, often in an upper quadrant, which is associated with pain in 20% of cases {1320}. Mammographically, osteosarcoma presents as a well-circumscribed mass with focal to extensive coarse calcification. Because of the usually circumscribed nature of these lesions, they may be misinterpreted as being benign {91}.

Macroscopy
Osteosarcomas vary in size from 1.4 to 13 cm; most are about 5 cm in size and are sharply delineated. The consistency varies from firm to stony hard depending on the proportion of osseous differentiation. Cavitation and necrosis are seen in larger tumours.

Histopathology
Histological features are similar to those of extraosseous osteosarcoma at other

sites of the body. Despite the predominantly circumscribed margins, at least focal infiltration is characteristically present. The tumour is composed of variably pleomorphic spindle or ovoid cells associated with varying amounts of osteoid or osseous tissue; cartilage is present in more than one third of cases {1320}.
Most of the known histological variants of osteosarcoma, including fibroblastic, osteoclast-rich, osteoblastic, and even telangiectatic subtypes, have been reported in the breast.

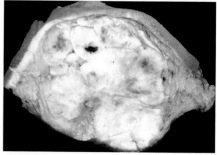

Fig. 10.26 Osteosarcoma. The sectioned surface shows a well-delineated, solid mass with focal haemorrhage.

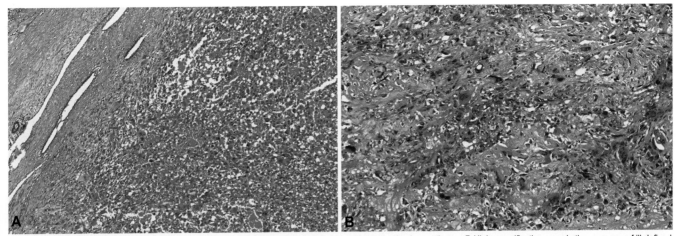

Fig. 10.27 Osteosarcoma. **A** Low magnification shows juxtapositioning of the tumour with adjacent benign breast tissue. **B** High magnification reveals the presence of ill-defined pink osteoid among malignant tumour cells that contain markedly pleomorphic nuclei.

Genetics
Complex genetic alterations have been observed in osteosarcoma, with variable expression of multiple cell-signalling ligands and receptors that include VEGF, IGF, EGF, AKT, PDGF, MAPK, and p70S6 kinase, which may have an impact on prognosis and therapy {5,513}.

Prognosis and predictive factors
Mammary osteosarcomas are highly aggressive lesions with an overall 5-year survival rate of 38% {1320}. Recurrences develop in more than two thirds of patients treated by local excision and in 11% of those treated by mastectomy. Metastases to the lungs and absence of axillary-node involvement are typical of osteosarcomas. Many of the patients who develop metastases die within 2 years of the initial diagnosis {1320}. Large tumour size at presentation, prominent infiltrating margins and necrosis are associated with more aggressive behaviour, while fibroblastic differentiation is said to be associated with a better prognosis.

Leiomyoma and leiomyosarcoma

C.D.M. Fletcher
V. Eusebi

Definition
Leiomyoma and leiomyosarcoma are, respectively, morphologically benign and malignant tumours that show distinct smooth-muscle differentiation.

ICD-O code
Leiomyoma	8890/0
Leiomyosarcoma	8890/3

Epidemiology
Benign and malignant smooth-muscle tumours of the breast are rare and represent < 1% of breast neoplasms. Most occur superficially in the skin, especially around the nipple–areola complex, and these may affect either sex, while deeper parenchymal lesions are extremely infrequent and seem to affect only females {380}. Myofibroblastomas were often mislabelled as (deeper) leiomyomas in the past. Leiomyomas and leiomyosarcomas occur mostly in adults in the fourth and seventh decades of life.

Clinical features
Leiomyoma and leiomyosarcoma both present most often as slowly growing palpable masses that may be painful and tender. Incidental leiomyomas of the nipple may be discovered in mastectomy specimens {965}. The rare deeper lesions are often somewhat larger and otherwise clinically non-distinctive.

Macroscopy
Cutaneous or nipple leiomyomas and leiomyosarcomas tend to be small and range from 0.5 to 1.5 cm in diameter with indistinct margins. The rare leiomyomas located in the breast parenchyma are well-circumscribed and range in size from 1 to 14 cm in diameter {380}. Leiomyosarcoma in breast parenchyma is no different from leiomyosarcoma at other soft-tissue locations and may show necrosis and haemorrhage.

Histopathology
The histology and immunophenotype of these lesions are identical to those of smooth-muscle tumours elsewhere in the body. Dermal or nipple lesions may be well-circumscribed {965}, but more commonly have irregular infiltrative borders {983}. Both are composed of spindle cells arranged in interlacing fascicles. In leiomyoma, cells have elongated cigar-shaped nuclei and eosinophilic cytoplasm with absent or minimal nuclear atypia. Mitoses are sparse. In leiomyosarcoma, nuclear atypia and mitotic activity are more prominent {415}. Tumour necrosis may also be observed. Cutaneous and nipple lesions are almost always immunopositive for smooth-muscle actin and desmin, whereas staining in leiomyosarcomas is less consistent. As many as 40% of smooth muscle tumours are reported to be reactive for keratin and/or epithelial membrane antigen {199,924}.
Smooth-muscle differentiation can also be

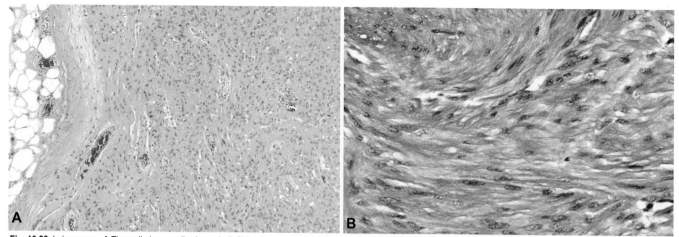

Fig. 10.28 Leiomyoma. **A** The well-circumscribed margin (left) is apparent. **B** The bland smooth-muscle cells proliferate in whorls and fascicles.

seen in the stroma of occasional fibro-adenomas {393,512} and as limited areas in hamartomas {443,1020}. Myofibroblast-oma and spindle cell metaplastic carci-noma need to be distinguished from leiomyoma and leiomyosarcoma.

Genetics
Soft-tissue leiomyosarcomas show mole-cular heterogeneity with reported losses of 16q and and 1p {111}.

Prognosis and predictive factors
Leiomyoma and cutaneous leiomyosarc-oma are best treated by complete excision, whereas mastectomy is appropriate for leiomyosarcoma arising in breast parenchyma {415}. Mammary leiomyosarc-oma does not metastasize to the lymph nodes. No prognostic parameters have been validated for the rare leiomyosarco-mas arising in the breast, but cutaneous les-ions virtually never metastasize.

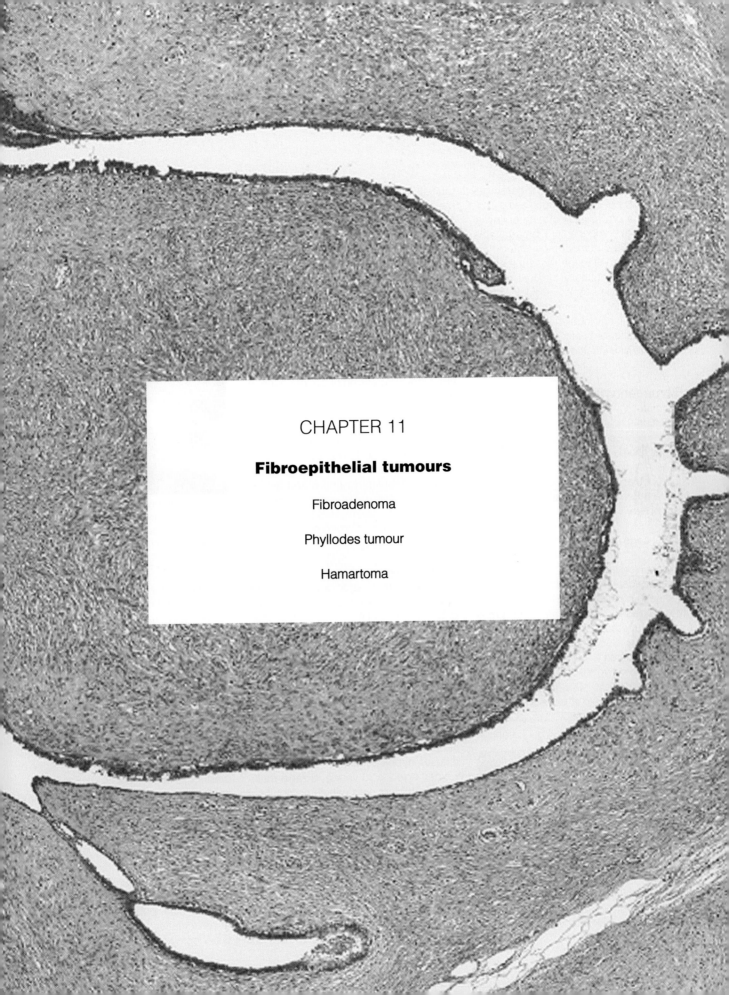

CHAPTER 11

Fibroepithelial tumours

Fibroadenoma

Phyllodes tumour

Hamartoma

Fibroepithelial tumours

P.H. Tan
G. Tse
A. Lee

J.F. Simpson
A.M. Hanby

Fibroepithelial tumours are a heterogeneous group of biphasic neoplasms consisting of a proliferation of both epithelial and stromal components. Fibroadenoma and phyllodes tumours constitute the major entities. Although hamartomas are not strictly fibroepithelial tumours, they resemble neoplasms clinicoradiologically and also have histological similarity to fibroadenomas with incorporation of both stromal and glandular elements; for these reasons they have been included in this chapter.

Fibroadenoma

Definition
A common benign biphasic tumour, the fibroadenoma consists of a circumscribed breast neoplasm arising from the terminal-duct lobular unit (TDLU), and featuring a proliferation of both epithelial and stromal elements.

ICD-O code   9010/0

Epidemiology
The fibroadenoma occurs most frequently in women of childbearing age, especially those aged < 30 years, although it may be encountered at any age.

Clinical features
Fibroadenoma typically presents as a painless, solitary, firm, slow-growing, mobile, well-defined nodule of up to 3 cm in diameter. Less frequently, it may occur as

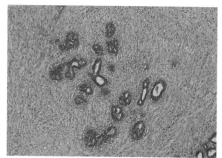

Fig. 11.02 Cellular fibroadenoma shows a pericanalicular growth pattern with a mild and diffuse increase in stromal cellularity.

multiple nodules arising synchronously or metachronously in the same or in both breasts and may grow very large (up to 20 cm), mainly when it occurs in adolescents. With screening mammography, small impalpable fibroadenomas are being discovered as radiological nodular densities or as calcified lesions. An increased likelihood of developing these lesions has been observed in female transplant recipients treated with cyclosporine for immunosuppression {677}, but changing the immunosuppressant may arrest the progression of cyclosporine-induced fibroadenoma {619}.

Macroscopy
Grossly, fibroadenomas are ovoid and well-circumscribed. The cut surface is grey or white, solid, rubbery, bulging, with a slightly lobulated pattern and slit-like spaces. Variations depend on the amount of hyalinization and myxoid change in the stromal component. Calcification of sclerotic lesions is common.

Histopathology
The admixture of stromal and epithelial proliferation gives rise to two distinct growth patterns of no clinical significance. The pericanalicular pattern is the result of proliferation of stromal cells around ducts in a circumferential fashion; this pattern is observed most frequently during the second and third decades of life. The intracanalicular pattern is caused by compression of the ducts into clefts by the proliferating stromal cells. The stromal component may sometimes exhibit focal or diffuse hypercellularity (especially in women aged < 20 years), bizarre multinucleated giant cells (which do not have any biological significance), extensive myxoid changes or hyalinization with dystrophic calcification and, rarely, ossification (especially in postmenopausal women). Myxoid fibroadenomas resembling myxomas have been described in association with Carney syndrome {226}. Foci of lipomatous, smooth muscle, and osteochondroid metaplasia may rarely occur. Mitotic figures are uncommon, but

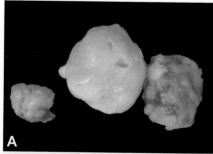

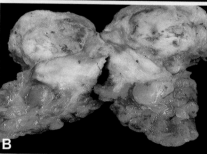

Fig. 11.01 Macroscopic appearance. **A** Fibroadenoma with lobulated contours and a whitish-grey cut surface. **B** Ossified fibroadenoma with yellowish gritty areas representing the bony calcified portions.

may be present, particularly in young or pregnant patients. Total infarction has rarely been reported, although it can occur during pregnancy.

Cellular fibroadenomas, as defined by prominent cellular stroma, may show histological features that overlap with those of benign phyllodes tumour.

The epithelial component of fibroadenoma can show varying degrees of usual ductal hyperplasia, which can be especially prominent in adolescents, and metaplastic changes such as apocrine or squamous metaplasia {730}. Foci of fibrocystic change, sclerosing adenosis and even extensive myoepithelial proliferation can also occur.

"Complex" fibroadenoma contains cysts > 3 mm in size, sclerosing adenosis, epithelial calcifications, or papillary apocrine hyperplasia. It accounts for about 16% to 23% of all fibroadenomas, tending to occur in older patients, with smaller sizes at presentation {358, 1337}. The diagnosis of complex fibroadenoma is reported

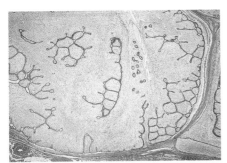

Fig. 11.03 Fibroadenoma with intracanalicular growth pattern.

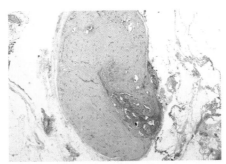

Fig. 11.04 Low-power magnification of a hyalinized fibroadenoma with part of its epithelial component affected by ductal carcinoma in situ.

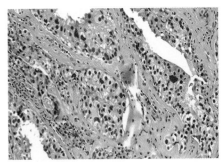

Fig. 11.05 Higher magnification of ductal carcinoma in situ, high nuclear grade, within the hyalinized fibroadenoma.

to be associated with a slightly higher relative risk (3.1 times that of the general population) of subsequent development of breast cancer {358}.

"Juvenile" fibroadenomas occur predominantly in adolescents and are characterized by increased stromal cellularity with a fascicular stromal arrangement, a pericanalicular epithelial growth pattern and usual ductal hyperplasia that often features delicate micropapillary epithelial projections, occasionally described as "gynaecomastoid"-like due to its resemblance to epithelial changes in gynaecomastia. They can sometimes assume enormous sizes, causing breast distortion, and these are referred to by some as "giant" fibroadenomas. However, other authors have restricted the term "giant fibroadenoma" to massive fibroadenomas with usual histology, with sizes often > 5 cm {24,895}.

Atypical ductal or atypical lobular hyperplasia may involve a fibroadenoma, but when confined to the fibroadenoma without involvement of surrounding non-fibroadenoma breast epithelium, the relative risk for subsequent development of breast cancer is apparently not increased {229}. Lobular carcinoma in situ or ductal carcinoma in situ occasionally develops within fibroadenomas. Invasive carcinoma may also affect a fibroadenoma, often as a result of carcinoma in adjacent tissue extending into the fibroadenoma.

Differential diagnosis

Intracanalicular fibroadenoma with increased stromal cellularity closely mimics benign phyllodes tumour, with the distinction based on the finding of well-developed fronds resulting from a markedly exaggerated intracanalicular growth pattern accompanied by stromal cellularity,

usually diffuse, but sometimes accentuated around epithelial clefts, in the phyllodes tumour. Cellular fibroadenomas and benign phyllodes tumours fall into the same spectrum of benign fibroepithelial lesions, sharing similar histological features, with both possessing a low pot-ential for local recurrence {516,999, 1040,1406}. This differentiation is particularly difficult when considering core biopsies, and if the differential diagnosis includes phyllodes tumour, the lesion would be best classified after excision {632,643,771}.

Genetics

Numerical abnormalities of chromosomes 16, 18 and 21 with one case of deletion of 17p have been reported in fibroadenomas {102}. Comparative genomic hybridization did not discover any alterations in DNA copy numbers in 20 fibroadenomas analysed {236}. Clonality studies of fibroadenomas found predominant polyclonality of both epithelium and stroma, although monoclonality was observed in areas of stromal expansion, suggesting stromal progression {729}. The DNA of fibroadenomas is less frequently methylated than that of phyllodes tumours {606}.

Prognosis and predictive factors

Most fibroadenomas do not recur after complete surgical excision. In adolescents, there is a tendency for one or more new lesions to develop at another site or even close to the site of the previous surgical treatment. In one study, fibroadenomas without complex features are not associated with an increase in risk of subsequent development of breast cancer, with presence of these complex features being associated with only a slight increase in relative risk {358}.

Phyllodes tumours

Definition

A group of generally circumscribed fibroepithelial neoplasms, histologically resembling intracanalicular fibroadenomas, characterized by a double-layered epithelial component arranged in clefts surrounded by a hypercellular stromal/mesenchymal component which in combination elaborate leaf-like structures. Phyllodes tumours (PTs) are classified into benign, borderline and malignant categories on the basis of a combination of histological features, including the degree of stromal hypercellularity, mitoses and cytological atypia, stromal overgrowth and nature of the tumour borders/margins. Most PTs are benign, but recurrences are not uncommon and a relatively small number of patients will develop haematogenous metastases, particularly following a diagnosis of malignant PT. Depending on the bland or overtly sarcomatous characteristics of their stromal component, PTs display a morphological spectrum mimicking cellular fibroadenomas and pure stromal sarcomas.

ICD-O code

Phyllodes tumour, not otherwise specified (NOS)	9020/1
Phyllodes tumour, benign	9020/0
Phyllodes tumour, borderline	9020/1
Phyllodes tumour, malignant	9020/3
Periductal stromal tumour, low grade	9020/3

Synonyms

Still widespread in the literature, the generic term "cystosarcoma phyllodes" is currently considered inappropriate and potentially dangerous since most of these tumours follow a benign course and may not display a sarcomatous stroma. It is

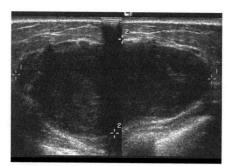

Fig. 11.06 Phyllodes tumour. Ultrasonography shows a relatively well-defined hypoechoic mass with macrolobulations and internal shadows.

highly preferable to use the neutral term "phyllodes tumour", according to the view already expressed in the WHO histological classification of 1981{1599A}, with the prefix of benign, borderline or malignant, as a reflection of putative behaviour based on histological characteristics.

The terms "giant fibroadenoma," "juvenile fibroadenoma" and "cellular fibroadenoma" have sometimes been used inappropriately as synonyms for benign PT; however, these are distinct entities and ought to be separately classified.

Epidemiology

In "Western" countries, PTs account for 0.3–1% of all primary tumours of the breast and for 2.5% of all fibroepithelial

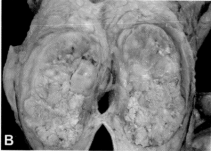

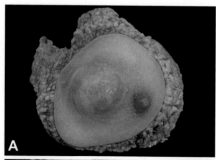

Fig. 11.07 Malignant phyllodes tumour. **A** Right mastectomy with a tumour mass protruding against the skin, located lateral to the nipple. **B** Cut section through the breast mass reveals a fleshy solid beige-coloured tumour with areas appearing whitish and whorled.

tumours of the breast. They occur predominantly in middle-aged women (average age at presentation, 40–50 years) about 15–20 years later than for fibroadenomas. In Asian countries, PTs may occur at a younger age (average age, 25–30 years) {267A}, and account for a higher proportion of primary breast tumours {1404}. Malignant PTs develop on average 2–5 years later than benign PTs. Malignant PT is more frequent among Hispanics, especially those born in Central and South America. Isolated examples of PTs in men have been recorded.

Histogenesis

PTs are thought to be derived from intralobular or periductal stroma. They most likely develop de novo, although there have been reports of progression of fibroadenoma to PT {1009}, with rare cases in which the presence of a pre-existing fibroadenoma adjacent to a PT can be demonstrated.

Clinical features

Usually, patients present with a unilateral, firm, painless breast mass, not attached to the skin. Very large tumours (> 10 cm) may stretch the skin with striking distension of superficial veins, but ulceration is very rare. Owing to mammographic screening, tumours of 2–3 cm in diameter are becoming more common, but the average size remains around 4–5 cm. Bloody nipple discharge caused by spontaneous infarction of the tumour has been described. Multifocal or bilateral lesions are rare {1404}.

Imaging reveals a rounded, usually sharply defined mass containing clefts or cysts and sometimes coarse calcifications {1401,1608}. Intraductal growth with PT projecting into a cystically dilated large duct has been reported on ultrasound imaging {803}.

Macroscopy

PTs form well-circumscribed firm, bulging masses. Because of their often clearly defined margins, they can be "shelled out" surgically. The cut surface is tan or pink to grey in colour and may be mucoid and fleshy. The characteristic whorled pattern with curved clefts resembling leaf buds is best seen in large lesions, but smaller lesions may have a homogeneous appearance. Haemorrhage or necrosis may be present in large lesions.

Histopathology

PTs typically exhibit an enhanced intracanalicular growth pattern with leaf-like projections into variably dilated elongated lumina. The epithelial component consists of luminal epithelial and myoepithelial cells stretched into arc-like clefts surmounting stromal fronds. Apocrine or squamous metaplasia is occasionally present and usual ductal hyperplasia is not rare.

In *benign PTs*, the stroma is usually more cellular than in fibroadenomas. The spindle-cell stromal nuclei are monomorphic and mitoses are rare, usually < 5 per 10 high-power fields (HPF) {1404}. Stromal cellularity may be higher in the zone immediately adjacent to the epithelium, sometimes referred to as peri-epithelial or subepithelial accentuation of stromal cellularity. Areas of sparse stromal cellularity, hyalinization or myxoid changes are not uncommon, reflecting stromal heterogeneity. Necrotic areas may be seen in very large tumours. The presence of occasional bizarre stromal giant cells should not be taken as a mark of malignancy {616}. Benign lipomatous, cartilagenous and osseous metaplasia have been reported. The margins are usually well-delimited and pushing, although very small tumour buds may protrude into the surrounding tissue. Such protrusive expansions may be left behind after surgical removal and are a source of local recurrence.

Malignant PTs are diagnosed when the tumour shows a combination of marked nuclear pleomorphism of stromal cells, stromal overgrowth defined as absence of epithelial elements in one low-power microscopic field containing only stroma, increased mitoses (≥ 10 per 10 HPF), increased stromal cellularity which is usually diffuse, and infiltrative borders. Malignant PTs are also diagnosed when malignant heterologous elements are present even in the absence of other features. Owing to overgrowth of sarcomatous components, the epithelial component may only be identified after examining multiple sections with diligent sampling of the tumour.

Borderline PT is diagnosed when the the tumour does not possess all the adverse histological characteristics found in malignant PTs. While borderline PTs have the potential for local recurrence, they usually do not metastasize.

Any PT that has recognizable epithelial elements may harbour ductal carcinoma in situ (DCIS), lobular neoplasia, or their invasive counterparts, although this is an uncommon finding. Adequate and extensive sampling of all PTs should be performed as the histological features characteristic of higher-grade tumours may be very focal.

Differential diagnosis

The main differential diagnosis for benign PT is fibroadenoma having a pronounced intracanalicular growth pattern, and this distinction is sometimes arguably arbitrary and a matter of judgement. A PT should have more cellular stroma along with the formation of leaf-like processes. The degree of stromal hypercellularity that is required to qualify a PT at its lower limit is difficult to define, but the stromal cellularity should be mostly present throughout the lesion, or closely accompanying the leafy fronds, to qualify as benign PT. Increased stromal cellularity adjacent to epithelium, at the epithelial–stromal interface, is often noticed in PT. Leaf-like processes may be found in intracanalicular fibroadenomas with uniformly hypocellular and oedematous stroma, but they are few in number and often poorly formed. The precise distinction between benign PT and fibroadenoma may be problematic in instances, especially in separating a cellular fibroadenoma from

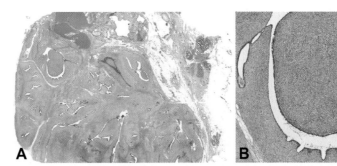

Fig. 11.08 Benign phyllodes tumour. **A** Low-power magnification demonstrating the characteristic leafy architecture with deep epithelium-lined clefts. **B** Higher magnification of a leafy stromal frond capped by epithelium.

a benign PT. As this differentiation may not be significant because of similar clinical outcomes in terms of reported recurrences {516,999,1040,1406}, a diagnosis of fibroadenoma is preferable when there is histological ambiguity, to avoid overtreatment. Some authors advocate using the term "benign fibroepithelial neoplasm", with explanation of the diagnostic difficulty as needed.

Malignant PTs may be confused with pure sarcomas of the breast. In such cases, diagnosis depends on finding residual epithelial structures. However, the clinical impact of these two entities appears to be similar {1626A}.

Periductal stromal tumour (also referred to by some authors as periductal stromal "sarcoma", although the neutral term "tumour" is preferred) is an entity that histologically overlaps with PT, the main

difference being the absence of leaf-like processes. It is non-circumscribed, consisting of a spindle-cell proliferation localized around open tubules. Progression to classic PT has been documented, suggesting that it may be part of the same spectrum of disease {210}.

Metaplastic carcinoma is also in the differential diagnosis, but immunohistochemical demonstration of epithelial differentiation helps resolve the diagnosis, although caution must be exercised in interpreting very focal keratin expression in limited samples {262B}.

Grading

Several grading systems have been proposed, but the use of a three-tiered system, to include benign, borderline, and malignant PT is preferred, because this approach leads to greater certainty at the

Table 11.01 Histological features of fibroadenoma, benign, borderline and malignant phyllodes tumours

Histological feature	Fibroadenoma	Phyllodes tumour		
		Benign	Borderline	Malignant[a]
Tumour border	Well-defined	Well-defined	Well-defined, may be focally permeative	Permeative
Stromal cellularity	Variable, scanty to uncommonly cellular, usually uniform	Cellular, usually mild, may be non-uniform or diffuse	Cellular, usually moderate, may be non-uniform or diffuse	Cellular, usually marked and diffuse
Stromal atypia	None	Mild or none	Mild or moderate	Marked
Mitotic activity	Usually none, rarely low	Usually few (< 5 per 10 HPF)	Usually frequent (5–9 per 10 HPF)	Usually abundant (≥ 10 per 10 HPF)
Stromal overgrowth	Absent	Absent	Absent, or very focal	Often present
Malignant heterologous elements	Absent	Absent	Absent	May be present
Distribution relative to all breast tumours	Common	Uncommon	Rare	Rare
Relative proportion of all phyllodes tumours	—	60–75%	15–20%	10–20%

HPF, high-power fields.

[a] While these features are often observed in combination, they may not always be present simultaneously. Presence of a malignant heterologous element qualifies designation as a malignant phyllodes tumour, without requirement for other histological criteria.

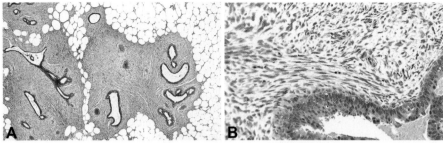

Fig. 11.09 Periductal stromal tumour, low grade. **A** An infiltrative hypercellular spindle cell proliferation surrounds ducts with open lumina. **B** At higher magnification, the neoplastic spindle cells contain at least 3 mitotic figures per 10 HPF.

ends of the spectrum of these fibroepithelial lesions. Grading is based on semi-quantitative assessment of stromal cellularity, cellular pleomorphism, mitotic activity, tumour margin/border appearance and stromal distribution/overgrowth.

The histological features used to distinguish benign, borderline, and malignant PT should be considered together, because emphasizing an individual feature may result in over-diagnosis, especially in the case of mitotic activity. Because of the structural variability of PTs, the selection of one block for every 1 cm of maximal tumour dimension is appropriate. Moreover, because the interface with normal breast tissue is critically important, histological examination of this area is essential. In rare examples, adjacent fibroadenomatoid change or periductal stromal hyperplasia can be difficult to distinguish from the infiltrative border of a phyllodes tumour. PTs should be graded according to the areas of highest stromal cellular activity and most florid architectural pattern. Since the size of HPFs is variable among different microscope brands, it has been suggested that the mitotic count be related to the size of the field diameter (×40 objective and ×10 eyepiece, 0.196 mm^2). Stromal overgrowth has been defined as stromal proliferation to the point where epithelial elements are absent in at least one

low-power field (×4 objective and ×10 eyepiece, 22.9 mm^2) {1404}. Several biological markers, including p53, Ki67, CD117, EGFR, VEGF, microvessel density {1405, 1461,1462,1462A}, p16, pRb and HOXB13 {267, 679A}, among others, have been reported to show increasing expression with PT grade, although these molecular markers have not as yet been proven to be of clinical utility.

As the histological features of PTs fall within a continuum, some of these lesions are difficult to grade precisely. Since malignant PTs are those most likely to cause metastasis and death, it is important to identify this group. So-defined, one study revealed that malignant PTs are associated with a metastatic and death rate of 22%, while no distant metastases were seen in borderline and benign PTs over the same duration of follow-up {1406}. Strict histological criteria for diagnosing malignant PT should be used in order to avoid overtreatment.

Genetics

Benign and borderline PTs are a paradigm of epithelial–stromal cross-talk, with the epithelium influencing stromal growth, e.g. via the Wnt signalling pathway, upregulation of transcriptionally active beta-catenin and downstream effectors such as cyclin D1 {644,656,657,1270}. The stroma in turn is

able to influence the epithelium, e.g. via *IGF* and *IGFR1* {656}. Evidence for loss of this feedback mechanism is given by loss of nuclear beta-catenin in many malignant PTs, some of which show heterogeneous, extensive cytogenetic abnormalities including amplification of *MYC* and aberrant expression of *TP53* {1271,1405}.

Other described cytogenetic changes include gains in chromosome 1q and losses at chromosome 13, reported to be associated with malignant progression {741}, with an increasing number of chromosomal abnormalities with increasing tumour grade {50}. Preliminary data from array comparative genomic hybridization (CGH) demonstrate interstitial deletion of 9p21 involving the *CDKN2A* locus and 9p deletion in malignant and some borderline PTs {657}.

Prognosis and predictive factors

Most PTs behave in a benign fashion, with local recurrences occurring in a small proportion of cases. Very rarely (about 2% or less overall), the tumour may metastasize, mainly in the cases of tumours of malignant grade. Local recurrences can occur in all PTs, at an overall rate of 21%, with ranges of 10–17%, 14–25% and 23–30% for benign, borderline and malignant PTs, respectively. These recurrences may mirror the microscopic pattern of the original tumour or show dedifferentiation with microscopic upgrading (in 25–75% of cases) {1400,1406}.

Many histological features have been reported to possess predictive value for local recurrences in PT, and status of surgical margins at previous excision appears to be the most reliable. Other less consistent predictors include stromal overgrowth, classification/grade and necrosis {106,1404}. A recent study found that, apart from surgical margins, histological parameters that had an independent impact on recurrence were stromal overgrowth and atypia, with mitotic activity being almost significant {1406}.

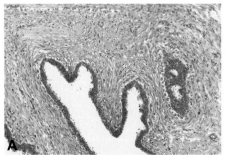
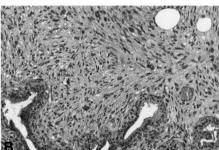
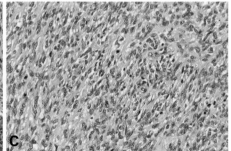

Fig. 11.10 Phyllodes tumour. **A** Stromal cellularity is accentuated in the peri-epithelial zones of a borderline phyllodes tumour. **B** Malignant phyllodes tumour shows marked pleomorphism of stromal cells. **C** Brisk mitotic activity is observed in the stromal cells of a malignant phyllodes tumour.

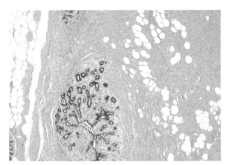

Fig. 11.11 A hamartoma showing a rounded border, inter-lobular fibrosis and a fibroadipose stroma.

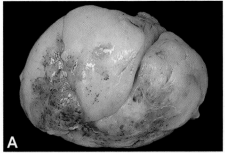

Fig. 11.12 Adenolipoma. **A** Macroscopic appearance of adenolipoma shows a well circumscribed, slightly lobulated fatty tumour with fibrous areas. **B** Histology shows mature adipose tissue with admixed breast lobules.

Distant metastases, seen almost exclusively in malignant PTs, have been reported in nearly all internal organs, but the lungs and skeleton are the most common sites of spread {1289,1406}. Most metastases consist of stromal elements only. Axillary lymph-node metastases are rare, but have been recorded {434,551}.

Local recurrences generally develop within 2–3 years, while most deaths from tumour occur within 5–8 years of diagnosis {76A, 324A}, sometimes after mediastinal compression through direct chest-wall invasion.

Hamartoma

Definition
A well-demarcated, generally encapsulated mass composed of all breast-tissue components.

Epidemiology
Hamartomas comprise 4.8% of benign breast tumours {247}. These lesions occur predominantly in women in their 40s, but may be found at any age, from teenagers to women in their 80s.

Clinical features
Hamartoma may present as a soft palpable mass {569,1460} or be asymptomatic and detected by mammography {319, 1538}. Imaging shows a circumscribed rounded mass, sometimes with intralesional heterogeneous echogenicity on ultrasonography {145}.

Owing to their well-defined borders, hamartomas are easily enucleated.

Macroscopy
Hamartomas are round or oval, measuring up to 20 cm in diameter. The cut surface may resemble normal breast tissue, lipomas or fibroadenomas.

Histopathology
Generally encapsulated, hamartomas are lobulated and show ducts, lobules with interlobular fibrous tissue and adipose tissue in varying proportions. Pseudoangiomatous stromal hyperplasia and smooth muscle may be present {247, 443, 1460}. Both the epithelial and stromal components may express hormone receptors {569}. Differentiation of hamartomas from fibroadenomas may be difficult on needle biopsy and is often impossible on fine-needle aspiration {570, 1460}. The adenolipoma is considered a hamartoma as it incorporates normal breast ducts and lobules within adipose tissue {662A}.

Genetics
Hamartomas can be seen in Cowden syndrome {1286}. Genetic data are limited, but aberrations involving chromosomal regions 12q12–15 and 6p21 have been described {306,1197}.

Prognosis and predictive factors
Hamartoma is benign and recurs rarely {1460}.

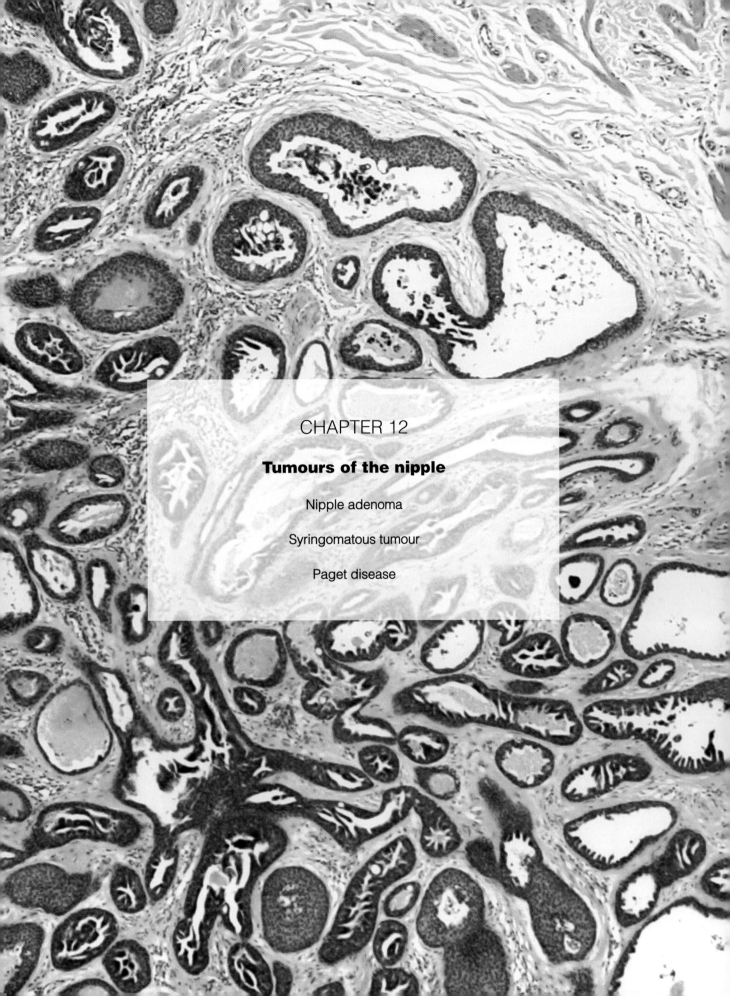

CHAPTER 12

Tumours of the nipple

Nipple adenoma

Syringomatous tumour

Paget disease

Nipple adenoma

V. Eusebi
S. Lester

Definition
A benign epithelial proliferation localized within and around the collecting ducts.

ICD-O code   8506/0

Synonyms
Nipple duct adenoma; papillary adenoma of the nipple; erosive adenomatosis; florid papillomatosis; papillomatosis of the nipple.

Epidemiology
Nipple adenoma is found in < 1% of breast specimens {1093}. Patient age ranges from 20 to 87 years (average, 43 years) {1424}. One case in a female infant aged 5 months has been reported {274}. Fewer than 5% of nipple adenomas affect males {1153,1212}.

Clinical features
About two thirds of patients present with nipple discharge and one third with either nipple erosion or a nodule {1093}. The duration of symptoms is extremely variable and may be up to 15 years {1414}. The clinical impression of Paget disease is frequent.

Macroscopy
There may be no macroscopic abnormalities although a mass lesion or nipple erosion may be seen.

Histopathology
Several morphological lesions (of which some overlap) characterize nipple adenoma {1416}. In the most common type, sclerosing adenosis, proliferating glands sprout from and compress collecting ducts, which then undergo cystic dilatation resulting in a discrete nodule on palpation. Rarely, the adenosis expands to cause erosion of the epidermis. The tubules present within the sclerosing adenosis are composed of luminal and myoepithelial cells.

When a pseudoinfiltrative pattern is prominent, the proliferating epithelium streams into the stroma featuring "infiltrating epitheliosis" {84,397}.

In the epithelial hyperplasia type, usual duct hyperplasia (florid epitheliosis) is mainly located within the collecting ducts. Sometimes the proliferation has a polypoid pattern resulting in the enlargement of the galactophore (lactiferous duct) ostia and exposure of the epithelial proliferation to the exterior in a fashion reminiscent of "ectropion" of the uterine cervix {1416}. Necrosis may be observed {347}. Toker cells are sometimes increased in number {1416} and, in the context of clinical skin changes, can easily be mistaken for Paget disease {866}.

Genetics
There are no molecular data on nipple adenoma per se. The molecular data on proliferative preinvasive disease are discussed in the genetics sections for individual subtypes of the proliferation, e.g. hyperplasia of usual type.

Prognosis and predictive factors
Nipple adenomas are benign lesions that may recur if incompletely excised, hence the ideal, but cosmetically unpleasant, treatment is removal of the lesion {1215}. Overall, twenty-four of 173 cases (14%) of nipple adenoma have been reported to be associated with carcinoma in the literature {1212}. The carcinoma is most often present at the time of excision, but can also develop later in the same area {663}.

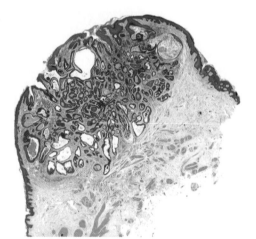
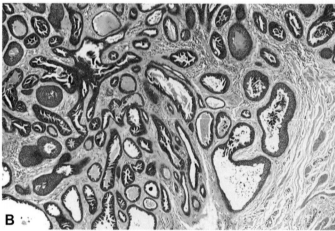

Fig. 12.01 Nipple adenoma. **A** A compact aggregate of tubules replaces the nipple stroma. **B** There is no significant proliferation in many of the tubules in this case.

Syringomatous tumour

V. Eusebi
S. Lester

Definition
Syringomatous tumour (SyT) is a non-metastasizing, locally invasive tumour of the nipple/areolar region that shows sweat-duct differentiation. Although originally named "syringomatous adenoma" {1202}, "syringomatous tumour" is favoured owing to the invasion into stroma and occasional local recurrence exhibited by these lesions {1416}.

ICD-O code   8407/0

Synonyms
Syringomatous adenoma of the nipple; infiltrating syringomatous adenoma of the nipple.

Epidemiology
Patients diagnosed with this lesion are aged between 11 and 67 years (average, 40 years).

Clinical features
SyT presents as a firm discrete mass (diameter, 1–3 cm) situated in the nipple and subareolar region and limited to the dermis {662}.

Macroscopy
The lesion appears grossly as a firm, ill-defined, dermal nodule.

Histopathology
SyT consists of nests and branching cords of cells, glandular structures and small keratinous cysts containing well-developed lamellar keratin. The proliferating epithelium surrounds the galactophore (lactiferous) ducts and penetrates the smooth muscle of the nipple and can be seen in perineural spaces. The margin of the lesion is difficult to assess because foci of tumour can be present at a great distance from the main tumour with intervening normal tissue.

Most of the tumour cells have a bland appearance with scant eosinophilic cytoplasm and regular round nuclei. The cells lining the gland lumina are cuboidal or flat. Frequently, the glandular structures display inner luminal and outer cuboidal basal cells that may occasionally contain smooth muscle actin. Mitoses are rare and necrotic areas are absent. The stroma is usually sclerotic, but myxoid areas containing spindle cells are frequent.

SyT must be distinguished from low-grade adenosquamous carcinoma and tubular carcinoma {1038,1416}.

Genetics
There are no available data on the genetic features of these lesions.

Prognosis and predictive factors
Five out of eleven lesions (45%) reported by Jones et al. {662} recurred between 1.5 months to 4 years after diagnosis, but no metastases developed. Optimal treatment is excision with generous margins.

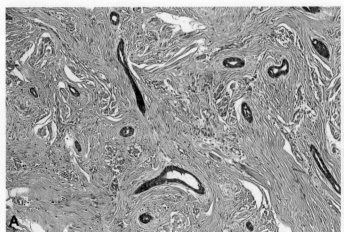 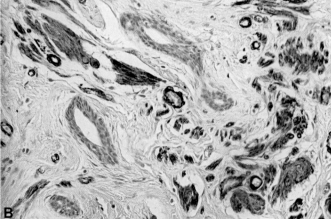

Fig. 12.02 Syringomatous tumour of the nipple. **A** Irregularly shaped glandular structures are present between smooth muscle bundles. **B** Immunostaining for actin delineates the fascicles of smooth muscle but the syringomatous tumour is unstained.

Paget disease of the nipple

S. Shousha
V. Eusebi
S. Lester

Definition
A breast cancer characterized by the presence of malignant glandular epithelial cells (Paget cells) within the squamous epithelium of the nipple that may extend into the areola and adjacent skin. It is usually associated with underlying carcinoma, which is mostly high-grade invasive carcinoma of no special type (53–60%) or ductal carcinoma in situ (DCIS) (24–43%) that can be central, peripheral or multicentric. Paget disease of the nipple (PD) without underlying carcinoma is rare, with a reported incidence of 1.4–13% of all PD cases {217,251,718, 1334}.

ICD-O code   8540/3

Epidemiology
PD represents 1–4% of all breast cancers {249,307}. It can be bilateral and affects men as well as women. The age range is 27–88 years (mean, 54–63 years). Between 20% and 30% of patients are premenopausal. There are published data suggesting that the incidence of PD associated with underlying carcinoma has decreased since 1988 {251}.

Etiology
There are two main theories as to the origin of PD. The first postulates that Paget cells originate in underlying or intraepidermal lactiferous or deeper ducts, then migrate into the epidermis. The second theory implicates Toker cells as precursors of Paget cells {887}, particularly in cases not associated with an underlying DCIS. Toker cells are benign cells present within the nipple epidermis, adjacent to duct orifices. They are seen in about 10% of haematoxylin and eosin (H&E)-stained nipple sections, and in > 80% of sections stained for keratin 7. They resemble Paget cells in having a clear cytoplasm and being positive for keratin 7 and CAM5.2, but differ from Paget cells in lacking malignant nuclear features and in being HER2-negative. Toker cells are usually scattered singly, but can occur in clusters {339,1007}, show nuclear atypia {339} and occasionally form glands {1446}.

Clinical features
Most patients (85–98%) present with eczematous or erythematous changes of the nipple. There may be also nipple discharge, bloody or non-bloody, ulceration or inversion. A prolonged period of symptoms, sometimes extending to 1 year or more, is common in up to one third of patients {307}. The presence of a palpable mass in the breast usually indicates an underlying invasive carcinoma. Mammography reveals malignant suspicious abnormalities in 32–49% of cases {307,718, 1618}. Magnetic resonance imaging (MRI) identifies lesions that may not be visible by conventional imaging {1334}. Subclinical PD, discovered incidentally after mastectomy for invasive carcinoma, represented 15% of cases of PD in one series {709}. PD can also be the presentation of a recurrence in the breast {1318}.

Macroscopy
The nipple may appear normal, or there may be redness, scaling, crusting or frank ulceration that may extend into the areola and adjacent skin.

Histopathology
Preoperative diagnosis is established by a punch biopsy. The histological hallmark of the disease is the presence of Paget cells within the epidermis. These are large cells with abundant pale stained cytoplasm and large nuclei with prominent nucleoli. They may be present singly in the peripheral and superficial parts of the lesion, or occur in closely packed clusters within the lower parts of the epidermis. Rarely, they may form glandular structures at the dermo-epidermal junction {1315,1445}. Paget cells contain mucin in 40% of cases {1516} and may contain melanin pigment as a result of phagocytosis. Three histological variants are recognized: classical, bowenoid and pemphigus-like {1416}. Rare cases of PD invading the dermis have been described. Axillary lymph-node metastases are detected in 26–59% of patients with underlying invasive or microinvasive carcinoma and in none with underlying DCIS {217,1334}.

Immunoprofile
Paget cells are almost always positive for keratin 7 and CAM5.2, and positive for HER2 in 80–90% of cases {133,1294}. Estrogen and progesterone receptors are expressed in about 40% and 30% of cases, respectively {217,307}. Carcinoembryonic

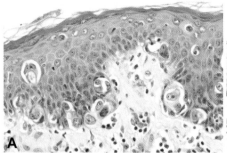 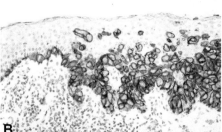 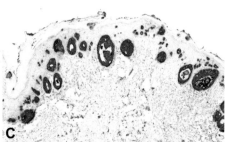

Fig. 12.04 Paget disease of the nipple. **A** Nipple epidermis containing Paget cells with pale stained cytoplasm and large irregular nuclei with prominent nucleoli. **B** HER2 immunostaining showing strong positive membrane staining of Paget cells. **C** Glandular Paget disease showing positive immunostaining for keratin 7.

antigen (CEA), epithelial membrane antigen (EMA), GCDFP-15 and p53 are positive in about 50% of cases. The underlying carcinoma usually has the same immuno-profile as PD.

Differential diagnosis

This includes malignant melanoma and Bowen disease of the skin. Both are negative for keratin 7. Malignant melanoma is positive for S100 protein, which is negative in PD and Bowen disease. Paget cells also have to be distinguished from Toker cells, as described above, and from breast carcinoma invading the skin and nipple from behind.

Genetics

In a series of 86 cases of PD, 8 out of 74 patients with known family hisory (11%) had a first-degree relative with breast cancer {1618}. No association with a specific gene mutation has been reported. Paget cells are genetically similar to the underlying carcinoma cells in 80% of cases {946}.

Prognosis and predictive factors

The prognosis depends on the presence or absence of an underlying carcinoma and on the stage of the disease. Reported 5-year recurrence-free survival is 75–90% for cases associated with DCIS and 63–75% for cases associated with invasive carcinoma. The 5-year overall survival is 94–98% in the presence of DCIS and 73–93% in the presence of invasive carcinoma {217,1334}.

CHAPTER 13

Lymphoid and haematopoietic tumours

Diffuse large B-cell lymphoma

Burkitt lymphoma

T-cell lymphoma

Extranodal marginal zone lymphomas of
mucosa-associated lymphoid tissue (MALT lymphoma)

Follicular lymphoma

Lymphoid and haematopoietic tumours

Introduction

N.L. Harris
E.S. Jaffe

General features

Lymphoma may arise in the breast as a primary tumour, while systemic lymphomas may involve the breast secondarily {65,192,893}. Primary lymphoma of the breast is often defined as a tumour limited to the breast and regional lymph nodes in a patient with no prior history of lymphoma {1425,1590}. However, it has also been suggested that primary lymphoma of the breast should be defined in the same way as other extranodal lymphomas: initial presentation with the dominant mass or symptom in the extranodal site in a patient without a prior history of lymphoma elsewhere, even if distant involvement is discovered at staging {202, 609,864,893,1396}. The lymphoma should be seen in close proximity to breast tissue, not confined to an intramammary lymph node.

Clinical features

Primary lymphomas of the breast are rare and have been estimated to comprise < 0.5% of primary breast tumours {1590}. Most patients are postmenopausal women, although younger patients have been reported, including pregnant or lactating women presenting with massive bilateral breast swelling due to Burkitt lymphoma {864,1301}. There is at least one case report of lymphoma of the breast in a man {1263}.

Patients usually present with a painless lump, which may be multinodular, and is bilateral in approximately 10% of cases. Occasional cases are asymptomatic and detected by imaging studies {806,1080}. Regional lymph nodes are involved in up to 50% of cases {893}. Treatment and prognosis depends on the specific histological type of lymphoma {883,1243}. Relapses in all histological subtypes are often extranodal.

Histopathology

Lymphomas of the breast most commonly appear as well-circumscribed tumours of varying size; on cut surface, the neoplastic tissue is similar to that of lymphomas in other sites, fleshy tan-white, with occasional haemorrhagic or necrotic foci in higher-grade tumours. Although grossly circumscribed, the majority of breast lymphomas have an infiltrating border, with permeation around lobules and ducts.

The majority of primary breast lymphomas in most series fall into the category of diffuse large B-cell lymphoma, not otherwise specified (DLBCL) {470,1388,1396,1482}, with the remainder including predominantly extranodal marginal-zone lymphoma of mucosa-associated lymphoid tissue (MALT) type and follicular lymphoma {470,488,609,883,893,1180,1396}. Rare cases of Burkitt lymphoma, lymphoblastic lymphoma of either B-cell or T-cell type, and peripheral T-cell lymphomas are reported, the latter including anaplastic large-cell lymphoma, anaplastic lymphoma kinase (ALK)-negative, and associated with breast implants {321,801,1193, 1592}.

Diffuse large B-cell lymphoma

E.S. Jaffe
L.J. Medeiros

ICD-O code   9680/3

Epidemiology

Diffuse large B-cell lymphoma (DLBCL), not otherwise specified, is the most common type of lymphoma presenting in the breast, accounting for approximately 50–65% of all breast lymphomas {470,1396, 1482}.

Histopathology

Histologically, DLBCL is composed of a diffuse infiltrate of large lymphoid cells re not a prominent feature. There may be preferential involvement of lobular structures, imparting a nodular or pseudofollicular appearance. Adjacent breast tissue may show evidence of lymphocytic mastopathy.

Immunoprofile

By immunohistochemistry, DLBCL of the breast has a mature B-cell phenotype, expressing CD20, CD79a, and PAX5. A higher proportion of cases appears to have an activated B-cell phenotype than a germinal-centre B-cell phenotype, when examined by immunohistochemistry and

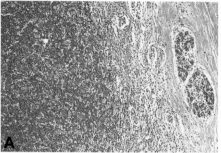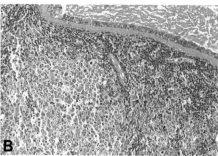

Fig. 13.01 Diffuse large B-cell lymphoma. **A** Medullary carcinoma-like appearance. **B** Neoplastic lymphoid cells infiltrate to the duct but do not invade the duct.

classified according to the Hans algorithm {550,1610}.

Prognosis and predictive factors

Most patients present with unilateral disease, but there is a risk of recurrence in the opposite breast. Patients are also more likely to relapse with disease in other extranodal sites, suggesting that DLBCL of the breast may have distinctive features {1243}. Relapse involving the central nervous system is seen in approximately 5–10% of patients. The breast may also be a site of involvement in patients with disseminated disease {1396}.

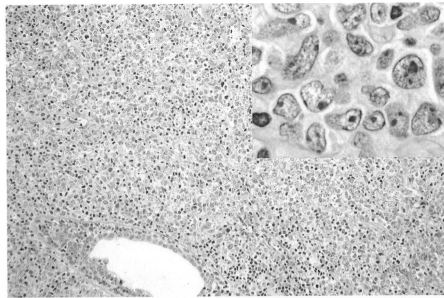

Fig. 13.02 Diffuse large B-cell lymphoma. Sheets of large lymphoid cells displace normal elements and surround residual duct. Inset shows atypical lymphoid cells with features of centroblasts, having peripherally-placed basophilic nucleoli.

Burkitt lymphoma

E.S. Jaffe
L.J. Medeiros

ICD-O code   9687/3

Clinical features

Burkitt lymphoma (BL) is characterized by three clinical variants: endemic BL, sporadic BL and immunodeficiency-associated BL {192}.
Presentation of BL in the breast is most common in endemic BL. Sporadic BL uncommonly involves the breast {852}. Patients are usually pregnant or lactating women, but presentation during puberty is also seen. Patients present with massive bilateral breast swelling, rather than discrete tumour masses, as more often seen in diffuse large B-cell lymphoma (DLBCL). The presence of Epstein-Barr virus (EBV) sequences correlates with the clinical variant, being most common in endemic BL (> 95%) and less frequent in sporadic BL (15–25%).

Histopathology

The histological features of BL of the breast are identical to those seen at other anatomical sites. The tumour is composed of sheets of uniform, medium sized cells, with round nuclei, multiple basophilic nucleoli, coarse chromatin and a rim of basophilic cytoplasm, best observed in Wright–Giemsa-stained smears

{522}. Cytoplasmic lipid vacuoles can be observed in touch imprints. Mitoses are very numerous. Numerous tingible-body macrophages produce a "starry sky" pattern. The breast tissue usually shows evidence of secretory activity.

Immunoprofile

By immunohistochemistry, BL has a mature B-cell phenotype, expressing CD20, CD79a, and PAX5. Staining for CD10 and BCL6 is positive and BCL2 is negative. The proliferation rate as measured by Ki67 is virtually 100%. Terminal deoxynucleotidyl transferase (Tdt) is negative. EBV sequences are detected by EBV-encoded RNA (EBER) in situ hybridization.

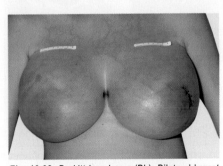

Fig. 13.03 Burkitt lymphoma (BL). Bilateral breast involvement may be the presenting manifestation during pregnancy and puberty. BL cells have prolactin receptors.

LMP-1 is negative, as BL has a latency I pattern when EBV is positive, and does not express the other EBV latency proteins.

Genetics

BL cells have translocations involving the *MYC* gene and one of the immunoglobulin genes, most often *IGH@*, and less often *IGK@* or *IGL@*.

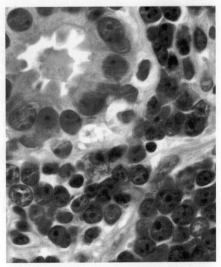

Fig. 13.04 Burkitt lymphoma involving the breast in a pregnant woman. Neoplastic cells diffusely infiltrate the breast tissue. Note evidence of secretion in duct.

T-cell lymphoma

E.S. Jaffe   L.J. Medeiros
N.L. Harris

ICD-O code
Anaplastic large cell lymphoma, anaplastic lymphoma kinase-negative   9702/3

Epidemiology
T-cell lymphomas rarely involve the breast as a primary site, but can secondarily involve the breast as part of disseminated disease. In one study the most common types of T-cell lymphoma to involve the breast were anaplastic large cell lymphoma (ALCL), either positive or negative for anaplastic lymphoma kinase (ALK), in patients with a history of systemic or cutaneous ALCL {316, 926}, peripheral T-cell lymphoma, not otherwise specified, and T-lymphoblastic leukaemia/lymphoma. In most of these cases, the patients had widely disseminated disease. Rare cases of subcutaneous panniculitis-like T-cell lymphoma have been reported {1287}, but the differential diagnosis with lupus mastitis can be challenging {697}.

A series of individual case reports and small series have described ALK-negative ALCL arising in association with breast implants placed for cosmetic purposes or as part of reconstruction following surgery for carcinoma {321,801,1193, 1437,1592}. Approximately 50 cases have been reported. The median time from placement of the implant to development of ALCL is 8 years. Both silicone- and saline-filled implants have been implicated, with a higher proportion of cases involving silicone.

Clinical features
Patients affected with ALCL ALK-negative of the breast most often present with a seroma, hence the designation "seroma-associated ALCL." Other common presentations include a mass in the fibrous capsule or severe contracture of the fibrous capsule surrounding the implant. All cases to date have been unilateral.

Histopathology
In seroma-associated ALCL, the neoplastic cells are confined to the fibrous capsule and, in many cases are predominantly identified within the seroma cavity. Extension beyond the fibrous capsule with infiltration of the breast parenchyma is rare. Cytologically the neoplastic cells are large, pleomorphic cells with basophilic cytoplasm, best identified in cytological specimens obtained from the seroma fluid. In histological sections, the tumour cells are generally adherent to the fibrous capsule. The cells are non-cohesive and lack an inflammatory background.

Immunoprofile
By immunohistochemistry, the cells of seroma-associated ALCL tumours are strongly positive for CD30, usually positive for cytotoxic granule-associated proteins, epithelial membrane antigen (EMA), and clusterin, and negative for CD15 and CD20 {1193}. The cells express T-cell-associated markers, most commonly CD3 and CD2, with variable expression of other T-cell-associated antigens. In situ hybridization for Epstein Barr virus-encoded RNA (EBER) is negative.

Genetics
Most cases of seroma-associated ALCL show clonal rearrangement of the T-cell receptor genes.

Prognosis and predictive factors
Seroma-associated ALCL has a good prognosis. The optimal therapeutic management has not yet been determined, and some patients have done well with limited local therapy, including removal of the implant with watchful waiting {1437}.

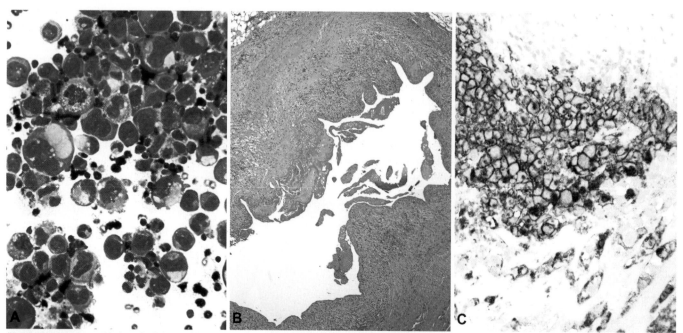

Fig. 13.05 Seroma-associated anaplastic large cell lymphoma, anaplastic lymphoma kinase-negative. **A** Cytological examination of the seroma fluid is the optimal diagnostic method, as tissue involvement is frequently limited in extent. The lymphoma cells are large and pleomorphic with deeply basophilic cytoplasm. Mitotic figures are often seen (Wright-Giemsa staining). **B** The seroma cavity is frequently lined by a fibrinous exudate, with the atypical cells adherent to the wall, and embedded within the exudate. **C** Immunostaining shows that the tumour cells are strongly positive for CD30.

Extranodal marginal zone lymphomas of mucosa-associated lymphoid tissue (MALT lymphoma)

A. Dogan
F. Fend

ICD-O code   9699/3

Epidemiology

Extranodal marginal zone lymphomas of mucosa-associated lymphoid tissue (MALT lymphoma) involving the breast are rare, accounting for < 0.5% of all breast malignancies. Most cases arise primarily in the breast, but secondary involvement of the breast by MALT lymphomas arising at other sites can be seen {893,1396}. Most cases occur in female adults in their sixth or seventh decade of life {883,893}.

The etiology of MALT lymphoma of the breast is not known; however, an association with an underlying autoimmune disorder has been implicated in rare cases {675}.

Clinical features

The patients generally present with a unilateral solitary breast mass that can be detected either by palpation or by mammography. However, involvement of regional lymph nodes may be present in a quarter of cases, and stage IV disease with involvement of the bone marrow can be seen rarely {883}.

Histopathology

Morphologically the MALT lymphoma shows the spectrum of changes well-described at other sites {626}. The tumour is composed of medium-sized lymphoid cells containing irregular nuclei with dispersed chromatin and inconspicuous nucleoli and, pale, abundant cytoplasm. The characteristic cytology of these cells is often described as "monocytoid" or "centrocyte-like." Additionally, scattered large transformed immunoblasts with prominent nucleoli

can be present. Plasma cell differentiation, sometimes with Dutcher bodies, can be seen in up to 75% of cases {1159}. Architecturally, the neoplastic infiltrate is frequently associated with hyperplastic B-cell follicles, and occupies the marginal zone at the periphery of B-cell follicle mantle zone. Lymphoepithelial lesions, a characteristic feature of MALT lymphoma, may be seen if breast acini or ducts are present; however, these are often absent or if present, inconspicuous in contrast to MALT lymphomas at some other sites. In advanced cases, the tumour cells may overrun and colonize the reactive B-cell follicles, mimicking follicular lymphoma. Transformation into a large B-cell lymphoma, characterized by the presence of diffuse sheets of large cells has been described {421}.

Immunoprofile

Immunophenotypically, the neoplastic cells show phenotypical properties of normal marginal zone/memory B-cells, and express CD20, CD79a, PAX5, BCL2, and sometimes aberrantly CD43, but not CD5, CD10, CD23, BCL6, IgD or cyclin D1. If plasma-cell differentiation is present immunoglobulin light-chain restriction can be demonstrated by immunohistochemistry. In those cases with a more diffuse growth pattern, underlying follicular infrastructure overrun by MALT lymphoma can be identified by markers of follicular dendritic cells, such as CD21 or CD23.

Genetics

Genetically, MALT lymphomas of the breast show clonal rearrangement of immunoglobulin genes. Fluorescence in situ

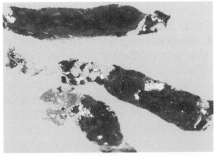

Fig. 13.07 MALT lymphoma. A breast core biopsy showing relatively well-circumscribed, nodular, dense lymphoid infiltrate.

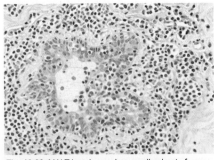

Fig. 13.08 MALT lymphoma. In a small subset of cases, lympho-epithelial lesions may be evident.

hybridization (FISH) studies have identified trisomy 3, 12 and 18 in a subset of cases; however, other cytogenetic abnormalities characteristic of MALT lymphoma such as t(11;18)(q21;q21) have not been reported {421}.

Prognosis and predictive factors

Clinically, primary MALT lymphomas of the breast are indolent with a 5-year overall survival of > 90%. Most cases respond to locally directed therapy such as radiotherapy or surgical excision {883}.

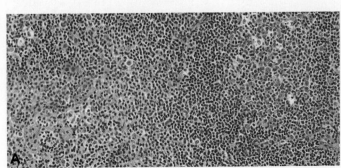
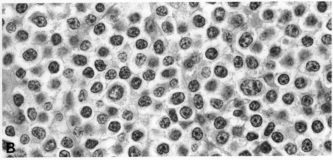

Fig. 13.09 MALT lymphoma. **A** The infiltrate is polymorphic, containing a reactive follicle (right) and a perifollicular/marginal zone component of "monocytoid"-appearing lymphoid cells. **B** The neoplastic cells have round uniform nuclei and pale abundant cytoplasm. Occasional larger transformed immunoblasts are also present.

Follicular lymphoma

F. Fend
N.L. Harris
A. Dogan

ICD-O code 9690/3

Epidemiology

A variety of low-grade B-cell lymphomas other than MALT lymphoma can occur in the breast. Among these, follicular lymphoma is the most common, accounting for 5–46% of all non-Hodgkin lymphomas (NHL) in recent series {470,488,609,883, 893,1180,1396}.

Clinical features

Follicular lymphoma may present as primary disease in the breast, with or without involvement of axillary lymph nodes, but the percentage of cases with primary versus secondary involvement of the breast varies widely in different series. Some cases may arise from intramammary lymph nodes.

Histopathology

The morphology of follicular lymphoma is comparable to nodal and other extranodal sites, with both follicular and diffuse growth patterns and a predominance of histological grade 1 or 2 over grade 3A or 3B. The neoplastic follicles show a monotonous pattern and vague borders and contain centrocytes with various proportions of centroblasts, depending on grade. Lymphoepithelial lesions are usually absent.

Low-grade B-cell NHL other than follicular and MALT lymphomas encountered in the breast are usually a manifestation of disseminated disease.

Immunoprofile

The neoplastic follicles of follicular lymphoma show expression of pan-B-cell markers CD20 and CD79a, as well as CD10, BCL6 and BCL2 in most cases. Follicular dendritic-cell networks can be demonstrated by stains for CD21 or CD23, but disappear in areas with a diffuse pattern. Follicular lymphoma commonly contains a high percentage of reactive T-cells.

Differential diagnosis

The differential diagnosis includes other low-grade B-cell lymphoma subtypes, mainly MALT lymphoma, and chronic mastitis with reactive follicular hyperplasia. The latter may present as so-called

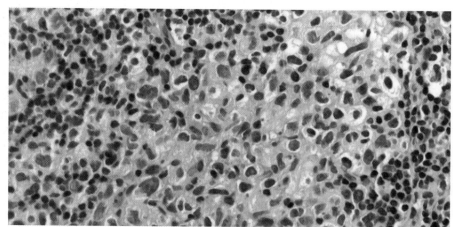

Fig. 13.10 Follicular lymphoma of the breast, grade 3A. A neoplastic follicle in a breast core biopsy contains many large, atypical centroblasts and centrocytes.

cutaneous pseudolymphoma, especially of the areolar region {172}. The presence of dense collagenous tissue, especially in core biopsies, may cause an "Indian file" pattern of infiltration and raise a differential diagnosis of lobular carcinoma. The diagnosis of these cases can easily be resolved by immunohistochemical analysis. From the presently available studies, it is unclear whether some cases of follicular lymphoma of the breast may represent examples of primary cutaneous follicle centre cell lymphoma, the morphology, immunophenotype and molecular genetics of which are distinct from those of conventional follicular lymphoma, and include predominance of large cells, a commonly diffuse growth pattern, lack of

expression of BCL2 protein and usually absence of *BCL2* rearrangement {1583}.

Genetics

The frequency of the characteristic t(14;18)(q32;q21) translocation or other cytogenetic or molecular alterations has not been assessed systematically for primary follicular lymphoma of the breast.

Prognosis and predictive factors

Relapse rates, patterns of spread and clinical behaviour of primary follicular lymphoma of the breast are comparable to those of conventional nodal disease, although a worse prognosis has been reported recently {883}.

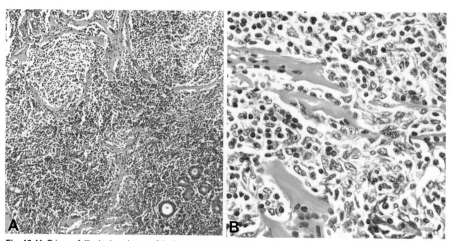

Fig. 13.11 Primary follicular lymphoma of the breast, grade 1/2. **A** The tumour shows a vaguely follicular pattern without formation of lymphoepithelial lesions. **B** High magnification reveals a mixture of centrocytes and rare centroblasts.

CHAPTER 14

Metastases of extramammary malignancies to the breast

Metastases of extramammary malignancies to the breast

A. Lee
A. Sahin

Definition
Metastasis to the breast from a malignancy arising outside the breast.

ICD-O code   8000/6

Origin of metastases
A wide range of extramammary malignancies can metastasize to the breast. Common types include haematological malignancies, melanoma, carcinomas of the lung, ovary, prostate, kidney and stomach and carcinoid tumours {39,1449, 1584}. In children, rhabdomyosarcoma and lymphoma are the most common {1100,1196}.

Epidemiology
In clinical series, metastases to the breast represent about 0.2% to 1.3% of malignant tumours in the breast {40,536,769}. The frequency is higher at examination post mortem. It is much more common in women {485}.

Clinical features
In about 30% of cases, the breast lesion is the first sign of malignancy {40,485,769}. In those with a history of malignancy, the interval between initial diagnosis and mammary metastasis varies between 1 month and 15 years {42,769,900,996}. A long interval is particularly seen in some tumour types, for example melanoma and ovarian carcinoma {769,900}. The patient usually presents with a rapidly growing, painless, firm, palpable mass {40,996, 1448}.
Mammography most commonly shows a well-defined rounded mass {40,776,1348, 1511}. Multiple masses are present in a minority. Calcification is rare, apart from metastases from serous papillary carcinoma of the ovary. Spiculation is much less common than in primary mammary carcinoma. Ultrasound typically shows a hypoechoic mass, sometimes heterogeneous or poorly defined {776}.
Since the appropriate treatment for most patients is systemic or palliative, non-operative diagnosis avoids unnecessary surgery. Diagnosis is easier with core biopsy

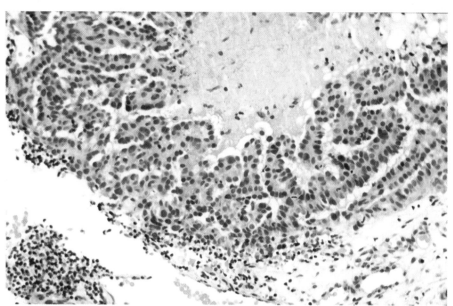

Fig. 14.01 Serous papillary carcinoma of the ovary metastatic to the breast. The papillary architecture is a useful clue to the diagnosis.

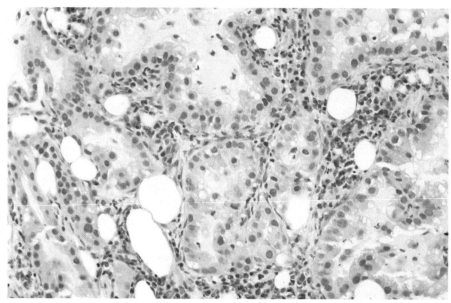

Fig. 14.02 Pulmonary adenocarcinoma metastatic to the breast. The growth pattern is unusual for a mammary primary. Immunostaining for thyroid transcription factor-1 was positive.

{769,777}, but fine-needle aspiration (FNA) can be used to diagnose some metastases, such as small cell carcinoma and melanoma {1268,1348,1594}.

Macroscopy
Typically, the tumour is well-circumscribed.

Histopathology

The pathologist should consider this diagnosis if the morphology is unusual for a primary mammary tumour. About two thirds of cases will have histological features raising the possibility of metastasis {769}. For the other third, the history is vital for diagnosis. Small cell carcinoma suggests pulmonary origin. Clear cell carcinoma suggests renal origin. Papillary carcinoma raises the possibility of ovarian serous papillary carcinoma {1161}. Pigment and intranuclear inclusions suggest melanoma {99}. The nuclear features are a useful clue to the diagnosis of lymphoma. Elastosis and carcinoma in situ suggest mammary origin {769}. Calcification is common in primary mammary carcinoma, but is rare in metastases, except serous papillary carcinoma of ovary.

If there is a known malignancy elsewhere, diagnosis is often possible by comparison with the previous tumour. It is important to consider which tumour is the primary. Immunohistochemistry is particularly helpful if there is no previous history {769,784}. Mammary origin is supported by expression of keratin 7, estrogen receptor, progesterone receptor and GCDFP-15 and absence of keratin 20 {769,784}. Thyroid transcription factor-1 (TTF1) is a useful marker of pulmonary adenocarcinoma {680}, and Wilms'

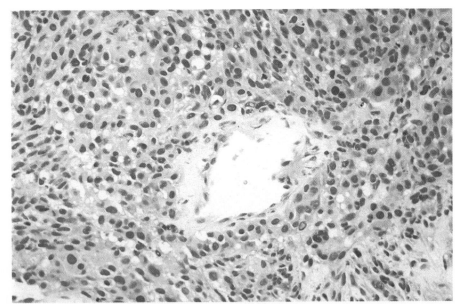

Fig. 14.03 Melanoma metastatic to the breast. The spindle cells and intra-nuclear inclusion are clues to the diagnosis.

tumour-1 (WT1) is a good marker of ovarian serous papillary carcinoma {1450}. S100 is a sensitive marker of melanoma, but is also expressed by some breast cancers, so keratins and other melanoma markers, such as HMB45 and melan-A, should be assessed {99}. It is important to use a panel of antibodies as no single marker is completely sensitive or specific.

Prognosis and predictive factors

In general the prognosis is poor as most patients have widely disseminated disease. While most patients die within a year {1584}, longer survival is described for some tumour types, such as lymphoma {238} and carcinoid tumours {1584}.

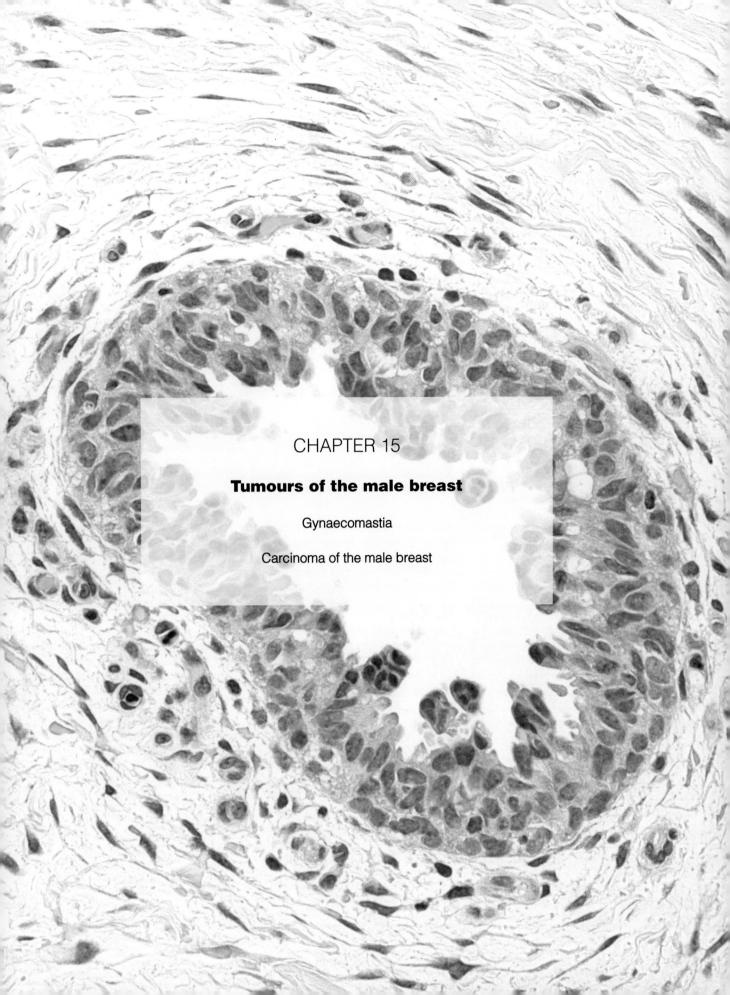

CHAPTER 15

Tumours of the male breast

Gynaecomastia

Carcinoma of the male breast

Gynaecomastia

A. Reiner
S. Badve

Definition
Gynaecomastia is a non-neoplastic, often reversible enlargement of the male breast associated with proliferation of ductal elements and mesenchymal components.

Synonyms
No other terms are used widely today.

Epidemiology
Gynaecomastia is a relatively common condition, occurring at any age, although it shows a bimodal age distribution with peaks during puberty and the sixth and seventh decades of life. Transient breast enlargement in male infants, attributable to exposure to maternal hormones, can be seen, but this usually regresses spontaneously within a few weeks. Similarly, an incidence of reversible breast enlargement of 50–70% in adolescent boys has been reported {963}. In adulthood, palpable breast tissue occurs in 30–65% of males, with autopsy studies documenting a frequency of up to 55% {44}.

Clinical features
Gynaecomastia presents as a palpable tender mass beneath the areola. It may be bilateral or unilateral. In cases of bilateral involvement, enlargement may predominate on one side. Clinical examination includes assessment of endocrine

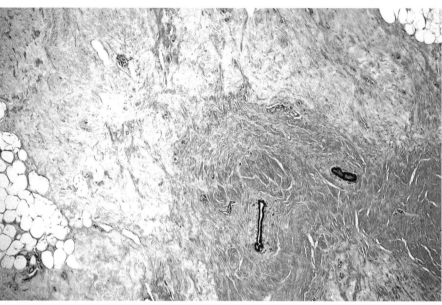

Fig. 15.01 Gynaecomastia of the male breast. Fibrous type.

status and possibly imaging technology {655}. Etiological factors are listed in Table 15.01. Patient history, particularly a detailed history of drug intake, may provide a clue to the etiology of disease.

Macroscopy
The gross appearance is generally not specific but differs significantly from that seen in breast carcinoma. The lesion consists of an either circumscribed or ill-defined greyish-white, firm tissue that merges with the adjacent fatty tissue.

Histopathology
The histological appearance varies according to the relative proportion of ducts and mesenchymal tissue. The ducts, increased in number, are lined by a bilayer of epithelial and myoepithelial cells and are surrounded by fibrous stroma admixed with adipose tissue.
Two main histological patterns are described that may co-exist in a given lesion. The florid pattern is characterized by irregular branching ducts that show proliferation of epithelial cells. These cells may be organized in small focal tufts and exhibit a micropapillary growth pattern. Proliferation is usually mild but can be prominent and mitotic figures may be visible. However, cellular anaplasia is not seen. The surrounding stroma is loose, oedematous, often cellular (fibroblastic) and composed of fibroblasts and myofibroblasts. The fibrous pattern is characterized by hyalinized, sparsely cellular periductal stroma and flat bilayered epithelial lining of the ducts. The architecture

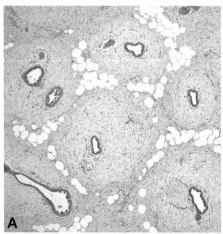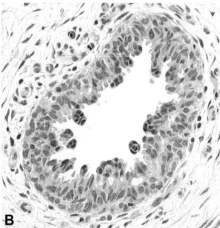

Fig. 15.02 Gynaecomastia of the male breast. Florid type. **A** Ducts within loose stroma. **B** Proliferation of ductal epithelium with tufts and micropapillary pattern.

can be similar to that seen in pseudoangiomatous stromal hyperplasia {89}. In rare cases, apocrine or even squamous metaplasia may be observed. Atypical ductal hyperplasia is an extremely rare event but has been described {1414}. Benign but atypical multi-nucleated stromal cells similar to those described in the fem-ale breast can be occasionally identified {89}. Lobules are very rare in the normal male breast but can be seen; their presence has been associated with hormonal co-stimulation by estrogens and progesterone. No relationship between histological type and cause of gynaecomastia exists.

Differential diagnosis
True gynaecomastia should be distinguished from pseudo-gynaecomastia, which consists of adipose tissue only, and from the rare cases of breast carcinoma.

Genetics
Klinefelter syndrome, characterized by karyotype 47,XXY, is the most common chromosomal disorder associated with gynaecomastia. Patients with Klinefelter syndrome show gynaecomastia in 50–70% of cases. In rare cases, genetic alterations of the androgen receptor resulting in decreased androgen sensitivity may play a role in development of gynaecomastia

{183}. In most cases, genetics does not play a role in this condition.

Prognosis and predictive factors
In most cases, gynaecomastia regresses within 2 years and therefore a "wait-and-watch" policy is often an appropriate clinical management strategy. Gynaecomastia is not considered to be a risk factor for the development of breast cancer in males, since the rates of gynaecomastia in male patients with breast cancer and in the general population are similar {1570}; however, some studies have reported a slightly increased risk of breast cancer in patients with gynaecomastia, which may be due to the fact that the same risk factors are associated with both conditions.

Table 15.01 Etiological factors involved in the pathogenesis of gynaecomastia

Hormonal imbalance	Cause[a]
Absolute excess of estrogens	Therapeutic administration (e.g. prostate cancer)
Increased endogenous production of estrogen	Tumours (e.g. Leydig cell tumour, feminizing adreno-cortical tumours)
	Increased aromatization of androgens to estrogens (e.g. obesity, ageing, alcoholic liver cirrhosis, hyperthyroidism)
Absolute deficiency of androgens	Hypogonadism (e.g. Klinefelter syndrome, testicular trauma, mumps, orchitis, drugs)
Altered ratio of serum androgen to estrogen	Puberty Ageing Liver cirrhosis Renal failure and dialysis Hyperthyroidism Drugs, including anabolic steroids
Decreased androgen action	Drugs Androgen-receptor defects

[a] Examples are given in parentheses and do not list causes completely. For a review see {963}

Carcinoma of the male breast

A. Reiner
S. Badve

Definition

Carcinoma of the male breast is a rare malignant epithelial tumour that is histologically identical to cancer of the female breast; both in situ and invasive variants can be seen.

ICD-O code   8500/3

Epidemiology

Breast cancer in males accounts for only < 1% of all cases of breast cancer and for 1% of cancers in males {647}. Globally, there is broad variation in the incidence of this disease. In the USA, with an estimated 1970 new cases of breast cancer being diagnosed in men in 2010, this disease represents 0.25% of all cancers in men and, with an estimated 390 deaths from breast cancer, 0.13% of all cancer deaths in men annually {1570}. In contrast, in the United Republic of Tanzania and areas of central Africa, breast cancer accounts for up to 6% of cancers in men {43}. Although it has been suggested that a slight increase occurred between 1975 and 2000, the incidence of male breast cancer seems to have remained stable or decreased slightly between 2000 and 2005.

Breast cancer tends to occur in a slightly older age group in men than in women (mean age, 67 versus 61 years), although younger males may also be affected. The bimodal age distribution observed in women with breast cancer is not seen in men.

Etiology

Relatively little is known about the etiology of this disease, except that hormonal imbalance and environmental conditions are major contributing factors.

Conditions that seem to be consistently associated with elevated risk of male breast cancer are obesity and testicular disorders like cryptorchidism, mumps orchitis and testicular trauma. Diseases with a variable contribution to risk are liver cirrhosis, diabetes and hyperthyroidism. Drugs that cause hormonal imbalance, such as those used for the treatment of prostate cancer, may increase risk.

An increased risk of male breast cancer is reportedly associated with radiation to the chest wall and occupational exposure to radiation or electromagnetic fields. Some reports suggest an increased risk of development of breast carcinoma after occupational exposure to petrol and airline fuels.

In most studies, gynaecomastia is not considered to be a risk factor for breast cancer; however, some studies have documented a slightly increased risk {184, 185,430}, which may be attributable to the fact that the two conditions share the same risk factors.

Clinical features

Clinically, breast cancer in men presents as a painless firm mass situated in the subareolar region. Unlike gynaecomastia, the lesion tends to be located eccentrically in relation to the nipple. It is usually unilateral, but may rarely (0–1.9% of cases) involve both breasts {169}. Bloody nipple discharge may occur at a fairly early stage and is associated in 75% of cases with malignancy. Compared with the female breast, changes in the nipple areolar complex, seen as fixation, retraction, inversion and ulceration, occur with greater frequency in males. Paget disease of the nipple has been documented. Tumour characteristics related to advanced stage (tumour size > 2 cm and positive axillary lymph nodes) are more common in men. Palpable axillary nodes are detected in approximately 50% of cases. The management of these patients is similar to that for postmenopausal women with breast cancer.

Macroscopy

Invasive carcinomas present as an irregular stellate or multinodular firm greyish-white mass with a mean diameter of 2–2.5 cm. Tumours tend to invade the nipple, overlying skin or pectoral muscle at a rather early stage. In situ carcinomas may present as partly cystic in appearance.

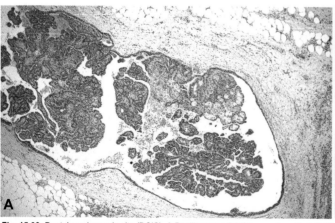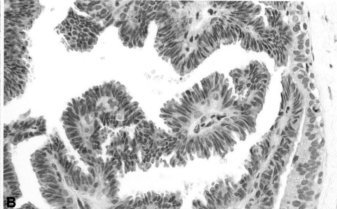

Fig. 15.03 Ductal carcinoma in situ (DCIS). **A** Papillary-type DCIS in a male patient. **B** The papillary structures are lined by atypical cylindrical epithelium.

Histopathology

Carcinoma in situ

Although both ductal and lobular carcinoma in situ can occur in males, lobular carcinoma in situ is an extremely rare finding. The incidence of ductal carcinoma in situ (DCIS) is reported in up to 10% of all cases of breast cancer in males. It is histologically similar to that seen in females and all architectural patterns have been identified. There seems to be a relatively greater incidence of papillary intraductal carcinoma, and Paget disease and a decreased incidence of comedo necrosis in males than in females {584}.

Grading and assessment of steroid hormone receptors for DCIS should be performed in the same way as for carcinoma in situ in females.

Invasive carcinoma

Invasive carcinoma of no special type (NST) is the most common type and is identical to that occurring in the female breast. Invasive papillary carcinoma is more common in males than in females, accounting for approximately for 2–4% of cases. Invasive lobular carcinoma is very rare, perhaps because of the lack of significant lobule formation in the male breast, and has been associated with exposure to estrogens and progesterone. Other histological types of tumour, such as medullary, mucinous or tubular carcinomas, are very rare. Histological grading should be applied as for invasive breast carcinoma in females. Carcinomas of grade 2 and 3 are reported in 80% of cases {430}. Currently no conclusive data exist on molecular subtypes.

Positivity for estrogen receptors is reported in > 90% of cases of breast cancer in men and for progesterone receptors in 80% of cases {19}. In order to select the optimal regimen of adjuvant therapy, assessment of hormone receptors and HER2 needs to be performed in the same manner as for breast cancer in women. National guidelines developed for the analysis of these markers in the female breast should be followed. Owing to the rarity of this disease, detailed data on HER2 expression are not available and a wide range of frequency of between 1% and 15% is reported in the literature {1236}. Molecular tests appear to yield results comparable to those for the female breast. Overall, robust analysis of large populations on biological markers is still needed.

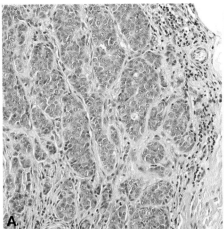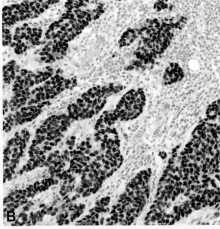

Fig. 15.04 Invasive carcinoma of no special type (NST). **A** Invasive carcinoma NST in a male patient. **B** Immunohistochemistry for estrogen receptor is strongly positive.

Metastasis to the breast

The ratio of primary to metastatic tumours is reported to be in the order of 25 : 1. The most frequent primary sites include prostate, colon, urinary bladder, malignant melanoma and lymphoma. Expression of markers such as prostate-specific antigen (PSA) has been reported in male breast cancers and should not be misinterpreted as indicating metastases from prostatic carcinoma {475,690}.

Genetics

As in women, only a small proportion of breast cancers in men can be explained by genetic mutations. Approximately 15–20% of men with breast cancer report a family history of breast or ovarian cancer. Risk is particularly increased in cases of an affected sister (relative risk, 2.25) or both mother and sister (relative risk, 9.73) {185}. Men who inherit germline mutations in *BRCA2* have an estimated lifetime risk of breast cancer of 5–10%, while risk in the general population is 0.1%. Male carriers of *BRCA2* mutations have a risk of 7.1% of developing breast cancer by the age of 70 years and 8.4% by the age of 80 years {404}. The reported frequencies of male patients with breast cancer carrying *BRCA2* mutations vary considerably and may be as high as almost 30% {344,461,492,1047,1048}. The association between germline mutations and breast cancer in men is weaker for *BRCA1* than for *BRCA2*. The lifetime risk of developing breast cancer for men with germline mutations in *BRCA1* is 1–5%. Breast cancer in men has also been associated with mutations in *CHEK2*, *TP53* and *PTEN* tumour suppressor genes {430,1570}.

Klinefelter syndrome is a hereditary condition consisting of 47,XXY karyotype. Patients suffer from hormonal imbalance with higher ratio of estrogen to testosterone. The relative risk of developing breast cancer for men with this condition is reported to be between 20- and 50-fold {612}. The incidence of Klinefelter syndrome is reported to be 3–7.5% in men with breast cancer.

Mutations of the androgen receptor gene and polymorphism of the cytochrome 450 enyzme (CYP17) have been associated with an increased incidence of breast cancer in males in some studies {1570}.

Prognosis and predictive factors

The duration of symptoms before diagnosis tends to be longer for males than for females, but might be declining. The disease is driven mainly by known prognostic factors as TNM stage, tumour grade and estrogen-receptor status and is comparable to breast cancer in postmenopausal females. In addition, age and race seem to influence prognosis {715}. However, the disease is often more advanced at diagnosis in men, with > 40% of men with breast cancer presenting with stages III or IV {493}. This adversely influences overall prognosis. However, when stage-matched disease is considered, the prognosis for male and female patients is similar. Approximately 40% of male patients with breast cancer will die of causes other than their cancer. This likely reflects the higher rate of intercurrent illness associated with the older mean age of patients at diagnosis {715}.

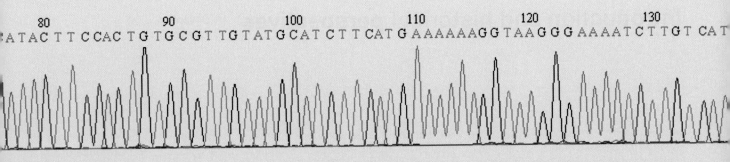

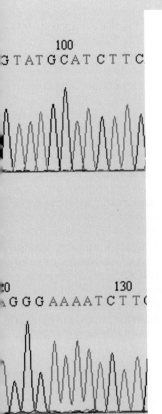

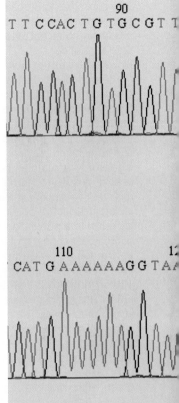

CHAPTER 16

Genetic susceptibility: inherited syndromes

Introduction and historical perspectives

Inherited syndromes associated with an increased risk of breast cancer: Introduction

BRCA1 and BRCA2 syndromes

Li-Fraumeni syndrome

Ataxia telangiectasia syndrome

Cowden syndrome

Lynch syndrome

Other breast cancer-predisposing genes

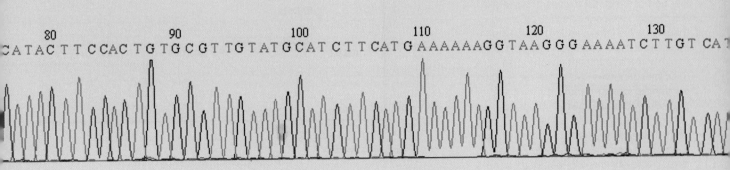

Introduction and historical perspectives

P. Devilee
D. Easton

In 1866, the French neurologist Paul Broca reported ten cases of breast cancer in four generations of his wife's family. Although familial clustering of breast cancer was observed by the ancient Greeks, this report still remains the first well-documented description of inherited breast cancer. Retrospectively, it is now easy to fully subscribe to Broca's conclusion that the very large excess of breast cancers in this family could not reasonably be attributed to chance.

However, it was not until the 1960s, when the search for risk factors for breast cancer began, that the importance of family history was appreciated. Many studies have since documented that if a woman's mother or sister has had breast cancer, she herself is more likely to develop the disease. Most studies reported relative risks of between 2 and 3 for first-degree relatives of patients with breast cancer selected irrespective of age at diagnosis or laterality. In a population-based study of 5559 breast-cancer probands diagnosed before age 80 years, the estimated relative risk of developing breast cancer was 1.8 for the 49 202 first-degree relatives {503}. This estimate was confirmed in a large meta-analysis involving 58 209 women with breast cancer and 101 986 women without this disease {282}.

A number of researchers have systematically ascertained and collected pedigrees with multiple cases of breast cancer. Analysis of these kindreds showed that familial breast cancer differed from its nonfamilial counterpart in several aspects, including: (1) a significantly earlier age of onset; (2) excess of bilaterality; (3) specific associations with other malignancies in the family; and (4) vertical transmission. These observations, and particularly the associations with other specific malignancies, led to the recognition of familial breast-cancer syndromes, or cancer syndromes in which breast cancer is a component (Table 16.01).

Mathematical analyses of breast-cancer pedigrees can define genetic models to explain the observed inheritance patterns in these families. In a sample of 1579 nuclear families ascertained through a population-based series of probands, Newman et al. found evidence for an autosomal-dominant model with a rare, but highly penetrant susceptibility allele {982}. Inherited susceptibility affected only 4% of families in the sample: multiple cases of this relatively common disease occurred in other families by chance. In conjunction with the emergence of more elaborate linkage maps of the human genome in the 1980s, this provided the basis for a genome-wide linkage search in a small set of families in which multiple cases of breast cancer displayed a clear autosomal-dominant pattern of inheritance. This led to the discovery of the *BRCA1* locus on chromosome 17 in 1990, and the identification of the *BRCA1* gene sequence a few years later {537,925}.

Initially, linkage to the *BRCA1* locus was suggested to be mainly restricted to families with multiple cases of early-onset breast cancer (i.e. at < 50 years). Subsequent work by a worldwide consortium of investigators not only confirmed this association with overwhelming statistical evidence, but also demonstrated significantly that mutations in *BRCA1* predispose strongly to the development of ovarian cancer {362}. The existence of a breast–ovarian cancer syndrome had already been suggested by Henry Lynch in 1978, and was given a formal genetic basis by this finding.

Linkage analysis was also instrumental in the discovery of the *BRCA2* gene in 1995 by a consortium of investigators led by Michael Stratton. First, it was shown that breast-cancer families with at least one case of male breast cancer did not show linkage to 17q21, the *BRCA1* locus. A subsequent linkage search in a small number of families with cases of male breast cancer then identified 13q12 as the location of *BRCA2* {1598}. The identification of the gene sequence {1597}, was greatly expedited by progress within the Human Genome Project, an international collaboration aimed at sequencing the entire human genome by the year 2000. The ability to select a specific familial "cancer phenotype", as was the case for *BRCA1* and *BRCA2*, was also important in the identification of the *PTEN* gene by linkage analysis, in 1997. Mutations in *PTEN* are found in the majority of families afflicted by Cowden syndrome {973,974}.

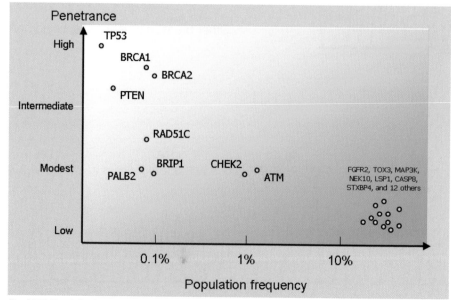

Fig. 16.01 Population frequency and penetrance of genes involved in susceptibility to breast cancer {1501}.

These families are characterized by the occurrence of multiple hamartomatous lesions, as well as an increased risk of neoplasms of the thyroid, breast, and female genitourinary tract. A similar story unfolded for ataxia telangiectasia, a recessive disorder characterized by cerebellar ataxia, telangiectases, immune defects, and a predisposition to malignancy. Patients' mothers, who are obligate heterozygote carriers, were found to have a moderately increased risk of developing breast cancer {1389}. Like *BRCA1*, *BRCA2*, and *PTEN*, the *ATM* gene (mutations in which underlie ataxia telangiectasia), was identified through "positional cloning" on the basis of linkage mapping to 11q23 in families with ataxia telangiectasia {1269}. Other genes predisposing to breast cancer were identified via investigation of interesting biological candidates. For example, many of the sporadic forms of cancers that are also found to cluster in families with the Li-Fraumeni syndrome acquire somatic mutations in the *TP53* gene. Therefore, it was postulated that Li-Fraumeni syndrome could be attributable to germline mutations in *TP53*, which was indeed found to be the case {861,1361}. Likewise, when it became clear that BRCA1, BRCA2 and ATM were all involved in an intricate network of proteins dealing with DNA-damage repair, it was logical to scan breast-cancer families for germline mutations in the genes encoding other DNA repair proteins. All the genes underlying the 14 complementation groups of Fanconi anaemia (FA), a recessive chromosome-breakage disorder, became attractive candidate breast cancer susceptibility genes when it was found that FA complementation group D1 is characterized by biallelic mutations in *BRCA2* {325}. Subsequently, small proportions (< 1%) of breast-cancer families were found to have mutations in *PALB2* (FANCN) {385,1132}, *BRIP1* (FANCJ) {1293}, *RAD51C* (FANCO) {909}, *NLRP2* {1373}, *CHEK2* {908,1481} or *BARD1* {320}. Table 16.02 presents an overview of the genes in which germline mutations have been detected that co-segregate with familial breast cancer, or that have been associated with moderately increased risks of breast cancer. Together, these genes constitute the genetic landscape of breast-cancer susceptibility. Since 2007, genome-wide association scans have yielded almost 20 new alleles associated with an increased risk of breast cancer

(e.g. *FGFR2*, *TOX3*) {1501}; these differ from those identified in families with respect to their high prevalence in the general population and the very low relative risks they confer (generally < 1.25). *BRCA1* and *BRCA2* jointly still account for the largest proportions of the familial risk (about 20%). *TP53* and *PTEN* mutations are too rare to make a significant contribution. The 20 common low-risk alleles account for < 5% of this risk. Because

linkage analyses in non-BRCA1/2 families have thus far failed to identify a third major locus, it is believed that the remainder of familial risk will be explained by a plethora of rare, high-risk variants and common low-risk variants (Table 16.02). We expect many more breast-cancer genes to be discovered over the next decade with the emergence of whole-genome sequencing.

Table 16.01 Inherited syndromes involving cancers of the breast

Syndrome	MIM No.	Gene	Location	Associated cancers
BRCA1 syndrome	113705	*BRCA1*	17q21	Breast, ovary, colon, liver, cervix, endometrium, fallopian tube, peritoneum
BRCA2 syndrome	600185	*BRCA2*	13q12	Breast (male and female), ovary, prostate, pancreas, gall bladder, fallopian tube, stomach, melanoma
Li-Fraumeni	151623	*TP53*	17p13	Breast, sarcoma, brain, adrenal, leukaemia
Cowden	158350	*PTEN*	10q24	Skin, thyroid, breast, cerebellum, colon
Peutz-Jeghers	175200	*STK11*	19p13.3	Hamartomatous intestinal polyposis, breast, ovary, cervix, testis, pancreas
Saethre-Chotzen	101400	*TWIST1*	7p	Breast (nonmalignant features: acrocephaly, mild syndactyly)
Ataxia telangiectasia	208900	*ATM*	11q23	Breast (in heterozygotes)

Table 16.02 Genes in which germline mutations have been associated with familial breast cancer

Gene (HGNC Symbol)	Description	Location	Proportion of families with a mutation
ATM	Ataxia telangiectasia mutated	11q22.3	Approx. 2% of *BRCA1/2*-negative breast cancer families (0.4% in healthy controls) {1175}
BRCA1	Breast cancer 1, early onset	17q21.3	Approx. 10% of breast cancer-only families and up to 40% of breast-ovarian cancer families
BRCA2 (FANCD1)	Breast cancer 2, early onset	13q13.1	Approx. 10% of breast cancer-only families and up to 25% of breast-ovarian cancer families
CHEK2	CHK2 checkpoint homologue (*S. pombe*)	22q12.1	Varies between countries; approx. 1.5% of familial breast cancer (0.5% in healthy controls) {1623}
BRIP1 (FANCJ, BACH1)	BRCA1-interacting protein C-terminal helicase 1	17q23.2	Approx. 0.7% of *BRCA1/2*-negative breast or breast-ovarian cancer families (0.1% in healthy controls) {1293}
NLRP2 (NBS1)	NLR family, pyrin domain-containing 2	19q13.4	Approx. 3% of Polish familial breast cancer, and 0.6% of healthy controls {514}; negligible outside eastern Europe
PALB2 (FANCN)	Partner and localizer of BRCA2	16p12.2	Approx. 1% of *BRCA1/2*-negative familial/early onset breast cancer {1441}
PTEN	Phosphatase and tensin homologue	10q23.3	Approx. 80% of families with Cowden syndrome {1042}
TP53	Tumour protein p53	17p13.1	Approx. 70% of families with classical Li-Fraumeni syndrome; 20–40% in Li-Fraumeni-like families {1240}
RAD51C	RAD51 homologue C (*S. cerevisiae*)	17q22	Approx. 1% of *BRCA1/2*-negative breast-ovarian cancer families {909}

HGNC, HUGO Gene Nomenclature Committee.

Inherited syndromes associated with an increased risk of breast cancer: Introduction

D. Easton
P. Devilee
G. Chenevix-Trench

Rare mutations in at least 11 genes are known to be associated with an increased risk of breast cancer. In the majority of cases, these mutations are also associated with nonmalignant features, or with an increased risk of multiple cancers, so that in at least in some families they form a recognizable syndrome. A major exception is *CHEK2*, for which there are no known features other than an increased risk of breast cancer. Clinically, the most important syndromes are associated with mutations in *BRCA1* and *BRCA2* (see *BRCA1 gene, BRCA2 gene,* and *BRCA1 and BRCA2 syndrome*) and *TP53* (which causes an increased risk of breast cancer in the context of Li-Fraumeni syndrome; see p. 183).

Highly increased risk of breast cancer

Cowden syndrome is a rare autosomal-dominant disorder characterized by hamartomas and an increased risk of multiple cancers, including breast, endometrial, thyroid, kidney and colorectal cancers, oral and skin papillomas, trichilemmomas, mixed polyposis including hamartomas, and Lhermitte Duclos disease. The lifetime risk of breast cancer is reported to be 25–50%, but this is has not been well-estimated {93}. More than 80% of families with Cowden syndrome segregate a mutation in *PTEN*.

Peutz-Jeghers syndrome is characterized by gastrointestinal polyposis and mucocutaneous pigmentation. Individuals with Peutz-Jeghers syndrome are at increased risk of a wide variety of epithelial malignancies, including colorectal, gastric, pancreatic, breast, and ovarian cancers. Almost all cases have deleterious mutations in *STK11* (*LKB1*).

Saethre-Chotzen syndrome is characterized by coronal synostosis (unilateral or bilateral), facial asymmetry (particularly in individuals with unilateral coronal synostosis), ptosis, and characteristic appearance of the ear (small pinna with a prominent crus). Syndactyly of digits two and three of the hand is variably present. One study has reported a high risk of breast cancer in this syndrome {1249}

Hereditary diffuse gastric cancer

Germline mutations in *CDH1* predispose to hereditary diffuse gastric cancer (HDGC) {480,524}. Women have a 39–52% risk of developing lobular breast cancer.

Moderately increased risk of breast cancer

In addition to *BRCA1* and *BRCA2*, deleterious mutations in five other DNA repair genes (*ATM, BRIP1, PALB2, CHEK2* and, more equivocally, *RAD51C*) have been shown to be associated with an increased risk of breast cancer (Table 16.05). Four of these genes are responsible for recessive syndromes, but the increased risk of breast cancer is also present in heterozygous carriers.

Homozygous carriers of *ATM* mutations are the cause of ataxia telangiectasia (AT), a rare recessive condition characterized by cerebellar ataxia, telangiectases, radiation hypersensitivity, immunodeficiency and increased risk of cancer, particularly lymphoma. Biallelic mutations in two of these genes, *BRIP1* and *PALB2*, are the cause of Fanconi anaemia (*FANCJ* and *FANCN* respectively). Biallelic mutations in *RAD51C* are associated with a Fanconi anaemia-like disorder {1507}. Uniquely, biallelic *CHEK2* mutations do not appear to be associated with any particular phenotype.

Table 16.04 Syndromes and genes associated with a highly increased risk of breast cancer

Syndrome	MIM No.	Gene	Location	Frequency	Relative risk of breast cancer	Risk of breast cancer by age 70 years	Other associated cancers	Phenotypic features (homozygotes)
BRCA1	113705	*BRCA1*	17q21.3	1 in 860 {58}	—	65% {54}	Ovary, colon, liver, cervix, endometrium, fallopian tube, peritoneum	Lethal?
BRCA2	600185	*BRCA2*	13q13.1	1 in 740 {58}	—	45% {54}	Male breast, ovary, prostate, pancreas, gall bladder, fallopian tube, stomach, melanoma	Fanconi anaemia, AML, Wilms' tumour, medulloblastoma
Li-Fraumeni	151623	*TP53*	17p13	1 in 5 000 {753}	—	Approx. 60–80% {266}	Sarcoma, brain, adrenal, leukaemia	—
Cowden	158350	*PTEN*	10q24	1 in 250 000 {93}	—	25–50% {93}	Skin, thyroid, cerebellum, colon	—
Peutz-Jeghers	175200	*STK11*	19p13.3	1 in 25 000 to 1 in 300 000 {1495}	—	32–54% {1495}	Hamartomatous intestinal polyposis, ovary, cervix, testes, pancreas	—
Saethre-Chotzen	—	—	—	—	17× {1249}	—	—	Acrocephaly, mild syndactyly
AML, acute myeloid leukaemia								

Table 16.05 Syndromes and genes associated with a moderately increased risk of breast cancer

Syndrome	MIM No.	Gene	Location	Frequency (heterozygotes)	Relative risk of breast cancer	Risk of breast cancer by age 70 years (heterozygotes)	Other associated cancers (heterozygotes)	Phenotypic features (homozygotes)
Ataxia telangiectasia	208900	ATM	11q22.3	0.6% {1433}	Approx. 2.3× {235,1037,1433}	23%	—	Cerebellar ataxia, telangiectases, immuno-deficiency, lymphomas
Fanconi anaemia (J)	609054	BRIP1	17q23.2	1 in 1000 {1293}	Approx. 2× {1293}	Approx. 13%	—	Fanconi anaemia (not childhood cancer)
Fanconi anaemia (N)	610832	PALB2	16p12.2	< 1 in 1000 {1132}	Approx. 2–4× {1132,385}	13–24%	—	Fanconi anaemia, AML, Wilms tumour, medulloblastoma
—	604373	CHEK2	22q12.1	1 in 100[a] {250}	Approx. 2.3× {250}	15%[b]	Prostate? Colorectal?	None known
Fanconi anaemia (O)[c]	613390	RAD51C	17q22	?	?	?	Ovary	Fanconi anaemia-like (no haematological symptoms or malignancy)

AML, acute myeloid leukaemia

[a] Population-specific (highest in the Netherlands and Finland).

[b] A lower risk has been associated with the missense substitution I157T.

[c] Although RAD51C mutations have been found in families with breast and ovarian cancer, the evidence for an increased risk of breast cancer is weak.

In each case, the increased risk to hetero-zygous carriers is typically two- to three-fold, although the relative risk is higher at young ages. The estimates are most ac-curate for CHEK2 (where a single founder variant, 1100delC, is responsible for the majority of carriers in western Europe) and ATM. Certain mutations in ATM (no-tably c.7271A>G, which is associated with a milder AT phenotype) appear to be associated with a higher risk of breast cancer {504}. There is some evidence that nontruncating mutations in CHEK2 and ATM may also be associated with in-creased risk of breast cancer, which may substantially alter the proportion of breast cancers attributable to these genes {762,1422}.

Mutations in RAD51C have been found in families with breast and ovarian cancer {909}. However, while the evidence for an association with ovarian cancer is clear, there is no clear evidence of an increased frequency of mutations in breast cancer cases with no family history of ovarian cancer, hence the evidence for RAD51C being a breast-cancer susceptibility gene is currently equivocal {909,1087}. Muta-tions in RAD51D have also been found in such families, but only the risk of ovarian cancer appears to be clearly associated with RAD51D mutations {833}.

BRCA1 and BRCA2 syndromes

D. Goldgar
P. Devilee

Definitions

The BRCA1 and BRCA2 syndromes are inherited in an autosomal-dominant fashion and are associated with a markedly increased susceptibility to breast and ovarian tumours, which is attributable to pathogenic germline mutations in the BRCA1 or BRCA2 genes.

The BRCA1 syndrome comprises the subset of familial breast and ovarian tumours that are attributable to germline pathogenic mutations in the BRCA1 gene on chromosome 17q, while the BRCA2 syndrome can be defined as the corresponding subset of breast and ovarian tumours attributable to germline pathogenic mutations in the BRCA2 gene.

MIM Nos

BRCA1 syndrome, 113705   {902}
BRCA2 syndrome, 600185   {902}

Synonyms

BRCA1 syndrome: breast cancer 1; early-onset breast-ovarian cancer syndrome.
BRCA2 syndrome: site-specific early-onset breast-cancer syndrome; Fanconi anaemia FANCD1

Incidence

Estimates of the frequency of carriers of pathogenic mutations in BRCA1 in admixed European origin populations have varied between 0.12%, corresponding to a carrier frequency of 1/833 {456}, and 0.32% {1188}; however, it should be noted that both these estimates were not based on direct observation in a population-based study but were inferred from the frequency of mutations in patients with breast and ovarian cancer respectively, and the estimated relative risks (RR). The frequency of specific mutations is much higher in certain populations due to the effects of "bottlenecks" whereby a large reduction in population size is followed by rapid expansion, and/or long periods of geographical or cultural isolation. The frequency of pathogenic mutations in BRCA2 in the general population has not been well-studied. However, the same study that estimated a carrier frequency of pathogenic mutations in BRCA1

of 3/1000 estimated a frequency for BRCA2 of 7/1000, similar to that of Whittemore et al. {1579}. However a study based on the UK population and fitting a comprehensive model to a population-based data-set reported considerably lower frequencies of 0.10% and 0.14% respectively, {58}. In all studies that have estimated both, the frequency of BRCA2 mutations is estimated to be higher than that of BRCA1 in admixed European populations.

There have been direct estimates of the frequency of specific mutations in some founder populations, most notably the c.67_68delAG (185delAG) mutation which has been found in approximately 1% of Jewish individuals, the BRCA2 c.5946delT (6174delT) which has also been estimated to have a prevalence of 1% in Ashkenazi Jews {1191}, and the c.771del5 (999del5) Icelandic founder mutation which has an estimated frequency of 0.6% in that population {1439}. In both BRCA1 and BRCA2, de novo mutations are extremely rare.

Diagnostic criteria

Diagnosis of BRCA1 and BRCA2 syndromes is made through genetic testing by sequencing of patient DNA samples in a clinically-approved diagnostic laboratory. Criteria for such testing vary across countries, although many centres use criteria based on a predicted probability from a risk-prediction program such as Boadicea {56,60}, BRCAPRO {124,1074}, or empirical methods such as those proposed by Evans et al. {400,402}. Typically, a probability threshold of 10–20% of carrying

a mutation in BRCA1 or BRCA2 on the basis of personal and family history is used in many settings. In the USA, where all testing is done by a single laboratory, criteria are left to the discretion of individual providers. In the UK, the National Institute for Health and Clinical Excellence (NICE) guidelines for testing specify that an individual should have an estimated probability of > 20% from such a program in order to have BRCA1/2 genetic testing covered by the National Health Service. Antoniou et al. have compared several such prediction programs in a set of 1934 families with breast cancer in the UK and found them to all provide reasonably good predictions, but only Boadicea accurately predicted the number of mutations in various subclasses of risk {57}.

Once testing has been performed, any sequence variants identified are classified as benign/low clinical significance, pathogenic, or a variant of uncertain significance (VUS). When a pathogenic mutation is identified in an individual, the individual can be said to have BRCA1 syndrome and at-risk family members could be tested. The finding of a VUS in a patient sample greatly hinders the clinical utility and for this reason much research has been undertaken in the last 10 years to classify such variants using a variety of approaches {363,1191}

Penetrance for breast and ovarian cancer

Although pathogenic mutations in BRCA1 or BRCA2 are known to confer a substantial risk of breast cancer, the estimated

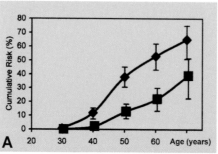
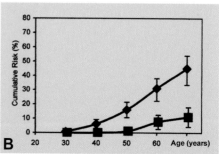

Fig. 16.02 **A** Cumulative risk of breast (♦) and ovarian (■) cancer in BRCA1-mutation carriers. **B** Cumulative risk of breast (♦) and ovarian (■) cancer in BRCA2-mutation carriers {1517}.

penetrance varies widely across different studies depending on the study design and analytical method. A summary of these early studies can be found in Table 1 in Antoniou et al. {54}. To address the huge range of variation in estimation of cumulative risk (penetrance), Antoniou et al. conducted a combined analysis of risk of breast and ovarian cancer associated with BRCA mutations, using data from 22 international studies involving 8139 cases of breast cancer, of which 500 were carriers of mutations in BRCA1 or BRCA2 {54}. Importantly, these cases were not selected on the basis of family history. It was estimated from this study that the cumulative risk of breast cancer or ovarian cancer by the age of 70 years for carriers of BRCA1 mutations was 65% (95% CI, 44–78%) and 39% (95% CI, 18–54%), respectively, whereas the corresponding estimates for carriers of BRCA2 mutations were 45% (95% CI, 31–56%) and 11% (95% CI, 2.4–19%), respectively. More recently, a meta-analysis of 10 studies estimating risks of cancer associated with mutations in BRCA {254} reported a similar cumulative risk of breast and ovarian cancer for BRCA1 and for BRCA2 mutation-carriers, with risks of breast cancer to age 70 years of 57% (BRCA1) and 49% (BRCA2) and risks of ovarian cancer of 40% (BRCA1) and 18% (BRCA2). Some studies have shown that the founder mutations in the Ashkenazi Jewish population were associated with higher-than-average risks of breast and ovarian cancer {695}, while others have disputed this finding {59}. There have been consistent findings that mutations in certain regions of the BRCA1 and BRCA2 genes are associated with different risks compared with others, although studies do not always agree on the exact boundaries of these regions. For example, regions in the central portions of both BRCA1 {1435} and BRCA2 {481,1434} have been associated with higher risks of ovarian cancer and lower risks of breast cancer.

In males, pathogenic mutations in BRCA1 or BRCA2 are associated with increased risks of breast cancer, although all studies to date have shown that RR of male breast cancer is considerably higher in carriers of mutations in BRCA2. In Ontario, Canada, for example, Tai et al. {1392} estimated cumulative risks of male breast cancer to age 70 years of 1.8% and 6.8%, for BRCA1 and BRCA2 respectively, compared with a risk for the general population of 0.07%, with particularly high RR of breast cancer in young male carriers of BRCA2 mutations. In an analysis of a series of 115 unselected men with breast cancer, Ding et al. {344} found 18 pathogenic mutations in BRCA2 (16%), while Basham et al. {108} estimated that 8% of breast cancers in men were attributable to BRCA2 mutations.

Other cancers in carriers of mutations in BRCA1 or BRCA2

A number of studies have examined the risk of other cancers in carriers of BRCA1 mutations and the evidence to date suggests that there may be slight increased risks of prostate cancer, pancreatic cancer, and cervical cancer {1436}. It should be noted that there are also very high RRs for ovarian cancer-related sites such as the fallopian tube and peritoneum, although in many studies these are included with ovarian cancer. An early study by the Breast Cancer Linkage Consortium (BCLC) examined a variety of cancers in a series of 173 families collected from 20 different centres in Europe, the USA and Canada found a statistically significant excess risk of prostate cancer (RR, 4.65), pancreatic cancer (RR, 3.51), gallbladder and bile duct cancer (RR, 4.97), stomach cancer (RR, 2.59), and malignant melanoma (RR, 2.58) {1430}. A more recent study of a cohort of families in the Netherlands confirmed the increased risks of prostate and pancreatic cancer and also found potential associations with pharyngeal cancer and bone cancer {1483}. Another early study of two large families with BRCA2 mutations noted an association with laryngeal cancer as well as a suggestion of increased risk of ocular/uveal melanoma {365}. Studies of case series have estimated that 1–2% of prostate cancers diagnosed before age 65 years are attributable to mutations in BRCA2 {367} as well as a small fraction of ocular melanoma {627,1333}. In general, the risk of cancers other than breast and ovarian appears lower in BRCA1 carriers than in BRCA2 carriers, although the risks of breast and ovarian cancer are higher, suggesting that the overall burden of cancer may be similar for the two genes.

Risk modifiers in carriers of mutations in BRCA1/BRCA2

The risk figures cited above reflect the risk to an average woman at a given age. However, the risk to an individual woman will depend on many additional factors, both environmental/lifestyle, and other genetic factors. The fact that penetrance estimates derived from multiple-case families, even when correctly accounting for ascertainment, are generally higher than those from population-based studies or studies of cases unselected for family

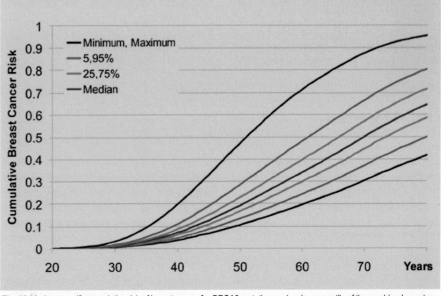

Fig. 16.03 Age-specific cumulative risk of breast cancer for BRCA2-mutation carriers by percentile of the combined genotype distribution at single-nucleotide polymorphisms (SNPs) rs2981582 in FGFR2, rs3803662 in TOX3/TNRC9, rs889312 in MAP3K1, rs3817198 in LSP1, rs13387042 in 2q35 region, rs4973768 in SLC4A7/NEK10 and rs10941679 in the 5p12 region {1543}.

history, provides evidence for such modifying effects. Genetic modelling of family data has shown evidence for a polygenic risk that explains familial aggregation even after accounting for BRCA1/2 status {58}.

Lifestyle factors

Thus far, the primary risk factors that have been examined as modifiers of risk in carriers of mutations in BRCA1/2 are those that are known to influence risk of breast cancer in the general population. In general, the role of these factors in carriers are similar in magnitude to those found in the general population, but the power of some studies has not been sufficient to derive statistically meaningful conclusions. Most studies have shown, however, that parity is a protective factor with effects similar to those seen in the general population {905}, although at least two studies have found parity to increase risk of breast cancer in carriers of BRCA2 mutations but reduce risk among carriers of BRCA1 mutations {300,905}. Perhaps the most consistent finding across studies is that use of oral contraceptives (OC) significantly reduces the risk of ovarian cancer in carriers of BRCA1 and BRCA2 mutations by about 50% {61,962}. For this reason, the effect of OC use on breast-cancer risk is important since risks of breast cancer are higher than those for ovarian cancer, particularly for BRCA2 carriers, this large protective effect for ovarian cancer could be offset by a more modest increase in breast cancer risk. Some studies have suggested that OC use is associated with a significant 40% increased risk of breast cancer {194}, while others have found smaller or no increased risks {961}.

A recent meta-analysis of 18 studies examining the role of OC use in BRCA1/2 carriers confirmed the 50% reduction in risk for ovarian cancer and found that there was an increased risk of breast cancer only for use of OC formulations prior to 1975 {624}.

There is some evidence that the effect of low-dose ionizing radiation such as chest X-rays before age 20 years in carriers is significantly larger than that in the general population {49}. There are now a number of ongoing prospective studies of carriers that should give more precise estimates, but this will require independent prospective validation.

Genetic factors

With the advent of large genome-wide association studies (GWAS) and large validation cohorts in breast cancer there are now at least 20 common genetic variants that have been shown convincingly to be associated with modest increases (odds ratio of 1.1–1.2) in breast cancer risk in the general population {1501}. It is reasonable to hypothesize that these variants may also influence the risk of breast and/or ovarian cancer in BRCA1 carriers. Because of the small effect sizes, it was recognized that large-scale collaborative studies were needed to address these questions; this provided the impetus for the formation of the CIMBA (Consortium of Investigators of Modifiers of BRCA1/2) consortium in 2005 {260}. This consortium now has a database of > 27 000 women with a pathogenic BRCA1 or BRCA2 mutation from research and clinical-genetics centres from all over the world, which can be used to test the effects of specific

genetic variants in BRCA1 and BRCA2 carriers. Thus far, most of the variants from GWAS studies of breast cancer in the general population have shown similar effects in BRCA2 carriers to that observed in the general population but, with one or two exceptions, do not seem to affect the risk of breast cancer in BRCA1 carriers {62}. Further analysis demonstrated that much of this difference could be explained by stratification by hormone-receptor status of the tumours. There have also been recent GWAS studies in subsets of the carriers in CIMBA for both BRCA1 and BRCA2. The BRCA1 GWAS {63} identified a novel locus on chromosome 19 that was also associated with ER-negative breast cancer in the general population and was also shown to be important in sporadic ovarian cancer, while the BRCA2 GWAS {479} identified two novel loci but largely identified loci that had been previously identified in studies in sporadic breast cancer. The utility of these common low-penetrance alleles in terms of risk prediction in BRCA2 carriers has been examined by Antoniou et al. {55} who demonstrated that using eight such single-nucleotide polymorphisms (SNPs) provides a potentially clinically useful refinement to risk prediction with the top 5% of the risk distribution having a cumulative risk of 80% compared with 50% for the bottom 5%. As more SNPs are incorporated into the model and with the addition of other factors, such as mutation prediction and lifestyle factors, even greater risk differentials can be achieved in the prediction of an individual woman's risk of developing breast (and ovarian) cancer.

BRCA1 gene

P. Devilee
G. Chenevix-Trench
D. Goldgar

Chromosomal location and gene structure

The BRCA1 gene maps to cytoband 17q21, and contains 23 coding exons spanning about 81 kb of genomic DNA {1344}. The BRCA1 transcript is 7094 bp long and encodes a nuclear protein of 1863 amino acids (about 210 kDa). The promotor region of BRCA1 contains a tandem duplication of approximately 30 kb, which thus produces two copies of BRCA1 exons 1 and 2, and two copies of exons 1–5 of an adjacent gene that has been designated

NBR1. It was suggested {1098} that these duplicated exons are non-processed pseudogenes, which could confound the analysis of BRCA1 mutations and have implications for the normal and abnormal regulation of BRCA1 transcription, translation, and function. The genomic region encompassing BRCA1 has an unusually high density of Alu repetitive DNA (41.5%), but a relatively low density (4.8%) of other repetitive sequences {1344}. These features have been proposed to have contributed

to the unusual high frequency of large genomic rearrangements detected in families with breast cancer {410}.

The BRCA1 protein shares no sequence homology with any other protein, but several structural domains have been recognized. A RING finger domain at the N-terminus mediates the interaction with BARD1, which confers an E3-ubiquitin ligase activity on the complex. Besides the nuclear localization signal, encoded by exon 11, BRCA1 contains two copies of a sequence of approximately 95 amino-acid residues that are organized as a tandem repeat at the carboxyl terminus, the so-called "BRCT domains". This domain occurs in a large family of nonorthologous proteins that are predominantly involved in cell-cycle checkpoint functions related to the DNA damage response, such as 53BP1 and RAD9.

Gene expression

Mutations in *BRCA1* have been shown to strongly predispose to breast and ovarian cancer and, to a lesser extent, to cancers of the colon, cervix, uterus, prostate and pancreas. In accordance with this, many different tissues express BRCA1 at the mRNA level, and this expression is strongly cell-cycle dependent, peaking at the G1/S boundary; expression is upregulated in differentiating mammary epithelial cells in response to glucocorticoids {1133}. Paradoxically, BRCA1-deficient tumour cells proliferate rapidly in situ.

More than 30 *BRCA1* splice variants have been observed in different tissues, but their regulation and possible functions are poorly understood at the moment {1039}. The most important, which maintain the open reading frame, are splice-variants lacking exons 9–10, exon 11, or exons 9–11. Of note, exon 11 encodes

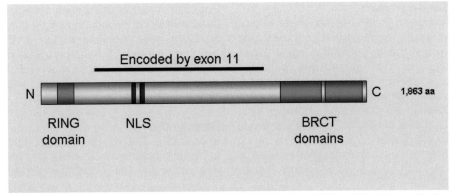

Fig. 16.04 Functional domains in the BRCA1 protein. The RING domain contains a C3HC4 motif that interacts with other proteins. NLS, nuclear localization signal; BRCT, BRCA-1-related C-terminal.

almost 60% of the full-length BRCA1 protein.

Gene function

The exact cellular function of BRCA1 is still unexplained, as is its specific connection to breast and ovarian cancer. Thus, it is not known which proteins are targeted by the ubiquitination activity of the BRCA1/BARD1 complex, nor which genes are regulated by the transcriptional-regulation and chromatin-remodelling activities that have been ascribed to the BRCT domain. Nonetheless, it is clear that BRCA1 is important in the regulation of the cellular response to

DNA damage {608}. The protein becomes associated with DNA-damage foci in a manner that is modulated by its phosphorylation by damage-associated kinases. Mutations in *BRCA1* have been shown to sensitize cells to a variety of DNA-damaging agents, and to specifically disrupt the G2/M cell-cycle checkpoint. Through its interaction with FANCJ (BRIP1), BRCA1 has become linked to the DNA-damage response network of Fanconi anaemia proteins {1548}. It has been proposed that BRCA1 is a signal integrator, linking sensors and response mechanisms for several types of DNA damage {608}.

BRCA2 gene

P. Devilee
G. Chenevix-Trench
M. Stratton

Chromosomal location and gene structure

The *BRCA2* gene maps to chromosome 13, band q13.1, and consists of 27 coding exons spanning about 84 kb of genomic DNA {1423}. The *BRCA2* mRNA is 10 930 bp in length, and encodes a protein of 3418 amino acids. Like *BRCA1*, the *BRCA2* gene has a large central exon 11, a translational start-site in exon 2, and AT-rich coding sequences.

The BRCA2 protein shares no sequence homology with any other protein. The C-terminal one third of the protein corresponds to the best-conserved portion of BRCA2 across dog, mouse, rat, and chicken orthologues. This region can be subdivided into a helical domain and three oligonucleotide/oligosaccharide-binding (OB) folds, the second of which contains a 130-amino acid insertion that adopts a

tower-like structure protruding away from the OB fold {1605}. The tower contains a helix-turn-helix motif that is similar to the DNA-binding domains of bacterial site-specific recombinases.

The middle 1100-residue region of *BRCA2* contains eight evolutionarily conserved motifs of approximately 35 residues each, termed BRC repeats, which all have the capacity to bind RAD51.

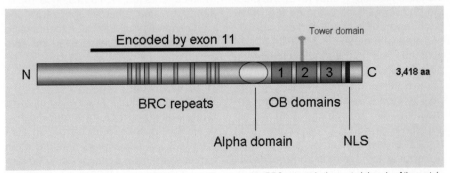

Fig. 16.05 Functional domains in the BRCA2 protein. There are eight BRC repeats in the central domain of the protein that interact with RAD51. The OB domains have a strong affinity for single-stranded DNA. OB domain, oligonucleotide/-oligosaccharide-binding domain

Gene expression

Mutations in BRCA2 have been shown to strongly predispose to breast and ovarian cancer, and to a lesser extent to cancers of the prostate, pancreas and stomach {1483}. Many different tissues express BRCA2 at the mRNA level, in a pattern that is strikingly similar to that of BRCA1. The highest levels of expression are observed in breast and thymus, with slightly lower levels in the lung, ovary, and spleen {1423}.

Both BRCA1 and BRCA2 show upregulated mRNA expression in rapidly proliferating cells, peaking at the G1/S boundary; expression is also upregulated in differentiating mammary epithelial cells in response to glucocorticoids {1133}.

Gene function

In contrast to BRCA1, BRCA2 is thought to be more directly involved in the error-free repair of DNA double-stranded breaks through homologous recombination. At the site of this type of DNA damage, the BRC repeat-domain of BRCA2 promotes the assembly of RAD51 nucleoprotein filaments on single-stranded DNA, whilst concurrently impeding loading onto double-stranded DNA {1509}, thereby stimulating strand invasion. Thus BRCA2 directly controls the availability and activity of RAD51.

Histopathological features of BRCA1- and BRCA2-associated breast cancers

S.R. Lakhani
M.J. van de Vijver
J. Jacquemier
A.L. Richardson
S.B. Fox
F. O'Malley

Histological type

Most hereditary breast cancers (approx. 70–80%) are invasive carcinomas of no special type (NST); however, carcinomas with medullary features are over-represented in patients with germ-line mutations in the BRCA1 gene (13% BRCA1 versus 2% controls) {181,747}. Multivariate analysis has demonstrated that features predictive of BRCA1 phenotype include pushing margins, lymphocytic infiltrate and high mitotic counts, but not the medullary phenotype per se – hence BRCA1 tumours are high-grade, "medullary-like" cancers {747}.

Unlike BRCA1, currently no specific morphological type has been clearly associated with either BRCA2 or non-BRCA1/2 (BRCAX) – which appear to be morphologically heterogeneous. Multivariate analysis of morphological features suggests that pushing margins, lack of tubule formation and high grade are significantly associated with BRCA2 tumours {96}. Lobular, tubular and tubulo-lobular carcinomas (collectively called the tubulo-lobular group) {878} and pleomorphic lobular carcinomas {68} have been reported in small studies to be associated with mutations in BRCA2; however, this has not been substantiated in other much larger studies {96,747}. There is some evidence that BRCA2 may play a role in the etiology of some sporadic lobular carcinomas {1329}. An association of lobular carcinoma with familial breast-cancer patients who do not appear to have mutations in BRCA1 or BRCA2 (i.e. BRCAX) has also been reported {746}.

Histological grade

Overall, both BRCA1- and BRCA2-associated tumours are of higher grade than are sporadic breast cancers. Tumours associated with mutations in BRCA1 have a higher score for all three parameters assessed (tubule formation, pleomorphism, mitotic counts), while tumours associated with mutations in BRCA2 appear to lack tubules, have higher mitotic counts, but may not be more pleomorphic. BRCAX tumours resemble sporadic breast cancers.

Steroid hormone receptors

BRCA1-associated breast cancers are more likely to be negative for estrogen and progesterone receptors (ER and PR) (approx. 70–90% of cases) compared with sporadic breast cancers (approx. 30% of cases). It is worth highlighting that ER-positive tumours can arise in patients with germline mutations in BRCA1, (approximately 10–30% of cases). In contrast, the frequency of ER and PR expression in BRCA2- and BRCAX-associated cancers is not significantly different to that in sporadic cancers {69,77, 750,752,808,1061}, although when adjusted for grade, one study showed that BRCA2 tumours were more often ER-positive than were the controls {96}.

HER2 and TP53

BRCA1- and BRCA2-associated cancers rarely overexpress or show amplification of HER2 (approx. 3% of cases). In contrast, BRCA1-associated tumours often express and have mutations in TP53 (approx. 90% of cases) {590}, while this is not a feature of BRCA2 cancers {752,1061, 1127}.

Other biological markers

BRCA1-associated cancers do not usually express BCL2 or cyclin D1 (ER-associated genes) and do not show amplification of CCND1. They do, however, overexpress p27 and cyclin E1, like other high-grade and "basal-like" cancers. Proliferation as measured by the Ki67 index is high, and EGFR overexpression and MYC amplification have also been described.

Association with the "basal" and triple negative phenotype

BRCA1-associated cancers are often triple-negative (ER-negative, PR-negative, HER2-negative) and a high proportion (60–70%) demonstrate a "basal-like" phenotype (expression of basal/myoepithelial markers such as keratin 5/6, keratin 14, smooth-muscle actin, EGFR, P-cadherin, caveolin 1) {71,460,750,1111}. In both ER-positive and ER-negative BRCA1-associated cancers, those with loss of the wildtype BRCA1 allele were more likely to express basal keratins {1467}. This is not a significant feature of BRCA2-/BRCAX-related breast cancers and the frequency is not higher than in sporadic cancers. Conversely, the BRCA1 pathway appears to be altered in a large proportion of sporadic breast cancers with a "basal" phenotype.

In a study investigating the incidence of BRCA1/2 mutations in an unselected series of triple negative breast cancers, approx. 15% had BRCA1 and 4% BRCA2 mutations {511}

Can pathology aid clinical decision-making?

Unlike tumours associated with BRCA2

mutations or *BRCAX*, the morphology of tumours associated with mutations in *BRCA1* is fairly distinct and it has been postulated that this may help to identify potential carriers of a germline mutation and hence triage patients towards testing. Current risk-estimation models are not very specific or accurate and new parameters that aid this process would be beneficial. Several studies have demonstrated that the addition of pathology to models of risk estimation improves the ability to predict the BRCA status {401,423,639,750}. Similarly, there is some evidence that pathology may add to the ability to identify unclassified sequence variants that are pathogenic {259,1088}. Since BRCA1 function is required for homology-directed repair of DNA double-strand breaks, identifying a tumour with a BRCA1/BRCA2 phenotype could help the clinician in the decision whether to use anti-PARP (poly ADP-ribose polymerase), anthracyclines, cisplatin or taxanes. Tumours carrying mutations in *BRCA1* or *BRCA2* are very sensitive to PARP inhibitors, a concept that has been validated in clinical trials {1473}.

Genetic alterations and gene-expression profiles of BRCA1- and BRCA2-associated breast cancers

J.S. Reis-Filho
A.L. Richardson
M.J. van de Vijver
D. Goldgar
D. Easton

Tumours arising in carriers of mutations in the *BRCA1* and *BRCA2* genes have been the subject of numerous research endeavours aiming to characterize their transcriptomic profiles and patterns of copy-number aberrations by microarray-based gene-expression profiling and microarray-based comparative genomic hybridization (aCGH), respectively.

Transcriptomic analysis of BRCA1 and BRCA2 cancers have initially suggested that these tumours would have fundamentally different patterns of gene expression. Gene signatures that distinguish between BRCA1 and BRCA2 cancers and between BRCA1 and BRCA2 and sporadic breast cancers have been identified {566}. Subsequent studies, however, have demonstrated that a reliable distinction between tumours from patients harbouring germline mutations in *BRCA1* or *BRCA2* cannot be achieved solely on the basis of their gene-expression profiles {436,592,1496,1536} and that the main transcriptomic differences between BRCA1 and other types of breast cancer are related to lack of estrogen-receptor (ER) expression and high proliferation of these tumours {97, 592, 1536}.

As a group, tumours arising in carriers of *BRCA1* mutations have been shown to be remarkably similar to sporadic triple-negative and basal-like breast cancers in terms of their gene-expression profiles {1357,1536}. The similarities are such that some have suggested that sporadic basal-like breast cancers may be phenocopies of tumours arising in carriers of germline mutations in *BRCA1* {1470, 1471}. Importantly, however, approximately 15% of all tumours arising in carriers of *BRCA1* mutations are ER-positive; these BRCA1 breast cancers have been shown to display preferentially a luminal B phenotype (i.e. ER-positive and high proliferation) {1467,1468,1536}. It has recently been posited that breast cancers arising in carriers of *BRCA1* mutations may also be classified as claudin-low subtype {1123}, a subgroup reported to be enriched for the so-called cancer stem cells {1122}. It should be noted, however, that the clinical and biological significance of this molecular subtype is yet to be fully established. The vast majority of tumours arising in carriers of germline mutations in *BRCA2*, on the other hand, are classified as luminal A or luminal B breast cancers {1357,1536}, consistent with the high prevalence of ER-positive tumours in this group of hereditary cancers {752}.

Chromosomal and aCGH analyses of breast tumours arising in carriers of *BRCA1* and *BRCA2* mutations have yielded conflicting results {41,664,665, 667,910–912,1372,1484,1536,1575}. Some have observed remarkably similar patterns of gene copy-number aberrations between (i) BRCA1 cancers and sporadic triple-negative and basal-like breast cancers; and (ii) BRCA2 cancers and sporadic breast cancers of matching molecular subtype, ER status and histological grade {910–912,1372,1536}. In fact, several studies have now suggested that the patterns of gene copy-number aberrations in both sporadic and hereditary breast cancers largely segregate with the ER status and histological grade of the tumour {912,1001}. On the other hand, aCGH signatures to identify breast cancers arising in carriers of germline mutations in *BRCA1* or *BRCA2* have been developed {665,667,1484}. It has been suggested that these signatures identify BRCA1 or BRCA2 tumours with substantial levels of accuracy (91% and 86.5% for BRCA1 and BRCA2 cancers, respectively {665,667}). Importantly, these aCGH predictors also classify a subgroup of sporadic breast cancers as BRCA1-like or BRCA2-like {41,665–667,1527}. It has been suggested that HER2-negative sporadic breast cancers with a BRCA1-like profile have a significantly better response to a non-standard regimen of platinum-based chemotherapy {1527}.

Despite the controversies as to whether tumours arising in carriers of germline mutations in *BRCA1* or *BRCA2* do harbour distinct patterns of genetic aberrations, it is now accepted that BRCA1 tumours often display a complex pattern of low-level gene copy-number gains and losses affecting multiple chromosomal regions (i.e. the so-called "complex sawtooth" pattern {463,574}), with recurrent changes affecting gains of 3q, 7p, 8q, 10p, 12p and 17q, and losses of 4p, 4q, 5q and 18q {41,664,665,667,910–912, 1372,1484,1536,1575}. BRCA2 cancers are more heterogeneous; however, they often display a complex pattern of genomic aberrations and are characterized by recurrent gains of 8q, 17q and 20q and losses of 8p, 13q and 11q {41,664, 665,667,910–912,1372,1484,1536,1575}. Importantly, these aberrations reported in BRCA1 and BRCA2 cancers are also found in sporadic cancers of similar molecular subtype {911,1372,1536}. In addition, BRCA1 tumours, in a way akin to sporadic basal-like breast cancers, often display chromosome X isodisomy {1182}. A "mutator" phenotype, characterized by multiple tandem duplications, has been reported in ER-negative breast cancers, but is not a common denominator of

BRCA1 mutant breast cancers {1375}. It has been suggested that frequent intragenic chromosome breaks, inversions, deletions and copy number aberrations affecting the tumour suppressor gene *PTEN* may constitute a remarkably common denominator of BRCA1 breast cancers {1245}. This finding certainly merits additional investigation, given its therapeutic implications and the reported low prevalence of *PTEN* mutations in sporadic breast cancers, even those of basal-like and triple-negative phenotype {886,1374}.

Targeted sequencing and loss-of-heterozygosity analysis of BRCA1 and BRCA2 breast cancers have revealed that *TP53* mutations are found in > 90% of BRCA1 cancers {296,591,868}, and that the pattern of *TP53* mutations in BRCA1 tumours differs from that of sporadic ER-positive and ER-negative breast cancers {868}. *TP53* mutations, however, appear not to be a common feature of BRCA1 ER-positive cancers {868}. Likewise, *TP53* mutations in BRCA2 breast cancers, which are predominantly ER-positive, are not as prevalent (29–64%). Importantly, several

studies have now demonstrated that in the vast majority of hereditary BRCA1 and BRCA2 breast cancers, the wild-type *BRCA1* or *BRCA2* allele is lost {868, 1362, 1467}. This observation also holds true for ER-positive BRCA1 breast cancers {868, 1467}, providing strong circumstantial evidence to demonstrate that most of these tumours are unlikely to constitute sporadic ER-positive breast cancers developing in a background of *BRCA1* germline mutations. Additional recurrent genetic aberrations found in BRCA1 and

BRCA2 hereditary breast cancers are summarized in Table 16.03. It should be emphasized that with the advent of massively parallel sequencing, it is likely that in the next few years the complete landscape of genetic and epigenetic aberrations in tumours arising in carriers of mutations in *BRCA1* and *BRCA2* will be available. These findings are likely to answer the question of whether hereditary BRCA1 and BRCA2 cancers are in fact distinct from sporadic breast cancers of similar phenotype.

Table 16.03 Characteristics of hereditary breast cancers associated with BRCA1 and BRCA2 syndromes

Characteristic	BRCA1 cancers	BRCA2 cancers
"Intrinsic" molecular subtype	> 80% basal-like; rarely of luminal and normal-like subtype. A proportion of the basal-like subtype can be reclassified as claudin-low subtype	Preferentially of luminal phenotype
TP53 gene mutations	> 90%	29–64%
HER2 gene amplification	< 5%	< 5%
CCND1 gene amplification	0–22%	24–60%
MYB gene amplification	29%	0%

Li-Fraumeni syndrome

J. Birch
J. Garber

Definition

Li-Fraumeni syndrome (LFS) is an autosomal dominant heritable condition predisposing to a broad spectrum of cancers. It is caused by germline mutations in the *TP53* gene. The main cancers that characterize LFS are sarcomas of soft tissue and bone, breast cancers, brain tumours and adrenocortical carcinomas. Multiple primary neoplasms are frequent in carriers of mutations.

MIM Nos

Li-Fraumeni syndrome   151623
TP53 mutations
(germline and sporadic)   191170

Synonym

Sarcoma family syndrome of Li and Fraumeni

Incidence

The R15 (November 2010) version of the International Agency for Research on Cancer (IARC) *TP53* germline mutation database {1097} includes 597 germline mutations reported in the world literature from 1990 onwards. The estimated birth prevalence of germline *TP53* mutations is 1 in 20 000 to 1 in 5000 {510,753} but 1 in 300 for a specific mutation in Southern Brazil {13}. There may be a high frequency of de novo mutations {509}.

Diagnostic criteria

LFS and Li-Fraumeni-like syndrome (LFL) were originally defined by clinical criteria {143,798,861}. Germline mutations in *TP53* have been found with frequencies of 56–74% in patients with LFS and 16–33% in those with LFL {142,510,1239}. Chompret et al. proposed criteria for selecting patients for clinical genetic testing (revised in 2009) that yield a detection rate of around 30% {174,265,510,1440}.

Breast tumours

Breast tumours are by far the most frequent tumours associated with LFS. The IARC database records 301 breast tumours (26%) in mutation carriers and their families.

Early studies on LFS noted the very young age of diagnosis of breast cancer with around 30% of patients aged < 30 years {143,798}. Subsequent studies of cases of breast cancer diagnosed at age < 30 years with no family history and no *BRCA1/2* mutations found germline *TP53* mutations in 4%, 3% and 0% of cases, respectively {491,754,951}. Combining these results, there were 4 mutations among 209 cases (2%). Among 22 cases aged < 30 years with a family history of breast cancer or who met the criteria for LFS or LFL, *TP53* mutations were detected in 2 (9%) {754}. These findings were supported by other studies {148,1545}. It seems that the rate of germline mutations in *TP53* among women with breast cancer aged < 30 years is very low in the absence of a relevant family history.

Little information on the histopathological types of breast tumours found with germline mutations in *TP53* is available in the literature. To address this, 73 breast tumours among 50 families with germline mutations in *TP53* have been reviewed (JM Birch, AM Kelsey & DGR Evans, unpublished data). In 29 cases, the diagnosis was carcinoma/adenocarcinoma of no special type (NST). In the remaining 44 cases, pathology reports and/or tissue blocks were available for review. These were classified as: invasive carcinoma NST, 26 cases; ductal carcinoma in situ (DCIS), 5 cases; phyllodes tumour, 5 cases; invasive lobular carcinoma, 2 cases; 1 case each of mucinous carcinoma, medullary carcinoma, Paget disease, intraductal carcinoma and spindle cell sarcoma (probably radiation-induced); and fibroadenoma, 2 cases.

This distribution is similar to that for sporadic tumours, except phyllodes tumour: 7% of total cases compared with < 1% in most series. We previously suggested that phyllodes tumour was a component of the LFS/TP53 syndrome {141}. The age distribution is striking and shows a major peak at age 27–32 years, most of these tumours being invasive carcinoma NST. The histologies of tumours arising in the second peak of incidence at age 36–47 years are more mixed. Only two cases occurred in women aged > 59 years.

An immunohistochemical study of breast tumours associated with germline mutations in *TP53* found an excess of cases with amplification of HER2, 9 of 12 (83%) vs 16% in a comparison cohort of 231 early-onset breast cancers. However,

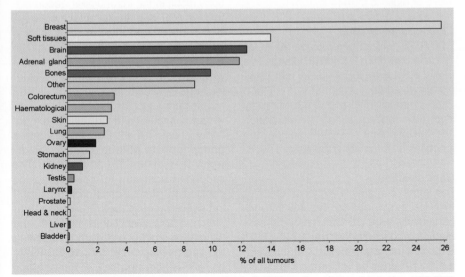

Fig. 16.06 Percentage distribution of 1165 tumours associated with *TP53* germline mutations. Adapted from IARC *TP53* Database, R15 release, November 2010 {1097}.

hormone receptor status (estrogen and progesterone receptors, ER and PR) was similar in both groups {1585}.

Further work is required to define the morphological, immunohistochemical and molecular characteristics of breast cancers in carriers of germline mutations of *TP53*.

Other tumours

Soft tissue (14.0%), brain (12.4%), adrenal gland (11.9%) and bones (9.9%) account for > 48% of tumours in patients/families with germline mutations in *TP53*. The majority of papers reporting families with germline mutations in *TP53* do not record specific morphologies.

A report on 236 sarcomas recorded in the IARC database included 158 in women aged < 20 years at diagnosis. Among these, 80% were osteosarcoma (73 cases) or rhabdomyosarcoma (53 cases). Among the 78 cases in older women, osteo-sarcoma (18 cases), leiomyosarcoma (18 cases) and liposarcoma (11 cases) were the most frequent {1022}. Given the age and cancer-type restrictions imposed by the LFS, LFL and Chompret criteria used to select families for mutation analysis, the age distribution and consequently the frequencies of morphological types are likely to be biased. These considerations also apply to the interpretation of distribution of other tumours by age and morphology. Adrenocortical tumours are exceedingly rare in the general population but are remarkably frequent in LFS. A special situation exists in southern Brazil where a recurrent mutation in *TP53*, R337H, is found in association with a high incidence of adrenocortical tumours. Carriers of this mutation are likely to be descended from a single founder {474}. In other populations, up to 80% of incident adrenocortical tumours may be associated with germline mutations in *TP53*, regardless of family history {371,1502}.

There is little systematic information on the frequency of specific morphological types of brain tumours in LFS. In the series of 50 families with *TP53* mutations described above, there were 18 cases of glioblastoma multiforme/high-grade astrocytoma, 10 other high-grade tumours including 3 choroid plexus carcinomas, but only 3 low-grade astrocytomas. Choroid plexus tumours in young children are a recognized component of LFS {1067}.

Tumours at all other sites represent 3% or less of the total. To what extent these are associated with *TP53* carrier status is un-

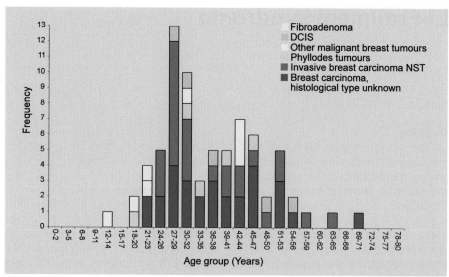

Fig. 16.07 Frequency distribution of 73 breast tumours in 50 families with germline *TP53* mutations by 3-year age group and histological type.

certain. Furthermore, mutation carriers may be more vulnerable to exogenous carcinogens, possibly giving rise to international variations in the incidence of minor components of this syndrome.

Genetics

It is now accepted that presence of a germline mutation in *TP53* is synonymous with LFS {1067}. It had been suggested that germline mutations in *CHEK2* were a cause of the LFS phenotype, but this has since been refuted {399,1067,1238}. Mutations in certain genes, including *BRCA2*, other Fanconi genes and DNA mismatch repair (MMR) genes can give rise to Li-Fraumeni-like patterns of cancer in monoallelic or biallelic form {405,1557}.

Chromosomal location

The *TP53* gene encompasses 20 kb on chromosome 17p12.1. *TP53* belongs to a family of growth suppressors that comprises two additional members, *TP73* and *TP63*. Whereas *TP73* and *TP63* are mostly involved in the regulation of differentiation and development, *TP53* has specialized functions as a tumour suppressor {786}.

Gene structure

The gene contains 11 exons, the first exon being non-coding. The first intron is particularly large (10 kb). The coding sequence is concentrated over 1.3 kb. *TP53* is ubiquitously expressed, mostly as a single mRNA species (although rare alternatively spliced variants have been reported). The promoter does not contain a

classical TATA box, but shows binding elements for several common transcription factors, including c-Jun and NF-kappaB {533A}.

Gene expression

The p53 protein is constitutively expressed in most cell types but, in normal circumstances, does not accumulate to a significant level due to rapid degradation by the proteasome machinery. In response to various types of cellular stress, the p53 protein undergoes a number of post-translational modifications that release p53 from the negative control of MDM2, a protein that binds to p53 and mediates it degradation. These modifications result in the intranuclear accumulation of p53 and in its activation as a transcription factor. Two major signalling pathways can trigger *TP53* activation. The first, and best characterized, is the pathway of response to DNA damage, including large kinases of the phosphoinositol-3 kinase family such as ATM (ataxia telangiectasia mutated) and the cell-cycle regulatory kinase CHEK2. Both these kinases phosphorylate p53 at the extreme *N*-terminus (serines 15, 20 and 37). The second is activated in response to the constitutive stimulation of growth-promoting signalling cascades. The central regulator in this pathway is p14ARF, the alternative product of the locus encoding the cyclin-kinase inhibitor p16/CDKN2A. p14ARF is activated by E2F transcription factors, and binds MDM2, thus neutralizing its capacity to induce p53 degradation.

This pathway may be part of a normal feedback-control loop in which p53 is activated as a cell-cycle brake in cells exposed to hyperproliferative stimuli {1113}.

Gene function

After accumulation, the p53 protein acts as a transcriptional regulator for a panel of genes that differ according to the nature of the stimulus, its intensity and the cell type considered. Broadly speaking, the genes controlled by p53 fall into three main categories, including cell regulatory genes (*CDKN1A/WAF1, GADD45, SFN/14-3-3S, CCNG1/CYCLING*), pro-apoptotic genes (*FAS/APO1/CD95, KILLER/DR5/TNFRSF10B, AIF1, PUMA/BBC3, BAX*) and genes involved in DNA repair (*MGMT,MLH1*). The p53 protein also binds to components of the transcription, replication and repair machinery and may exert additional controls on DNA stability through the modulation of these mechanisms. Collectively, the genes targeted by p53 mediate two types of cellular responses: cell-cycle arrest, followed by DNA repair in cells exposed to mild forms of genotoxic stress, and apoptosis, in cells exposed to levels of damage that cannot be efficiently repaired. Both responses contribute to the transient or permanent suppression of cells that contain damaged, potentially oncogenic DNA. In the mouse, inactivation of *TP53* by homologous recombination does not prevent normal growth, but results in a strong predisposition to early, multiple cancers, illustrating the crucial role of this gene as a tumour suppressor {352}.

Mutation spectrum

Missense mutations, mainly in the DNA-binding domain, account for 73% of germline mutations. Nonsense and frameshift mutations comprise a further 17%. The frequency distribution follows a similar pattern to that for somatic mutations {1097}, but there is a relatively higher proportion of splicing mutations in the germline, 8%, compared with 2% of somatic mutation. In the germline, 50% of mutations are GC to AT transitions at CpG sites compared with 25% of somatic mutations, but there is a higher proportion of transversions in somatic mutations (31%)

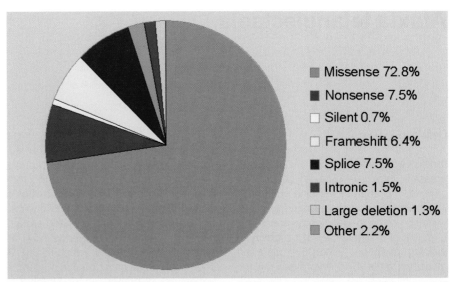

Fig. 16.08 Distribution of 579 *TP53* germline mutations by mutation effect. Adapted from IARC *TP53* Database, R15 release, November 2010 {1097}.

compared with germline mutations (18%). This pattern suggests that a higher proportion of germline mutations are attributable to spontaneous endogenous processes {1035}. Somatic and germline mutations cluster at specific codons. The major mutation hotspots are in the DNA-binding domain at codons 175, 245, 248, and 282. These coincide with residues that directly contact DNA or are important in stabilizing the protein structure {1067}.

Genotype–phenotype correlations

Some correlations between classes of mutation and cancer phenotype have been demonstrated. Alleles associated with severe loss of transactivation function and dominant-negative effects confer a more highly penetrant cancer phenotype than partial deficiency alleles. Brain tumours appear to be associated with missense mutations in the DNA binding loop that contacts the minor groove (codons 175, 245, 248). Missense mutations in the loops opposing the DNA-binding surface (codons 151, 152, 219, 220) were associated with adrenocortical tumours. These latter mutations probably exert a milder effect on protein function. Mutations outside the DNA-binding surface appeared to confer a later age of onset in breast cancer {142,943,1034,1097}. Studies suggest that the *MDM2* SNP309 polymorph-ism

and certain polymorphisms within *TP53* have an impact on cancer risk and age of onset in carriers of *TP53* mutations {165,173,418,872}. However, a recent study suggests only a modest association between *MDM2* SNP309 and increased risk of cancer {1601}.

Prognosis and predictive factors

There have been no formal studies of survival from LFS-associated cancers in carriers of *TP53* mutations. However, cancer survivors are frequently struck by second and subsequent cancers. Although anecdotal cases exist, it is not clear whether carriers of *TP53* mutations are particularly sensitive to radiation carcinogenesis {573,581,810,1251}. The estimated risk of cancer in male carriers is 73% and approaches 100% in females {266}.

Pre-symptomatic testing for germline mutations in TP53 is carried out in many centres worldwide. Guidelines have been developed for the testing itself and for screening for early diagnosis and clinical management in mutation carriers {403, 755,1518}. Given the limited clinical benefits, testing and follow-up of families raises a number of ethical and medical considerations, especially in children {860}.

Ataxia telangiectasia

G. Chenevix-Trench
R. Balleine

Definition

Ataxia telangiectasia (AT) is an autosomal-recessive syndrome characterized by progressive cerebellar ataxia, oculomotor apraxia, choreoathetosis, sino-pulmonary infections, oculocutaneous telangiectasia, variable immune deficiency, sterility, a high risk of malignancy and sensitivity to ionizing radiation {901,1063}. Germline mutations in the *ATM* gene (ataxia telangiectasia mutated) are the cause of this autosomal-recessive disorder.

MIM No.   208900

Synonyms

Louis-Bar syndrome

Incidence

AT is a rare condition with an estimated prevalence of 1–2.5 per 100 000 {1063}.

Tumours in AT patients

AT patients show a high incidence of malignancy, in particular, leukaemias and lymphomas {1036,1365}.

Breast cancer in *ATM* mutation carriers

An increased incidence of breast cancer in the order of two- to threefold compared with the general population has consistently been observed in female relatives of AT patients {235,1037,1433}.

This led to the hypothesis that carriers of mutations in the *ATM* gene were at increased risk of breast cancer, and that the risk might be higher for carriers of missense mutations because of a dominant-negative effect on protein function {478}. Bernstein et al. reported a high risk of breast cancer in heterozygous carriers of the c.7271T>G (p.Val2424Gly) mutation, with an estimated hazard ratio of 8.6 (95% CI, 3.9–18.9) {121}. Furthermore, this mutation has been shown to act as a dominant-negative in terms of its associated expression profile in lymphoblastoid cell lines {1537}. However, ascribing pathogenicity to rarer missense variants of *ATM* has been a challenge. Tavtigian et al. pooled published data with data from their own mutation screening of breast-

cancer cases and controls {1421}. Using an in silico missense-substitution analysis, they carried out analyses of protein-truncating, splice-junction, and rare missense variants. This showed that a subset of rare, evolutionarily unlikely missense substitutions, falling in and around the FAT (a conserved sequence in FRAP, ATM and TRRAP), kinase, and FATC (FAT C-terminal) domains, appear to confer the highest risk of breast cancer. Fletcher et al. compared five *ATM* missense variants, that occur with a frequency of about 1% in controls, in > 26 000 cases of breast cancer and 29 000 controls and reported an overall trend odds ratio of 1.06 {453}. These studies suggest that a subset of missense mutations in *ATM* confer a moderate increased risk of breast cancer, and that some polymorphic missense variants may be associated with a very small increase in risk, analogous to the effect of other low-risk alleles that have been identified in genome-wide association studies {364}. However, the rarity of individual variants of *ATM* poses an ongoing challenge to studies seeking to elucidate precise genotype–phenotype correlates of breast-cancer incidence, features and outcome.

Clinical and pathological features

Heterozygous mutations in *ATM* have been associated with young age of breast-cancer onset {235,1037,1433}. there is limited information on the pathology of breast cancers occurring in carriers of *ATM* variants, and no distinctive tumour phenotype has been identified {95}.

Response to therapy and prognosis

Heterozygous carriers of *ATM* variants do not show the severe toxic effects of radiation therapy that can occur in AT patients {1381}, but a recent report found an increased risk of contralateral breast cancer in heterozygous carriers of deleterious *ATM* mutations treated with radiotherapy {120}.

There is evidence that inhibition of PARP1 is synthetically lethal with mutation or loss

of *ATM* and that the effect is mediated through mitotic catastrophe independently of apoptosis {1577}. *ATM* mutation carriers affected with breast cancer might therefore be candidates for treatment with PARP inhibitors, in a manner similar to carriers of mutations in *BRCA1* and *BRCA2*.

ATM expression in breast cancer

In the normal breast, immunohistochemical studies have identified strong nuclear staining of ATM protein in the ducto-lobular epithelium, with a lower level of staining in myoepithelial cells {51,1447}. In a tissue microarray-based study, Tommiska et al. reported that the level of ATM expression in breast cancers was usually comparable to that in normal breast epithelium. Relative reduction in ATM expression was more common in breast cancers occurring in carriers of *BRCA1/BRCA2* mutations. In non-BRCA1/BRCA2 cases, a reduction in ATM expression was associated with higher grade, negativity for estrogen receptor (ER) and progesterone receptor (PR), and the "triple-negative" (negative for ER, PR and HER2) tumour type {1447}.

Genetics

Classic AT is a monogenic disease caused by mutations in the *ATM* gene. Most AT patients are compound heterozygotes for mutations in *ATM*.

Chromosomal location

ATM is located on chromosome 11q22–23.

Gene structure

ATM extends over 150 kb of DNA and has 66 exons. The *ATM* transcript is 13 kb, encoding a 3056 amino-acid protein of 350 kDa. The initiating codon is within exon 4 {1480}

Gene expression

ATM is expressed in all normal tissues {1269}.

Gene function

ATM is a serine/threonine kinase that belongs to the PI3-kinase-related kinase

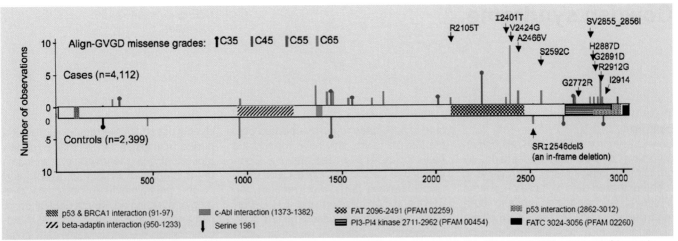

Fig. 16.09 The domain organization of the ATM protein and distribution of breast cancer-associated C65 missense substitutions falling from Ile1960 until the end of the protein. Reprinted from {1421} with permission from Elsevier.

(PIKK) family, with conserved kinase and regulatory domains in the C-terminal region {781}. ATM has a large number of phosphorylation targets, including major human tumour suppressor genes such as *TP53* and *BRCA1*.

In response to DNA damage, in particular double-strand DNA breaks, ATM is activated by autophosphorylation. Many of its known functions relate to the activation of cell-cycle checkpoints that impede progression of the cell cycle in cells with damaged DNA. For example, at the G1/S phase cell-cycle checkpoint, ATM phosphorylates p53 and its binding partner MDM2, leading to activation and stabilization of p53. ATM also phosphorylates CHK2, leading to upregulation, activation and ultimately inhibition of cyclin dependent kinase 2 (CDK2) via degradation of CDC25A (cell division cycle 25A). ATM functions to slow S-phase progression via phosphorylation of components of the MRN complex, direct phosphorylation of BRCA1,

FANCD2 and SMC1. Phosphorylation of CHK2, BRCA1 and RAD17 contribute to the G2/M checkpoint {688,1306}.

ATM is also known to contribute to DNA repair through CHK2-mediated phosphorylation of BRCA1 and regulation of chromatin dynamics, and it has been implicated in the maintenance of telomere length {688,1306}.

Mutation spectrum in AT patients

Over 500 unique mutations in *ATM* have been reported that are distributed throughout the gene, with no mutation hotspots {477}. *ATM* mutations can be broadly categorized as: (1) protein-truncating, non-expressing; (2) in-frame deletions encoding mutant protein without kinase activity; or (3) missense mutations encoding mutant protein with reduced kinase activity {1433}. Most AT patients carry protein-truncating non-expressing mutations. Approximately 90% of AT patients have no detectable ATM protein, 10% have trace amounts and 1% express a

normal amount of protein without kinase activity. Detection of ATM protein and in vitro assays for radiosensitivity and ATM kinase activity may form part of diagnostic testing for AT {477}.

Genotype–phenotype correlations

The major characteristics of AT are generally consistent, but there is variability in the age of onset, progression and severity of symptoms as well as the occurrence of cancer. In particular, it has been observed that *ATM* missense mutations resulting in some protein expression and residual kinase activity may result in an attenuated phenotype {269}. In this regard, the c.7271T>G missense mutation has been of interest since rare homozygotes for this mutation showed a less severe form of AT and normal levels of ATM protein. In addition, elevated rates of breast cancer have been observed in homozygote and heterozygote carriers {1365}.

Cowden syndrome

C. Eng
J. Garber

Definition

Cowden syndrome (CS) is an autosomal-dominant disorder mainly caused by germline mutations of the *PTEN* gene. It is characterized by a high risk of cancers of the breast, endometrium and non-medullary thyroid, as well as multiple hamartomas most typically involving the gastrointestinal, neurological and muco-cutaneous systems. As *PTEN* mutations also underpin the paediatric syndrome Bannyan-Riley-Ruvalcaba syndrome and Proteus syndrome, these syndromes are collectively referred to as "PTEN hamartoma tumour syndrome" {585}.

MIM No.   158350

Synonyms

PTEN hamartoma tumour syndrome; Cowden disease; multiple hamartoma syndrome

Incidence

Limited estimates of prevalence has been permitted since the identification of the CS susceptibility gene {804}, with an estimate of 1 : 250 000 {972} based on one national series. This is almost certainly an underestimate, because of the challenging nature of CS diagnosis, with its breadth and subtlety of features {382}.

Diagnostic criteria

The diagnosis of CS represents a considerable clinical challenge. The International Cowden Consortium (ICC) {973} first compiled operational diagnostic criteria for CS, based on clinical experience and the published literature in 1996. These clinical criteria have been regularly updated over the last 15 years, and have formed the basis for the USA-based National Comprehensive Cancer Network (NCCN) Practice Guidelines {381}. Most recently, the Cleveland Clinic, where the ICC is currently centred, has released the first scoring system for practical use in an adult clinical setting, on the basis of a prospective multicentre global study involving probands recruited from centres in North America, Europe and Asia {1402}. The Cleveland Clinic score has been externally validated, and demonstrated to provide superior predictions relative to the most recent NCCN criteria.

The Cleveland Clinic score for an individual adult patient is the sum of specific weights allocated to the presence of key phenotypical features (Table 16.06). The individual score of a subject corresponds to a specific probability of a *PTEN* mutation being identified for that subject. The Cleveland Clinic score is available on the internet for risk evaluation and patient counselling (http://lerner.ccf.org/gmi/cc-score). On a community level, selecting individuals with a threshold score of 10 and higher for *PTEN* mutation testing would correspond to an expected sensitivity of 90–93%, and a specificity of 62–75%, and is thus recommended as a practice guideline in a specialist genetics setting.

Since the clinical presentation of a germline *PTEN* mutation in the paediatric setting is distinct from that in adults, Cleveland Clinic paediatric criteria for testing for mutations in *PTEN* in individuals aged < 18 years have been developed separately (Table 16.07) {1402}.

Overall, for adults, the most commonly reported manifestations are macrocephaly (specifically, megaencephaly), carcinoma of the breast, endometrium, thyroid and colon, gastrointestinal polyposis syndrome (often including, but not limited to, hamartomas or ganglioneuromas), fibrocystic breast disease, multiple early-onset uterine leiomyomas and characteristic mucocutaneous features. Paediatric patients usually present with macrocephaly and at least one other feature, including autism or developmental delay, characteristic dermatological features, vascular features such as arteriovenous malformations, or gastrointestinal polyps.

Breast tumours

Age distribution and penetrance

Invasive carcinomas of the breast have been diagnosed as early as age 14 years and as late as in the 60s {826}. The average age of diagnosis of breast cancer for females with CS is between 38 and 46 years {201,1367,1402}. A single population-based clinical study suggested that benign breast disease can occur in two thirds of affected women, while CS females have a 25–50% lifetime risk of developing invasive breast cancer {381, 1367}. Male breast cancer can also occur in CS, but the frequency is unknown {411, 879}.

Clinical features

It is believed that the clinical presentation of breast cancer in CS is no different from that of the general population. However, no formal data are currently available.

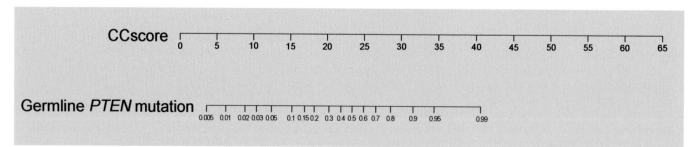

Fig. 16.10 The Cleveland Clinic (CC) score nomogram showing correlation between total score (upper line) and probability of a germline mutation of *PTEN* (lower line) {1402}.

Histopathology

A systematic study of 59 cases of breast histopathology from 19 women with CS has been performed {1286}. Thirty-five specimens had some form of malignant pathology. Of these, 31 (90%) had invasive carcinoma NST, one tubular carcinoma and one lobular carcinoma in situ. Sixteen of the 31 had both invasive and in situ components of ductal carcinoma, while 12 had ductal carcinoma in situ (DCIS) only and two invasive carcinoma NST only. The authors noted that 19 of these carcinomas appeared to have arisen in the midst of densely fibrotic hamartomatous tissue. Multifocality and bilaterality of breast cancer is common in patients with CS. To date, 34% of CS patients with breast cancer as reported in the literature had bilateral disease, which was approximately evenly split between metachronous and synchronous status {1185}. Of note, a recent report has suggested that apocrine differentiation is common in breast cancers from patients with germline mutations in *PTEN* {100}. However, the relatively small number of samples in this study, as well as the absence of corresponding amplification of *HER2* (*ERBB2*), as would ordinarily be expected in apocrine carcinoma, suggests that additional validation is required.

Certainly, benign breast disease is more common than malignant, with the former believed to occur in 75% of affected females. Fibrocystic disease of the breast and breast hamartomas are commonly seen {1286}. A small radiological study has reported an association between CS and multiple tubular adenomas of the breast {1246}. Given the dense breasts of patients with CS, and their high risk of breast cancer, magnetic resonance imaging is a standard recommendation for screening for breast cancer in these individuals.

Prognosis and predictive factors

Whether the prognosis differs from sporadic cases, after matching for bilaterality, has not been established. Although prophylactic risk-reducing mastectomies have been performed in the setting of CS {28}, it remains unclear whether this approach is superior to surveillance. Typically, prophylactic mastectomies are performed when clinical surveillance can no longer distinguish benign from malignant disease.

Other tumours

Uterine tumours

Age distribution and penetrance

The frequency of endometrial cancer in females with CS is about 10%, an estimate not based on rigorous study. These individuals have a median age of presentation in their 40s, and even patients presenting at age < 30 years are recognized {1402}. Benign tumours of the uterus are also common in CS. Uterine leiomyomas occur in almost half of affected women {826,1402}. They are usually multifocal and occur at a young age.

Clinical features

There have been no systematic studies of uterine tumours in CS. Clinical observation and anecdotal reports suggest that the leiomyomas can become quite symptomatic, presenting with bleeding and pain. It is unclear if the clinical presentation of the endometrial carcinomas is different from that of sporadic cases.

Histopathology

There have been no systematic studies of uterine tumours in CS, although it is believed that the histopathology is no different from that of typical sporadic cases.

Prognosis and prognostic factors

Whether the prognosis differs from that for sporadic cases is unknown.

Thyroid tumours

Age of distribution and penetrance

Non-medullary thyroid carcinomas occur at a frequency of 8–18% of affected individuals, regardless of sex {826,1367, 1402}. Median age of presentation is in the 30s, with patients recognized in the paediatric age group. Benign thyroid disease occurs in approximately 70% of affected individuals {1402}. Component features include multinodular goitre and follicular adenomas.

Clinical features

Many of the benign tumours in CS individuals remain asymptomatic. However, the most common presenting sign or symptom would be a neck mass. Like many inherited syndromes, CS thyroid lesions can be multifocal and bilobar.

Histopathology

No systematic studies have been performed to examine the thyroid in CS.

Gastrointestinal tumours

Colorectal adenocarcinoma is a newly reported component cancer for CS, and is relatively uncommon, with an estimated prevalence of 13% {565}. All patients presented at age < 50 years, consistent with a genetic association. In terms of benign gastrointestinal disease, gastrointestinal polyps were found in 93% of CS individuals

Table 16.06 Component features and weights of the Cleveland Clinic scoring system for the diagnosis of Cowden syndrome {1402}

Component feature	Scoring weight[a]
Neurological	
Macrocephaly, presence	6
Extreme (male, OFC ≥ 63 cm)	10
Extreme (female, OFC ≥ 60 cm)	10
Lhermitte Duclos disease	10
Autism or developmental delay	1
Breast and gynaecological	
Breast cancer, age of onset	
< 30 years	4
30–39 years	4
40–49 years	2
≥ 50 years	1
Fibrocystic breast disease	1
Endometrial cancer, age of onset	
20–29 years	10
30–39 years	6
40–49 years	6
≥ 50 years	1
Fibroids	1
Gastrointestinal	
Polyposis syndrome (five or more polyps, any type)	6
Intestinal hamartoma or ganglioneuroma, any number	10
Glycogenic acanthosis	10
Skin	
Trichilemmomas, biopsy-proven	10
Oral papillomas	6
Penile freckling	6
Acral keratoses	1
Arteriovenous malformations	6
Skin lipomas	1
Endocrine	
Thyroid cancer, age of onset	
< 20 years	10
20–29 years	4
30–39 years	4
40–49 years	4
≥ 50 years	1
Thyroid goitre, nodules or adenomas or Hashimoto thyroiditis	4
Genitourinary	
Renal cell carcinoma	1

[a] The sum of corresponding weights of positive features is obtained for a predictor.
OFC, occipitofrontal circumference

Table 16.07 Cleveland Clinic paediatric criteria for the diagnosis of Cowden syndrome[a]

PTEN testing should be considered for paediatric individuals with the following criteria:	% prevalence in patients with PTEN mutations
1. Macrocephaly (≥ 2 SD)	100%
2. At least one of the following four additional criteria should be present:	
A. Autism or developmental delay	82%
B. Dermatological features, including lipomas, trichilemmomas, oral papillomas, penile freckling	60%
C. Vascular features, such as arteriovenous malformations, or haemangiomas	29%
D. Gastrointestinal polyps	14%
SD, standard deviation.	
[a] Other clinical diagnoses that should lead to evaluation for these clinical features include paediatric-onset thyroid cancer and germ cell tumours.	

who underwent endoscopy {565}. Hyperplastic polyps represented the most common type identified, although all types were represented. While less common, intestinal hamartomas and ganglioneuromas are highly specific for PTEN mutation {565,1402}.

Other hamartomatous tumours

Dysplastic cerebellar gangliocytoma (Lhermitte-Duclos disease) is a rare hamartomatous disorder that is the major neoplastic manifestation of CS in the central nervous system.

Genetics

Chromosomal location and mode of transmission

CS is an autosomal-dominant disorder, with age-related penetrance and variable expression. The primary gene for CS susceptibility, PTEN, resides on 10q23.3 {1042}. Germline variants of SDHB (locus 1p36.13) and SDHD (locus 11q23) that encode subunits of the succinate dehydrogenase (SDH) complex have also been implicated in 10% of cases of CS without germline PTEN mutations {991}. Recently, 30% of CS without germline PTEN mutations were found to have germline epimutation of the KILLIN gene, localized to 10q23.31 {115}.

Gene structure

PTEN (also known as MMAC1 or TEP1) comprises 9 exons spanning 105 kb of genomic distance {797,799,804,1370}. PTEN encodes a transcript of 9027 bp. SDHB comprises 8 exons spanning 35 kb, with a transcript length of 1153 bp. SDHD is composed of 4 exons spanning 9 kb, with a transcript length of 1313 bp. KILLIN shares the same transcription

start-site as PTEN, but is transcribed in the opposite direction. KILLIN comprises a single exon with a transcript length of 537 bp.

Gene expression

PTEN is expressed almost ubiquitously in the adult human. In normal human embryonic and fetal development, PTEN protein is also expressed ubiquitously, although levels may change throughout development {490}. PTEN is very highly expressed in the developing central nervous system as well as in the neural crest and its derivatives, e.g. enteric ganglia {490}. KILLIN is a newly discovered protein that is almost ubiquitously expressed but at varying levels.

Gene function

PTEN encodes a dual specificity lipid and protein phosphatase. It can dephosphorylate phosphatidylinositol-3,4,5-triphosphate (PIP3), the product of phosphatidyl inositol-3-kinase (PI3K), which activates phosphoinositide-dependent kinase (PDK1), which in turn activates Akt/PKB by phosphorylation {851, 1364}. This results in G1 arrest and/or apoptosis. The protein phosphatase is involved in the inhibition of cell migration, and also in downregulating several cell cyclins {382}. To date, the majority of naturally occurring missense mutations tested are functionally null, result in haploinsufficiency, or act as dominant-negatives, abrogating both lipid and protein phosphatase activity {1539}. In addition to these mechanisms, there is also evidence that subcellular localization of PTEN protein, particularly in terms of nuclear-cytoplasmic distribution and shuttling, may be a key mechanism for regulation of its activity and function {1112}. This localization

may be mediated by post-translational modifications {1456} and regulated by ATP, which is required for PTEN protein subcellular localization {822,823}. The observation that mutation of the ATP-binding motifs of PTEN result in oxidative nuclear DNA damage {564} supports the view that nucleo-cytoplasmic shuttling of PTEN is an important mechanism for investigation. The final common result of the mechanisms described above is a reduction of PTEN protein activity. With this loss of PTEN protein activity, a corresponding increase in phosphorylation of Akt and dysregulation of the MAPK pathway results in failure to activate cell-cycle arrest or initiate apoptosis. Interestingly, these downstream effects may be highly sensitive to the dose of PTEN protein; there is evidence that subtle variations in PTEN protein dosage may affect cancer susceptibility in both clinical {1402} and animal models {31}, a phenomenon that is currently unique among known tumour-suppressor genes. Apart from a direct effect on proliferation, PTEN mutation has also been observed to cause disruption of chromosomal integrity using in vitro models {1300}.

Mutation spectrum

Both germline and somatic mutations of PTEN have been identified in breast cancer. As with most other tumour-suppressor genes, the germline mutations found in PTEN are scattered throughout all nine exons. They comprise loss-of-function mutations, including missense, nonsense, frameshift and splice-site mutations. In addition, promoter mutations and large exon deletions have also been identified. Hotspots for mutations are found in exons 5, 7 and 8. For SDHB and SDHD, all mutations identified to date have been missense mutations {991}. Epigenetic alterations, such as the germline methylation of the 10q23.31 bidirectional promoter CpG island, silencing KILLIN expression {115}, are also associated with patients with the CS phenotype.

Genotype–phenotype correlations

There has been considerable interest in genotype–phenotype correlation in CS, particularly with the elucidation of the crystal structure of the PTEN protein {775}. However, to date, this work has been primarily exploratory, because of limited numbers of CS patients. One early study was unable to identify any such association {972}; a second suggested that the presence of missense mutations and/or mutations 5' of the phosphatase core motif seem to be associated with a surrogate for disease severity (multi-organ involvement) {879}. Following these studies, accumulating data in recent years have suggested an association between *PTEN*-promoter mutations and breast cancer {1426,1628}. A preliminary association between mutation of ATP-binding motifs of *PTEN* and breast cancer has also been reported {823}. There is a striking recent observation that the frequency of breast and kidney cancer is higher in subjects with *SDHB* and *SDHD* variants {991} and *KILLIN* promoter methylation {115} even relative to subjects with germline mutations in *PTEN*.

The clinical spectrum of PTEN hamartoma tumour syndrome encompasses allelic disorders such as Bannayan-Riley-Ruvalcaba syndrome (BRRS, MIM No. 153480) {585,880} (which is characterized by macrocephaly, lipomatosis, haemangiomatosis and speckled penis), and subsets of Proteus syndrome and Proteus-like (non-CS, non-BRRS) syndromes {1627}. Germline mutations in *PTEN* in one case of macrocephaly and autism and hydrocephaly-associated with VATER association have been reported {1160}.

Lynch syndrome

P. Peltomaki
J. Garber

Definition

Lynch syndrome is an autosomal-dominant disorder caused by a defect in one of the DNA mismatch repair (MMR) genes. The syndrome is characterized by the development of colorectal carcinoma, endometrial carcinoma and other cancers.

MIM No.   120435-6

Synonyms

Hereditary nonpolyposis colorectal cancer (HNPCC) {158}

Incidence

Lynch syndrome accounts for approximately 2–5% of all cases of colorectal cancer {1}. The estimated frequency of carriers of a mutation in an MMR gene is 1 in 1000.

Diagnostic criteria

Before the discovery of the DNA MMR gene defects responsible for Lynch syndrome in the 1990s, clinical diagnostic criteria (the Amsterdam II criteria) {1506} (Table 16.08) were used to identify families likely to have Lynch syndrome. Other widely used criteria are the revised Bethesda guidelines, which are less stringent {1478} (Table 16.08). Individuals that meet at least one of the Bethesda criteria are considered to have suspected Lynch syndrome, and investigating tumours for microsatellite instability (MSI) is warranted as a prescreening method before testing for germline mutations.

Currently, the term "Lynch syndrome" is restricted to families with an identified pathogenic germline mutation in one of the DNA MMR genes {158}. In addition, patients with inactivation of *MSH2* due to a deletion of the 3' exons of the *EPCAM/TACSTD1* gene are considered to have Lynch syndrome {807}. Also patients with constitutional hypermethylation ("epimutation") of the *MLH1* promoter {583,945} may be designated as having Lynch syndrome, although segregation and penetrance of *MLH1* epimutations in subsequent generations remain unclear.

Breast tumours

With the main exception of a single investigation {1291}, no excess of breast carcinoma has been observed in families with Lynch syndrome compared with the general population {2,90,482,1504,1559}. This would suggest that breast carcinoma is not part of the spectrum of tumours associated with Lynch syndrome. There is some molecular evidence both in support of and against the scenario that inherited MMR deficiency drives breast tumorigenesis in Lynch syndrome (see below). The mean age at diagnosis reported for Lynch syndrome-associated breast cancer varies from 46 {1504} to 66 years {1298}. Molecular findings combined with epidemiological observations of early age at onset in the absence of any excess in relative risk have been interpreted to suggest that MMR defects may accelerate tumorigenesis, but are unlikely to be the initiating event. No specific histological phenotype is recognized (most are invasive carcinomas of no special type [NST]); however, recent studies suggest that MMR-deficient breast cancers were more likely to be poorly differentiated with a high mitotic index, steroid hormone receptor-negative and frequent lymphocytic reactions similar to their colorectal counterparts {649, 1543,1576}.

Other tumours

Carriers of a pathogenic DNA MMR gene mutation have a lifetime risk of 10–53% for developing colorectal carcinoma, 15–44% for developing endometrial carcinoma, and < 15% for other cancers {90,255, 1296,1558}. The risk of developing cancer depends on the predisposing gene, sex and environmental factors. Among extracolonic tumours from patients with Lynch syndrome, the relative risk is highest for carcinoma of the endometrium, ovaries, ureter, renal pelvis, and small bowel, which are therefore the most specific for Lynch syndrome {1558}. Colorectal carcinomas are often diagnosed at an early age (mean, 45–50 years) and the same also applies to many extracolonic tumours, at least when compared to the corresponding sporadic tumours {1503}.

Genetics

Germline mutations

Lynch syndrome is transmitted as an autosomal-dominant trait. It is associated with heterozygous germline mutations in one

---

Table 16.08 Amsterdam II and revised Bethesda criteria for the diagnosis of Lynch syndrome

Amsterdam criteria II

There should be at least three relatives with a Lynch syndrome-associated cancer (colorectal cancer, cancer of the endometrium, small bowel, ureter or renal pelvis); all of the following criteria should be present:

(1) One should be a first-degree relative of the other two;
(2) At least two successive generations should be affected;
(3) At least one should be diagnosed before age 50 years;
(4) Familial adenomatous polyposis should be excluded in the colorectal cancer case(s), if any;
(5) Tumours should be verified by pathological examination.

Revised Bethesda criteria

(1) Colorectal cancer diagnosed in a patient aged < 50 years;
(2) Presence of synchronous, metachronous colorectal, or other Lynch syndrome-related tumours[a], regardless of age;
(3) Colorectal cancer with MSI-H phenotype diagnosed in a patient aged < 60 years;
(4) Patient with colorectal cancer and a first-degree relative with a Lynch syndrome-related tumour, with one of the cancers diagnosed at < 50 years;
(5) Patient with colorectal cancer with two or more first-degree or second-degree relatives with a Lynch syndrome-related tumour, regardless of age.

MSI-H, high degree of microsatellite instability.

[a] Lynch syndrome related tumours include colorectal, endometrial, stomach, ovarian, pancreas, ureter, renal pelvis, biliary tract, and brain tumours, sebaceous gland adenomas, keratoacanthomas and carcinoma of the small bowel.

Table 16.09 Characteristics of human DNA mismatch repair genes associated with Lynch syndrome

Gene	Chromosomal location	Length of cDNA (kb)	Number of exons	Genomic size (kb)	References
MLH1	3p21–p23	2.3	19	58–100	{195,544,710,813,817,1072}
MSH2	2p21	2.8	16	73	{12,440,711,766,818,1085}
MSH6	2p21	4.2	10	20	{993,1068,1278}
PMS2	7p22	2.6	15	16	{992,994}
MLH3	14q24	4.4	12	36	{816}

of five genes with a verified or putative function in DNA MMR, namely *MLH1* (mutL homologue 1), *MSH2* (mutS homologue 2), *MSH6* (mutS homologue 6), *PMS2* (postmeiotic segregation 2), and *MLH3* (mutL homologue 3). The structural characteristics of these genes are given in Table 16.09.

The International Society for Gastrointestinal Hereditary Tumours (InSiGHT) maintains a central database for Lynch syndrome-associated mutations, variants, and polymorphisms (http://www.insight-group.org). The great majority of the presently known 3000 unique mutations and variants occur in *MLH1* and *MSH2*, with fewer changes in *MSH6*, *PMS2* and *MLH3*. While > 80% of mutations are specific to each family, prevalent founder mutations occur in certain populations {1086}. As a rule, the mutations are scattered throughout the genes. Most *MSH2* and *MLH1* mutations are truncating {1086,1595}. However, one third of MMR gene alterations are of missense type, and functional testing is often mandatory for a proper assignment of pathogenicity for such changes. Characteristics of variants with reported results of functional and/or in silico testing are available in a database (http://www.mmruv.info) {1049}. The mechanism behind constitutional inactivation of a DNA MMR gene is not always genetic (point mutation or large rearrangement) but may be epigenetic (germline epimutation {582A,807}.

Mutations in DNA MMR genes account for two thirds of all classical Lynch syndrome

families meeting the Amsterdam criteria and showing MSI in tumours {817A}. Occurrence of these mutations is clearly lower (< 30%) in kindreds not meeting the Amsterdam criteria {1013,1582}.

Acquired genetic changes in cancers associated with Lynch syndrome

MMR gene mutations are dominant at the pedigree level (inactivation of one copy of a given MMR gene by germline mutation causes cancer predisposition), but recessive at a cellular level (cancer initiation additionally requires inactivation of the respective wild-type copy). Tumour tissues from patients with Lynch syndrome typically show the absence of the respective MMR protein by immunohistochemical analysis (and occasionally, additional MMR proteins in a defined pattern {568}). This has been shown to apply to almost all colorectal carcinomas and extracolonic cancers of the Lynch-syndrome spectrum {531}. A significant proportion of breast carcinomas from families with Lynch syndrome (44–75%) have also been found to lack the MMR protein corresponding to the germline mutation {649,1298,1543}, suggesting that the loss of MMR protein(s) is important in the etiopathogenesis of these tumours.

Parallel to the lack of MMR protein, the demonstration of MSI serves as an important biomarker for Lynch-syndrome cancers. A panel of five markers (BAT25, BAT26, D2S123, D5S346 and D17S250) was recommended for screening purposes

{159}. Size shifts at two or more microsatellite loci indicate a high degree of MSI (MSI-H). The mononucleotide repeats BAT26 and BAT25 are particularly sensitive for MSI-H in both familial and sporadic colorectal cancers, but their performance in extracolonic cancers is less well known. An investigation of different cancers from a nationwide cohort of families with Lynch syndrome showed that, despite origin from verified MMR gene mutation carriers, the frequency of MSI-H in tumours varied between high (96–100% for ureter, stomach, and colon), intermediate (60–63% for endometrium and bladder), and low (0–25% for kidney and brain) {531}. Breast carcinomas from carriers of MMR gene mutations have been reported to show MSI-H with frequencies ranging from 0% {953} to 64% {323}.

Prognosis and predictive factors

Mutations in *MLH1* and *MSH2* have a high penetrance, with > 80% of carriers developing some form of cancer during their lifetime {1505}. There is no clear-cut correlation between the involved gene, mutation site within the gene, or mutation type vs clinical features. *MSH2* mutations may confer a higher risk for extracolonic cancer than *MLH1* mutations, whereas *MSH6* mutations may be associated with atypical clinical features, including an elevated occurrence of endometrial cancer relative to colorectal cancer as well as late age of onset {568}. *PMS2* mutations are associated with a lower penetrance and variable clinical phenotypes ranging from early or late onset, apparently sporadic colorectal cancer (heterozygosity for germline mutation {1296,1458}) to Turcot syndrome or a distinct childhood cancer syndrome (homozygosity or compound heterozygosity for germline mutation; {1586}). Breast cancer has not been specifically linked to any particular MMR gene or mutation.

Other breast-cancer predisposing genes

D. Easton
P. Devilee

Variants in known high-penetrance susceptibility genes, principally *BRCA1* and *BRCA2*, account for < 20% of the familial risk of breast cancer {361}. Genetic linkage analyses in families with multiple cases of breast cancer not attributable to mutations in *BRCA1* or *BRCA2* have failed to identify further high-penetrance loci, and have led to the hypothesis that the residual familial risk may be due to multiple loci conferring lower risks. Formal segregation analyses have demonstrated that the pattern of familial risks of breast cancer can be modelled by the effects of mutations in *BRCA1*, *BRCA2* and a "polygenic" component, consistent with the effects of many loci of small effect whose risks combine multiplicatively {60}.

Linkage studies lack the power to identify common lower-penetrance variants, and these have been sought through case–control association studies. Early studies concentrated on polymorphisms in genes though to be functionally relevant, such as genes involved in hormone synthesis and metabolism, but this approach has generally proved ineffective {1102}. The strongest evidence for a susceptibility locus identified through this approach is for the coding single-nucleotide polymorphism (SNP) D302H (rs1045485) in *CASP8* {290}.

The major impetus for the identification of common low-penetrance susceptibility alleles has been provided by the development of array technologies for genotyping SNPs affordably on a genome-wide scale. By genotyping 300 000 to 1 million markers, it is possible to capture most of the common variation in the genome. Although the risks conferred by common loci are modest, genotyping in very large collaborative studies can provide definite evidence of association, and more than 1300 loci for more than 200 common diseases or traits have been identified by this approach (www.genome.gov/gwastudies). To date, six genome-wide association studies (GWAS) have been published for breast cancer, and have reliably identified 19 susceptibility loci (Table 16.10). The strongest associations are conferred by alleles at the *FGFR2* and *TOX3* loci, for which the per-allele relative risks are 1.2–1.3-fold {364}. Taken together, these loci explain about 8% of the familial risk of breast cancer. It is likely, however, that many further loci have been missed owing to lack of statistical power, so the overall contribution of common variants to breast-cancer susceptibility is probably much greater.

The majority of the loci confer higher relative risks of estrogen receptor-positive (ER-positive) than ER-negative breast cancer {189,473}. The chief exceptions are the 6q25 locus, upstream of *ESR1*, and the 19p13 locus, for which the association is predominantly with ER-negative disease. The 2q35 locus confers similar risks of both ER-positive and ER-negative disease. None of the SNPs have been definitely associated with any other cancer type, with the exception of the 19p13 SNPs, which are also associated with ovarian cancer.

Most of the susceptibility loci have been assessed for their association with breast-cancer risk in carriers of *BRCA1* and *BRCA2* mutations. The majority of the loci

Table 16.10 Low-penetrance loci associated with an increased risk of breast cancer

Locus	Chromosome	SNP	RAF	OR per allele	P-value[a]	Reference
1p11.2	1	rs11249433	0.39	1.16	7×10^{-10}	{1431}
2q35	2	rs13387042	0.50	1.20	1×10^{-13}	{1361A, 1925A}
NEK10/SLC4A7	3	rs4973768	0.46	1.11	4×10^{-23}	{20A}
MAP3K1	5	rs889312	0.28	1.13	7×10^{-20}	{364}
MRPS30	5	rs10941679	0.24	1.19	3×10^{-11}	{925A,1361B}
ESR1	6	rs2046210	0.36	1.29	2×10^{-15}	{1626B}
8q24	8	rs13281615	0.40	1.08	5×10^{-12}	{364}
9p31.2	9	rs865686	0.61	1.15	2×10^{-10}	{453A}
FGFR2	10	rs2981582	0.38	1.26	2×10^{-76}	{364,613B}
LSP1	11	rs3817198	0.30	1.07	3×10^{-9}	{364}
RAD51L1	14	rs999737	0.76	1.06	2×10^{-7}	{1431A}
TOX3	16	rs3803662	0.25	1.20	1×10^{-36}	{364,1361A}
COX11	17	rs6504950	0.73	1.05	1×10^{-8}	{20A}
19p13[b]	19	rs8170	0.17	1.26	2×10^{-9}	{63}
		rs2363956	0.49	0.84	5×10^{-9}	
CDKNA/B	9	rs1011970	0.17	1.09	3×10^{-8}	{1469A}
ANKRD16	10	rs2380205	0.57	1.06	5×10^{-7}	{1469A}
ZNF365	10	rs10995190	0.15	0.86	5×10^{-15}	{1469A}
ZMIZ1	10	rs704010	0.39	1.07	4×10^{-9}	{1469A}
11p13	11	rs614367	0.15	1.15	3×10^{-15}	{1469A}

OR, odds ratio; RAF, risk allele frequency; SNP, single nucleotide polymorphism
[a] P for trend, from the first study reporting the replication (not necessarily the current combined evidence)
[b] Identified as a modifier of breast-cancer risk in carriers of *BRCA1* mutations, but also associated with estrogen-receptor-negative breast cancer in population-based studies.

have shown evidence of association in *BRCA2* mutation carriers, whereas few of the loci are associated with risk in *BRCA1* mutation carriers. This difference appears to be related to the difference in tumour pathology between *BRCA1* and *BRCA2* mutation carriers: it is notable that the loci associated with risk in *BRCA1* mutation carriers (*TOX3*, 6q25, 19p13 and 2q35) are also associated with the risk of ER-negative breast cancer in the general population.

It is important to note that, in almost all cases, the gene(s) driving the association are still unknown. The major exception is *FGFR2*, for which the associated SNPs have been shown to be associated with changes in FGFR2 expression in breast tissue and fibroblasts {610,918}. The 8q24 locus is presumed to regulate *MYC* expression. Other likely causative genes include *TOX3*, *CCND1* and *MAP3K1*. Identification of the causal variant is also problematic, owing to the strong linkage disequilibrium among neighbouring markers. Again the strongest evidence is for *FGFR2*, where the most plausible causative variant (rs2981578), in intron 2 of the gene, alters binding of transcription factors Oct-1/Runx2 {918,1476}. The causal variants may be associated with higher risks of breast cancer than the markers identified.

While the risks associated with the common low-penetrance alleles are modest, these risks appear to combine multiplicatively, so that the total effect on risk can be substantial. For example, based on a risk profile of the known alleles, the top 5% of the population have a risk that is about twofold that of the population average. While discrimination is probably too poor to provide useful risk prediction in isolation, it may become more important as more alleles are identified, and may already be useful in women with a family history of the disease or in combination with other risk factors.

Contributors

Dr Craig ALLRED
Pathology and Immunology
Washington University School of Medicine
Campus Box 8118
660 South Euclid Avenue
St Louis, MO 63110
USA
Tel. +1 314 362 6313
dcallred@path.wustl.edu

Dr Sunil BADVE
Immunohistochemistry
Clarian Pathology Laboratory
Indiana University School of Medicine
350 West 11th Street, Room 4010
Indianapolis, IN 46202
USA
Tel. +1 317 491 6484/Fax +1 317 491 6419
sbadve@iupui.edu

Dr Rosemary BALLEINE
Translational Oncology, Sydney West Cancer
Network, Westmead Millennium Institute and
Sydney Medical School Westmead
Westmead Hospital, PO Box 533
Wentworthville, NSW 2145
AUSTRALIA
Tel. +61 2 9845 8086
Fax +61 2 9845 9102
rosemary.balleine@sydney.edu.au

Dr Jillian BIRCH
Cancer Research UK Paediatric and Familial
Cancer Research Group, The Medical School,
University of Manchester
Stopford Building, Room 1.900, Oxford Road
Manchester M13 9PT
ENGLAND
Tel. +44 (0)161 275 5404
Fax +44 (0)161 275 5348
jillian.m.birch@manchester.ac.uk

Dr Anita BORGES*
Histopathology & Cytopathology, Asian Institute
of Oncology & S.L. Raheja Hospital
400016 Mahim
Mumbai
INDIA
Tel. +91 9821873107
Fax +91 222 444 3893
anitaborges@gmail.com

Dr Peter BRITTON
Cambridge Breast Unit
Cambridge University Hospitals
NHS Foundation Trust, Hills Road
Cambridge CB2 0QQ
ENGLAND
Tel. +44 1223 586993
Fax +44 1223 217886
peter.britton@addenbrookes.nhs.uk

Dr Edi BROGI
Department of Pathology
Breast and Imaging Center
Memorial Sloan-Kettering Cancer Center
1275 York Avenue
New York, NY 10065
USA
Tel. +1 646 888 5486
brogie@mskcc.org

Dr Gianni BUSSOLATI
Istituto di Anatomia e Istologia Patologica
University of Turin
Via Santena 7
10126 Turin
ITALY
Tel. +39 011 670 65 05
Fax +39 011 663 52 67
gianni.bussolati@unito.it

Dr Benjaporn CHAIWUN
Department of Pathology
Faculty of Medicine, Chiang Mai University
110 Intravaroros street
50200 Chiang Mai
THAILAND
Tel. +66 81 992 5938
Fax +66 53 404829
bchaiwun_a@yahoo.co.th

Dr Emmanuelle CHARAFE-JAUFFRET
Centre de Recherche en Cancérologie de
Marseille, Laboratoire d'Oncologie Moléculaire
UMR891 INSERM/Institut Paoli-Calmettes
Marseille
FRANCE
Tel. +33 4 91 22 35 09
Fax +33 4 91 22 35 44
jauffrete@marseille.fnclcc.fr

Dr Georgia CHENEVIX-TRENCH
The Queensland Institute of Medical Research
300 Herston Road
Herston, QLD 4006
AUSTRALIA
Tel: +61 7 3362 0390
Fax +61 7 3362 0105
Georgia.Trench@qimr.edu.au

Dr Kee Seng CHIA
Department of Epidemiology and Public Health
and Centre for Molecular Epidemiology
Yong Loo Lin School of Medicine
National University of Singapore
Block MD3, 16 Medical Drive, 117597
SINGAPORE
Tel. +65 16 8203
Fax +65 6779 1489
ephcks@nus.edu.sg

Dr Graham COLDITZ
Department of Surgery, Washington University
School of Medicine, Siteman Cancer Center
660 S. Euclid Avenue, Suite 2306
St Louis, MO 63110
USA
Tel. +1 314 454 7940
Fax +1 314 454 7941
colditzg@wustl.edu

Dr Laura COLLINS
Division of Anatomic Pathology, Department of
Pathology, Beth Israel Deaconess Medical Center
330 Brookline Avenue
Boston, MA 02215
USA
Tel. +1 617 667 4344
Fax +1 617 975 5620
lcollins@bidmc.harvard.edu

Dr Gábor CSERNI
Department of Pathology
University of Szeged
Bács-Kiskun County Teaching Hospital
Nyíri út 38
H-6000 Kecskemét
HUNGARY
Tel. +36 76 516700
Fax +36 76 481219
cserni@freemail.hu

*The asterisk indicates participation in the
Working Group Meeting on the Classification
of Tumours of the Breast that was held in Lyon,
France, September 1–3, 2011

Dr David DABBS
Department of Pathology
Magee-Womens Hospital, UPMC.
300 Halket Street
Pittsburgh, PA 15213
USA
Tel. +1 412 641 4651
Fax +1 412 641 3069
ddabbs@upmc.edu

Dr Thomas DECKER
Department of Pathology
Dietrich-Bonhoeffer Medical Center
PF 400135
17022 Neubrandenburg
GERMANY
Tel. +49 395 775 3359
Fax +49 395 775 3358
thomas.decker@bonhoeffer-klinikum-neubrandenburg.de

Dr Peter DEVILEE
Departments of Human and Clinical Genetics
and Pathology
Leiden University Medical Center
2333 AL Leiden
THE NETHERLANDS
Tel. +31 71 526 9510/ 9404
Fax +31 71 526 8285
P.Devilee@lumc.nl

Dr Ahmet DOGAN
Department of Laboratory Medicine and
Pathology, Mayo Clinic
200 1st Street S.W.
Rochester, MN 55905
USA
Tel. +1 507 266 4802
Fax +1 507 284 1599
Dogan.Ahmet@mayo.edu

Dr Doug EASTON
Cancer Research UK
Genetic Epidemiology Unit
University of Cambridge
Cambridge CB1 8RN
ENGLAND
Tel. +44 122 374 0160
Fax +44 122 374 0159
douglas@srl.cam.ac.uk

Dr Ian O. ELLIS*
Department of Histopathology
University of Nottingham
Nottingham City Hospital NHS Trust
Hucknall Road
Nottingham NG5 1PB
ENGLAND
Tel. +44 115 9691169
Fax +44 115 962 7768
ian.ellis@nottingham.ac.uk

Dr Charis ENG
Genomic Medicine Institute Cleveland Clinic
9500 Euclid Avenue
NE-50 Cleveland
OH 44195
USA
Tel. +1 216 444 3440
Fax +1 216 636 0655
engc@ccf.org

Dr Vincenzo EUSEBI*
Anatomic Pathology
Bellaria Hospital University of Bologna
Via Altura, 3
40139 Bologna
ITALY
Tel. +39 0516225523
Fax +39 0516225759
vincenzo.eusebi@unibo.it

Dr Falko FEND
Institute of Pathology, University Hospital
Tübingen, Eberhard-Karls-University
Liebermeisterstrasse 8
72076 Tübingen
GERMANY
Tel. +49 7071 29 82266
Fax +49 7071 29 2258
falko.fend@med.uni-tuebingen.de

Dr Christopher D.M. FLETCHER
Harvard Medical School, Surgical Pathology,
Brigham and Women's Hospital
Dana-Farber Cancer Institute
75 Francis Street, Mailstop: Pathology
Boston, MA 02115
USA
Tel. +1 617 732 8558 / Fax +1 617 566 3897
cfletcher@partners.org

Dr Maria Pia FOSCHINI
Sezione Anatomia Patologica M. Malpigni
Universita di Bologna, Ospedale Bellaria
Via Altura 3
40139 Bologna
ITALY
Tel. +39 051 622 5750
Fax +39 051 622 5759
mariapia.foschini@ausl.bologna.it

Dr Stephen B. FOX
Pathology Department, Peter MacCallum
Cancer Centre, University of Melbourne
St Andrew's Place
East Melbourne, VIC 3002
AUSTRALIA
Tel. +61 3 9656 1529
Fax +61 3 9656 1460
stephen.fox@petermac.org

Dr Judy GARBER*
Cancer Risk and Prevention Program
Medical Oncology/Population Sciences
Harvard Medical School
Dana-Farber Cancer Institute
44 Binney Street, Smith 210
Boston, MA 02115
USA
Tel. +1 617 632 5770
judy_garber@dfci.harvard.edu

Dr Helenice GOBBI*
Departamento de Anatomia Patológica
Faculdade de Medicina da UFMG
Av. Alfredo Balena, 190
MG 30130-100 Belo Horizonte
BRAZIL
Tel. +55 31 9194 5772
Fax +55 31 3409 9664
helenicegobbi@gmail.com

Dr David GOLDGAR
Department of Dermatology, School of Medicine
University Health Care, School of Medicine
30 North 1900 E RM 4B454
Salt Lake City, UT 84132
USA
Tel.+1 801 581 6465
Fax +1 801 581 6484
david.goldgar@hsc.utah.edu

Dr Andrew M. HANBY
Section of Pathology and Tumour Biology
Leeds Institute of Molecular Medicine, St
James' University Hospital, Wellcome Trust
Brenner Building, Beckett Street
Leeds LS9 7TF
ENGLAND
Tel. +44 113 343 8433/ Fax +44 113 343 8431
a.m.hanby@leeds.ac.uk

Dr Nancy Lee HARRIS
Pathology-Warren 2
Massachusetts General Hospital
55 Fruit Street
Boston, MA 02114
USA
Tel. +1 617 726 5155
Fax +1 617 726 9353
nlharris@partners.org

Dr Malcolm HAYES
Department of Pathology & Laboratory Medicine
BC Cancer Research Agency
600 West 10th Avenue
Vancouver, BC V5Z 1L3
CANADA
Tel. +1 604 877 6098
Fax +1 604 877 6178
mhayes@bccancer.bc.ca

Dr Daniel HAYES
Department of Internal Medicine, University of
Michigan Comprehensive Cancer Center
Room 6312,1500 E. Medical Center Drive
SPC 5942, Ann Arbor, MI 48109-5942
USA
Tel. +1 734 615 6725
Fax +1 734 647 9271
hayesdf@umich.edu

Dr Shu ICHIHARA*
Department of Pathology
Nagoya Medical Center
4-1-1 Sannomaru, Naka-ku
460-0001 Nagoya
JAPAN
Tel. +81 52 951 1111
Fax +81 52 951 1323
shu-kkr@umin.ac.jp

Dr Jorma ISOLA
Laboratory of Cancer Biology
Institute of Medical Technology
Biokatu 6-8
33520 Tampere
FINLAND
Tel. +35 8503005609
jorma.isola@uta.fi

Dr Jocelyne JACQUEMIER
Department of Pathology
Institut Paoli Calmettes
232, Boulevard Sainte Marguerite
13009 Marseille
FRANCE
Tel. +33 4 91 22 34 57
Fax +33 4 91 22 35 73
jacquemierj@marseille.fnclcc.fr

Dr Elaine S. JAFFE
Hematopathology Section, Center for Cancer
Research, National Cancer Institute
10 Center Drive, MSC-1500, Room 2B42
Bethesda, MD 20892
USA
Tel. +1 301 496 0184
Fax +1 301 402 2415
elainejaffe@nih.gov

Dr Louise JONES
Institute of Cancer, Barts and The London
School of Medicine and Dentistry
Charterhouse Square
London EC1M 68BQ
ENGLAND
Tel. +44 20 7882 5555
Fax +44 20 7882 3888
l.j.jones@qmul.ac.uk

Dr Janina KULKA
2nd Department of Pathology
Semmelweis University Budapest
Ulloi út 93
1091 Budapest
HUNGARY
Tel. +36 1 215 6921
Fax +36 1 215 6921
kj@korb2.sote.hu

Dr Sunil R. LAKHANI*
Dept of Anatomical Pathology, Pathology
Queensland, Dept of Molecular and Cellular
Pathology, School of Medicine, University of
Queensland & UQ Centre for Clinical Research,
The Royal Brisbane & Women's Hospital
Herston 4029, Brisbane, QLD
AUSTRALIA
Tel. +61 7 3346 6052; Fax +61 7 3346 5596
s.lakhani@uq.edu.au

Dr Andrew LEE
Department of Histopathology
City Hospital Campus
Nottingham University Hospitals
Hucknall Road
Nottingham NG5 1PB
ENGLAND
Tel. +44 115 969 1169
Fax +44 115 962 7768
andrew.lee@nuh.nhs.uk

Dr Susan LESTER*
Breast Pathology Services, Harvard Medical
School, Brigham and Women's Hospital
Dana-Farber Cancer Institute
75 Francis Street
Boston, MA 02115
USA
Tel. +1 617 732 7510
Fax +1 617 264 5118
slester@partners.org

Dr Gaëtan MACGROGAN
Department of Pathology
Institut Bergonie
229, cours de l'argonne
33074 Bordeaux
FRANCE
Tel. +33 5 56 33 04 36
Fax +33 5 56 33 04 38
macgrogan@bergonie.org

Dr Gaetano MAGRO
Dipartimento GF INGRASSIA
Anatomia Patologica
Universita di Catania
95123 Catania
ITALY
Tel. +39 378 2024
Fax +39 378 2023
g.magro@unict.it

Dr L. Jeffrey MEDEIROS
Department of Hematopathology, The Univer-
sity of Texas MD Anderson Cancer Center,
1515 Holcombe Boulevard, Box 0072
Houston, TX 77030
USA
Tel. +1 713 794 5446
Fax +1 713 745 0736
ljmedeiros@mdanderson.org

Dr Michal MICHAL
Sikl's Department of Pathology
Laboratore Spec. Diagnostiky
Medical Faculty Hospital
Alej Svobody 80
Pilsen
CZECH REPUBLIC
Tel. +420 60 3886633
Fax +420 37 7104650
michal@fnplzen.cz

Dr Keith MILLER
UCL Advanced Diagnostics
1st floor Rockefeller Building
21 University Street
London WC1E 6JJ
ENGLAND
Tel. +44 20 7679 6039
Fax +44 20 7679 627
rmkdhkm@ucl.ac.uk

Dr Takuya MORIYA
Department of Pathology
Kawasaki Medical School
701-0192 Kurashiki City
JAPAN
Tel. +81 86 462 1111
Fax +81 86 462 1199
tmoriya@med.kawasaki-m.ac.jp

Dr Monica MORROW*
Department of Surgery, Anne Burnett
Windfohr Chair of Clinical Oncology
Memorial Sloan-Kettering Cancer Center
1275 York Avenue, MRI-1034
New York, NY 10065
USA
Tel. +1 212 639 7754
Fax +1 646 422 2092
morrowm@mskcc.org

Dr Yun NIU
Breast Pathology Department and Laboratory
Cancer Institute & Hospital
Tianjin Medical University
CHINA
Tel. +86 13 821228780
Fax +86 22 23359337
yunniu2000@126.com

Dr Hiroko OHGAKI*
Section of Molecular Pathology
International Agency for Research on Cancer
150 cours Albert Thomas
69372 Lyon
FRANCE
Tel. +33 4 72 73 85 34
Fax +33 4 72 73 86 98
ohgaki@iarc.fr

Dr Frances O'MALLEY
Department of Laboratory Medicine and
Pathobiology
University of Toronto
St Michael's Hospital, 30 Bond Street
Toronto, ON M5B 1W8
CANADA
omalleyf@smh.ca

Dr Jose PALACIOS*
Department of Pathology
Hospital Universitario Virgen del Rocío
Avda Manuel Siurot, s/n
41013 Seville
SPAIN
Tel. +34 9550 13029 / +34 651 78287
Fax +34 9550 13029
jose.palacios.sspa@juntadeandalucia.es

Dr Juan PALAZZO
Department of Pathology
Thomas Jefferson University Hospital
111 South 11th Street
Philadelphia, PA 19107
USA
Tel. +1 215 955 6352/4103
Fax +1 215 923 1969
Juan.Palazzo@jefferson.edu

Dr Paivi PELTOMAKI
Department of Medical Genetics
University of Helsinki
PO Box 63 (Haartmaninkatu 8)
FIN-00014 Helsinki
FINLAND
Tel. +358 919 125 092
Fax +358 919 125 105
paivi.peltomaki@helsinki.fi

Dr Charles M. PEROU
Department of Genetics
Linberger Comprehensive Cancer Center
University of North Carolina
450 West Drive, CB#7264
Chapel Hill, NC 27599-7264
USA
Tel. +1 919 843 5740
Fax +1 919 843 5717
cperou@med.unc.edu

Dr Sarah E. PINDER
Division of Cancer Studies, Bermondsey Wing
King's College London, Research Breast
Pathology, Research Oncology, Guy's Hospital
Great Maze Pond
London SE1 9RT
ENGLAND
Tel. +44 20 7188 4260
Fax +44 20 7188 0919
sarah.pinder@kcl.ac.uk

Dr Cecily QUINN
St Vincent's University Hospital
Elm Park Dublin 4
REPUBLIC OF IRELAND
Tel. +353 1 209 4658
Fax + 353 1 209 4840
c.quinn@st-vincents.ie

Dr Emad RAKHA
Department of Histopathology
City Hospital Campus
Nottingham University Hospitals
Hucknall Road
Nottingham NG5 1PB
ENGLAND
Tel. +44 0115 9691169
Fax +44 0115 9627768
emadrakha@yahoo.com

Dr Angelika REINER
Department of Pathology
Donauspital
Langobardenstrasse 122
A1220 Vienna
AUSTRIA
Tel. +43 1 28802 5200
Fax +43 1 28802 5280
angelika.reiner@wienkav.at

Dr Jorge S. REIS-FILHO*
The Breakthrough Breast Cancer Research
Centre
Institute of Cancer Research
237 Fulham Road
London SW3 6JB
ENGLAND
Tel. +44 20 71535529
Fax +44 20 71535533
Jorge.Reis-Filho@icr.ac.uk

Dr Carol REYNOLDS
Division of Anatomic Pathology
Mayo Clinic
200 1st Street SW
Rochester, MN 55905
USA
Tel. +1 507 266 5397
Fax +1 507 284 1875
reynolds.carol@mayo.edu

Dr Andrea L. RICHARDSON
Department of Pathology, Harvard Medical
School, Brigham and Women's Hospital
75 Francis Street, Amory, 3rd Floor
Boston, MA 02115
USA
Tel. +1 617 582 7352
Fax +1 617 632 3709
Andrea_Richardson@dcfi.harvard.edu

Dr Brian ROUS*
National Cancer Staging Panel for Registration
Eastern Cancer Registration & Information Centre
Unit C - Magog Court
Shelford Bottom
Cambridge CB22 3AD
ENGLAND
Tel. +1 223 213 625
Fax +1 223 213 571
brian.rous@ecric.nhs.uk

Dr Emiel RUTGERS
The Netherlands Cancer Institute
Antoni van Leeuwenhoek Hospital
Plesmanlaan 121
1066 CX Amsterdam
THE NETHERLANDS
Tel. +32 2 774 164
e.rutgers@nki.nl

Dr Aysegul SAHIN
Breast Pathology Section, The University of
Texas MD Anderson Cancer Center
1515 Holcombe Boulevard, Box 0085
Houston, TX 77030
USA
Tel. +1 713 794 1500
Fax +1 713 745 5704
asahin@mdanderson.org

Dr Anna SAPINO
Department of Biomedical Sciences and
Oncology
University of Turin
Via Santena 7
10126 Turin
ITALY
Tel. +39 011 6706510
Fax +39 011 6635267
anna.sapino@unito.it

Dr Fernando SCHMITT
Medical Faculty of Porto University
IPATIMUP-Institute of Molecular Pathology
and Immunology of Porto University
Rua Dr Roberto Frias S/N, 4200-465
Porto
PORTUGAL
Tel. +351 2255 70700
Fax +351 2255 70799
fernando.schmitt@ipatimup.pt

Dr Stuart J. SCHNITT*
Beth Israel Deaconess Medical Center
330 Brookline Avenue
Boston, MA, 02215
USA
Tel. +1 617 667 5773
Fax +1 617 975 5620
sschnitt@bidmc.harvard.edu

Dr Dennis SGROI
Molecular Pathology Unit
Massachusetts General Hospital
149 13th Street, Room 7139
Charlestown, MA 02129
USA
Tel. +1 617 726 5697
Fax +1 617 726 5684
dsgroi@partners.org

Dr Sandra J. SHIN*
Department of Pathology and Laboratory
Medicine, New York-Presbyterian Hospital
Weill Cornell Medical College
525 East 68th Street, Starr Pavilion, 1031
New York, NY 10065
USA
Tel. +1 212 746 6482
Fax +1 212 746 6484
sjshin@med.cornell.edu

Dr Sami SHOUSHA
Department of Histopathology
Charing Cross Hospital and Imperial College
Faculty of Medicine
London W6 8RF
ENGLAND
Tel. +44 20 3311 7144
Fax +44 20 3311 1364
s.shousha@imperial.ac.uk

Dr Peter T. SIMPSON
UQ Centre for Clinical Research
The University of Queensland
The Royal Brisbane & Women's Hospital
Building 71/918
Herston, Brisbane 4029, Queensland
AUSTRALIA
Tel. +61 7 3346 6048
Fax +61 7 3346 5596
p.simpson@uq.edu.au

Dr Jean F. SIMPSON*
Department of Pathology
Vanderbilt University Medical Center
1161 21st Avenue South, Room C-3318 MCN
Nashville, TN 37232-2561
USA
Tel. +1 615 322 3041
Fax +1 615 343 5137
jean.simpson@vanderbilt.edu

Dr Alena SKALOVA
Department of Pathology
Medical Faculty of Charles University
Ed. Beneše 13
305 99 Plzen
CZECH REPUBLIC
Tel. +420 377 402 545
Fax +420 377 402 634
skalova@fnplzen.cz

Dr Nour SNEIGE
Department of Pathology, The University of
Texas MD Anderson Cancer Center
1515 Holcombe Boulevard, Box 0053
Houston, TX 77030
USA
Tel. +1 713 794 5625
Fax +1 713 792 2499
nsneige@mdanderson.org

Dr Christos SOTIRIOU
Functional Genomics & Translational Research
Jules Bordet Institute
121 boulevard de Waterloo laan
1000 Brussels
BELGIUM
Tel. +32 2 541 3111
Fax +32 2 538 0858
christos.sotiriou@bordet.be

Dr Michael STRATTON
Cancer Genome Project
The Wellcome Trust Sanger Institute
Hinxton CB10 1SA
ENGLAND
Tel. +44 1223 494757
Fax +44 1223 494969
mrs@sanger.ac.uk

Dr Fraser SYMMANS
The University of Texas MD Anderson Cancer
Center
1515 Holcombe Boulevard, Box 0085
Houston, TX 77030
USA
Tel. +1 713 792 0918
fsymmans@mdanderson.org

Dr Puay Hoon TAN*
Department of Pathology
Singapore General Hospital
Outram Road
Singapore, 169608
SINGAPORE
Tel. +65 6321 4874
Fax +65 6222 6826
tan.puay.hoon@sgh.com.sg

Dr Tibor TOT
Laboratory Medicine
Central Hospital Falun
Uppsala University
S 791 82 Falun
SWEDEN
Tel. +46 23 492 696
Fax +46 23 492 389
tibor.tot@ltdalarna.se

Dr Gary TSE*
Department of Anatomical and Cellular Pathology
The Chinese University of Hong Kong
Prince of Wales Hospital, Ngan Shing Street
Hong Kong Special Administrative Region
CHINA
Tel. +852 2632 2359
Fax +852 2637 4858
garytse@cuhk.edu.hk

Dr Hitoshi TSUDA
Department of Pathology and Clinical Laboratories
National Cancer Center Hospital
5-1-1 Tsukiji, Chuo-ku
104-0045 Tokyo
JAPAN
Tel. +81 3 3542 2511 ext 5753
Fax +81 3 5565 7029
hstsuda@ncc.go.jp

Dr Andrew TUTT
Breakthrough Breast Cancer Research Unit,
Research Oncology, Guy's Hospital Campus,
King's College London School of Medicine
3rd Floor Bermondsey Wing
London SE1 9RT
ENGLAND
Tel. +44 207 188 9881
Fax +44 207 188 3666
andrew.tutt@icr.ac.uk

Dr Sitki TUZLALI
Department of Pathology
Istanbul Medical Faculty
Istanbul University
Topkapi 34390
TURKEY
Tel. +90 212 414 2400
Fax +90 212 631 1367
tuzlalips@turk.net

Dr Marc J. VAN DE VIJVER*
Department of Pathology
Academic Medical Centre
Meibergdreef 9
1105 AZ Amsterdam
THE NETHERLANDS
Tel. +31 20 566 4100
Fax +31 20 566 9523
m.j.vandevijver@amc.uva.nl

Dr Guiseppe VIALE
Divisione di Anatomia Patologica e di Medicina
di Laboratorio, Istituto Europeo di Oncologia
Università degli Studi di Milano
Via Ripamonti 435
20141 Milan
ITALY
Tel. +39 02 57 489 419
Fax +39 02 94 379 214
giuseppe.viale@ieo.it

Dr Anne VINCENT-SALOMON
Service de Pathologie et INSERM U830
Institut Curie
26 rue d'Ulm
75248 Paris cedex 05
FRANCE
Tel. +33 1 44 32 42 15 or 42 50
Fax +33 53 10 40 10
anne.salomon@curie.net

Dr Dan VISSCHER
Department of Pathology, 2G332 UH
University of Michigan Medical Center
1500 E. Medical Center Drive
Ann Arbor, Michigan 48109-0602
USA
Tel. +1 734 647 9125
Fax +1 734 763 4095
visscher.daniel@mayo.edu

Dr Donald WEAVER
Department of Pathology
Given Courtyard, Second Floor South
University of Vermont College of Medicine
89 Beaumont Avenue
Burlington , VT 05405-0068
USA
Tel. +1 802 847 3566
Fax +1 802 847 4155
Donald.Weaver@vtmednet.org

Dr Robin WILSON
Department of Clinical Radiology
Royal Marsden
Downs Road
Sutton SM2 5P
ENGLAND
Tel. +44 208 661 3216
robinwilson@nhs.net

IARC/WHO Committee for the International Classification of Diseases for Oncology (ICD-O)

Dr David FORMAN
Section of Cancer Information
International Agency for Research on Cancer
150 cours Albert Thomas
69372 Lyon cedex 08
FRANCE
Tel. +33 4 72 73 80 56
Fax +33 4 72 73 86 96
formand@iarc.fr

Mrs April FRITZ
A. Fritz and Associates, LLC
21361 Crestview Road
Reno, NV 89521
USA
Tel. +1 775 636 7243
Fax +1 888 891 3012
april@afritz.org

Dr Robert JAKOB
Classifications and Terminologies
Evidence and Information for Policy
World Health Organization (WHO)
20 Avenue Appia
1211 Geneva 27
SWITZERLAND
Tel. +41 22 791 58 77
Fax +41 22 791 48 94
jakobr@who.int

Dr Paul KLEIHUES
Department of Pathology
University Hospital
Schmelzbergstrasse 12
8091 Zurich
SWITZERLAND
Tel. +41 44 255 2502
Fax +41 44 255 2525
kleihues@pathol.uzh.ch

Dr Hiroko OHGAKI
Section of Molecular Pathology
International Agency for Research on Cancer
150 cours Albert Thomas
69372 Lyon cedex 08
FRANCE
Tel. +33 4 72 73 85 34
Fax +33 4 72 73 86 98
ohgaki@iarc.fr

Dr D. Maxwell PARKIN
Clinical Trials Service and Epidemiology
Studies Unit, University of Oxford
Richard Doll Building, Old Road Campus
Roosevelt Drive, Headington
Oxford OX3 7LF
ENGLAND
Tel. +44 1865 743663
Fax +44 1865 743985
ctsu0138@herald.ox.ac.uk

Dr Brian ROUS
Eastern Cancer Registry and Information Centre
Unit C - Magog Court
Shelford Bottom, Hinton Way
CB22 3AD Cambridge
ENGLAND
Tel. +1 223 213 625
Fax +1 223 213 571
brian.rous@ecric.nhs.uk

Dr Stuart J. SCHNITT
Beth Israel Deaconess Medical Center
330 Brookline Avenue
Boston, MA, 02215
USA
Tel. +1 617 667 5773
Fax +1 617 975 5620
sschnitt@bidmc.harvard.edu

Dr K. SHANMUGARATNAM
Department of Pathology
National University Hospital
5 Lower Kent Ridge Road
Singapore 119074
SINGAPORE
Tel. +65 6772 4312
Fax +65 6773 6021
k_shanmugaratnam@nuhs.edu.sg

Dr Leslie H. SOBIN
Frederick National Laboratory for Cancer Research
The Cancer Human Biobank
National Cancer Institute
11400 Rockville Pike, Suite 700
Rockville, MD 20852
USA
Tel. +1 301 827 4361
Fax +1 301 480 1069
leslie.sobin@nih.gov

Source of figures

1.01A,B	IARC
1.02	Wilson R.
1.03	Reprinted with permission from Churchill Livingsone Press, Edinburgh
1.04A-C	Tabàr L. Mammography Department, Central Hospital, Falun, Sweden
1.05A-C	Tabàr L.
1.06A-F	Adapted from {1949}
1.07A,B	Allred C.
1.08	Kulka J.
1.09	Kulka J.
1.10A,B	Kulka J.
1.12A-D	Dabbs D.
1.13A,B	Dabbs D.
1.11A,B	Dabbs D.
1.14A,B	Dabbs D.
2.01A-C	Tabàr L.
2.02	Caduff R. Department of Pathology, University Hospital USZ, Zürich, Switzerland
2.03A,B	Schnitt S.J.
2.03C	Ellis I.O.
2.04	Jacquemier J.
2.05A,B	Tavassoli F.A. Yale University School of Medicine, New Haven, U.S.A
2.06	Peterse J.L. Department of Pathology, Netherlands Cancer Institute , Amsterdam, The Netherlands
2.07A,B	Schnitt S.J.
2.08A,B	Tavassoli F.A.
3.01A,B	Tabàr L.
3.02	Sastre-Garau X. Service de Pathologie, Institut Curie, Paris, France
3.03	Sastre-Garau X.
3.04A-C	Sastre-Garau X.
3.05A,B	Tavassoli F.A.
3.06	Tabàr L.
3.07A,B	Tavassoli F.A.
3.08	Tavassoli F.A.
3.09A,B	Lakhani S.R.
3.10A-C	Lakhani S.R.
3.10D	Jacquemier J.
3.11	Jacquemier J.
3.12	Tavassoli F.A.
3.13A-D	Sneige N.
3.14A-D	Okcu Institut für Pathologie, Karl Franzens Universitat, Graz, Austria

3.15	Tavassoli F.A.
3.16	Tavassoli F.A.
3.17	Reis-Filho J.S.
3.18	Tavassoli F.A.
3.19A,B	Tavassoli F.A.
3.20A	Caduff R.
3.20B,C	Tavassoli F.A.
3.21	Reis-Filho J.S.
3.22A	O'Malley F.
3.22B	Eusebi V.
3.23A,B	Michal M.
3.24A,B	Michal M.
3.25A-D	Nour S.
3.26	Eusebi V.
3.27A	Tavassoli F.A.
3.27B	Eusebi V.
3.28A-D	Eusebi V.
3.29	Eusebi V.
3.30	Tavassoli F.A.
3.31A,B	Tavassoli F.A.
3.32	Tavassoli F.A.
3.33A	Schnitt S.J.
3.33B	Bussolati G.
3.34	Bussolati G.
3.35	Tse G.
3.36	Tse G.
3.37	Peterse J.L.
3.38A-C	Peterse J.L.
3.39A-F	Charafe-Jauffret E.
3.40A-C	Tot T.
3.41A,B	Eusebi V.
3.42	Eusebi V.
3.43	Eusebi V.
3.44A,B	Eusebi V.
3.45	Tavassoli F.A.
3.46	Hasebe T., Nishimura R., Fujii S. National Cancer Center, Japan
3.47A	Nakaguro M., Nagoya University Hospital, Japan
3.47B	Tsubura A. Kansai Medical University, Japan
3.47C	Tavassoli F.A.
3.48	Ono K. Tosei General Hospital, Japan
3.49A-C	Eusebi V.
4.01	Lakhani S.R.
4.02	Lakhani S.R.
4.03	Lakhani S.R.
4.04A-C	Lakhani S.R.
4.05	Lakhani S.R.
5.01A	Tavassoli F.A.
5.01B-D	Collins L.
5.02	Schnitt S.J.
5.03	Schnitt S.J.

5.04A,B	Schnitt S.J.
5.05A,B	Tavassoli F.A.
5.06	Britton P.
5.07	Britton P.
5.08A-D	Tavassoli F.A.
5.09A-F	Schnitt S.J.
5.10	Tabàr L.
5.11A-F	Schnitt S.J.
5.12A,B	Adapted from {1950}
6.01A,B	Tavassoli F.A.
6.02A-C	Tavassoli F.A.
7.01	Bukhanov K. Mount Sinai Hospital, Toronto, Canada
7.02	Tan P.H.
7.03	Pavel C. Mount Sinai Hospital, Toronto, Canada
7.04A,B	Ichihara S.
7.05	O'Malley F.
7.06	Tan P.H.
7.07A,B	Tan P.H.
7.08A,B	Ichihara S.
7.09A,B	Tan P.H.
7.10	Tan P.H.
7.11	MacGrogan G.
7.12A-D	MacGrogan G.
7.13A	Ichihara S.
7.13B	Tabàr L.
7.14	Ichihara S.
7.15	Ichihara S.
7.16A,B	Collins L.
7.17	Tan P.H.
7.18	Tan P.H.
7.19A,B	Tan P.H.
7.20	Tan P.H.
7.21	Tan P.H.
7.22A,B	Schnitt S.J.
7.23A	Tan P.H.
7.23B	Schnitt S.J.
7.23C	Tan P.H.
8.01A,B	Boecker W. Gerhard Domagk Institute of Pathology, University of Münster, Münster, Germany
8.02A	Nielsen B. B. Institute of Pathology, Randers Hospital, Randers, Denmark
8.02B	Schnitt S.J.
8.02C	Drijkoningen M. Department of Pathology, University Hospital St. Rafael, Leuven, Belgium
8.03	Shin S.J.
8.04	Shin S.J.

8.05	Hanselaar A.G.J.M.	10.17A	Tavassoli F.A.	13.01A,B	Lamovec J.
	Dutch Cancer Society,	10.17B	Tan P.H.		Department of Pathology,
	Amsterdam, The Netherlands,	10.18A	Tan P.H.		Institute of Oncology,
8.06	Boecker W.	10.18B	Bellocq J.P.		Ljubljana, Slovenia
8.07	Drijkoningen M.		Service d'Anatomie Pathologique,	13.02	Medeiros L.J.
8.08A,B	Foschini M. P.		Hôpitaux Universitaires de	13.03	Jaffe E.S.
8.09A,B	Foschini M. P.		Strasbourg,	13.04	Jaffe E.S.
8.10	Foschini M. P.		Strasbourg, France	13.05A,B	Jaffe E.S.
8.11	Foschini M. P.	10.19A,B	Tan P.H.	13.05C	Medeiros L.J.
8.12	Eusebi V.	10.20A,B	Tan P.H.	13.07	Dogan A.
		10.21	Peterse J.L.	13.08	Dogan A.
9.01	Tan P.H.	10.22A,B	Peterse J.L.	13.09A,B	Dogan A.
9.02	Tan P.H.	10.23A-C	Eusebi V.	13.10	Fend F.
9.03A,B	Dabbs D.	10.24	Fletcher C. D. M.	13.11A,B	Harris N.L.
9.04A,B	Dabbs D.	10.25A,B	Tan P.H.		
9.05	Lakhani S.R.	10.26	Tan P.H.	14.01	Lee A.
9.06	Tan P.H.	10.27A,B	Tan P.H.	14.02	Lee A.
9.07A,B	Tan P.H.	10.28A,B	Tavassoli F.A.	14.03	Lee A.
10.01	Fletcher C. D. M.	11.01A,B	Tan P.H.	15.01	Reiner A.
10.02	MacGrogan G.	11.02	Tan P.H.	15.02A,B	Reiner A.
10.03	MacGrogan G.	11.03	Bellocq J.P.	15.03A,B	Reiner A.
10.04A,B	MacGrogan G.	11.04	Tan P.H.	15.04A,B	Reiner A.
10.05	Peterse J.L.	11.05	Tan P.H.		
10.06	Schnitt S.J.	11.06	Tan P.H.	16.01	Varghese J.S.
10.07	Schnitt S.J.	11.07A,B	Tan P.H.	16.02A,B	Villa M.T.
10.08	Schnitt S.J.	11.08A-B	Tan P.H.	16.03	Walsh M.D.
10.09	Tan P.H.	11.09A,B	Tavassoli F.A.	16.04	Devilee P.
10.10	Michal M.	11.10A-C	Tan P.H.	16.05	Devilee P.
10.11	Tan P.H.	11.11	Tan P.H.	16.06	Adapted from {1097}
10.12	Tan P.H.	11.12A,B	Tan P.H.	16.07	Birch J.M.
10.13	Tan P.H.			16.08	Adapted from {1097}
10.14	Tan P.H.	12.01A,B	Eusebi V.	16.09	Tavtigian S.V.
10.15A,B	Magro G.	12.02A,B	Eusebi V.	16.10	Tan M.H.
10.16	Tan P.H.	12.04A,C	Shousha S.		

References

1. Aaltonen LA, Salovaara R, Kristo P, Canzian F, Hemminki A, Peltomaki P, Chadwick RB, Kaariainen H, Eskelinen M, Jarvinen H, Mecklin JP, de la Chapelle A (1998). Incidence of hereditary nonpolyposis colorectal cancer and the feasibility of molecular screening for the disease. N Engl J Med 338: 1481–1487.

2. Aarnio M, Sankila R, Pukkala E, Salovaara R, Aaltonen LA, de la Chapelle A., Peltomaki P, Mecklin JP, Jarvinen HJ (1999). Cancer risk in mutation carriers of DNA-mismatch-repair genes. Int J Cancer 81: 214–218.

3. Abati AD, Kimmel M, Rosen PP (1990). Apocrine mammary carcinoma. A clinicopathologic study of 72 cases. Am J Clin Pathol 94: 371–377.

4. Abd El-Rehim DM, Ball G, Pinder SE, Rakha E, Paish C, Robertson JF, Macmillan D, Blamey RW, Ellis IO (2005). High-throughput protein expression analysis using tissue microarray technology of a large well-characterised series identifies biologically distinct classes of breast cancer confirming recent cDNA expression analyses. Int J Cancer 116: 340–350.

5. Abdeen A, Chou AJ, Healey JH, Khanna C, Osborne TS, Hewitt SM, Kim M, Wang D, Moody K, Gorlick R (2009). Correlation between clinical outcome and growth factor pathway expression in osteogenic sarcoma. Cancer 115: 5243–5250.

6. Abdel-Fatah TM, Powe DG, Hodi Z, Lee AH, Reis-Filho JS, Ellis IO (2007). High frequency of coexistence of columnar cell lesions, lobular neoplasia, and low grade ductal carcinoma in situ with invasive tubular carcinoma and invasive lobular carcinoma. Am J Surg Pathol 31: 417–426.

7. Abdel-Fatah TM, Powe DG, Hodi Z, Reis-Filho JS, Lee AH, Ellis IO (2008). Morphologic and molecular evolutionary pathways of low nuclear grade invasive breast cancers and their putative precursor lesions: further evidence to support the concept of low nuclear grade breast neoplasia family. Am J Surg Pathol 32: 513–523.

8. Aboumrad MH, Horn RC, Jr, Fine G (1963). Lipid-secreting mammary carcinoma. Report of a case associated with Paget's disease of the nipple. Cancer 16: 521–525.

9. Abraham SC, Reynolds C, Lee JH, Montgomery EA, Baisden BL, Krasinskas AM, Wu TT (2002). Fibromatosis of the breast and mutations involving the APC/beta-catenin pathway. Hum Pathol 33: 39–46.

10. Abramowitz MC, Li T, Morrow M, Sigurdson ER, Anderson P, Nicolaou N, Freedman G (2009). Dermal lymphatic invasion and inflammatory breast cancer are independent predictors of outcome after postmastectomy radiation. Am J Clin Oncol 32: 30–33.

11. Abrial SC, Penault-Llorca F, Delva R, Bougnoux P, Leduc B, Mouret-Reynier MA, Mery-Mignard D, Bleuse JP, Dauplat J, Cure H, Chollet P (2005). High prognostic significance of residual disease after neoadjuvant chemotherapy: a retrospective study in 710 patients with operable breast cancer. Breast Cancer Res Treat 94: 255–263.

12. Acharya S, Wilson T, Gradia S, Kane MF, Guerrette S, Marsischky GT, Kolodner R, Fishel R (1996). hMSH2 forms specific mispair-binding complexes with hMSH3 and hMSH6. Proc Natl Acad Sci U S A 93: 13629–13634.

13. Achatz MI, Hainaut P, Ashton-Prolla P (2009). Highly prevalent TP53 mutation predisposing to many cancers in the Brazilian population: a case for newborn screening? Lancet Oncol 10: 920–925.

14. Acs G, Lawton TJ, Rebbeck TR, LiVolsi VA, Zhang PJ (2001). Differential expression of E-cadherin in lobular and ductal neoplasms of the breast and its biologic and diagnostic implications. Am J Clin Pathol 115: 85–98.

14A. Acs G, Simpson JF, Bleiweiss IJ, Hugh J, Reynolds C, Olson S, Page DL (2003). Microglandular adenosis with transition into adenoid cystic carcinoma of the breast. Am J Surg Pathol 27: 1052–1060.

15. Adami HO, Hansen J, Jung B, Lindgren A, Rimsten A (1981). Bilateral carcinoma of the breast. Epidemiology and histopathology. Acta Radiol Oncol 20: 305–309.

15A. Adem C, Reynolds C, Adlakha H, Roche PC, Nascimento AG (2002). Wide spectrum screening keratin as a marker of metaplastic spindle cell carcinoma of the breast: an immunohistochemical study of 24 patients. Histopathology 40: 556–562.

15B. Adelaide J, Finetti P, Bekhouche I, Repellini L, Geneix J, Sircoulomb F, Charafe-Jauffret E, Cervera N, Desplans J, Parzy D, Schoenmakers E, Viens P, Jacquemier J, Birnbaum D, Bertucci F, Chaffanet M (2007). Integrated profiling of basal and luminal breast cancers. Cancer Res 67: 11565–11575.

16. Adem C, Reynolds C, Ingle JN, Nascimento AG (2004). Primary breast sarcoma: clinicopathologic series from the Mayo Clinic and review of the literature. Br J Cancer 91: 237–241.

17. Adeniran A, Al-Ahmadie H, Mahoney MC, Robinson-Smith TM (2004). Granular cell tumor of the breast: a series of 17 cases and review of the literature. Breast J 10: 528–531.

18. Adrada B, Arribas E, Gilcrease M, Yang WT (2009). Invasive micropapillary carcinoma of the breast: mammographic, sonographic, and MRI features. AJR Am J Roentgenol 193: W58–W63.

19. Agrawal A, Ayantunde AA, Rampaul R, Robertson JF (2007). Male breast cancer: a review of clinical management. Breast Cancer Res Treat 103: 11–21.

20. Ahmed AA, Heller DS (2000). Malignant adenomyoepithelioma of the breast with malignant proliferation of epithelial and myoepithelial elements: a case report and review of the literature. Arch Pathol Lab Med 124: 632–636.

20A. Ahmed S, Thomas G, Ghoussaini M, Healey CS, Humphreys MK, Platte R, Morrison J, Maranian M, Pooley KA, Luben R, Eccles D, Evans DG, Fletcher O, Johnson N, dos Santos Silva I, Peto J, Stratton MR, Rahman N, Jacobs K, Prentice R et al. (2009). Newly discovered breast cancer susceptibility loci on 3p24 and 17q23.2. Nat Genet 41: 585–590.

21. Aida Y, Takeuchi E, Shinagawa T, Tadokoro M, Inoue S, Omata Y, Noro M (1993). Fine needle aspiration cytology of lipid-secreting carcinoma of the breast. A case report. Acta Cytol 37: 547–551.

22. Aktepe F, Kapucuoglu N, Pak I (1996). The effects of chemotherapy on breast cancer tissue in locally advanced breast cancer. Histopathology 29: 63–67.

23. Al Sarakbi W, Worku D, Escobar PF, Mokbel K (2006). Breast papillomas: current management with a focus on a new diagnostic and therapeutic modality. Int Semin Surg Oncol 3: 1. Abstract.

24. Alagaratnam TT, Ng WF, Leung EY (1995). Giant fibroadenomas of the breast in an oriental community. J R Coll Surg Edinb 40: 161–162.

25. Albonico G, Querzoli P, Ferretti S, Rinaldi R, Nenci I (1998). Biological profile of in situ breast cancer investigated by immunohistochemical technique. Cancer Detect Prev 22: 313–318.

26. Albores-Saavedra J, Heard SC, McLaren B, Kamino H, Witkiewicz AK (2005). Cylindroma (dermal analog tumor) of the breast: a comparison with cylindroma of the skin and adenoid cystic carcinoma of the breast. Am J Clin Pathol 123: 866–873.

27. Alexander DD, Morimoto LM, Mink PJ, Cushing CA (2010). A review and meta-analysis of red and processed meat consumption and breast cancer. Nutr Res Rev 23: 349–365.

28. Ali E, Athanasopoulos PG, Forouhi P, Malata CM (2010). Cowden syndrome and reconstructive breast surgery: Case reports and review of the literature. J Plast Reconstr Aesthet Surg 64: 545–549.

29. Ali S, Teichberg S, DeRisi DC, Urmacher C (1994). Giant myofibroblastoma of the male breast. Am J Surg Pathol 18: 1170–1176.

30. Ali-Fehmi R, Carolin K, Wallis T, Visscher DW (2003). Clinicopathologic analysis of breast lesions associated with multiple papillomas. Hum Pathol 34: 234–239.

31. Alimonti A, Carracedo A, Clohessy JG, Trotman LC, Nardella C, Egia A, Salmena L, Sampieri K, Haveman WJ, Brogi E, Richardson AL, Zhang J, Pandolfi PP (2010). Subtle variations in Pten dose determine cancer susceptibility. Nat Genet 42: 454–458.

32. Allred DC (2010). Biological features of human premalignant breast disease and the progression to cancer. In: Diseases of the breast, 4th edition. Harris JR, Lippman ME, Morrow M, Osborne CK, eds. Wolters Kluwer Lippincott Williams & Wilkins: Philadelphia: pp 323–334.

33. Allred DC (2010). Issues and updates: evaluating estrogen receptor-alpha, progesterone receptor, and HER2 in breast cancer. Mod Pathol 23 Suppl 2: S52–S59.

34. Allred DC, Anderson SJ, Paik S, Wickerham DL, Nagtegaal ID, Swain SM, Mamounas EP, Julian TB, Geyer CE Jr, Costantino JP, Land SR, Wolmark N (2012). Adjuvant tamoxifen reduces subsequent breast cancer in women with hormone receptor-positive DCIS: a study based on NSABP protocol B-24. J Clin Oncol. In press.

34A. Allred DC, Bryant J, Paik S, Fisher E, Julian T, Margolese R, Smith R, Mamounas T, Osborne CK, Fisher B, Wolmark N (2002). Estrogen receptor expression as a predictive marker of the effectiveness of tamoxifen in the treatment of DCIS: Findings from the NSABP Protocol B-24. Breast Cancer Res Treat 76 (Suppl 1): A30.

35. Allred DC, Carlson RW, Berry DA, Burstein HJ, Edge SB, Goldstein LJ, Gown A, Hammond ME, Iglehart JD, Moench S, Pierce LJ, Ravdin P, Schnitt SJ, Wolff AC (2009). NCCN Task Force Report: Estrogen receptor and progesterone receptor testing in breast cancer by immunohistochemistry. J Natl Compr Canc Netw 7 Suppl 6: S1–S21.

36. Allred DC, Wu Y, Mao S, Nagtegaal ID, Lee S, Perou CM, Mohsin SK, O'Connell P, Tsimelzon A, Medina D (2008). Ductal carcinoma in situ and the emergence of diversity during breast cancer evolution. Clin Cancer Res 14: 370–378.

37. Alpaugh ML, Tomlinson JS, Ye Y, Barsky SH (2002). Relationship of sialyl-Lewis(x/a) underexpression and E-cadherin overexpression in the lymphovascular embolus of inflammatory breast carcinoma. Am J Pathol 161: 619–628.

38. Altekruse SF, Kosary CL, Krapcho M, Neyman N, Aminou R, Waldron W, Ruhl J, Howlader N, Tatalovich Z, Cho H, Mariotto A, Eisner MP, Lewis DR, Cronin K, Chen HS, Feuer.E.J., Stinchcomb DG, Edwards BK, eds. SEER Cancer Statistics Review, 1975-2007. National Cancer Institute, Bethesda, MD (http://seer.cancer.gov/csr/1975_2007/).

39. Alva S, Shetty-Alva N (1999). An update of tumor metastasis to the breast data. Arch Surg 134: 450

40. Alvarado Cabrero I, Carrera Alvarez M., Perez Montiel D, Tavassoli FA (2003). Metastases to the breast. Eur J Surg Oncol 29: 854–855.

41. Alvarez S, Diaz-Uriarte R, Osorio A, Barroso A, Melchor L, Paz MF, Honrado E, Rodriguez R, Urioste M, Valle L, Diez O, Cigudosa JC, Dopazo J, Esteller M, Benitez J (2005). A predictor based on the somatic genomic changes of the BRCA1/BRCA2 breast cancer tumors identifies the non-BRCA1/BRCA2 tumors with BRCA1 promoter hypermethylation. Clin Cancer Res 11: 1146–1153.

42. Amichetti M, Perani B, Boi S (1990). Metastases to the breast from extramammary malignancies. Oncology 47: 257–260.

43. Amir H, Hirji KF (1992). Carcinoma of the male breast in Tanzania. J Natl Med Assoc 84: 337–340.

44. Andersen JA, Gram JB (1982). Male breast at autopsy. Acta Pathol Microbiol Immunol Scand A 90: 191–197.

45. Andersen JA, Vendelboe ML (1981).

Cytoplasmic mucous globules in lobular carcinoma in situ. Diagnosis and prognosis. Am J Surg Pathol 5: 251–255.
46. Anderson E (2002). The role of oestrogen and progesterone receptors in human mammary development and tumorigenesis. Breast Cancer Res 4: 197–201.
47. Anderson JA (1974). Lobular carcinoma in situ. A histological study of 52 cases. Acta Pathol Microbiol Scand A 82: 735–741.
48. Anderson WF, Pfeiffer RM, Dores GM, Sherman ME (2006). Comparison of age distribution patterns for different histopathologic types of breast carcinoma. Cancer Epidemiol Biomarkers Prev 15: 1899–1905.
49. Andrieu N, Easton DF, Chang-Claude J, Rookus MA, Brohet R, Cardis E, Antoniou AC, Wagner T, Simard J, Evans G, Peock S, Fricker JP, Nogues C, Van't Veer L, van Leeuwen FE, Goldgar DE (2006). Effect of chest X-rays on the risk of breast cancer among BRCA1/2 mutation carriers in the international BRCA1/2 carrier cohort study: a report from the EMBRACE, GENEPSO, GEO-HEBON, and IBCCS Collaborators' Group. J Clin Oncol 24: 3361–3366.
50. Ang MK, Ooi AS, Thike AA, Tan P, Zhang Z, Dykema K, Furge K, Teh BT, Tan PH (2010). Molecular classification of breast phyllodes tumors: validation of the histologic grading scheme and insights into malignant progression. Breast Cancer Res Treat 129: 319–329.
51. Angele S, Jones C, Reis Filho JS, Fulford LG, Treilleux I, Lakhani SR, Hall J (2004). Expression of ATM, p53, and the MRE11-Rad50-NBS1 complex in myoepithelial cells from benign and malignant proliferations of the breast. J Clin Pathol 57: 1179–1184.
52. Angele S, Jones C, Reis Filho JS, Fulford LG, Treilleux I, Lakhani SR, Hall J (2004). Expression of ATM, p53, and the MRE11-Rad50-NBS1 complex in myoepithelial cells from benign and malignant proliferations of the breast. J Clin Pathol 57: 1179–1184.
53. Antonescu CR, Yoshida A, Guo T, Chang NE, Zhang L, Agaram NP, Qin LX, Brennan MF, Singer S, Maki RG (2009). KDR activating mutations in human angiosarcomas are sensitive to specific kinase inhibitors. Cancer Res 69: 7175–7179.
53A. Ansquer Y, Delaney S, Santulli P, Salomon L, Carbonne B, Salmon R (2010). Risk of invasive breast cancer after lobular intra-epithelial neoplasia: review of the literature. Eur J Surg Oncol 36: 604–609.
54. Antoniou A, Pharoah PD, Narod S, Risch HA, Eyfjord JE, Hopper JL, Loman N, Olsson H, Johannsson O, Borg A, Pasini B, Radice P, Manoukian S, Eccles DM, Tang N, Olah E, Anton-Culver H, Warner E, Lubinski J, Gronwald J et al. (2003). Average risks of breast and ovarian cancer associated with BRCA1 or BRCA2 mutations detected in case series unselected for family history: a combined analysis of 22 studies. Am J Hum Genet 72: 1117–1130.
55. Antoniou AC, Beesley J, McGuffog L, Sinilnikova OM, Healey S, Neuhausen SL, Ding YC, Rebbeck TR, Weitzel JN, Lynch HT, Isaacs C, Ganz PA, Tomlinson G, Olopade OI, Couch FJ, Wang X, Lindor NM, Pankratz VS, Radice P, Manoukian S et al. (2010). Common breast cancer susceptibility alleles and the risk of breast cancer for BRCA1 and BRCA2 mutation carriers: implications for risk prediction. Cancer Res 70: 9742–9754.
56. Antoniou AC, Cunningham AP, Peto J, Evans DG, Lalloo F, Narod SA, Risch HA, Eyfjord JE, Hopper JL, Southey MC, Olsson H, Johannsson O, Borg A, Pasini B, Radice P, Manoukian S, Eccles DM, Tang N, Olah E, Anton-Culver H et al. (2008). The BOADICEA model of genetic susceptibility to breast and ovarian cancers: updates and extensions. Br J Cancer 98: 1457–1466.
57. Antoniou AC, Hardy R, Walker L, Evans DG, Shenton A, Eeles R, Shanley S, Pichert G, Izatt L, Rose S, Douglas F, Eccles D, Morrison PJ, Scott J, Zimmern RL, Easton DF, Pharoah PD (2008). Predicting the likelihood of carrying a BRCA1 or BRCA2 mutation: validation of BOADICEA, BRCAPRO, IBIS, Myriad and the Manchester scoring system using data from UK genetics clinics. J Med Genet 45: 425–431.
58. Antoniou AC, Pharoah PD, McMullan G, Day NE, Stratton MR, Peto J, Ponder BJ, Easton DF (2002). A comprehensive model for familial breast cancer incorporating BRCA1, BRCA2 and other genes. Br J Cancer 86: 76–83.
59. Antoniou AC, Pharoah PD, Narod S, Risch HA, Eyfjord JE, Hopper JL, Olsson H, Johannsson O, Borg A, Pasini B, Radice P, Manoukian S, Eccles DM, Tang N, Olah E, Anton-Culver H, Warner E, Lubinski J, Gronwald J, Gorski B et al. (2005). Breast and ovarian cancer risks to carriers of the BRCA1 5382insC and 185delAG and BRCA2 6174delT mutations: a combined analysis of 22 population based studies. J Med Genet 42: 602–603.
60. Antoniou AC, Pharoah PP, Smith P, Easton DF (2004). The BOADICEA model of genetic susceptibility to breast and ovarian cancer. Br J Cancer 91: 1580–1590.
61. Antoniou AC, Rookus M, Andrieu N, Brohet R, Chang-Claude J, Peock S, Cook M, Evans DG, Eeles R, Nogues C, Faivre L, Gesta P, van Leeuwen FE, Ausems MG, Osorio A, Caldes T, Simard J, Lubinski J, Gerdes AM, Olah E et al. (2009). Reproductive and hormonal factors, and ovarian cancer risk for BRCA1 and BRCA2 mutation carriers: results from the International BRCA1/2 Carrier Cohort Study. Cancer Epidemiol Biomarkers Prev 18: 601–610.
62. Antoniou AC, Spurdle AB, Sinilnikova OM, Healey S, Pooley KA, Schmutzler RK, Versmold B, Engel C, Meindl A, Arnold N, Hofmann W, Sutter C, Niederacher D, Deissler H, Caldes T, Kampjarvi K, Nevanlinna H, Simard J, Beesley J, Chen X et al. (2008). Common breast cancer-predisposition alleles are associated with breast cancer risk in BRCA1 and BRCA2 mutation carriers. Am J Hum Genet 82: 937–948.
63. Antoniou AC, Wang X, Fredericksen ZS, McGuffog L, Tarrell R, Sinilnikova OM, Healey S, Morrison J, Kartsonaki C, Lesnick T, Ghoussaini M, Barrowdale D, Peock S, Cook M, Oliver C, Frost D, Eccles D, Evans DG, Eeles R, Izatt L et al. (2010). A locus on 19p13 modifies risk of breast cancer in BRCA1 mutation carriers and is associated with hormone receptor-negative breast cancer in the general population. Nat Genet 42: 885–892.
63A. Aparicio SA, Huntsman DG (2010). Does massively parallel DNA resequencing signify the end of histopathology as we know it? J Pathol 220: 307–315.
64. Arbabi L, Warhol MJ (1982). Pleomorphic liposarcoma following radiotherapy for breast carcinoma. Cancer 49: 878–880.
65. Arber DA, Simpson JF, Weiss LM, Rappaport H (1994). Non-Hodgkin's lymphoma involving the breast. Am J Surg Pathol 18: 288–295.
66. Arce C, Cortes-Padilla D, Huntsman DG, Miller MA, Duennas-Gonzalez A, Alvarado A, Perez V, Gallardo-Rincon D, Lara-Medina F (2005). Secretory carcinoma of the breast containing the ETV6-NTRK3 fusion gene in a male: case report and review of the literature. World J Surg Oncol 3: 35
67. Arias-Stella J, Jr, Rosen PP (1988). Hemangiopericytoma of the breast. Mod Pathol 1: 98–103.
68. Armes JE, Egan AJ, Southey MC, Dite GS, McCredie MR, Giles GG, Hopper JL, Venter DJ (1998). The histologic phenotypes of breast carcinoma occurring before age 40 years in women with and without BRCA1 or BRCA2 germline mutations: a population-based study. Cancer 83: 2335–2345.
69. Armes JE, Trute L, White D, Southey MC, Hammet F, Tesoriero A, Hutchins AM, Dite GS, McCredie MR, Giles GG, Hopper JL, Venter DJ (1999). Distinct molecular pathogeneses of early-onset breast cancers in BRCA1 and BRCA2 mutation carriers: a population-based study. Cancer Res 59: 2011–2017.
70. Arnedos M, Nerurkar A, Osin P, A'Hern R, Smith IE, Dowsett M (2009). Discordance between core needle biopsy (CNB) and excisional biopsy (EB) for estrogen receptor (ER), progesterone receptor (PgR) and HER2 status in early breast cancer (EBC). Ann Oncol 20: 1948–1952.
71. Arnes JB, Brunet JS, Stefansson I, Begin LR, Wong N, Chappuis PO, Akslen LA, Foulkes WD (2005). Placental cadherin and the basal epithelial phenotype of BRCA1-related breast cancer. Clin Cancer Res 11: 4003–4011.
72. Aroner SA, Collins LC, Schnitt SJ, Connolly JL, Colditz GA, Tamimi RM (2010). Columnar cell lesions and subsequent breast cancer risk: a nested case-control study. Breast Cancer Res 12: R61
73. Arpino G, Bardou VJ, Clark GM, Elledge RM (2004). Infiltrating lobular carcinoma of the breast: tumor characteristics and clinical outcome. Breast Cancer Res 6: R149–R156.
74. Ashikaga T, Krag DN, Land SR, Julian TB, Anderson SJ, Brown AM, Skelly JM, Harlow SP, Weaver DL, Mamounas EP, Costantino JP, Wolmark N (2010). Morbidity results from the NSABP B-32 trial comparing sentinel lymph node dissection versus axillary dissection. J Surg Oncol 102: 111–118.
75. Ashikari R, Huvos AG, Urban JA, Robbins GF (1973). Infiltrating lobular carcinoma of the breast. Cancer 31: 110–116.
76. Asioli S, Marucci G, Ficarra G, Stephens M, Foschini MP, Ellis IO, Eusebi V (2006). Polymorphous adenocarcinoma of the breast. Report of three cases. Virchows Arch 448: 29–34.
76A. Asoglu O, Ugurlu MM, Blanchard K, Grant CS, Reynolds C, Cha SS, Donohue JH (2004). Risk factors for recurrence and death after primary surgical treatment of malignant phyllodes tumors. Ann Surg Oncol 11: 1011–1017.
77. Atchley DP, Albarracin CT, Lopez A, Valero V, Amos CI, Gonzalez-Angulo AM, Hortobagyi GN, Arun BK (2008). Clinical and pathologic characteristics of patients with BRCA-positive and BRCA-negative breast cancer. J Clin Oncol 26: 4282–4288.
78. Aubele MM, Cummings MC, Mattis AE, Zitzelsberger HF, Walch AK, Kremer M, Hofler H, Werner M (2000). Accumulation of chromosomal imbalances from intraductal proliferative lesions to adjacent in situ and invasive ductal breast cancer. Diagn Mol Pathol 9: 14–19.
79. Aulmann S, Elsawaf Z, Penzel R, Schirmacher P, Sinn HP (2009). Invasive tubular carcinoma of the breast frequently is clonally related to flat epithelial atypia and low-grade ductal carcinoma in situ. Am J Surg Pathol 33: 1646–1653.
80. Austin RM, Dupree WB (1986). Liposarcoma of the breast: a clinicopathologic study of 20 cases. Hum Pathol 17: 906–913.
81. Aydin O, Cinel L, Egilmez R, Ocal K, Ozer C (2001). Adenomyoepithelioma of the breast. Diagn Cytopathol 25: 194–196.
82. Azoulay S, Lae M, Freneaux P, Merle S, Al Ghuzlan A, Chnecker C, Rosty C, Klijanienko J, Sigal-Zafrani B, Salmon R, Fourquet A, Sastre-Garau X, Vincent-Salomon A (2005). KIT is highly expressed in adenoid cystic carcinoma of the breast, a basal-like carcinoma associated with a favorable outcome. Mod Pathol 18: 1623–1631.
83. Azumi N, Battifora H (1987). The cellular composition of adenoid cystic carcinoma. An immunohistochemical study. Cancer 60: 1589–1598.
84. Azzopardi JG, Ahmed A, Millis RR (1979). Problems in breast pathology. Major problems in pathology. Saunders: Phildelphia.
85. Azzopardi JG, Eusebi V (1977). Melanocyte colonization and pigmentation of breast carcinoma. Histopathology 1: 21–30.
86. Azzopardi JG, Salm R (1984). Ductal adenoma of the breast: a lesion which can mimic carcinoma. J Pathol 144: 15–23.
87. Bachmeier BE, Nerlich AG, Mirisola V, Jochum M, Pfeffer U (2008). Lineage infidelity and expression of melanocytic markers in human breast cancer. Int J Oncol 33: 1011–1015.
88. Baddoura FK, Judd RL (1990). Apocrine adenoma of the breast: report of a case with investigation of lectin binding patterns in apocrine breast lesions. Mod Pathol 3: 373–376.
89. Badve S, Sloane JP (1995). Pseudoangiomatous hyperplasia of male breast. Histopathology 26: 463–466.
90. Baglietto L, Lindor NM, Dowty JG, White DM, Wagner A, Gomez Garcia EB, Vriends AH, Cartwright NR, Barnetson RA, Farrington SM, Tenesa A, Hampel H, Buchanan D, Arnold S, Young J, Walsh MD, Jass J, Macrae F, Antill Y, Winship IM et al. (2010). Risks of Lynch syndrome cancers for MSH6 mutation carriers. J Natl Cancer Inst 102: 193–201.
91. Bahrami A, Resetkova E, Ro JY, Ibanez JD, Ayala AG (2007). Primary osteosarcoma of the breast: report of 2 cases. Arch Pathol Lab Med 131: 792–795.
92. Baker TP, Lenert JT, Parker J, Kemp B, Kushwaha A, Evans G, Hunt KK (2001). Lactating adenoma: a diagnosis of exclusion. Breast J 7: 354–357.
93. Ball S, Arolker M, Purushotham AD (2001). Breast cancer, Cowden disease and PTEN-MATCHS syndrome. Eur J Surg Oncol 27: 604–606.
94. Ballance WA, Ro JY, el-Naggar AK, Grignon DJ, Ayala AG, Romsdahl MG (1990). Pleomorphic adenoma (benign mixed tumor) of the breast. An immunohistochemical, flow cytometric, and ultrastructural study and review of the literature. Am J Clin Pathol 93: 795–801.
95. Balleine RL, Murali R, Bilous AM, Farshid G, Waring P, Provan P, Byth K, Thorne H, kConFab Investigators, Kirk JA (2006). Histopathological features of breast cancer in carriers of ATM gene variants. Histopathology 49: 523–532.
96. Bane AL, Beck JC, Bleiweiss I, Buys

SS, Catalano E, Daly MB, Giles G, Godwin AK, Hibshoosh H, Hopper JL, John EM, Layfield L, Longacre T, Miron A, Senie R, Southey MC, West DW, Whittemore AS, Wu H, Andrulis IL et al. (2007). BRCA2 mutation-associated breast cancers exhibit a distinguishing phenotype based on morphology and molecular profiles from tissue microarrays. Am J Surg Pathol 31: 121–128.

97. Bane AL, Pinnaduwage D, Colby S, Reedijk M, Egan SE, Bull SB, O'Malley FP, Andrulis IL (2009). Expression profiling of familial breast cancers demonstrates higher expression of FGFR2 in BRCA2-associated tumors. Breast Cancer Res Treat 117: 183–191.

98. Bane AL, Tjan S, Parkes RK, Andrulis I, O'Malley FP (2005). Invasive lobular carcinoma: to grade or not to grade. Mod Pathol 18: 621–628.

99. Banerjee SS, Harris M (2000). Morphological and immunophenotypic variations in malignant melanoma. Histopathology 36: 387–402.

99A. Banev SG , Filipovski VA (2006). Chondrolipoma of the breast--case report and a review of literature. Breast 15: 425–426.

100. Banneau G, Guedj M, MacGrogan G, de Mascarel I, Velasco V, Schiappa R, Bonadona V, David A, Dugast C, Gilbert-Dussardier B, Ingster O, Vabres P, Caux F, de Reynies A, Iggo R, Sevenet N, Bonnet F, Longy M (2010). Molecular apocrine differentiation is a common feature of breast cancer in patients with germline PTEN mutations. Breast Cancer Res 12: R63

101. Barbareschi M, Pecciarini L, Cangi MG, Macri E, Rizzo A, Viale G, Doglioni C (2001). p63, a p53 homologue, is a selective nuclear marker of myoepithelial cells of the human breast. Am J Surg Pathol 25: 1054–1060.

102. Barbosa ML, Ribeiro EM, Silva GF, Maciel ME, Lima RS, Cavalli LR, Cavalli IJ (2004). Cytogenetic findings in phyllodes tumor and fibroadenomas of the breast. Cancer Genet Cytogenet 154: 156–159.

103. Bardou VJ, Arpino G, Elledge RM, Osborne CK, Clark GM (2003). Progesterone receptor status significantly improves outcome prediction over estrogen receptor status alone for adjuvant endocrine therapy in two large breast cancer databases. J Clin Oncol 21: 1973–1979.

104. Barkley CR, Ligibel JA, Wong JS, Lipsitz S, Smith BL, Golshan M (2008). Mucinous breast carcinoma: a large contemporary series. Am J Surg 196: 549–551.

105. Barnes L, Pietruszka M (1978). Rhabdomyosarcoma arising within a cystosarcoma phyllodes. Case report and review of the literature. Am J Surg Pathol 2: 423–429.

105A. Barnes PJ, Boutilier R, Chiasson D, Rayson D (2005). Metaplastic breast carcinoma: clinical-pathologic characteristics and HER2/neu expression. Breast Cancer Res Treat 91: 173–178.

106. Barrio AV, Clark BD, Goldberg JI, Hoque LW, Bernik SF, Flynn LW, Susnik B, Giri D, Polo K, Patil S, Van Zee KJ (2007). Clinicopathologic features and long-term outcomes of 293 phyllodes tumors of the breast. Ann Surg Oncol 14: 2961–2970.

107. Bartlett JM, Ibrahim M, Jasani B, Morgan JM, Ellis I, Kay E, Magee H, Barnett S, Miller K (2007). External quality assurance of HER2 fluorescence in situ hybridisation testing: results of a UK NEQAS pilot scheme. J Clin Pathol 60: 816–819.

108. Basham VM, Lipscombe JM, Ward JM,

Gayther SA, Ponder BA, Easton DF, Pharoah PD (2002). BRCA1 and BRCA2 mutations in a population-based study of male breast cancer. Breast Cancer Res. 4: R2. Abstract.

109. Bassler R, Katzer B (1992). Histopathology of myoepithelial (basocellular) hyperplasias in adenosis and epitheliosis of the breast demonstrated by the reactivity of cytokeratins and S100 protein. An analysis of heterogenic cell proliferations in 90 cases of benign and malignant breast diseases. Virchows Arch A Pathol Anat Histopathol 421: 435–442.

110. Basu SK, Schwartz C, Fisher SG, Hudson MM, Tarbell N, Muhs A, Marcus KJ, Mendenhall N, Mauch P, Kun LE, Constine LS (2008). Unilateral and bilateral breast cancer in women surviving pediatric Hodgkin's disease. Int J Radiat Oncol Biol Phys 72: 34–40.

111. Beck AH, Lee CH, Witten DM, Gleason BC, Edris B, Espinosa I, Zhu S, Li R, Montgomery KD, Marinelli RJ, Tibshirani R, Hastie T, Jablons DM, Rubin BP, Fletcher CD, West RB, van de Rijn M (2010). Discovery of molecular subtypes in leiomyosarcoma through integrative molecular profiling. Oncogene 29: 845–854.

112. Bedard PL, Cardoso F, Piccart-Gebhart MJ (2009). Stemming resistance to HER-2 targeted therapy. J Mammary Gland Biol Neoplasia 14: 55–66.

113. Begum SM, Jara-Lazaro AR, Thike AA, Tse GM, Wong JS, Ho JT, Tan PH (2009). Mucin extravasation in breast core biopsies—clinical significance and outcome correlation. Histopathology 55: 609–617.

114. Bellezza G, Lombardi T, Panzarola P, Sidoni A, Cavaliere A, Giansanti M (2007). Schwannoma of the breast: a case report and review of the literature. Tumori 93: 308–311.

115. Bennett KL, Mester J, Eng C (2010). Germline epigenetic regulation of KILLIN in Cowden and Cowden-like syndrome. JAMA 304: 2724–2731.

116. Bentz JS, Yassa N, Clayton F (1998). Pleomorphic lobular carcinoma of the breast: clinicopathologic features of 12 cases. Mod Pathol 11: 814–822.

117. Beral V (2003). Breast cancer and hormone-replacement therapy in the Million Women Study. Lancet 362: 419–427.

118. Beral V, Reeves G, Bull D, Green J (2011). Breast cancer risk in relation to the interval between menopause and starting hormone therapy. J Natl Cancer Inst 103: 296–305.

118A. Bergamaschi A, Kim YH, Wang P, Sorlie T, Hernandez-Boussard T, Lonning PE, Tibshirani R, Borresen-Dale AL, Pollack JR (2006). Distinct patterns of DNA copy number alteration are associated with different clinicopathological features and gene-expression subtypes of breast cancer. Genes Chromosomes Cancer 45: 1033–1040.

119. Bergstraesser LM, Srinivasan G, Jones JC, Stahl S, Weitzman SA (1995). Expression of hemidesmosomes and component proteins is lost by invasive breast cancer cells. Am J Pathol 147: 1823–1839.

120. Bernstein JL, Haile RW, Stovall M, Boice JD, Jr, Shore RE, Langholz B, Thomas DC, Bernstein L, Lynch CF, Olsen JH, Malone KE, Mellemkjaer L, Borresen-Dale AL, Rosenstein BS, Teraoka SN, Diep AT, Smith SA, Capanu M, Reiner AS, Liang X et al. (2010). Radiation exposure, the ATM Gene, and contralateral breast cancer in the women's environmental cancer and radiation epidemiolo-

gy study. J Natl Cancer Inst 102: 475–483.

121. Bernstein JL, Teraoka S, Southey MC, Jenkins MA, Andrulis IL, Knight JA, John EM, Lapinski R, Wolitzer AL, Whittemore AS, West D, Seminara D, Olson ER, Spurdle AB, Chenevix-Trench G, Giles GG, Hopper JL, Concannon P (2006). Population-based estimates of breast cancer risks associated with ATM gene variants c.7271T>G and c.1066-6T>G (IVS10-6T>G) from the Breast Cancer Family Registry. Hum Mutat 27: 1122–1128.

122. Bernstein L (2002). Epidemiology of endocrine-related risk factors for breast cancer. J Mammary Gland Biol Neoplasia 7: 3–15.

123. Bernstein L, Patel AV, Ursin G, Sullivan-Halley J, Press MF, Deapen D, Berlin JA, Daling JR, McDonald JA, Norman SA, Malone KE, Strom BL, Liff J, Folger SG, Simon MS, Burkman RT, Marchbanks PA, Weiss LK, Spirtas R (2005). Lifetime recreational exercise activity and breast cancer risk among black women and white women. J Natl Cancer Inst 97: 1671–1679.

124. Berry DA, Iversen ES, Jr, Gudbjartsson DF, Hiller EH, Garber JE, Peshkin BN, Lerman C, Watson P, Lynch HT, Hilsenbeck SG, Rubinstein WS, Hughes KS, Parmigiani G (2002). BRCAPRO validation, sensitivity of genetic testing of BRCA1/BRCA2, and prevalence of other breast cancer susceptibility genes. J Clin Oncol 20: 2701–2712.

125. Bertelsen L, Bernstein L, Olsen JH, Mellemkjaer L, Haile RW, Lynch CF, Malone KE, Anton-Culver H, Christensen J, Langholz B, Thomas DC, Begg CB, Capanu M, Ejlertsen B, Stovall M, Boice JD, Jr, Shore RE, Bernstein JL (2008). Effect of systemic adjuvant treatment on risk for contralateral breast cancer in the Women's Environment, Cancer and Radiation Epidemiology Study. J Natl Cancer Inst 100: 32–40.

126. Bertucci F, Finetti P, Cervera N, Charafe-Jauffret E, Mamessier E, Adelaide J, Debono S, Houvenaeghel G, Maraninchi D, Viens P, Charpin C, Jacquemier J, Birnbaum D (2006). Gene expression profiling shows medullary breast cancer is a subgroup of basal breast cancers. Cancer Res 66: 4636–4644.

126A. Bertucci F, Orsetti B, Negre V, Finetti P, Rouge C, Ahomadegbe JC, Bibeau F, Mathieu MC, Treilleux I, Jacquemier J, Ursule L, Martinec A, Wang Q, Benard J, Puisieux A, Birnbaum D, Theillet C (2008). Lobular and ductal carcinomas of the breast have distinct genomic and expression profiles. Oncogene 27: 5359–5372.

127. Berx G, Becker KF, Hofler H, van Roy F (1998). Mutations of the human E-cadherin (CDH1) gene. Hum Mutat 12: 226–237.

128. Berx G, Cleton-Jansen AM, Nollet F, de Leeuw WJ, Van de Vijver M, Cornelisse C, van Roy F (1995). E-cadherin is a tumour/invasion suppressor gene mutated in human lobular breast cancers. EMBO J 14: 6107–6115.

129. Berx G, Cleton-Jansen AM, Strumane K, de Leeuw WJ, Nollet F, van Roy F, Cornelisse C (1996). E-cadherin is inactivated in a majority of invasive human lobular breast cancers by truncation mutations throughout its extracellular domain. Oncogene 13: 1919–1925.

130. Beute BJ, Kalisher L, Hutter RV (1991). Lobular carcinoma in situ of the breast: clinical, pathologic, and mammographic features. AJR Am J Roentgenol 157: 257–265.

131. Bezic J, Forempoher G, Poljicanin A, Gunjaca G (2007). Apocrine adenoma of the breast coexistent with invasive carcinoma.

Pathol Res Pract 203: 809–812.

132. Bhargava R, Beriwal S, Striebel JM, Dabbs DJ (2010). Breast cancer molecular class ERBB2: preponderance of tumors with apocrine differentiation and expression of basal phenotype markers CK5, CK5/6, and EGFR. Appl Immunohistochem Mol Morphol 18: 113–118.

133. Bhargava R, Dabbs DJ (2007). Use of immunohistochemistry in diagnosis of breast epithelial lesions. Adv Anat Pathol 14: 93–107.

134. Bhatia S, Robison LL, Oberlin O, Greenberg M, Bunin G, Fossati-Bellani F, Meadows AT (1996). Breast cancer and other second neoplasms after childhood Hodgkin's disease. N Engl J Med 334: 745–751.

135. Bhattacharya B, Dilworth HP, Iacobuzio-Donahue C, Ricci F, Weber K, Furlong MA, Fisher C, Montgomery E (2005). Nuclear beta-catenin expression distinguishes deep fibromatosis from other benign and malignant fibroblastic and myofibroblastic lesions. Am J Surg Pathol 29: 653–659.

136. Bianchi S, Vezzosi V (2008). Microinvasive carcinoma of the breast. Pathol Oncol Res 14: 105–111.

137. Bijker N, Meijnen P, Peterse JL, Bogaerts J, Van Hoorebeeck I, Julien JP, Gennaro M, Rouanet P, Avril A, Fentiman IS, Bartelink H, Rutgers EJ (2006). Breast-conserving treatment with or without radiotherapy in ductal carcinoma-in-situ: ten-year results of European Organisation for Research and Treatment of Cancer randomized phase III trial 10853—a study by the EORTC Breast Cancer Cooperative Group and EORTC Radiotherapy Group. J Clin Oncol 24: 3381–3387.

138. Bijker N, Peterse JL, Duchateau L, Julien JP, Fentiman IS, Duval C, Di PS, Simony-Lafontaine J, de Mascarel, I, Van de Vijver, MJ (2001). Risk factors for recurrence and metastasis after breast-conserving therapy for ductal carcinoma-in-situ: analysis of European Organization for Research and Treatment of Cancer Trial 10853. J Clin Oncol 19: 2263–2271.

139. Billings SD, McKenney JK, Folpe AL, Hardacre MC, Weiss SW (2004). Cutaneous angiosarcoma following breast-conserving surgery and radiation: an analysis of 27 cases. Am J Surg Pathol 28: 781–788.

140. Bilous M (2010). Breast core needle biopsy: issues and controversies. Mod Pathol 23 Suppl 2: S36–S45.

141. Birch JM, Alston RD, McNally RJ, Evans DG, Kelsey AM, Harris M, Eden OB, Varley JM (2001). Relative frequency and morphology of cancers in carriers of germline TP53 mutations. Oncogene 20: 4621–4628.

142. Birch JM, Blair V, Kelsey AM, Evans DG, Harris M, Tricker KJ, Varley JM (1998). Cancer phenotype correlates with constitutional TP53 genotype in families with the Li-Fraumeni syndrome. Oncogene 17: 1061–1068.

143. Birch JM, Hartley AL, Tricker KJ, Prosser J, Condie A, Kelsey AM, Harris M, Jones PH, Binchy A, Crowther D (1994). Prevalence and diversity of constitutional mutations in the p53 gene among 21 Li-Fraumeni families. Cancer Res 54: 1298–1304.

144. Birdsall SH, Shipley JM, Summersgill BM, Black AJ, Jackson P, Kissin MW, Gusterson BA (1995). Cytogenetic findings in a case of nodular fasciitis of the breast. Cancer Genet Cytogenet 81: 166–168.

145. Black J, Metcalf C, Wylie EJ (1996). Ultrasonography of breast hamartomas. Australas Radiol 40: 412–415.

146. Blamey RW, Pinder SE, Ball GR, Ellis IO, Elston CW, Mitchell MJ, Haybittle JL (2007). Reading the prognosis of the individual with breast cancer. Eur J Cancer 43: 1545–1547.

147. Blanchard DK, Reynolds CA, Grant CS, Donohue JH (2003). Primary nonphylloides breast sarcomas. Am J Surg 186: 359–361.

148. Blanco A, Grana B, Fachal L, Santamarina M, Cameselle-Teijeiro J, Ruiz-Ponte C, Carracedo A, Vega A (2010). Beyond BRCA1 and BRCA2 wild-type breast and/or ovarian cancer families: germline mutations in TP53 and PTEN. Clin Genet 77: 193–196.

149. Bleicher RJ, O'Sullivan MJ, Ciocca V, Ciocca RM, Perkins LA, Ross E, Li T, Patchefsky AS, Sigurdson ER, Joseph NE, Sesa L, Morrow M (2008). A prospective feasibility trial to determine the significance of the sentinel node gradient in breast cancer: a predictor of nodal metastasis location. Cancer 113: 3100–3107.

149A. Bleiweiss IJ, Nagi CS, Jaffer S (2006). Axillary sentinel lymph nodes can be falsely positive due to iatrogenic displacement and transport of benign epithelial cells in patients with breast carcinoma. J Clin Oncol 24: 2013–2018.

150. Bloch KE, Marincek B, Amann FW, Russi EW (1991). Pulmonary hypertension five years after left pneumonectomy for adenoid cystic carcinoma. Chest 99: 1018–1019.

151. Bloom HJ, Richardson WW (1957). Histological grading and prognosis in breast cancer; a study of 1409 cases of which 359 have been followed for 15 years. Br J Cancer 11: 359–377.

152. Bluemke DA, Gatsonis CA, Chen MH, DeAngelis GA, DeBruhl N, Harms S, Heywang-Kobrunner SH, Hylton N, Kuhl CK, Lehman C, Pisano ED, Causer P, Schnitt SJ, Smazal SF, Stelling CB, Weatherall PT, Schnall MD (2004). Magnetic resonance imaging of the breast prior to biopsy. JAMA 292: 2735–2742.

153. Bodian CA, Perzin KH, Lattes R, Hoffmann P (1993). Reproducibility and validity of pathologic classifications of benign breast disease and implications for clinical applications. Cancer 71: 3908–3913.

154. Boecker W, Buerger H (2004). Usual and atypical ductal hyperplasia - members of the same family? Current Diag Pathol 10: 175–182.

155. Boecker W, Moll R, Dervan P, Buerger H, Poremba C, Diallo RI, Herbst H, Schmidt A, Lerch MM, Buchwalow IB (2002). Usual ductal hyperplasia of the breast is a committed stem (progenitor) cell lesion distinct from atypical ductal hyperplasia and ductal carcinoma in situ. J Pathol 198: 458–467.

156. Boffetta P, Couto E, Wichmann J, Ferrari P, Trichopoulos D, Bueno-de-Mesquita HB, van Duijnhoven FJ, Buchner FL, Key T, Boeing H, Nothlings U, Linseisen J, Gonzalez CA, Overvad K, Nielsen MR, Tjonneland A, Olsen A, Clavel-Chapelon F, Boutron-Ruault MC, Morois S et al. (2010). Fruit and vegetable intake and overall cancer risk in the European Prospective Investigation into Cancer and Nutrition (EPIC). J Natl Cancer Inst 102: 529–537.

157. Boice JD, Jr, Harvey EB, Blettner M, Stovall M, Flannery JT (1992). Cancer in the contralateral breast after radiotherapy for breast cancer. N Engl J Med 326: 781–785.

158. Boland CR (2005). Evolution of the nomenclature for the hereditary colorectal cancer syndromes. Fam Cancer 4: 211–218.

159. Boland CR, Thibodeau SN, Hamilton SR, Sidransky D, Eshleman JR, Burt RW, Meltzer SJ, Rodriguez-Bigas MA, Fodde R, Ranzani GN, Srivastava S (1998). A National Cancer Institute Workshop on Microsatellite Instability for cancer detection and familial predisposition: development of international criteria for the determination of microsatellite instability in colorectal cancer. Cancer Res 58: 5248–5257.

160. Boldt V, Stacher E, Halbwedl I, Popper H, Hultschig C, Moinfar F, Ullmann R, Tavassoli FA (2010). Positioning of necrotic lobular intraepithelial neoplasias (LIN, grade 3) within the sequence of breast carcinoma progression. Genes Chromosomes Cancer 49: 463–470.

161. Bombonati A, Sgroi DC (2011). The molecular pathology of breast cancer progression. J Pathol 223: 307–317.

162. Bonadonna G, Valagussa P, Brambilla C, Ferrari L, Moliterni A, Terenziani M, Zambetti M (1998). Primary chemotherapy in operable breast cancer: eight-year experience at the Milan Cancer Institute. J Clin Oncol 16: 93–100.

163. Bonadonna G, Veronesi U, Brambilla C, Ferrari L, Luini A, Greco M, Bartoli C, Coopmans de Yoldi G, Zucali R, Rilke F (1990). Primary chemotherapy to avoid mastectomy in tumors with diameters of three centimeters or more. J Natl Cancer Inst 82: 1539–1545.

164. Bonaventure P, Guo H, Tian B, Liu X, Bittner A, Roland B, Salunga R, Ma XJ, Kamme F, Meurers B, Bakker M, Jurzak M, Leysen JE, Erlander MG (2002). Nuclei and subnuclei gene expression profiling in mammalian brain. Brain Res 943: 38–47.

165. Bond GL, Hu W, Bond EE, Robins H, Lutzker SG, Arva NC, Bargonetti J, Bartel F, Taubert H, Wuerl P, Onel K, Yip L, Hwang SJ, Strong LC, Lozano G, Levine AJ (2004). A single nucleotide polymorphism in the MDM2 promoter attenuates the p53 tumor suppressor pathway and accelerates tumor formation in humans. Cell 119: 591–602.

166. Bonnet M, Guinebretiere JM, Kremmer E, Grunewald V, Benhamou E, Contesso G, Joab I (1999). Detection of Epstein-Barr virus in invasive breast cancers. J Natl Cancer Inst 91: 1376–1381.

167. Bonnier P, Charpin C, Lejeune C, Romain S, Tubiana N, Beedassy B, Martin PM, Serment H, Piana L (1995). Inflammatory carcinomas of the breast: a clinical, pathological, or a clinical and pathological definition? Int J Cancer 62: 382–385.

168. Bonnier P, Romain S, Giacalone PL, Laffargue F, Martin PM, Piana L (1995). Clinical and biologic prognostic factors in breast cancer diagnosed during postmenopausal hormone replacement therapy. Obstet Gynecol 85: 11–17.

169. Borgen PI, Wong GY, Vlamis V, Potter C, Hoffmann B, Kinne DW, Osborne MP, McKinnon WM (1992). Current management of male breast cancer. A review of 104 cases. Ann Surg 215: 451–457.

170. Borst MJ, Ingold JA (1993). Metastatic patterns of invasive lobular versus invasive ductal carcinoma of the breast. Surgery 114: 637–641.

171. Botta G, Fessia L, Ghiringhello B (1982). Juvenile milk protein secreting carcinoma. Virchows Arch A Pathol Anat Histol 395: 145–152.

172. Boudova L, Kazakov DV, Sima R, Vanecek T, Torlakovic E, Lamovec J, Kutzner H, Szepe P, Plank L, Bouda J, Hes O, Mukensnabl P, Michal M (2005). Cutaneous lymphoid hyperplasia and other lymphoid infiltrates of the breast nipple: a retrospective clinicopathologic study of fifty-six patients. Am J Dermatopathol 27: 375–386.

173. Bougeard G, Baert-Desurmont S, Tournier I, Vasseur S, Martin C, Brugieres L, Chompret A, Bressac-de Paillerets B, Stoppa-Lyonnet D, Bonaiti-Pellie C, Frebourg T (2006). Impact of the MDM2 SNP309 and p53 Arg72Pro polymorphism on age of tumour onset in Li-Fraumeni syndrome. J Med Genet 43: 531–533.

174. Bougeard G, Sesboue R, Baert-Desurmont S, Vasseur S, Martin C, Tinat J, Brugieres L, Chompret A, de Paillerets BB, Stoppa-Lyonnet D, Bonaiti-Pellie C, Frebourg T (2008). Molecular basis of the Li-Fraumeni syndrome: an update from the French LFS families. J Med Genet 45: 535–538.

175. Boughey JC, Peintinger F, Meric-Bernstam F, Perry AC, Hunt KK, Babiera GV, Singletary SE, Bedrosian I, Lucci A, Buzdar AU, Pusztai L, Kuerer HM (2006). Impact of preoperative versus postoperative chemotherapy on the extent and number of surgical procedures in patients treated in randomized clinical trials for breast cancer. Ann Surg 244: 464–470.

176. Boulos FI, Dupont WD, Simpson JF, Schuyler PA, Sanders ME, Freudenthal ME, Page DL (2008). Histologic associations and long-term cancer risk in columnar cell lesions of the breast: a retrospective cohort and a nested case-control study. Cancer 113: 2415–2421.

177. Boussen H, Bouzaiene H, Ben HJ, Dhiab T, Khomsi F, Benna F, Gamoudi A, Mourali N, Hechiche M, Rahal K, Levine PH (2010). Inflammatory breast cancer in Tunisia: epidemiological and clinical trends. Cancer 116: 2730–2735.

178. Bowman K, Munoz A, Mahvi DM, Breslin TM (2007). Lobular neoplasia diagnosed at core biopsy does not mandate surgical excision. J Surg Res 142: 275–280.

179. Brain E, Garrino C, Misset JL, Carbonero IG, Itzhaki M, Cvitkovic E, Goldschmidt E, Burki F, Regensberg C, Pappo E, Hagipantelli R, Musset M (1997). Long-term prognostic and predictive factors in 107 stage II/III breast cancer patients treated with anthracycline-based neoadjuvant chemotherapy. Br J Cancer 75: 1360–1367.

180. Bratthauer GL, Miettinen M, Tavassoli FA (2003). Cytokeratin immunoreactivity in lobular intraepithelial neoplasia. J Histochem Cytochem 51: 1527–1531.

181. Breast Cancer Linkage Consortium (1997). Pathology of familial breast cancer: differences between breast cancers in carriers of BRCA1 or BRCA2 mutations and sporadic cases. Lancet 349: 1505–1510.

182. Brenn T, Fletcher CD (2005). Radiation-associated cutaneous atypical vascular lesions and angiosarcoma: clinicopathologic analysis of 42 cases. Am J Surg Pathol 29: 983–996.

183. Brinkmann AO (2001). Molecular basis of androgen insensitivity. Mol Cell Endocrinol 179: 105–109.

184. Brinton LA, Carreon JD, Gierach GL, McGlynn KA, Gridley G (2010). Etiologic factors for male breast cancer in the U.S. Veterans Affairs medical care system database. Breast Cancer Res Treat 119: 185–192.

185. Brinton LA, Richesson DA, Gierach GL, Lacey JV, Jr, Park Y, Hollenbeck AR, Schatzkin A (2008). Prospective evaluation of risk factors for male breast cancer. J Natl Cancer Inst 100: 1477–1481.

186. Britton P, Duffy SW, Sinnatamby R, Wallis MG, Barter S, Gaskarth M, O'Neill A, Caldas C, Brenton JD, Forouhi P, Wishart GC (2009). One-stop diagnostic breast clinics: how often are breast cancers missed? Br J Cancer 100: 1873–1878.

187. Britton PD (2011). Fine needle aspiration or core biopsy. The Breast 8: 1–4.

188. Brodie C, Provenzano E (2008). Vascular proliferations of the breast. Histopathology 52: 30–44.

189. Broeks A, Schmidt MK, Sherman ME, Couch FJ, Hopper JL, Dite GS, Apicella C, Smith LD, Hammet F, Southey MC, Van't Veer LJ, de Groot R, Smit VT, Fasching PA, Beckmann MW, Jud S, Ekici AB, Hartmann A, Hein A, Schulz-Wendtland R et al. (2011). Low penetrance breast cancer susceptibility loci are associated with specific breast tumor subtypes: findings from the Breast Cancer Association Consortium. Hum Mol Genet 20: 3289–3303.

190. Broet P, de la Rochefordiere A, Scholl SM, Fourquet A, Mosseri V, Durand JC, Pouillart P, Asselain B (1995). Contralateral breast cancer: annual incidence and risk parameters. J Clin Oncol 13: 1578–1583.

191. Brogi E (2004). Benign and malignant spindle cell lesions of the breast. Semin Diagn Pathol 21: 57–64.

192. Brogi E, Harris NL (1999). Lymphomas of the breast: pathology and clinical behavior. Semin Oncol 26: 357–364.

193. Brogi E, Oyama T, Koerner FC (2001). Atypical cystic lobules in patients with lobular neoplasia. Int J Surg Pathol 9: 201–206.

194. Brohet RM, Goldgar DE, Easton DF, Antoniou AC, Andrieu N, Chang-Claude J, Peock S, Eeles RA, Cook M, Chu C, Nogues C, Lasset C, Berthet P, Meijers-Heijboer H, Gerdes AM, Olsson H, Caldes T, van Leeuwen FE, Rookus MA (2007). Oral contraceptives and breast cancer risk in the international BRCA1/2 carrier cohort study: a report from EMBRACE, GENEPSO, GEO-HEBON, and the IBCCS Collaborating Group. J Clin Oncol 25: 3831–3836.

195. Bronner CE, Baker SM, Morrison PT, Warren G, Smith LG, Lescoe MK, Kane M, Earabino C, Lipford J, Lindblom A, . (1994). Mutation in the DNA mismatch repair gene homologue hMLH1 is associated with hereditary non-polyposis colon cancer. Nature 368: 258–261.

196. Brookes MJ, Bourke AG (2008). Radiological appearances of papillary breast lesions. Clin Radiol 63: 1265–1273.

197. Brown AC, Audisio RA, Regitnig P (2010). Granular cell tumour of the breast. Surg Oncol 20: 97–105.

198. Brown AS, Hunt KK, Shen J, Huo L, Babiera GV, Ross MI, Meric-Bernstam F, Feig BW, Kuerer HM, Boughey JC, Ching CD, Gilcrease MZ (2010). Histologic changes associated with false-negative sentinel lymph nodes after preoperative chemotherapy in patients with confirmed lymph node-positive breast cancer before treatment. Cancer 116: 2878–2883.

199. Brown DC, Theaker JM, Banks PM, Gatter KC, Mason DY (1987). Cytokeratin expression in smooth muscle and smooth muscle tumours. Histopathology 11: 477–486.

200. Brown V, Carty NJ (2005). A case of nodular fascitis of the breast and review of the literature. Breast 14: 384–387.

201. Brownstein MH, Wolf M, Bikowski JB (1978). Cowden's disease: a cutaneous marker of breast cancer. Cancer 41: 2393–2398.

202. Brustein S, Filippa DA, Kimmel M, Lieberman PH, Rosen PP (1987). Malignant lymphoma of the breast. A study of 53 patients. Ann Surg 205: 144–150.

203. Buchanan CL, Flynn LW, Murray MP, Darvishian F, Cranor ML, Fey JV, King TA, Tan LK, Sclafani LM (2008). Is pleomorphic lobular carcinoma really a distinct clinical entity? J Surg Oncol 98: 314–317.
204. Buerger H, Mommers EC, Littmann R, Simon R, Diallo R, Poremba C, Dockhorn-Dworniczak B, van Diest PJ, Boecker W (2001). Ductal invasive G2 and G3 carcinomas of the breast are the end stages of at least two different lines of genetic evolution. J Pathol 194: 165–170.
205. Buerger H, Otterbach F, Simon R, Poremba C, Diallo R, Decker T, Riethdorf L, Brinkschmidt C, Dockhorn-Dworniczak B, Boecker W (1999). Comparative genomic hybridization of ductal carcinoma in situ of the breast-evidence of multiple genetic pathways. J Pathol 187: 396–402.
206. Buerger H, Otterbach F, Simon R, Schafer KL, Poremba C, Diallo R, Brinkschmidt C, Dockhorn-Dworniczak B, Boecker W (1999). Different genetic pathways in the evolution of invasive breast cancer are associated with distinct morphological subtypes. J Pathol 189: 521–526.
207. Buley ID, Gatter KC, Kelly PM, Heryet A, Millard PR (1988). Granular cell tumours revisited. An immunohistological and ultrastructural study. Histopathology 12: 263–274.
208. Bult P, Verwiel JM, Wobbes T, Kooy-Smits MM, Biert J, Holland R (2000). Malignant adenomyoepithelioma of the breast with metastasis in the thyroid gland 12 years after excision of the primary tumor. Case report and review of the literature. Virchows Arch 436: 158–166.
209. Bur ME, Zimarowski MJ, Schnitt SJ, Baker S, Lew R (1992). Estrogen receptor immunohistochemistry in carcinoma in situ of the breast. Cancer 69: 1174–1181.
210. Burga AM, Tavassoli FA (2003). Periductal stromal tumor: a rare lesion with low-grade sarcomatous behavior. Am J Surg Pathol 27: 343–348.
211. Butler RS, Venta LA, Wiley EL, Ellis RL, Dempsey PJ, Rubin E (1999). Sonographic evaluation of infiltrating lobular carcinoma. AJR Am J Roentgenol 172: 325–330.
211A. Buyse M, Loi S, Van't VL, Viale G, Delorenzi M, Glas AM et al. (2006). Validation and clinical utility of a 70-gene prognostic signature for women with node-negative breast cancer. J Natl Cancer Inst 98: 1183–1192.
212. Buza N, Zekry N, Charpin C, Tavassoli FA (2010). Myoepithelial carcinoma of the breast: a clinicopathological and immunohistochemical study of 15 diagnostically challenging cases. Virchows Arch 457: 337–345.
213. Cabioglu N, Ozmen V, Kaya H, Tuzlali S, Igci A, Muslumanoglu M, Kecer M, Dagoglu T (2009). Increased lymph node positivity in multifocal and multicentric breast cancer. J Am Coll Surg 208: 67–74.
214. Cai RZ, Tan PH (2005). Adenomyoepithelioma of the breast with squamous and sebaceous metaplasia. Pathology 37: 557–559.
215. Calderaro J, Bayou EH, Castaigne D, Mathieu MC, Andreiuolo F, Suciu V, Delaloge S, Vielh P (2010). Tubular adenoma of the breast with associated mucinous features: a cytological diagnostic trap. Cytopathology 21: 191–193.
216. Calderaro J, Espie M, Duclos J, Giachetti S, Wehrer D, Sandid W, Cahen-Doidy L, Albiter M, Janin A, de Roquancourt A (2009). Breast intracystic papillary carcinoma: an update. Breast J 15: 639–644.
217. Caliskan M, Gatti G, Sosnovskikh I, Rotmensz N, Botteri E, Musmeci S, Rosali dos Santos G, Viale G, Luini A (2008). Paget's disease of the breast: the experience of the European Institute of Oncology and review of the literature. Breast Cancer Res Treat 112: 513–521.
218. Camelo-Piragua SI, Habib C, Kanumuri P, Lago CE, Mason HS, Otis CN (2009). Mucoepidermoid carcinoma of the breast shares cytogenetic abnormality with mucoepidermoid carcinoma of the salivary gland: a case report with molecular analysis and review of the literature. Hum Pathol 40: 887–892.
219. Capella C, Eusebi V, Mann B, Azzopardi JG (1980). Endocrine differentiation in mucoid carcinoma of the breast. Histopathology 4: 613–630.
220. Capella C, Usellini L, Papotti M, Macri L, Finzi G, Eusebi V, Bussolati G (1990). Ultrastructural features of neuroendocrine differentiated carcinomas of the breast. Ultrastruct Pathol 14: 321–334.
221. Carey LA, Metzger R, Dees EC, Collichio F, Sartor CI, Ollila DW, Klauber-DeMore N, Halle J, Sawyer L, Moore DT, Graham ML (2005). American Joint Committee on Cancer tumor-node-metastasis stage after neoadjuvant chemotherapy and breast cancer outcome. J Natl Cancer Inst 97: 1137–1142.
222. Carley AM, Chivukula M, Carter GJ, Karabakhtsian RG, Dabbs DJ (2008). Frequency and clinical significance of simultaneous association of lobular neoplasia and columnar cell alterations in breast tissue specimens. Am J Clin Pathol 130: 254–258.
223. Carlson JW, Fletcher CD (2007). Immunohistochemistry for beta-catenin in the differential diagnosis of spindle cell lesions: analysis of a series and review of the literature. Histopathology 51: 509–514.
224. Carney JA, Stratakis CA (1996). Ductal adenoma of the breast and the Carney complex. Am J Surg Pathol 20: 1154–1155.
225. Carney JA, Toorkey BC (1991). Ductal adenoma of the breast with tubular features. A probable component of the complex of myxomas, spotty pigmentation, endocrine overactivity, and schwannomas. Am J Surg Pathol 15: 722–731.
226. Carney JA, Toorkey BC (1991). Myxoid fibroadenoma and allied conditions (myxomatosis) of the breast. A heritable disorder with special associations including cardiac and cutaneous myxomas. Am J Surg Pathol 15: 713–721.
227. Carstens PH, Greenberg RA, Francis D, Lyon H (1985). Tubular carcinoma of the breast. A long term follow-up. Histopathology 9: 271–280.
228. Cartagena N, Jr, Cabello-Inc, Willis I, Poppiti R, Jr (1988). Clear cell myoepithelial neoplasm of the breast. Hum Pathol 19: 1239–1243.
228A. Carter BA, Jensen RA, Simpson JF, Page DL (2000). Benign transport of breast epithelium into axillary lymph nodes after biopsy. Am J Clin Pathol 113: 259–265.
229. Carter BA, Page DL, Schuyler P, Parl FF, Simpson JF, Jensen RA, Dupont WD (2001). No elevation in long-term breast carcinoma risk for women with fibroadenomas that contain atypical hyperplasia. Cancer 92: 30–36.
230. Carter CL, Allen C, Henson DE (1989). Relation of tumor size, lymph node status, and survival in 24,740 breast cancer cases. Cancer 63: 181–187.
231. Carter D (1977). Intraductal papillary tumors of the breast: a study of 78 cases. Cancer 39: 1689–1692.
232. Carter D, Orr SL, Merino MJ (1983). Intracystic papillary carcinoma of the breast. After mastectomy, radiotherapy or excisional biopsy alone. Cancer 52: 14–19.
233. Carter MR, Hornick JL, Lester S, Fletcher CD (2006). Spindle cell (sarcomatoid) carcinoma of the breast: a clinicopathologic and immunohistochemical analysis of 29 cases. Am J Surg Pathol 30: 300–309.
233A. Caruso G, Ienzi R, Piovana G, Ricotta V, Cirino A, Salvaggio G, Lagalla R (2004). High-frequency ultrasound in the study of male breast palpable masses. Radiol Med 108: 185–193.
234. Catalina-Fernandez I, Saenz-Santamaria J (2009). Lipid-rich carcinoma of breast: a case report with fine needle aspiration cytology. Diagn Cytopathol 37: 935–936.
235. Cavaciuti E, Lauge A, Janin N, Ossian K, Hall J, Stoppa-Lyonnet D, Andrieu N (2005). Cancer risk according to type and location of ATM mutation in ataxia-telangiectasia families. Genes Chromosomes Cancer 42: 1–9.
236. Cavalli LR, Cornelio DA, Lima RS, Urban CA, Rone JD, Cavalli IJ, Haddad BR (2004). Lack of DNA copy number alterations revealed with comparative genomic hybridization in fibroadenomas of the breast. Cancer Genet Cytogenet 153: 173–176.
237. Cawson JN, Law EM, Kavanagh AM (2001). Invasive lobular carcinoma: sonographic features of cancers detected in a BreastScreen Program. Australas Radiol 45: 25–30.
238. Chaignaud B, Hall TJ, Powers C, Subramony C, Scott-Conner CE (1994). Diagnosis and natural history of extramammary tumors metastatic to the breast. J Am Coll Surg 179: 49–53.
239. Chaiwun B, Nakrungsee S, Sukhamwang N, Srisukho S (2010). A study of high-nuclear-grade breast cancer in Thailand: subclassification and correlation with prognostic factors and immunohistochemical study. Breast Cancer 17: 35–41.
240. Chan KW, Ghadially FN, Alagaratnam TT (1984). Benign spindle cell tumour of breast—a variant of spindled cell lipoma or fibroma of breast? Pathology 16: 331–336.
241. Chang HY, Nuyten DS, Sneddon JB, Hastie T, Tibshirani R, Sorlie T, Dai H, He YD, Van't Veer LJ, Bartelink H, van de Rijn, M, Brown PO, Van de Vijver, MJ (2005). Robustness, scalability, and integration of a wound-response gene expression signature in predicting breast cancer survival. Proc Natl Acad Sci U S A 102: 3738–3743.
242. Chang JC, Hilsenbeck SG (2010). Prognostic and predictive markers. In: Diseases of the breast, 4th edition.Harris JR, Lippman ME, Morrow M, Osbourne CK, eds. Wolters Kluwer Lippincott Williams & Wilkins: Philadelphia: pp 443–457.
243. Chapellier C, Balu-Maestro C, Bleuse A, Ettore F, Bruneton JN (2000). Ultrasonography of invasive lobular carcinoma of the breast: sonographic patterns and diagnostic value: report of 102 cases. Clin Imaging 24: 333–336.
244. Charafe-Jauffret E, Ginestier C, Iovino F, Tarpin C, Diebel M, Esterni B, Houvenaeghel G, Extra JM, Bertucci F, Jacquemier J, Xerri L, Dontu G, Stassi G, Xiao Y, Barsky SH, Birnbaum D, Viens P, Wicha MS (2010). Aldehyde dehydrogenase 1-positive cancer stem cells mediate metastasis and poor clinical outcome in inflammatory breast cancer. Clin Cancer Res 16: 45–55.
245. Charafe-Jauffret E, Mrad K, Intidhar LS, Ben HA, Ben RK, Ben AM, Ginestier C, Esterni B, Birnbaum D, Ben AF, Xerri L, Viens P, Mezlini A, Jacquemier J (2007). Inflammatory breast cancers in Tunisia and France show similar immunophenotypes. Breast 16: 352–358.
246. Charafe-Jauffret E, Tarpin C, Bardou VJ, Bertucci F, Ginestier C, Braud AC, Puig B, Geneix J, Hassoun J, Birnbaum D, Jacquemier J, Viens P (2004). Immunophenotypic analysis of inflammatory breast cancers: identification of an 'inflammatory signature'. J Pathol 202: 265–273.
247. Charpin C, Mathoulin MP, Andrac L, Barberis J, Boulat J, Sarradour B, Bonnier P, Piana L (1994). Reappraisal of breast hamartomas. A morphological study of 41 cases. Pathol Res Pract 190: 362–371.
248. Chaudary MA, Millis RR, Hoskins EO, Halder M, Bulbrook RD, Cuzick J, Hayward JL (1984). Bilateral primary breast cancer: a prospective study of disease incidence. Br J Surg 71: 711–714.
249. Chaudary MA, Millis RR, Lane EB, Miller NA (1986). Paget's disease of the nipple: a ten year review including clinical, pathological, and immunohistochemical findings. Breast Cancer Res Treat 8: 139–146.
250. CHEK2 Breast Cancer Case-Control Consortium (2004). CHEK2*1100delC and susceptibility to breast cancer: a collaborative analysis involving 10,860 breast cancer cases and 9,065 controls from 10 studies. Am J Hum Genet 74: 1175–1182.
250A. Chen AM, Meric-Bernstam F, Hunt KK, Thames HD, Oswald MJ, Outlaw ED, Strom EA, McNeese MD, Kuerer HM, Ross MI, Singletary SE, Ames FC, Feig BW, Sahin AA, Perkins GH, Schechter NR, Hortobagyi GN, Buchholz TA (2004). Breast conservation after neoadjuvant chemotherapy: the MD Anderson cancer center experience. J Clin Oncol 22: 2303–2312.
251. Chen CY, Sun LM, Anderson BO (2006). Paget disease of the breast: changing patterns of incidence, clinical presentation, and treatment in the U.S. Cancer 107: 1448–1458.
252. Chen KT (1990). Pleomorphic adenoma of the breast. Am J Clin Pathol 93: 792–794.
253. Chen PC, Chen CK, Nicastri AD, Wait RB (1994). Myoepithelial carcinoma of the breast with distant metastasis and accompanied by adenomyoepitheliomas. Histopathology 24: 543–548.
254. Chen S, Parmigiani G (2007). Meta-analysis of BRCA1 and BRCA2 penetrance. J Clin Oncol 25: 1329–1333.
255. Chen S, Wang W, Lee S, Nafa K, Lee J, Romans K, Watson P, Gruber SB, Euhus D, Kinzler KW, Jass J, Gallinger S, Lindor NM, Casey G, Ellis N, Giardiello FM, Offit K, Parmigiani G (2006). Prediction of germline mutations and cancer risk in the Lynch syndrome. JAMA 296: 1479–1487.
256. Chen WY, Manson JE, Hankinson SE, Rosner B, Holmes MD, Willett WC, Colditz GA (2006). Unopposed estrogen therapy and the risk of invasive breast cancer. Arch Intern Med 166: 1027–1032.
257. Chen Y, Thompson W, Semenciw R, Mao Y (1999). Epidemiology of contralateral breast cancer. Cancer Epidemiol Biomarkers Prev 8: 855–861.
258. Chen YY, Hwang ES, Roy R, DeVries S, Anderson J, Wa C, Fitzgibbons PL, Jacobs TW, MacGrogan G, Peterse H, Vincent-Salomon A, Tokuyasu T, Schnitt SJ, Waldman FM (2009).

Genetic and phenotypic characteristics of pleomorphic lobular carcinoma in situ of the breast. Am J Surg Pathol 33: 1683–1694.
259. Chenevix-Trench G, Healey S, Lakhani S, Waring P, Cummings M, Brinkworth R, Deffenbaugh AM, Burbidge LA, Pruss D, Judkins T, Scholl T, Bekessy A, Marsh A, Lovelock P, Wong M, Tesoriero A, Renard H, Southey M, Hopper JL, Yannoukakos K et al. (2006). Genetic and histopathologic evaluation of BRCA1 and BRCA2 DNA sequence variants of unknown clinical significance. Cancer Res 66: 2019–2027.
260. Chenevix-Trench G, Milne RL, Antoniou AC, Couch FJ, Easton DF, Goldgar DE (2007). An international initiative to identify genetic modifiers of cancer risk in BRCA1 and BRCA2 mutation carriers: the Consortium of Investigators of Modifiers of BRCA1 and BRCA2 (CIMBA). Breast Cancer Res 9: 104
261. Cheng J, Saku T, Okabe H, Furthmayr H (1992). Basement membranes in adenoid cystic carcinoma. An immunohistochemical study. Cancer 69: 2631–2640.
262. Chevallier B, Roche H, Olivier JP, Chollet P, Hurteloup P (1993). Inflammatory breast cancer. Pilot study of intensive induction chemotherapy (FEC-HD) results in a high histologic response rate. Am J Clin Oncol 16: 223–228.
262A. Chhieng C, Cranor M, Lesser ME, Rosen PP (1998). Metaplastic carcinoma of the breast with osteocartilaginous heterologous elements. Am J Surg Pathol 22: 188–194.
262B. Chia Y, Thike AA, Cheok PY, Yong-Zheng CL, Man-Kit TG, Tan PH (2012). Stromal keratin expression in phyllodes tumours of the breast: a comparison with other spindle cell breast lesions. J Clin Pathol.
262C. Chin K, DeVries S, Fridlyand J, Spellman PT, Roydasgupta R, Kuo WL, Lapuk A, Neve RM, Qian Z, Ryder T, Chen F, Feiler H, Tokuyasu T, Kingsley C, Dairkee S, Meng Z, Chew K, Pinkel D, Jain A, Ljung BM et al. (2006). Genomic and transcriptional aberrations linked to breast cancer pathophysiologies. Cancer Cell 10: 529–541.
262D. Chin SF, Teschendorff AE, Marioni JC, Wang Y, Barbosa-Morais NL, Thorne NP, Costa JL, Pinder SE, van de Wiel MA, Green AR, Ellis IO, Porter PL, Tavare S, Brenton JD, Ylstra B, Caldas C (2007). High-resolution aCGH and expression profiling identifies a novel genomic subtype of ER negative breast cancer. Genome Biol 8: R215.
263. Chlebowski RT, Anderson GL, Gass M, Lane DS, Aragaki AK, Kuller LH, Manson JE, Stefanick ML, Ockene J, Sarto GE, Johnson KC, Wactawski-Wende J, Ravdin PM, Schenken R, Hendrix SL, Rajkovic A, Rohan TE, Yasmeen S, Prentice RL (2010). Estrogen plus progestin and breast cancer incidence and mortality in postmenopausal women. JAMA 304: 1684–1692.
264. Chlebowski RT, Hendrix SL, Langer RD, Stefanick ML, Gass M, Lane D, Rodabough RJ, Gilligan MA, Cyr MG, Thomson CA, Khandekar J, Petrovitch H, McTiernan A (2003). Influence of estrogen plus progestin on breast cancer and mammography in healthy postmenopausal women: the Women's Health Initiative Randomized Trial. JAMA 289: 3243–3253.
265. Chompret A, Abel A, Stoppa-Lyonnet D, Brugieres L, Pages S, Feunteun J, Bonaiti-Pellie C (2001). Sensitivity and predictive value of criteria for p53 germline mutation screening. J Med Genet 38: 43–47.
266. Chompret A, Brugieres L, Ronsin M, Gardes M, Dessarps-Freichey F, Abel A, Hua D, Ligot L, Dondon MG, Bressac-de Paillerets B, Frebourg T, Lemerle J, Bonaiti-Pellie C, Feunteun J (2000). P53 germline mutations in childhood cancers and cancer risk for carrier individuals. Br J Cancer 82: 1932–1937.
267 Chong LY, Cheok PY, Tan WJ, Thike AA, Allen G, Ang MK, Ooi AS, Tan P, Teh BT, Tan PH (2011). Keratin 15, transcobalamin I and homeobox gene Hox-B13 expression in breast phyllodes tumors: novel markers in biological classification. Breast Cancer Res Treat.
267A. Chua CL, Thomas A, Ng BK (1988). Cystosarcoma phyllodes--Asian variations. Aust N Z J Surg 58: 301–305.
268. Chuba PJ, Hamre MR, Yap J, Severson RK, Lucas D, Shamsa F, Aref A (2005). Bilateral risk for subsequent breast cancer after lobular carcinoma-in-situ: analysis of surveillance, epidemiology, and end results data. J Clin Oncol 23: 5534–5541.
269. Chun HH, Gatti RA (2004). Ataxia-telangiectasia, an evolving phenotype. DNA Repair (Amst) 3: 1187–1196.
270. Clarke C, Sandle J, Lakhani SR (2005). Myoepithelial cells: pathology, cell separation and markers of myoepithelial differentiation. J Mammary Gland Biol Neoplasia 10: 273–280.
271. Clarke M, Collins R, Darby S, Davies C, Elphinstone P, Evans E, Godwin J, Gray R, Hicks C, James S, MacKinnon E, McGale P, McHugh T, Peto R, Taylor C, Wang Y (2005). Effects of radiotherapy and of differences in the extent of surgery for early breast cancer on local recurrence and 15-year survival: an overview of the randomised trials. Lancet 366: 2087–2106.
272. Clarke RB (2003). Steroid receptors and proliferation in the human breast. Steroids 68: 789–794.
272A. Clement PB, Azzopardi JG (1983). Microglandular adenosis of the breast--a lesion simulating tubular carcinoma. Histopathology 7: 169–180.
273. Clement PB, Young RH, Azzopardi JG (1987). Collagenous spherulosis of the breast. Am J Surg Pathol 11: 411–417.
273A. Cleton-Jansen AM (2002). E-cadherin and loss of heterozygosity at chromosome 16 in breast carcinogenesis: different genetic pathways in ductal and lobular breast cancer? Breast Cancer Res 4: 5–8.
273B. Cleton-Jansen AM, Buerger H, Haar N, Philippo K, Van der Vijver MJ, Boecker W, Smit VT, Cornelisse CJ (2004). Different mechanisms of chromosome 16 loss of heterozygosity in well- versus poorly differentiated ductal breast cancer. Genes Chromosomes Cancer 41: 109–116.
274. Clune JE, Kozakewich HP, VanBeek CA, Labow BI, Greene AK (2009). Nipple adenoma in infancy. J Pediatr Surg 44: 2219–2222.
275. Coarasa-Cerdan A, Palomo-Jimenez M, Montero-Montero A, Alegre-Bernal N, Guadano-Salvadores V (1998). Hemangiopericytoma of the breast: mammographic and sonographic findings. J Clin Ultrasound 26: 155–158.
276. Coffin CM, Hornick JL, Fletcher CD (2007). Inflammatory myofibroblastic tumor: comparison of clinicopathologic, histologic, and immunohistochemical features including ALK expression in atypical and aggressive cases. Am J Surg Pathol 31: 509–520.
277. Coffin CM, Humphrey PA, Dehner LP (1998). Extrapulmonary inflammatory myofibroblastic tumor: a clinical and pathological survey. Semin Diagn Pathol 15: 85–101.
278. Colditz GA, Hankinson SE, Hunter DJ, Willett WC, Manson JE, Stampfer MJ, Hennekens C, Rosner B, Speizer FE (1995). The use of estrogens and progestins and the risk of breast cancer in postmenopausal women. N Engl J Med 332: 1589–1593.
279. Colditz GA, Rosner B (2000). Cumulative risk of breast cancer to age 70 years according to risk factor status: data from the Nurses' Health Study. Am J Epidemiol 152: 950–964.
280. Collaborative Group on Hormonal Factors in Breast Cancer (1996). Breast cancer and hormonal contraceptives: further results. Contraception 54: 1S–106S.
281. Collaborative Group on Hormonal Factors in Breast Cancer (1997). Breast cancer and hormone replacement therapy: collaborative reanalysis of data from 51 epidemiological studies of 52,705 women with breast cancer and 108,411 women without breast cancer. Lancet 350: 1047–1059.
282. Collaborative Group on Hormonal Factors in Breast Cancer (2001). Familial breast cancer: collaborative reanalysis of individual data from 52 epidemiological studies including 58,209 women with breast cancer and 101,986 women without the disease. Lancet 358: 1389–1399.
283. Collins LC, Baer HJ, Tamimi RM, Connolly JL, Colditz GA, Schnitt SJ (2006). The influence of family history on breast cancer risk in women with biopsy-confirmed benign breast disease: results from the Nurses' Health Study. Cancer 107: 1240–1247.
284. Collins LC, Carlo VP, Hwang H, Barry TS, Gown AM, Schnitt SJ (2006). Intracystic papillary carcinomas of the breast: a reevaluation using a panel of myoepithelial cell markers. Am J Surg Pathol 30: 1002–1007.
285. Collins LC, Connolly JL, Page DL, Goulart RA, Pisano ED, Fajardo LL, Berg WA, Caudry DJ, McNeil BJ, Schnitt SJ (2004). Diagnostic agreement in the evaluation of image-guided breast core needle biopsies: results from a randomized clinical trial. Am J Surg Pathol 28: 126–131.
286. Collins LC, Schnitt SJ (2008). Papillary lesions of the breast: selected diagnostic and management issues. Histopathology 52: 20–29.
286A. Collins LC, Tamimi RM, Baer HJ, Connolly JL, Colditz GA, Schnitt SJ (2005). Outcome of patients with ductal carcinoma in situ untreated after diagnostic biopsy: results from the Nurses' Health Study. Cancer 103: 1778–1784.
287. Collishaw N, Boyd NF, Hammond SK, Johnson KC, Millar J, Miller B (2009). Canadian Expert Panel on Tobacco Smoke and Breast Cancer Risk. Ontario Tobacco Research Unit: Toronto, Canada.
288. Concannon P, Haile RW, Borresen-Dale AL, Rosenstein BS, Gatti RA, Teraoka SN, Diep TA, Jansen L, Atencio DP, Langholz B, Capanu M, Liang X, Begg CB, Thomas DC, Bernstein L, Olsen JH, Malone KE, Lynch CF, Anton-Culver H, Bernstein JL (2008). Variants in the ATM gene associated with a reduced risk of contralateral breast cancer. Cancer Res 68: 6486–6491.
289. Corradi D, Bosio S, Maestri R, Mormandi F, Curry A, Eyden B (2008). A giant myxoid mammary myofibroblastoma: evidence for a myogenic/synthetic phenotype and an extracellular matrix rich in fibronectin. Histopathology 52: 396–399.
290. Cox A, Dunning AM, Garcia-Closas M, Balasubramanian S, Reed MW, Pooley KA, Scollen S, Baynes C, Ponder BA, Chanock S, Lissowska J, Brinton L, Peplonska B, Southey MC, Hopper JL, McCredie MR, Giles GG, Fletcher O, Johnson N, dos Santos Silva I et al. (2007). A common coding variant in CASP8 is associated with breast cancer risk. Nat Genet 39: 352–358.
291. Cox CE, Nguyen K, Gray RJ, Salud C, Ku NN, Dupont E, Hutson L, Peltz E, Whitehead G, Reintgen D, Cantor A (2001). Importance of lymphatic mapping in ductal carcinoma in situ (DCIS): why map DCIS? Am Surg 67: 513–519.
292. Coyne JD (2001). Apocrine ductal carcinoma in-situ with an unusual morphological presentation. Histopathology 38: 280
293. Crisi GM, Marconi SA, Makari-Judson G, Goulart RA (2005). Expression of c-kit in adenoid cystic carcinoma of the breast. Am J Clin Pathol 124: 733–739.
294. Cristofanilli M (2010). Novel targeted therapies in inflammatory breast cancer. Cancer 116: 2837–2839.
295. Cristofanilli M, Buchholz TA (2010). Proceedings of the First International Inflammatory Breast Cancer Conference. Cancer 116: 2729.
296. Crook T, Brooks LA, Crossland S, Osin P, Barker KT, Waller J, Philp E, Smith PD, Yulug I, Peto J, Parker G, Allday MJ, Crompton MR, Gusterson BA (1998). p53 mutation with frequent novel condons but not a mutator phenotype in B. Oncogene 17: 1681–1689.
297. Cserni G (2007). Pathological evaluation of sentinel lymph nodes. Surg Oncol Clin N Am 16: 17–34.
298. Cserni G, Amendoeira I, Apostolikas N, Bellocq JP, Bianchi S, Boecker W, Borisch B, Connolly CE, Decker T, Dervan P, Drijkoningen M, Ellis IO, Elston CW, Eusebi V, Faverly D, Heikkila P, Holland R, Kerner H, Kulka J, Jacquemier J et al. (2004). Discrepancies in current practice of pathological evaluation of sentinel lymph nodes in breast cancer. Results of a questionnaire based survey by the European Working Group for Breast Screening Pathology. J Clin Pathol 57: 695–701.
299. Cserni G, Bianchi S, Vezzosi V, Peterse H, Sapino A, Arisio R, Reiner-Concin A, Regitnig P, Bellocq JP, Marin C, Bori R, Penuela JM, Iturriagagoitia AC (2006). The value of cytokeratin immunohistochemistry in the evaluation of axillary sentinel lymph nodes in patients with lobular breast carcinoma. J Clin Pathol 59: 518–522.
300. Cullinane CA, Lubinski J, Neuhausen SL, Ghadirian P, Lynch HT, Isaacs C, Weber B, Moller P, Offit K, Kim-Sing C, Friedman E, Randall S, Pasini B, Ainsworth P, Gershoni-Baruch R, Foulkes WD, Klijn J, Tung N, Rennert G, Olopade O et al. (2005). Effect of pregnancy as a risk factor for breast cancer in BRCA1/BRCA2 mutation carriers. Int J Cancer 117: 988–991.
301. d'Amore ES, Terrier-Lacombe MJ, Travagli JP, Friedman S, Contesso G (1988). Invasive apocrine carcinoma of the breast: a long term follow-up study of 34 cases. Breast Cancer Res Treat 12: 37–44.
302. D'Angelo P, Carli M, Ferrari A, Manzitti C, Mura R, Miglionico L, Di CA, Grigoli A, Cecchetto G, Bisogno G (2010). Breast metastases in children and adolescents with rhabdomyosarcoma: Experience of the Italian Soft Tissue Sarcoma Committee. Pediatr Blood Cancer 55: 1306–1309.
303. Da Silva L, Parry S, Reid L, Keith P,

Waddell N, Kossai M, Clarke C, Lakhani SR, Simpson PT (2008). Aberrant expression of E-cadherin in lobular carcinomas of the breast. Am J Surg Pathol 32: 773–783.

304. Dabbs DJ, Bhargava R, Chivukula M (2007). Lobular versus ductal breast neoplasms: the diagnostic utility of p120 catenin. Am J Surg Pathol 31: 427–437.

305. Dahlen A, Debiec-Rychter M, Pedeutour F, Domanski HA, Hoglund M, Bauer HC, Rydholm A, Sciot R, Mandahl N, Mertens F (2003). Clustering of deletions on chromosome 13 in benign and low-malignant lipomatous tumors. Int J Cancer 103: 616–623.

306. Dal Cin P, Wanschura S, Christiaens MR, Van den Berghe I, Moerman P, Polito P, Kazmierczak B, Bullerdiek J, Van den Berghe H (1997). Hamartoma of the breast with involvement of 6p21 and rearrangement of HMGIY. Genes Chromosomes Cancer 20: 90–92.

307. Dalberg K, Hellborg H, Warnberg F (2008). Paget's disease of the nipple in a population based cohort. Breast Cancer Res Treat 111: 313–319.

308. Daling JR, Malone KE, Doody DR, Voigt LF, Bernstein L, Coates RJ, Marchbanks PA, Norman SA, Weiss LK, Ursin G, Berlin JA, Burkman RT, Deapen D, Folger SG, McDonald JA, Simon MS, Strom BL, Wingo PA, Spirtas R (2002). Relation of regimens of combined hormone replacement therapy to lobular, ductal, and other histologic types of breast carcinoma. Cancer 95: 2455–2464.

309. Damera A, Evans AJ, Cornford EJ, Wilson AR, Burrell HC, James JJ, Pinder SE, Ellis IO, Lee AH, Macmillan RD (2003). Diagnosis of axillary nodal metastases by ultrasound-guided core biopsy in primary operable breast cancer. Br J Cancer 89: 1310–1313.

310. Damiani S, Chiodera P, Guaragni M, Eusebi V (2002). Mammary angiomyolipoma. Virchows Arch 440: 551–552.

311. Damiani S, Eusebi V (2001). Gynecomastia in type-1 neurofibromatosis with features of pseudoangiomatous stromal hyperplasia with giant cells. Report of two cases. Virchows Arch 438: 513–516.

312. Damiani S, Eusebi V, Losi L, D'Adda T, Rosai J (1998). Oncocytic carcinoma (malignant oncocytoma) of the breast. Am J Surg Pathol 22: 221–230.

313. Damiani S, Miettinen M, Peterse JL, Eusebi V (1994). Solitary fibrous tumour (myofibroblastoma) of the breast. Virchows Arch 425: 89–92.

314. Damiani S, Pasquinelli G, Lamovec J, Peterse JL, Eusebi V (2000). Acinic cell carcinoma of the breast: an immunohistochemical and ultra-structural study. Virchows Arch 437: 74–81.

315. Dammers JW (1991). [Carpal tunnel syndrome]. Ned Tijdschr Geneeskd 135: 193–194.

316. Daneshbod Y, Oryan A, Khojasteh HN, Rasekhi A, Ahmadi N, Mohammadianpanah M (2010). Primary ALK-positive anaplastic large cell lymphoma of the breast: a case report and review of the literature. J Pediatr Hematol Oncol 32: e75–e78.

317. Daniel BL, Gardner RW, Birdwell RL, Nowels KW, Johnson D (2003). Magnetic resonance imaging of intraductal papilloma of the breast. Magn Reson Imaging 21: 887–892.

317A. Davis WG, Hennessy B, Babiera G, Hunt K, Valero V, Buchholz TA, Sneige N, Gilcrease MZ (2005). Metaplastic sarcomatoid carcinoma of the breast with absent or minimal overt invasive carcinomatous component: a misnomer. Am J Surg Pathol 29: 1456–1463.

318. Dawood S, Ueno NT, Valero V, Woodward WA, Buchholz TA, Hortobagyi GN, Gonzalez-Angulo AM, Cristofanilli M (2010). Differences in survival among women with stage III inflammatory and noninflammatory locally advanced breast cancer appear early: a large population-based study. Cancer

319. Daya D, Trus T, D'Souza TJ, Minuk T, Yemen B (1995). Hamartoma of the breast, an underrecognized breast lesion. A clinicopathologic and radiographic study of 25 cases. Am J Clin Pathol 103: 685–689.

320. De Brakeleer S., De Greve J., Loris R, Janin N, Lissens W, Sermijn E, Teugels E (2010). Cancer predisposing missense and protein truncating BARD1 mutations in non-BRCA1 or BRCA2 breast cancer families. Hum Mutat 31: E1175–E1185.

321. de Jong D, Vasmel WL, de Boer JP, Verhave G, Barbe E, Casparie MK, van Leeuwen FE (2008). Anaplastic large-cell lymphoma in women with breast implants. JAMA 300: 2030–2035.

322. de Leeuw WJ, Berx G, Vos CB, Peterse JL, Van de Vijver M, Litvinov S, van Roy F, Cornelisse CJ, Cleton-Jansen AM (1997). Simultaneous loss of E-cadherin and catenins in invasive lobular breast cancer and lobular carcinoma in situ. J Pathol 183: 404–411.

323. de Leeuw WJ, van Puijenbroek M, Tollenaar RA, Cornelisse CJ, Vasen HF, Morreau H (2003). Correspondence re: A. Muller et al., Exclusion of breast cancer as an integral tumor of hereditary nonpolyposis colorectal cancer. Cancer Res., 62: 1014-1019, 2002. Cancer Res 63: 1148–1149.

324. de Mascarel I, Bonichon F, Durand M, Mauriac L, MacGrogan G, Soubeyran I, Picot V, Avril A, Coindre JM, Trojani M (1998). Obvious peritumoral emboli: an elusive prognostic factor reappraised. Multivariate analysis of 1320 node-negative breast cancers. Eur J Cancer 34: 58–65.

324A. de Roos WK, Kaye P, Dent DM (1999). Factors leading to local recurrence or death after surgical resection of phyllodes tumours of the breast. Br J Surg 86: 396–399.

325. de Winter JP, Joenje H (2009). The genetic and molecular basis of Fanconi anemia. Mutat Res 668: 11–19.

326. Dean-Colomb W, Esteva FJ (2008). Her2-positive breast cancer: herceptin and beyond. Eur J Cancer 44: 2806–2812.

327. Decorsiere JB, Thibaut I, Bouissou H (1988). [Adeno-myoepithelial proliferation in the breast]. Ann Pathol 8: 311–316.

328. delli Santi G, Bellioni M, Loreti A, Stagnitto D, La Pinta M, Dell'Osso A (2006). Giant breast lipoma: a rare cause of breast asymmetry. Plast Reconstr Surg 117: 1068–1069.

329. Dendale R, Vincent-Salomon A, Mouret-Fourme E, Savignoni A, Medioni J, Campana F, Vilcoq JR, de la Rochefordiere A, Soussi T, Asselain B, De Cremoux P, Fourquet A (2003). Medullary breast carcinoma: prognostic implications of p53 expression. Int J Biol Markers 18: 99–105.

330. Deng G, Lu Y, Zlotnikov G, Thor AD, Smith HS (1996). Loss of heterozygosity in normal tissue adjacent to breast carcinomas. Science 274: 2057–2059.

331. Denley H, Pinder SE, Tan PH, Sim CS, Brown R, Barker T, Gearty J, Elston CW, Ellis IO (2000). Metaplastic carcinoma of the breast arising within complex sclerosing lesion: a report of five cases. Histopathology 36: 203–209.

331A. Desmedt C, Giobbie-Hurder A, Neven P, Paridaens R, Christiaens MR, Smeets A et al. (2009). The Gene expression Grade Index: a potential predictor of relapse for endocrine-treated breast cancer patients in the BIG 1-98 trial. BMC Med Genomics 2: 40.

331B. Derksen PW, Liu X, Saridin F, van der Gulden H, Zevenhoven J, Evers B, van Beijnum Jr, Griffioen AW, Vink J, Krimpenfort P, Peterse JL, Cardiff RD, Berns A, Jonkers J (2006). Somatic inactivation of E-cadherin and p53 in mice leads to metastatic lobular mammary carcinoma through induction of anoikis resistance and angiogenesis. Cancer Cell 10: 437–449.

332. Desmedt C, Haibe-Kains B, Wirapati P, Buyse M, Larsimont D, Bontempi G, Delorenzi M, Piccart M, Sotiriou C (2008). Biological processes associated with breast cancer clinical outcome depend on the molecular subtypes. Clin Cancer Res 14: 5158–5165.

333. Devouassoux-Shisheboran M, Schammel MD, Man YG, Tavassoli FA (2000). Fibromatosis of the breast: age-correlated morphofunctional features of 33 cases. Arch Pathol Lab Med 124: 276–280.

334. Dewar R, Fadare O, Gilmore H, Gown AM (2011). Best practices in diagnostic immunohistochemistry: myoepithelial markers in breast pathology. Arch Pathol Lab Med 135: 422–429.

335. Dhingra KK, Mandal S, Roy S, Khurana N (2007). Malignant peripheral nerve sheath tumor of the breast: case report. World J Surg Oncol 5: 142

336. Di Cristofano C, Mrad K, Zavaglia K, Bertacca G, Aretini P, Cipollini G, Bevilacqua G, Ben Romdhane K, Cavazzana A (2005). Papillary lesions of the breast: a molecular progression? Breast Cancer Res Treat 90: 71–76.

337. Di Saverio S, Gutierrez J, Avisar E (2008). A retrospective review with long term follow up of 11,400 cases of pure mucinous breast carcinoma. Breast Cancer Res Treat 111: 541–547.

338. Di Tommaso L, Foschini MP, Ragazzini T, Magrini E, Fornelli A, Ellis IO, Eusebi V (2004). Mucoepidermoid carcinoma of the breast. Virchows Arch 444: 13–19.

339. Di Tommaso L, Franchi G, Destro A, Broglia F, Minuti F, Rahal D, Roncalli M (2008). Toker cells of the breast. Morphological and immunohistochemical characterization of 40 cases. Hum Pathol 39: 1295–1300.

340. Diab SG, Clark GM, Osborne CK, Libby A, Allred DC, Elledge RM (1999). Tumor characteristics and clinical outcome of tubular and mucinous breast carcinomas. J Clin Oncol 17: 1442–1448.

341. DiCostanzo D, Rosen PP, Gareen I, Franklin S, Lesser M (1990). Prognosis in infiltrating lobular carcinoma. An analysis of «classical» and variant tumors. Am J Surg Pathol 14: 12–23.

342. Dietzel M, Baltzer PA, Vag T, Groschel T, Gajda M, Camara O, Kaiser WA (2010). Magnetic resonance mammography of invasive lobular versus ductal carcinoma: systematic comparison of 811 patients reveals high diagnostic accuracy irrespective of typing. J Comput Assist Tomogr 34: 587–595.

343. Dina R, Eusebi V (1997). Clear cell tumors of the breast. Semin Diagn Pathol 14: 175–182.

343A. Ding L, Ellis MJ, Li S, Larson DE, Chen K, Wallis JW, Harris CC, McLellan MD, Fulton RS, Fulton LL, Abbott RM, Hoog J, Dooling DJ, Koboldt DC, Schmidt H, Kalicki J, Zhang Q, Chen L, Lin L, Wendl MC et al. (2010). Genome

remodelling in a basal-like breast cancer metastasis and xenograft. Nature 464: 999–1005.

344. Ding YC, Steele L, Kuan CJ, Greilac S, Neuhausen SL (2010). Mutations in BRCA2 and PALB2 in male breast cancer cases from the United States. Breast Cancer Res Treat

345. Dixon JM, Anderson TJ, Page DL, Lee D, Duffy SW (1982). Infiltrating lobular carcinoma of the breast. Histopathology 6: 149–161.

346. Dixon JM, Sainsbury JRC (1998). Handbook of diseases of the breast, 2nd edition. Churchill Livingstone: Edinburgh.

346A. Doane AS, Danso M, Lal P, Donaton M, Zhang L, Hudis C et al. (2006). An estrogen receptor-negative breast cancer subset characterized by a hormonally regulated transcriptional program and response to androgen. Oncogene 25: 3994–4008.

347. Doctor VM, Sirsat MV (1971). Florid papillomatosis (adenoma) and other benign tumours of the nipple and areola. Br J Cancer 25: 1–9.

348. Domagala W, Harezga B, Szadowska A, Markiewski M, Weber K, Osborn M (1993). Nuclear p53 protein accumulates preferentially in medullary and high-grade ductal but rarely in lobular breast carcinomas. Am J Pathol 142: 669–674.

349. Domfeh AB, Carley AL, Striebel JM, Karabakhtsian RG, Florea AV, McManus K, Beriwal S, Bhargava R (2008). WT1 immunoreactivity in breast carcinoma: selective expression in pure and mixed mucinous subtypes. Mod Pathol 21: 1217–1223.

350. Dominici LS, Negron G, V, Buzdar AU, Lucci A, Mittendorf EA, Le-Petross HT, Babiera GV, Meric-Bernstam F, Hunt KK, Kuerer HM (2010). Cytologically proven axillary lymph node metastases are eradicated in patients receiving preoperative chemotherapy with concurrent trastuzumab for HER2-positive breast cancer. Cancer 116: 2884–2889.

351. Domoto H, Terahata S, Sato K, Tamai S (1998). Nodular hidradenoma of the breast: report of two cases with literature review. Pathol Int 48: 907–911.

352. Donehower LA, Harvey M, Slagle BL, McArthur MJ, Montgomery CA, Jr, Butel JS, Bradley A (1992). Mice deficient for p53 are developmentally normal but susceptible to spontaneous tumours. Nature 356: 215–221.

353. Douglas-Jones AG, Pace DP (1997). Pathology of R4 spiculated lesions in the breast screening programme. Histopathology 30: 214–220.

353A. Dowsett M, Cuzick J, Wale C, Forbes J, Mallon EA, Salter J et al. (2010). Prediction of risk of distant recurrence using the 21-gene recurrence score in node-negative and node-positive postmenopausal patients with breast cancer treated with anastrozole or tamoxifen: a TransATAC study. J Clin Oncol 28: 1829–1834.

353B. Downs-Kelly E, Nayeemuddin KM, Albarracin C, Wu Y, Hunt KK, Gilcrease MZ (2009). Matrix-producing carcinoma of the breast: an aggressive subtype of metaplastic carcinoma. Am J Surg Pathol 33: 534–541.

354. Droufakou S, Deshmane V, Roylance R, Hanby A, Tomlinson I, Hart IR (2001). Multiple ways of silencing E-cadherin gene expression in lobular carcinoma of the breast. Int J Cancer 92: 404–408.

354A. Drudis T, Arroyo C, Van HK, Cordon-Cardo C, Rosen PP (1994). The pathology of low-grade adenosquamous carcinoma of the breast. An immunohistochemical study. Pathol Annu 29 (Pt 2): 181–197.

355. du Toit RS, Locker AP, Ellis IO, Elston CW, Nicholson RI, Blamey RW (1989). Invasive lobular carcinomas of the breast—the prognosis of histopathological subtypes. Br J Cancer 60: 605–609.

356. Dunne B, Lee AH, Pinder SE, Bell JA, Ellis IO (2003). An immunohistochemical study of metaplastic spindle cell carcinoma, phyllodes tumor and fibromatosis of the breast. Hum Pathol 34: 1009–1015.

356A. Dunning MJ, Curtis C, Barbosa-Morais NL, Caldas C, Tavare S, Lynch AG (2010). The importance of platform annotation in interpreting microarray data. Lancet Oncol 11: 717.

357. Dupont WD, Page DL (1985). Risk factors for breast cancer in women with proliferative breast disease. N Engl J Med 312: 146–151.

358. Dupont WD, Page DL, Parl FF, Vnencak-Jones CL, Plummer WD, Jr, Rados MS, Schuyler PA (1994). Long-term risk of breast cancer in women with fibroadenoma. N Engl J Med 331: 10–15.

359. Dupont WD, Parl FF, Hartmann WH, Brinton LA, Winfield AC, Worrell JA, Schuyler PA, Plummer WD (1993). Breast cancer risk associated with proliferative breast disease and atypical hyperplasia. Cancer 71: 1258–1265.

359A. Duprez R, Wilkerson PM, Lacroix-Triki M, Lambros MB, Mackay A, Hern RA, Gauthier A, Pawar V, Colombo PE, Daley F, Natrajan R, Ward E, MacGrogan G, Arbion F, Michenet P, Weigelt B, Vincent-Salomon A, Reis-Filho JS (2012). Immunophenotypic and genomic characterization of papillary carcinomas of the breast. J Pathol 226: 427–441.

360. Early Breast Cancer Trialists' Collaborative Group (EBCTCG) (2005). Effects of chemotherapy and hormonal therapy for early breast cancer on recurrence and 15-year survival: an overview of the randomised trials. Lancet 365: 1687–1717.

361. Easton DF (1999). How many more breast cancer predisposition genes are there? Breast Cancer Res 1: 14–17.

362. Easton DF, Bishop DT, Ford D, Crockford GP (1993). Genetic linkage analysis in familial breast and ovarian cancer: results from 214 families. The Breast Cancer Linkage Consortium. Am J Hum Genet 52: 678–701.

363. Easton DF, Deffenbaugh AM, Pruss D, Frye C, Wenstrup RJ, Ien-Brady K, Tavtigian SV, Monteiro AN, Iversen ES, Couch FJ, Goldgar DE (2007). A systematic genetic assessment of 1,433 sequence variants of unknown clinical significance in the BRCA1 and BRCA2 breast cancer-predisposition genes. Am J Hum Genet 81: 873–883.

364. Easton DF, Pooley KA, Dunning AM, Pharoah PD, Thompson D, Ballinger DG, Struewing JP, Morrison J, Field H, Luben R, Wareham N, Ahmed S, Healey CS, Bowman R, the SEARCH collaborators, Meyer KB, Haiman CA, Kolonel LK, Henderson BE, Le Marchand L, Brennan P et al. (2007). Genome-wide association study identifies novel breast cancer susceptibility loci. Nature 447: 1087–1093.

365. Easton DF, Steele L, Fields P, Ormiston W, Averill D, Daly PA, McManus R, Neuhausen SL, Ford D, Wooster R, Cannon-Albright LA, Stratton MR, Goldgar DE (1997). Cancer risks in two large breast cancer families linked to BRCA2 on chromosome 13q12-13. Am J Hum Genet 61: 120–128.

366. Edge SB, Byrd DR, eds (2010). AJCC cancer staging manual. 7th Edition. Springer: New York.

367. Edwards SM, Kote-Jarai Z, Meitz J, Hamoudi R, Hope Q, Osin P, Jackson R, Southgate C, Singh R, Falconer A, Dearnaley DP, Ardern-Jones A, Murkin A, Dowe A, Kelly J, Williams S, Oram R, Stevens M, Teare DM, Ponder BA et al. (2003). Two percent of men with early-onset prostate cancer harbor germline mutations in the BRCA2 gene. Am J Hum Genet 72: 1–12.

368. Eisinger F, Jacquemier J, Charpin C, Stoppa-Lyonnet D, Bressac-de Paillerets B, Peyrat JP, Longy M, Guinebretiere JM, Sauvan R, Noguchi T, Birnbaum D, Sobol H (1998). Mutations at BRCA1: the medullary breast carcinoma revisited. Cancer Res 58: 1588–1592.

369. Eisinger F, Nogues C, Birnbaum D, Jacquemier J, Sobol H (1998). BRCA1 and medullary breast cancer. JAMA 280: 1227–1228.

370. El Aouni N, Laurent I, Terrier P, Mansouri D, Suciu V, Delaloge S, Vielh P (2007). Granular cell tumor of the breast. Diagn Cytopathol 35: 725–727.

371. El Wakil A, Doghman M, Latre De Late P, Zambetti GP, Figueiredo BC, Lalli E (2011). Genetics and genomics of childhood adrenocortical tumors. Mol Cell Endocrinol 336: 169–173.

372. El-Sayed ME, Rakha EA, Reed J, Lee AH, Evans AJ, Ellis IO (2008). Predictive value of needle core biopsy diagnoses of lesions of uncertain malignant potential (B3) in abnormalities detected by mammographic screening. Histopathology 53: 650–657.

373. Eliassen AH, Colditz GA, Rosner B, Willett WC, Hankinson SE (2006). Adult weight change and risk of postmenopausal breast cancer. JAMA 296: 193–201.

374. Eliassen AH, Missmer SA, Tworoger SS, Spiegelman D, Barbieri RL, Dowsett M, Hankinson SE (2006). Endogenous steroid hormone concentrations and risk of breast cancer among premenopausal women. J Natl Cancer Inst 98: 1406–1415.

375. Ellis DL, Teitelbaum SL (1974). Inflammatory carcinoma of the breast. A pathologic definition. Cancer 33: 1045–1047.

376. Ellis IO, Galea M, Broughton N, Locker A, Blamey RW, Elston CW (1992). Pathological prognostic factors in breast cancer. II. Histological type. Relationship with survival in a large study with long-term follow-up. Histopathology 20: 479–489.

376A. Ellis MJ, Suman VJ, Hoog J, Lin L, Snider J, Prat A et al. (2011). Randomized phase II neoadjuvant comparison between letrozole, anastrozole, and exemestane for postmenopausal women with estrogen receptor-rich stage 2 to 3 breast cancer: clinical and biomarker outcomes and predictive value of the baseline PAM50-based intrinsic subtype--ACOSOG Z1031. J Clin Oncol 29: 2342–2349.

377. Elston CW, Ellis IO (1991). Pathological prognostic factors in breast cancer. I. The value of histological grade in breast cancer: experience from a large study with long-term follow-up. Histopathology 19: 403–410.

378. Elston CW, Ellis IO, eds (1998). The breast. Volume 13, Systemic pathology, 3rd edition. Churchill Livingstone: Edinburgh, New York.

379. Elston CW, Sloane JP, Amendoeira I, Apostolikas N, Bellocq JP, Bianchi S, Boecker W, Bussolati G, Coleman D, Connolly CE, Dervan P, Drijkoningen M, Eusebi V, Faverly D, Holland R, Jacquemier J, Lacerda M, Martinez-Penuela J, De MC, Mossi S et al. (2000). Causes of inconsistency in diagnosing and classifying intraductal proliferations of the breast. European Commission Working Group on Breast Screening Pathology. Eur J Cancer 36: 1769–1772.

380. Ende L, Mercado C, Axelrod D, Darvishian F, Levine P, Cangiarella J (2007). Intraparenchymal leiomyoma of the breast: a case report and review of the literature. Ann Clin Lab Sci 37: 268–273.

381. Eng C (2000). Will the real Cowden syndrome please stand up: revised diagnostic criteria. J Med Genet 37: 828–830.

382. Eng C (2003). PTEN: one gene, many syndromes. Hum Mutat 22: 183–198.

383. Epstein M, Ma Y, Press MF (2010). ERBB2 testing: assessment of status for targeted therapies. In: Diseases of the breast, 4th edition.Harris JR, Lippman ME, Morrow M, Osbourne CK, eds. Wolters Kluwer Lippincott Williams & Wilkins: Philadelphia: pp 431–442.

384. Erhan Y, Erhan Y, Zekioglu O (2005). Pure invasive micropapillary carcinoma of the male breast: report of a rare case. Can J Surg 48: 156–157.

384A. Erickson-Johnson MR, Chou MM, Evers BR, Roth CW, Seys AR, Jin L, Ye Y, Lau AW, Wang X, Oliveira AM (2011). Nodular fasciitis: a novel model of transient neoplasia induced by MYH9-USP6 gene fusion. Lab Invest 91: 1427–1433.

385. Erkko H, Xia B, Nikkila J, Schleutker J, Syrjakoski K, Mannermaa A, Kallioniemi A, Pylkas K, Karppinen SM, Rapakko K, Miron A, Sheng Q, Li G, Mattila H, Bell DW, Haber DA, Grip M, Reiman M, Jukkola-Vuorinen A, Mustonen A et al. (2007). A recurrent mutation in PALB2 in Finnish cancer families. Nature 446: 316–319.

386. Ernster VL, Ballard-Barbash R, Barlow WE, Zheng Y, Weaver DL, Cutter G, Yankaskas BC, Rosenberg R, Carney PA, Kerlikowske K, Taplin SH, Urban N, Geller BM (2002). Detection of ductal carcinoma in situ in women undergoing screening mammography. J Natl Cancer Inst 94: 1546–1554.

387. Ernster VL, Barclay J, Kerlikowske K, Wilkie H, Ballard-Barbash R (2000). Mortality among women with ductal carcinoma in situ of the breast in the population-based surveillance, epidemiology and end results program. Arch Intern Med 160: 953–958.

388. Esposito NN, Dabbs DJ, Bhargava R (2009). Are encapsulated papillary carcinomas of the breast in situ or invasive? A basement membrane study of 27 cases. Am J Clin Pathol 131: 228–242.

389. Etzell JE, DeVries S, Chew K, Florendo C, Molinaro A, Ljung BM, Waldman FM (2001). Loss of chromosome 16q in lobular carcinoma in situ. Hum Pathol 32: 292–296.

390. Eusebi V, Betts C, Haagensen DE, Jr, Gugliotta P, Bussolati G, Azzopardi JG (1984). Apocrine differentiation in lobular carcinoma of the breast: a morphologic, immunologic, and ultrastructural study. Hum Pathol 15: 134–140.

391. Eusebi V, Casadei GP, Bussolati G, Azzopardi JG (1987). Adenomyoepithelioma of the breast with a distinctive type of apocrine adenosis. Histopathology 11: 305–315.

392. Eusebi V, Cattani MG, Ceccarelli C, Lamovec J (1989). Sarcomatoid carcinomas of the breast: an immunocytochemical study of 14 cases. Recent Progr Surg Pathol 9: 83–99.

393. Eusebi V, Cunsolo A, Fedeli F, Severi B, Scarani P (1980). Benign smooth muscle cell metaplasia in breast. Tumori 66: 643–653.

394. Eusebi V, Feudale E, Foschini MP, Micheli A, Conti A, Riva C, Di Palma S, Rilke F (1994). Long-term follow-up of in situ carcinoma of the breast. Semin Diagn Pathol 11: 223–235.

395. Eusebi V, Foschini MP, Bussolati G, Rosen PP (1995). Myoblastomatoid (histiocytoid) carcinoma of the breast. A type of apocrine carcinoma. Am J Surg Pathol 19: 553–562.

396. Eusebi V, Magalhaes F, Azzopardi JG (1992). Pleomorphic lobular carcinoma of the breast: an aggressive tumor showing apocrine differentiation. Hum Pathol 23: 655–662.

397. Eusebi V, Millis RR (2010). Epitheliosis, infiltrating epitheliosis, and radial scar. Semin Diagn Pathol 27: 5–12.

398. Eusebi V, Millis RR, Cattani MG, Bussolati G, Azzopardi JG (1986). Apocrine carcinoma of the breast. A morphologic and immunocytochemical study. Am J Pathol 123: 532–541.

398A. Eusebi V, Lamovec J, Cattani MG, Fedeli F, Millis RR (1986). Acantholytic variant of squamous-cell carcinoma of the breast. Am J Surg Pathol 10: 855–861.

399. Evans DG, Birch JM, Narod SA (2008). Is CHEK2 a cause of the Li-Fraumeni syndrome? J Med Genet 45: 63–64.

400. Evans DG, Eccles DM, Rahman N, Young K, Bulman M, Amir E, Shenton A, Howell A, Lalloo F (2004). A new scoring system for the chances of identifying a BRCA1/2 mutation outperforms existing models including BRCAPRO. J Med Genet 41: 474–480.

401. Evans DG, Lalloo F, Cramer A, Jones EA, Knox F, Amir E, Howell A (2009). Addition of pathology and biomarker information significantly improves the performance of the Manchester scoring system for BRCA1 and BRCA2 testing. J Med Genet 46: 811–817.

402. Evans DG, Lalloo F, Wallace A, Rahman N (2005). Update on the Manchester Scoring System for BRCA1 and BRCA2 testing. J Med Genet 42: e39

403. Evans DG, Lunt P, Clancy T, Eeles R (2010). Childhood predictive genetic testing for Li-Fraumeni syndrome. Fam Cancer 9: 65–69.

404. Evans DG, Susnerwala I, Dawson J, Woodward E, Maher ER, Lalloo F (2010). Risk of breast cancer in male BRCA2 carriers. J Med Genet 47: 710–711.

405. Evans DG, Wu CL, Birch JM (2008). BRCA2: a cause of Li-Fraumeni-like syndrome. J Med Genet 45: 62–63.

406. Evans H, Bridge J (2002). Nodular fasciitis. In: Pathology and genetics of tumours of soft tissue and bone.Fletcher CDM, Unni KK, Mertens F, eds. WHO Classification of Tumours, 3rd edition. IARCPress: Lyon: pp 48–49.

407. Evans HL, Batsakis JG (1984). Polymorphous low-grade adenocarcinoma of minor salivary glands. A study of 14 cases of a distinctive neoplasm. Cancer 53: 935–942.

408. Evans HL, Luna MA (2000). Polymorphous low-grade adenocarcinoma: a study of 40 cases with long-term follow up and an evaluation of the importance of papillary areas. Am J Surg Pathol 24: 1319–1328.

409. Evans N, Lyons K (2000). The use of ultrasound in the diagnosis of invasive lobular carcinoma of the breast less than 10 mm in size. Clin Radiol 55: 261–263.

410. Ewald IP, Ribeiro PLI, Palmero EI, Cossio SL, Giugliani R, Ashton-Prolla P (2009). Genomic rearrangements in BRCA1 and BRCA2: A literature review. Genetics and Molecular Biology 32: 437–446.

411. Fackenthal JD, Marsh DJ, Richardson AL, Cummings SA, Eng C, Robinson BG, Olopade OI (2001). Male breast cancer in

Cowden syndrome patients with germline PTEN mutations. J Med Genet 38: 159–164.
412. Fadare O (2006). Pleomorphic lobular carcinoma in situ of the breast composed almost entirely of signet ring cells. Pathol Int 56: 683–687.
413. Fadare O, Wang SA, Hileeto D (2008). The expression of cytokeratin 5/6 in invasive lobular carcinoma of the breast: evidence of a basal-like subset? Hum Pathol 39: 331–336.
414. Faille A, De CP, Extra JM, Linares G, Espie M, Bourstyn E, De RA, Giacchetti S, Marty M, Calvo F (1994). p53 mutations and overexpression in locally advanced breast cancers. Br J Cancer 69: 1145–1150.
415. Falconieri G, Della LD, Zanconati F, Bittesini L (1997). Leiomyosarcoma of the female breast: report of two new cases and a review of the literature. Am J Clin Pathol 108: 19–25.
416. Fan C, Oh DS, Wessels L, Weigelt B, Nuyten DS, Nobel AB, Van't Veer LJ, Perou CM (2006). Concordance among gene-expression-based predictors for breast cancer. N Engl J Med 355: 560–569.
417. Fan F, Smith W, Wang X, Jewell W, Thomas PA, Tawfik O (2007). Myoepithelial carcinoma of the breast arising in an adenomyoepithelioma: mammographic, ultrasound and histologic features. Breast J 13: 203–204.
418. Fang S, Krahe R, Lozano G, Han Y, Chen W, Post SM, Zhang B, Wilson CD, Bachinski LL, Strong LC, Amos CI (2010). Effects of MDM2, MDM4 and TP53 codon 72 polymorphisms on cancer risk in a cohort study of carriers of TP53 germline mutations. PLoS One 5: e10813
419. Fang ZM, Tse RV, Marjoniemi VM, Kozlov S, Lavin MF, Chen H, Kearsley JH, Graham PH, Clarke RA (2009). Radioresistant malignant myoepithelioma of the breast with high level of ataxia telangiectasia mutated protein. J Med Imaging Radiat Oncol 53: 234–239.
420. Fangfang L, Danhua S, Songlin L, Yanfeng Z (2010). An unusual breast malignant peripheral nerve sheath tumour and review of the literature. J Clin Pathol 63: 663–664.
421. Farinha P, Andre S, Cabecadas J, Soares J (2002). High frequency of MALT lymphoma in a series of 14 cases of primary breast lymphoma. Appl Immunohistochem Mol Morphol 10: 115–120.
422. Farmer P, Bonnefoi H, Becette V, Tubiana-Hulin M, Fumoleau P, Larsimont D, MacGrogan G, Bergh J, Cameron D, Goldstein D, Duss S, Nicoulaz AL, Brisken C, Fiche M, Delorenzi M, Iggo R (2005). Identification of molecular apocrine breast tumours by microarray analysis. Oncogene 24: 4660–4671.
423. Farshid G, Balleine RL, Cummings M, Waring P (2006). Morphology of breast cancer as a means of triage of patients for BRCA1 genetic testing. Am J Surg Pathol 30: 1357–1366.
424. Farshid G, Moinfar F, Meredith DJ, Peiterse S, Tavassoli FA (2001). Spindle cell ductal carcinoma in situ. An unusual variant of ductal intra-epithelial neoplasia that simulates ductal hyperplasia or a myoepithelial proliferation. Virchows Arch 439: 70–77.
425. Fayette J, Martin E, Piperno-Neumann S, Le Cesne A, Robert C, Bonvalot S, Ranchere D, Pouillart P, Coindre JM, Blay JY (2007). Angiosarcomas, a heterogeneous group of sarcomas with specific behavior depending on primary site: a retrospective study of 161 cases. Ann Oncol 18: 2030–2036.
426. Fechner RE (1972). Infiltrating lobular carcinoma without lobular carcinoma in situ. Cancer 29: 1539–1545.
427. Fechner RE (1975). Histologic variants of infiltrating lobular carcinoma of the breast. Hum Pathol 6: 373–378.
428. Fedko MG, Scow JS, Shah SS, Reynolds C, Degnim AC, Jakub JW, Boughey JC (2010). Pure tubular carcinoma and axillary nodal metastases. Ann Surg Oncol 17 Suppl 3: 338–342.
429. Fehr A, Kovacs A, Loning T, Frierson H, Jr, van den Oord J, Stenman G (2011). The MYB-NFIB gene fusion-a novel genetic link between adenoid cystic carcinoma and dermal cylindroma. J Pathol 224: 322–327.
430. Fentiman IS, Fourquet A, Hortobagyi GN (2006). Male breast cancer. Lancet 367: 595–604.
431. Fentiman IS, Millis RR, Smith P, Ellul JP, Lampejo O (1997). Mucoid breast carcinomas: histology and prognosis. Br J Cancer 75: 1061–1065.
432. Ferlay J, Shin HR, Bray F, Forman D, Mathers C, Parkin DM, eds. GLOBOCAN 2008 v1.2, Cancer incidence and mortality worldwide: IARC CancerBase No. 10 [Internet]. Lyon, France: International Agency for Research on Cancer (http://globocan.iarc.fr).
433. Ferlicot S, Vincent-Salomon A, Medioni J, Genin P, Rosty C, Sigal-Zafrani B, Freneaux P, Jouve M, Thiery JP, Sastre-Garau X (2004). Wide metastatic spreading in infiltrating lobular carcinoma of the breast. Eur J Cancer 40: 336–341.
434. Fernandez BB, Hernanzez FJ, Spindler W (1976). Metastatic cystosarcoma phyllodes: a light and electron microscopic study. Cancer 37: 1737–1746.
435. Fernandez-Aguilar S, Simon P, Buxant F, Simonart T, Noel JC (2005). Tubular carcinoma of the breast and associated intra-epithelial lesions: a comparative study with invasive low-grade ductal carcinomas. Virchows Arch 447: 683–687.
436. Fernandez-Ramires R, Gomez G, Munoz-Repeto I, de Cecco L, Llort G, Cazorla A, Blanco I, Gariboldi M, Pierotti MA, Benitez J, Osorio A (2011). Transcriptional characteristics of familial non-BRCA1/BRCA2 breast tumors. Int J Cancer 128: 2635–2644.
437. Ferreira M, Albarracin CT, Resetkova E (2008). Pseudoangiomatous stromal hyperplasia tumor: a clinical, radiologic and pathologic study of 26 cases. Mod Pathol 21: 201–207.
438. Finck FM, Schwinn CP, Keasbey LE (1968). Clear cell hidradenoma of the breast. Cancer 22: 125–135.
439. Fineberg S, Rosen PP (1994). Cutaneous angiosarcoma and atypical vascular lesions of the skin and breast after radiation therapy for breast carcinoma. Am J Clin Pathol 102: 757–763.
440. Fishel R, Lescoe MK, Rao MR, Copeland NG, Jenkins NA, Garber J, Kane M, Kolodner R (1993). The human mutator gene homolog MSH2 and its association with hereditary nonpolyposis colon cancer. Cell 75: 1027–1038.
441. Fisher B, Bryant J, Wolmark N, Mamounas E, Brown A, Fisher ER, Wickerham DL, Begovic M, DeCillis A, Robidoux A, Margolese RG, Cruz AB, Jr, Hoehn JL, Lees AW, Dimitrov NV, Bear HD (1998). Effect of preoperative chemotherapy on the outcome of women with operable breast cancer. J Clin Oncol 16: 2672–2685.
442. Fisher B, Dignam J, Wolmark N, Wickerham DL, Fisher ER, Mamounas E, Smith R, Begovic M, Dimitrov NV, Margolese RG, Kardinal CG, Kavanah MT, Fehrenbacher L, Oishi RH (1999). Tamoxifen in treatment of intraductal breast cancer: National Surgical Adjuvant Breast and Bowel Project B-24 randomised controlled trial. Lancet 353: 1993–2000.
443. Fisher CJ, Hanby AM, Robinson L, Millis RR (1992). Mammary hamartoma—a review of 35 cases. Histopathology 20: 99–106.
444. Fisher ER, Gregorio R, Kim WS, Redmond C (1977). Lipid in invasive cancer of the breast. Am J Clin Pathol 68: 558–561.
445. Fisher ER, Gregorio RM, Fisher B, Redmond C, Vellios F, Sommers SC (1975). The pathology of invasive breast cancer. A syllabus derived from findings of the National Surgical Adjuvant Breast Project (protocol no. 4). Cancer 36: 1–85.
446. Fisher ER, Gregorio RM, Redmond C, Fisher B (1977). Tubulolobular invasive breast cancer: a variant of lobular invasive cancer. Hum Pathol 8: 679–683.
447. Fisher ER, Land SR, Fisher B, Mamounas E, Gilarski L, Wolmark N (2004). Pathologic findings from the National Surgical Adjuvant Breast and Bowel Project: twelve-year observations concerning lobular carcinoma in situ. Cancer 100: 238–244.
448. Fisher ER, Palekar AS, Gregorio RM, Paulson JD (1983). Mucoepidermoid and squamous cell carcinomas of breast with reference to squamous metaplasia and giant cell tumors. Am J Surg Pathol 7: 15–27.
449. Fisher ER, Wang J, Bryant J, Fisher B, Mamounas E, Wolmark N (2002). Pathobiology of preoperative chemotherapy: findings from the National Surgical Adjuvant Breast and Bowel (NSABP) protocol B-18. Cancer 95: 681–695.
450. Fitzgibbons PL, Henson DE, Hutter RV (1998). Benign breast changes and the risk for subsequent breast cancer: an update of the 1985 consensus statement. Cancer Committee of the College of American Pathologists. Arch Pathol Lab Med 122: 1053–1055.
451. Flagiello D, Gerbault-Seureau M, Sastre-Garau X, Padoy E, Vielh P, Dutrillaux B (1998). Highly recurrent der(1;16)(q10;p10) and other 16q arm alterations in lobular breast cancer. Genes Chromosomes Cancer 23: 300–306.
452. Fletcher CDM (2007). Soft tissue tumors. In: Diagnostic histopathology of tumors, 3rd edition. Fletcher CDM, ed. Churchill-Livingstone Elsevier: Edinburgh: pp 1527–1592.
453. Fletcher O, Johnson N, dos Santos Silva I, Orr N, Ashworth A, Nevanlinna H, Heikkinen T, Aittomaki K, Blomqvist C, Burwinkel B, Bartram CR, Meindl A, Schmutzler RK, Cox A, Brock I, Elliott G, Reed MW, Southey MC, Smith L, Spurdle AB et al. (2010). Missense variants in ATM in 26,101 breast cancer cases and 29,842 controls. Cancer Epidemiol Biomarkers Prev 19: 2143–2151.
453A. Fletcher O, Johnson N, Orr N, Hosking FJ, Gibson LJ, Walker K, Zelenika D, Gut I, Heath S, Palles C, Coupland B, Broderick P, Schoemaker M, Jones M, Williamson J, Chilcott-Burns S, Tomczyk K, Simpson G, Jacobs KB, Chanock SJ et al. (2011). Novel breast cancer susceptibility locus at 9q31.2: results of a genome-wide association study. J Natl Cancer Inst 103: 425–435.
454. Flint A, Oberman HA (1984). Infarction and squamous metaplasia of intraductal papilloma: a benign breast lesion that may simulate carcinoma. Hum Pathol 15: 764–767.
455. Foote FW, Jr, Stewart FW (1946). A histologic classification of carcinoma of the breast. Surgery 19: 74–99.
456. Ford D, Easton DF, Peto J (1995). Estimates of the gene frequency of BRCA1 and its contribution to breast and ovarian cancer incidence. Am J Hum Genet 57: 1457–1462.
457. Foschini MP, Dina RE, Eusebi V (1993). Sarcomatoid neoplasms of the breast: proposed definitions for biphasic and monophasic sarcomatoid mammary carcinomas. Semin Diagn Pathol 10: 128–136.
458. Foschini MP, Eusebi V (1998). Carcinomas of the breast showing myoepithelial cell differentiation. A review of the literature. Virchows Arch 432: 303–310.
459. Foschini MP, Krausz T (2010). Salivary gland-type tumors of the breast: a spectrum of benign and malignant tumors including «triple negative carcinomas» of low malignant potential. Semin Diagn Pathol 27: 77–90.
459A. Foschini MP, Pizzicannella G, Peterse JL, Eusebi V (1995). Adenomyoepithelioma of the breast associated with low-grade adenosquamous and sarcomatoid carcinomas. Virchows Arch 427: 243–250.
460. Foulkes WD, Stefansson IM, Chappuis PO, Begin LR, Goffin JR, Wong N, Trudel M, Akslen LA (2003). Germline BRCA1 mutations and a basal epithelial phenotype in breast cancer. J Natl Cancer Inst 95: 1482–1485.
461. Frank TS, Deffenbaugh AM, Reid JE, Hulick M, Ward BE, Lingenfelter B, Gumpper KL, Scholl T, Tavtigian SV, Pruss DR, Critchfield GC (2002). Clinical characteristics of individuals with germline mutations in BRCA1 and BRCA2: analysis of 10,000 individuals. J Clin Oncol 20: 1480–1490.
462. Friberg F, Andersson EP, Bengtsson J (2007). Pedagogical encounters between nurses and patients in a medical ward—a field study. Int J Nurs Stud 44: 534–544.
463. Fridlyand J, Snijders AM, Ylstra B, Li H, Olshen A, Segraves R, Dairkee S, Tokuyasu T, Ljung BM, Jain AN, McLennan J, Ziegler J, Chin K, DeVries S, Feiler H, Gray JW, Waldman F, Pinkel D, Albertson DG (2006). Breast tumor copy number aberration phenotypes and genomic instability. BMC Cancer 6: 96.
463A. Friedrich RE, Hagel C (2010). Appendices of the nipple and areola of the breast in Neurofibromatosis type 1 patients are neurofibromas. Anticancer Res 30: 1815–1817.
463B. Fritz A, Percy C, Jack A, Shanmugaratnam K, Sobin L, Parkin DM, Whelan S (2000) International Classification of Diseases for Oncology, 3rd edition. World Health Organization: Geneva.
464. Frykberg ER (1999). Lobular carcinoma in situ of the breast. Breast J 5: 296–303.
465. Fukunaga M, Ushigome S (1997). Myofibroblastoma of the breast with diverse differentiations. Arch Pathol Lab Med 121: 599–603.
466. Fukuoka K, Hirokawa M, Shimizu M, Sadahira Y, Manabe T, Kurebayashi J, Sonoo H (1999). Basaloid type adenoid cystic carcinoma of the breast. APMIS 107: 762–766.
467. Fulford LG, Easton DF, Reis-Filho JS, Sofronis A, Gillett CE, Lakhani SR, Hanby A (2006). Specific morphological features predictive for the basal phenotype in grade 3 invasive ductal carcinoma of breast. Histopathology 49: 22–34.
468. Gallego Melcon S, Sanchez de Toledo Codina J (2007). Molecular biology of rhabdomyosarcoma. Clin Transl Oncol 9: 415–419.
469. Gamallo C, Palacios J, Suarez A,

Pizarro A, Navarro P, Quintanilla M, Cano A (1993). Correlation of E-cadherin expression with differentiation grade and histological type in breast carcinoma. Am J Pathol 142: 987–993.

469A. Gallager HS (1984). Pathologic types of breast cancer: their prognoses. Cancer 53: 623–629.

470. Ganjoo K, Advani R, Mariappan MR, McMillan A, Horning S (2007). Non-Hodgkin lymphoma of the breast. Cancer 110: 25–30.

471. Gao X, Fisher SG, Emami B (2003). Risk of second primary cancer in the contralateral breast in women treated for early-stage breast cancer: a population-based study. Int J Radiat Oncol Biol Phys 56: 1038–1045.

472. Gapstur SM, Morrow M, Sellers TA (1999). Hormone replacement therapy and risk of breast cancer with a favorable histology: results of the Iowa Women's Health Study. JAMA 281: 2091–2097.

473. Garcia-Closas M, Hall P, Nevanlinna H, Pooley K, Morrison J, Richesson DA, Bojesen SE, Nordestgaard BG, Axelsson CK, Arias JI, Milne RL, Ribas G, Gonzalez-Neira A, Benitez J, Zamora P, Brauch H, Justenhoven C, Hamann U, Ko YD, Bruening T et al. (2008). Heterogeneity of breast cancer associations with five susceptibility loci by clinical and pathological characteristics. PLoS Genet 4: e1000054.

474. Garritano S, Gemignani F, Palmero EI, Olivier M, Martel-Planche G, Le Calvez-Kelm F, Brugieres L, Vargas FR, Brentani RR, Ashton-Prolla P, Landi S, Tavtigian SV, Hainaut P, Achatz MI (2010). Detailed haplotype analysis at the TP53 locus in p.R337H mutation carriers in the population of Southern Brazil: evidence for a founder effect. Hum Mutat 31: 143–150.

475. Gatalica Z, Norris BA, Kovatich AJ (2000). Immunohistochemical localization of prostate-specific antigen in ductal epithelium of male breast. Potential diagnostic pitfall in patients with gynecomastia. Appl Immunohistochem Mol Morphol 8: 158–161.

476. Gatalica Z, Velagaleti G, Kuivaniemi H, Tromp G, Palazzo J, Graves KM, Guigneaux M, Wood T, Sinha M, Luxon B (2005). Gene expression profile of an adenomyoepithelioma of the breast with a reciprocal translocation involving chromosomes 8 and 16. Cancer Genet Cytogenet 156: 14–22.

477. Gatti R, ed (1993). Ataxia-telangiectasia. Gene reviews [Internet]. Seattle: University of Washington.

478. Gatti RA, Tward A, Concannon P (1999). Cancer risk in ATM heterozygotes: a model of phenotypic and mechanistic differences between missense and truncating mutations. Mol Genet Metab 68: 419–423.

479. Gaudet MM, Kirchhoff T, Green T, Vijai J, Korn JM, Guiducci C, Segre AV, McGee K, McGuffog L, Kartsonaki C, Morrison J, Healey S, Sinilnikova OM, Stoppa-Lyonnet D, Mazoyer S, Gauthier-Villars M, Sobol H, Longy M, Frenay M, GEMO Study Collaborators et al. (2010). Common genetic variants and modification of penetrance of BRCA2-associated breast cancer. PLoS Genet 6: e1001183

480. Gayther SA, Gorringe KL, Ramus SJ, Huntsman D, Roviello F, Grehan N, Machado JC, Pinto E, Seruca R, Halling K, MacLeod P, Powell SM, Jackson CE, Ponder BA, Caldas C (1998). Identification of germ-line E-cadherin mutations in gastric cancer families of European origin. Cancer Res 58: 4086–4089.

481. Gayther SA, Mangion J, Russell P, Seal S, Barfoot R, Ponder BA, Stratton MR, Easton D (1997). Variation of risks of breast and ovarian cancer associated with different germline mutations of the BRCA2 gene. Nat Genet 15: 103–105.

482. Geary J, Sasieni P, Houlston R, Izatt L, Eeles R, Payne SJ, Fisher S, Hodgson SV (2008). Gene-related cancer spectrum in families with hereditary non-polyposis colorectal cancer (HNPCC). Fam Cancer 7: 163–172.

483. Geddes DT (2009). Ultrasound imaging of the lactating breast: methodology and application. Int Breastfeed J 4: 4. Abstract.

484. Gengler C, Guillou L (2006). Solitary fibrous tumour and haemangiopericytoma: evolution of a concept. Histopathology 48: 63–74.

485. Georgiannos SN, Chin J, Goode AW, Sheaff M (2001). Secondary neoplasms of the breast: a survey of the 20th Century. Cancer 92: 2259–2266.

485A. Gersell DJ, Katzenstein AL (1981). Spindle cell carcinoma of the breast. A clinocopathologic and ultrastructural study. Hum Pathol 12: 550–561.

485B. Geyer FC, Lambros MB, Natrajan R, Mehta R, Mackay A, Savage K, Parry S, Ashworth A, Badve S, Reis-Filho JS (2010). Genomic and immunohistochemical analysis of adenosquamous carcinoma of the breast. Mod Pathol 23: 951–960.

485C. Geyer FC, Weigelt B, Natrajan R, Lambros MB, de Biase D, Vatcheva R, Savage K, Mackay A, Ashworth A, Reis-Filho JS (2010). Molecular analysis reveals a genetic basis for the phenotypic diversity of metaplastic breast carcinomas. J Pathol 220: 562–573.

486. Ghabach B, Anderson WF, Curtis RE, Huycke MM, Lavigne JA, Dores GM (2010). Adenoid cystic carcinoma of the breast in the United States (1977 to 2006): a population-based cohort study. Breast Cancer Res 12: R54.

487. Giannotti FO, Miiji LN, Vainchenker M, Gordan AN (2001). Breast cancer with choriocarcinomatous and neuroendocrine features. Sao Paulo Med J 119: 154–155.

488. Giardini R, Piccolo C, Rilke F (1992). Primary non-Hodgkin's lymphomas of the female breast. Cancer 69: 725–735.

489. Gibbons D, Leitch M, Coscia J, Lindberg G, Molberg K, Ashfaq R, Saboorian MH (2000). Fine needle aspiration cytology and histologic findings of granular cell tumor of the breast: review of 19 cases with clinical/radiologic correlation. Breast J 6: 27–30.

489A. Gilbert JA, Goetz MP, Reynolds CA, Ingle JN, Giordano KF, Suman VJ, Blair HE, Jenkins RB, Lingle WL, Reinholz MM, Adjei AA, Ames MM (2008). Molecular analysis of metaplastic breast carcinoma: high EGFR copy number via aneusomy. Mol Cancer Ther 7: 944–951.

489B. Gillett CE, Bobrow LG, Millis RR (1990). S100 protein in human mammary tissue--immunoreactivity in breast carcinoma, including Paget's disease of the nipple, and value as a marker of myoepithelial cells. J Pathol 160: 19–24.

490. Gimm O, Attie-Bitach T, Lees JA, Vekemans M, Eng C (2000). Expression of the PTEN tumour suppressor protein during human development. Hum Mol Genet 9: 1633–1639.

491. Ginsburg OM, Akbari MR, Aziz Z, Young R, Lynch H, Ghadirian P, Robidoux A, Londono J, Vasquez G, Gomes M, Costa MM, Dimitrakakis C, Gutierrez G, Pilarski R, Royer R, Narod SA (2009). The prevalence of germ-line TP53 mutations in women diagnosed with breast cancer before age 30. Fam Cancer 8: 563–567.

492. Giordano SH, Buzdar AU, Hortobagyi GN (2002). Breast cancer in men. Ann Intern Med 137: 678–687.

493. Giordano SH, Cohen DS, Buzdar AU, Perkins G, Hortobagyi GN (2004). Breast carcinoma in men: a population-based study. Cancer 101: 51–57.

494. Giri DD, Dundas SA, Nottingham JF, Underwood JC (1989). Oestrogen receptors in benign epithelial lesions and intraduct carcinomas of the breast: an immunohistological study. Histopathology 15: 575–584.

495. Giuliano AE, Hunt KK, Ballman KV, Beitsch PD, Whitworth PW, Blumencranz PW, Leitch AM, Saha S, McCall LM, Morrow M (2011). Axillary dissection vs no axillary dissection in women with invasive breast cancer and sentinel node metastasis: a randomized clinical trial. JAMA 305: 569–575.

496. Glazebrook KN, Reynolds C, Smith RL, Gimenez EI, Boughey JC (2010). Adenoid cystic carcinoma of the breast. AJR Am J Roentgenol 194: 1391–1396.

497. Gleason BC, Hornick JL (2008). Inflammatory myofibroblastic tumours: where are we now? J Clin Pathol 61: 428–437.

498. Gobbi H, Jensen RA, Simpson JF, Olson SJ, Page DL (2001). Atypical ductal hyperplasia and ductal carcinoma in situ of the breast associated with perineural invasion. Hum Pathol 32: 785–790.

499. Gobbi H, Simpson JF, Borowsky A, Jensen RA, Page DL (1999). Metaplastic breast tumors with a dominant fibromatosis-like phenotype have a high risk of local recurrence. Cancer 85: 2170–2182.

499A. Gobbi H, Simpson JF, Jensen RA, Olson SJ, Page DL (2003). Metaplastic spindle cell breast tumors arising within papillomas, complex sclerosing lesions, and nipple adenomas. Mod Pathol 16: 893–901.

500. Gobbi H, Tse G, Page DL, Olson SJ, Jensen RA, Simpson JF (2000). Reactive spindle cell nodules of the breast after core biopsy or fine-needle aspiration. Am J Clin Pathol 113: 288–294.

501. Gocht A, Bosmuller HC, Bassler R, Tavassoli FA, Moinfar F, Katenkamp D, Schirrmacher K, Luders P, Saeger W (1999). Breast tumors with myofibroblastic differentiation: clinico-pathological observations in myofibroblastoma and myofibrosarcoma. Pathol Res Pract 195: 1–10.

502. Gokaslan ST, Carlile B, Dudak M, Albores-Saavedra J (2001). Solitary cylindroma (dermal analog tumor) of the breast: a previously undescribed neoplasm at this site. Am J Surg Pathol 25: 823–826.

503. Goldgar DE, Easton DF, Cannon-Albright LA, Skolnick MH (1994). Systematic population-based assessment of cancer risk in first-degree relatives of cancer probands. J Natl Cancer Inst 86: 1600–1608.

504. Goldgar DE, Healey S, Dowty JG, Da Silva L, Chen X, Spurdle AB, Terry MB, Daly MJ, Buys SM, Southey MC, Andrulis I, John EM, Khanna KK, Hopper JL, Oefner PJ, Lakhani S, Chenevix-Trench G (2011). Rare variants in the ATM gene and risk of breast cancer. Breast Cancer Res 13: R73

505. Goldhirsch A, Ingle JN, Gelber RD, Coates AS, Thurlimann B, Senn HJ (2009). Thresholds for therapies: highlights of the St Gallen International Expert Consensus on the primary therapy of early breast cancer 2009. Ann Oncol 20: 1319–1329.

506. Goldstein NS, O'Malley BA (1997). Cancerization of small ectatic ducts of the breast by ductal carcinoma in situ cells with apocrine snouts: a lesion associated with tubular carcinoma. Am J Clin Pathol 107: 561–566.

507. Gong G, DeVries S, Chew KL, Cha I, Ljung BM, Waldman FM (2001). Genetic changes in paired atypical and usual ductal hyperplasia of the breast by comparative genomic hybridization. Clin Cancer Res 7: 2410–2414.

508. Gonzalez CA, Riboli E (2010). Diet and cancer prevention: Contributions from the European Prospective Investigation into Cancer and Nutrition (EPIC) study. Eur J Cancer 46: 2555–2562.

509. Gonzalez KD, Buzin CH, Noltner KA, Gu D, Li W, Malkin D, Sommer SS (2009). High frequency of de novo mutations in Li-Fraumeni syndrome. J Med Genet 46: 689–693.

510. Gonzalez KD, Noltner KA, Buzin CH, Gu D, Wen-Fong CY, Nguyen VQ, Han JH, Lowstuter K, Longmate J, Sommer SS, Weitzel JN (2009). Beyond Li Fraumeni Syndrome: clinical characteristics of families with p53 germline mutations. J Clin Oncol 27: 1250–1256.

511. Gonzalez-Angulo AM, Timms KM, Liu S, Chen H, Litton JK, Potter J, Lanchbury JS, Stemke-Hale K, Hennessy BT, Arun BK, Hortobagyi GN, Do KA, Mills GB, Meric-Bernstam F (2011). Incidence and outcome of BRCA mutations in unselected patients with triple receptor-negative breast cancer. Clin Cancer Res 17: 1082–1089.

512. Goodman ZD, Taxy JB (1981). Fibroadenomas of the breast with prominent smooth muscle. Am J Surg Pathol 5: 99–101.

513. Gorlick R (2009). Current concepts on the molecular biology of osteosarcoma. Cancer Treat Res 152: 467–478.

514. Gorski B, Debniak T, Masojc B, Mierzejewski M, Medrek K, Cybulski C, Jakubowska A, Kurzawski G, Chosia M, Scott R, Lubinski J (2003). Germline 657del5 mutation in the NBS1 gene in breast cancer patients. Int J Cancer 106: 379–381.

515. Grabau D, Jensen MB, Rank F, Blichert-Toft M (2007). Axillary lymph node micrometastases in invasive breast cancer: national figures on incidence and overall survival. APMIS 115: 828–837.

516. Grady I, Gorsuch H, Wilburn-Bailey S (2008). Long-term outcome of benign fibroadenomas treated by ultrasound-guided percutaneous excision. Breast J 14: 275–278.

517. Granier G, Lemoine MC, Mares P, Pignodel C, Marty-Double C (2005). [Primary angiosarcoma of the male breast]. Ann Pathol 25: 235–239.

518. Green DM (1990). Mucoid carcinoma of the breast with choriocarcinoma in its metastases. Histopathology 16: 504–506.

519. Green I, McCormick B, Cranor M, Rosen PP (1997). A comparative study of pure tubular and tubulolobular carcinoma of the breast. Am J Surg Pathol 21: 653–657.

519A. Greenman C, Stephens P, Smith R, Dalgliesh GL, Hunter C, Bignell G, Davies H, Teague J, Butler A, Stevens C, Edkins S, O'Meara S, Vastrik I, Schmidt EE, Avis T, Barthorpe S, Bhamra G, Buck G, Choudhury B, Clements J et al. (2007). Patterns of somatic mutation in human cancer genomes. Nature 446: 153–158.

520. Gresik CM, Godellas C, Aranha GV, Rajan P, Shoup M (2010). Pseudoangiomatous stromal hyperplasia of the breast: a contemporary approach to its clinical and radiologic features and ideal management. Surgery 148: 752–757.

520A. Gruel N, Lucchesi C, Raynal V, Rodrigues MJ, Pierron G, Goudefroye R, Cottu P, Reyal F, Sastre-Garau X, Fourquet A, Delattre O, Vincent-Salomon A (2010). Lobular invasive carcinoma of the breast is a molecular entity distinct from luminal invasive ductal carcinoma. Eur J Cancer 46: 2399–2407.
521. Gu F, Schumacher FR, Canzian F, Allen NE, Albanes D, Berg CD, Berndt SI, Boeing H, Bueno-de-Mesquita HB, Buring JE, Chabbert-Buffet N, Chanock SJ, Clavel-Chapelon F, Dumeaux V, Gaziano JM, Giovannucci EL, Haiman CA, Hankinson SE, Hayes RB, Henderson BE et al. (2010). Eighteen insulin-like growth factor pathway genes, circulating levels of IGF-I and its binding protein, and risk of prostate and breast cancer. Cancer Epidemiol Biomarkers Prev 19: 2877–2887.
522. Gualco G, Weiss LM, Harrington WJ, Jr, Bacchi CE (2009). Nodal diffuse large B-cell lymphomas in children and adolescents: immunohistochemical expression patterns and c-MYC translocation in relation to clinical outcome. Am J Surg Pathol 33: 1815–1822.
523. Guerin M, Gabillot M, Mathieu MC, Travagli JP, Spielmann M, Andrieu N, Riou G (1989). Structure and expression of c-erbB-2 and EGF receptor genes in inflammatory and non-inflammatory breast cancer: prognostic significance. Int J Cancer 43: 201–208.
524. Guilford P, Hopkins J, Harraway J, McLeod M, McLeod N, Harawira P, Taite H, Scoular R, Miller A, Reeve AE (1998). E-cadherin germline mutations in familial gastric cancer. Nature 392: 402–405.
525. Gump FE, Sternschein MJ, Wolff M (1981). Fibromatosis of the breast. Surg Gynecol Obstet 153: 57–60.
526. Gunhan-Bilgen I, Oktay A (2007). Tubular carcinoma of the breast: mammographic, sonographic, clinical and pathologic findings. Eur J Radiol 61: 158–162.
527. Gunhan-Bilgen I, Zekioglu O, Ustun EE, Memis A, Erhan Y (2002). Invasive micropapillary carcinoma of the breast: clinical, mammographic, and sonographic findings with histopathologic correlation. AJR Am J Roentgenol 179: 927–931.
528. Gunther K, Merkelbach-Bruse S, Amo-Takyi BK, Handt S, Schroder W, Tietze L (2001). Differences in genetic alterations between primary lobular and ductal breast cancers detected by comparative genomic hybridization. J Pathol 193: 40–47.
529. Guo X, Chen L, Lang R, Fan Y, Zhang X, Fu L (2006). Invasive micropapillary carcinoma of the breast: association of pathologic features with lymph node metastasis. Am J Clin Pathol 126: 740–746.
530. Guo X, Fan Y, Lang R, Gu F, Chen L, Cui L, Pringle GA, Zhang X, Fu L (2008). Tumor infiltrating lymphocytes differ in invasive micropapillary carcinoma and medullary carcinoma of breast. Mod Pathol 21: 1101–1107.
531. Gylling AH, Nieminen TT, bdel-Rahman WM, Nuorva K, Juhola M, Joensuu EI, Jarvinen HJ, Mecklin JP, Aarnio M, Peltomaki PT (2008). Differential cancer predisposition in Lynch syndrome: insights from molecular analysis of brain and urinary tract tumors. Carcinogenesis 29: 1351–1359.
532. Haagensen CD, ed. (1986). Diseases of the breast. 3rd Edition. Saunders: Philadelphia.
533. Haagensen CD, Lane N, Lattes R, Bodian C (1978). Lobular neoplasia (so-called lobular carcinoma in situ) of the breast. Cancer 42: 737–769.
533A. Hainaut P, Hollstein M (2000). p53 and human cancer: the first ten thousand mutations. Adv Cancer Res 77: 81–137.
534. Haj M, Weiss M, Loberant N, Cohen I (2003). Inflammatory pseudotumor of the breast: case report and literature review. Breast J 9: 423–425.
535. Hajdu M, Singer S, Maki RG, Schwartz GK, Keohan ML, Antonescu CR (2010). IGF2 over-expression in solitary fibrous tumours is independent of anatomical location and is related to loss of imprinting. J Pathol 221: 300–307.
536. Hajdu SI, Urban JA (1972). Cancers metastatic to the breast. Cancer 29: 1691–1696.
537. Hall JM, Lee MK, Newman B, Morrow JE, Anderson LA, Huey B, King MC (1990). Linkage of early-onset familial breast cancer to chromosome 17q21. Science 250: 1684–1689.
537A. Halpert B, Young MO (1948). Carcinosarcoma of the mammary gland. Surgery 23: 289–292.
538. Hamajima N, Hirose K, Tajima K, Rohan T, Calle EE, Heath CW, Jr, Coates RJ, Liff JM, Talamini R, Chantarakul N, Koetsawang S, Rachawat D, Morabia A, Schuman L, Stewart W, Szklo M, Bain C, Schofield F, Siskind V, Band P et al. (2002). Alcohol, tobacco and breast cancer—collaborative reanalysis of individual data from 53 epidemiological studies, including 58,515 women with breast cancer and 95,067 women without the disease. Br J Cancer 87: 1234–1245.
539. Hamele-Bena D, Cranor ML, Rosen PP (1996). Mammary mucocele-like lesions. Benign and malignant. Am J Surg Pathol 20: 1081–1085.
540. Hamele-Bena D, Cranor ML, Sciotto C, Erlandson R, Rosen PP (1996). Uncommon presentation of mammary myofibroblastoma. Mod Pathol 9: 786–790.
541. Hammond ME, Hayes DF, Dowsett M, Allred DC, Hagerty KL, Badve S, Fitzgibbons PL, Francis G, Goldstein NS, Hayes M, Hicks DG, Lester S, Love R, Mangu PB, McShane L, Miller K, Osborne CK, Paik S, Perlmutter J, Rhodes A et al. (2010). American Society of Clinical Oncology/College of American Pathologists guideline recommendations for immunohistochemical testing of estrogen and progesterone receptors in breast cancer. J Clin Oncol 28: 2784–2795.
542. Hammond ME, Hayes DF, Dowsett M, Allred DC, Hagerty KL, Badve S, Fitzgibbons PL, Francis G, Goldstein NS, Hayes M, Hicks DG, Lester S, Love R, Mangu PB, McShane L, Miller K, Osborne CK, Paik S, Perlmutter J, Rhodes A et al. (2010). American Society of Clinical Oncology/College of American Pathologists guideline recommendations for immunohistochemical testing of estrogen and progesterone receptors in breast cancer. Arch Pathol Lab Med 134: 907–922.
543. Han B, Mori I, Nakamura M, Wang X, Ozaki T, Nakamura Y, Kakudo K (2006). Myoepithelial carcinoma arising in an adenomyoepithelioma of the breast: case report with immunohistochemical and mutational analysis. Pathol Int 56: 211–216.
544. Han HJ, Maruyama M, Baba S, Park JG, Nakamura Y (1995). Genomic structure of human mismatch repair gene, hMLH1, and its mutation analysis in patients with hereditary non-polyposis colorectal cancer (HNPCC). Hum Mol Genet 4: 237–242.
545. Hance KW, Anderson WF, Devesa SS, Young HA, Levine PH (2005). Trends in inflammatory breast carcinoma incidence and survival: the surveillance, epidemiology, and end results program at the National Cancer Institute. J Natl Cancer Inst 97: 966–975.
546. Hankey BF, Curtis RE, Naughton MD, Boice JD, Jr, Flannery JT (1983). A retrospective cohort analysis of second breast cancer risk for primary breast cancer patients with an assessment of the effect of radiation therapy. J Natl Cancer Inst 70: 797–804.
547. Hankinson SE, Colditz GA, Hunter DJ, Manson JE, Willett WC, Stampfer MJ, Longcope C, Speizer FE (1995). Reproductive factors and family history of breast cancer in relation to plasma estrogen and prolactin levels in postmenopausal women in the Nurses' Health Study (United States). Cancer Causes Control 6: 217–224.
548. Hankinson SE, Willett WC, Colditz GA, Hunter DJ, Michaud DS, Deroo B, Rosner B, Speizer FE, Pollak M (1998). Circulating concentrations of insulin-like growth factor-I and risk of breast cancer. Lancet 351: 1393–1396.
549. Hanna W, Kahn HJ (1985). Ultrastructural and immunohistochemical characteristics of mucoepidermoid carcinoma of the breast. Hum Pathol 16: 941–946.
550. Hans CP, Weisenburger DD, Greiner TC, Gascoyne RD, Delabie J, Ott G, Muller-Hermelink HK, Campo E, Braziel RM, Jaffe ES, Pan Z, Farinha P, Smith LM, Falini B, Banham AH, Rosenwald A, Staudt LM, Connors JM, Armitage JO, Chan WC (2004). Confirmation of the molecular classification of diffuse large B-cell lymphoma by immunohistochemistry using a tissue microarray. Blood 103: 275–282.
551. Harada S, Fujiwara H, Hisatsugu T, Sugihara H (1987). Malignant cystosarcoma phyllodes with lymph node metastasis—a case report. Jpn J Surg 17: 174–177.
552. Harris GC, Denley HE, Pinder SE, Lee AH, Ellis IO, Elston CW, Evans A (2003). Correlation of histologic prognostic factors in core biopsies and therapeutic excisions of invasive breast carcinoma. Am J Surg Pathol 27: 11–15.
553. Harris KP, Faliakou EC, Exon DJ, Nasiri N, Sacks NP, Gui GP (1999). Treatment and outcome of intracystic papillary carcinoma of the breast. Br J Surg 86: 1274
554. Harris M, Howell A, Chrissohou M, Swindell RI, Hudson M, Sellwood RA (1984). A comparison of the metastatic pattern of infiltrating lobular carcinoma and infiltrating duct carcinoma of the breast. Br J Cancer 50: 23–30.
555. Hartman M, Czene K, Reilly M, Adolfsson J, Bergh J, Adami HO, Dickman PW, Hall P (2007). Incidence and prognosis of synchronous and metachronous bilateral breast cancer. J Clin Oncol 25: 4210–4216.
556. Hartman M, Hall P, Edgren G, Reilly M, Lindstrom L, Lichtenstein P, Kaprio J, Skytthe A, Peto J, Czene K (2008). Breast cancer onset in twins and women with bilateral disease. J Clin Oncol 26: 4086–4091.
557. Hartmann LC, Sellers TA, Frost MH, Lingle WL, Degnim AC, Ghosh K, Vierkant RA, Maloney SD, Pankratz VS, Hillman DW, Suman VJ, Johnson J, Blake C, Tlsty T, Vachon CM, Melton LJ, III, Visscher DW (2005). Benign breast disease and the risk of breast cancer. N Engl J Med 353: 229–237.
558. Harvey JM, Clark GM, Osborne CK, Allred DC (1999). Estrogen receptor status by immunohistochemistry is superior to the ligand-binding assay for predicting response to adjuvant endocrine therapy in breast cancer. J Clin Oncol 17: 1474–1481.
559. Hastrup N, Sehested M (1985). High-grade mucoepidermoid carcinoma of the breast. Histopathology 9: 887–892.
559A. Hayes MJ, Thomas D, Emmons A, Giordano TJ, Kleer CG (2008). Genetic changes of Wnt pathway genes are common events in metaplastic carcinomas of the breast. Clin Cancer Res 14: 4038–4044.
560. Hayes MM (2011). Adenomyoepithelioma of the breast: a review stressing its propensity for malignant transformation. J Clin Pathol 64: 477–484.
561. Hayes MM, Lesack D, Girardet C, Del Vecchio M, Eusebi V (2005). Carcinoma ex-pleomorphic adenoma of the breast. Report of three cases suggesting a relationship to metaplastic carcinoma of matrix-producing type. Virchows Arch 446: 142–149.
562. Hayes MM, Seidman JD, Ashton MA (1995). Glycogen-rich clear cell carcinoma of the breast. A clinicopathologic study of 21 cases. Am J Surg Pathol 19: 904–911.
563. Hays DM, Donaldson SS, Shimada H, Crist WM, Newton WA, Jr, Andrassy RJ, Wiener E, Green J, Triche T, Maurer HM (1997). Primary and metastatic rhabdomyosarcoma in the breast: neoplasms of adolescent females, a report from the Intergroup Rhabdomyosarcoma Study. Med Pediatr Oncol 29: 181–189.
564. He X, Ni Y, Wang Y, Romigh T, Eng C (2011). Naturally occurring germline and tumor-associated mutations within the ATP-binding motifs of PTEN lead to oxidative damage of DNA associated with decreased nuclear p53. Hum Mol Genet 20: 80–89.
565. Heald B, Mester J, Rybicki L, Orloff MS, Burke CA, Eng C (2010). Frequent gastrointestinal polyps and colorectal adenocarcinomas in a prospective series of PTEN mutation carriers. Gastroenterology 139: 1927–1933.
566. Hedenfalk I, Duggan D, Chen Y, Radmacher M, Bittner M, Simon R, Meltzer P, Gusterson B, Esteller M, Kallioniemi OP, Wilfond B, Borg A, Trent J, Raffeld M, Yakhini Z, Ben-Dor A, Dougherty E, Kononen J, Bubendorf L, Fehrle W et al. (2001). Gene-expression profiles in hereditary breast cancer. N Engl J Med 344: 539–548.
567. Hegyi L, Thway K, Newton R, Osin P, Nerurkar A, Hayes AJ, Fisher C (2009). Malignant myoepithelioma arising in adenomyoepithelioma of the breast and coincident multiple gastrointestinal stromal tumours in a patient with neurofibromatosis type 1. J Clin Pathol 62: 653–655.
568. Hendriks YM, de Jong AE, Morreau H, Tops CM, Vasen HF, Wijnen JT, Breuning MH, Brocker-Vriends AH (2006). Diagnostic approach and management of Lynch syndrome (hereditary nonpolyposis colorectal carcinoma): a guide for clinicians. CA Cancer J Clin 56: 213–225.
568A. Hennessy BT, Giordano S, Broglio K, Duan Z, Trent J, Buchholz TA, Babiera G, Hortobagyi GN, Valero V (2006). Biphasic metaplastic sarcomatoid carcinoma of the breast. Ann Oncol 17: 605–613.
568B. Hennessy BT, Gonzalez-Angulo AM, Stemke-Hale K, Gilcrease MZ, Krishnamurthy S, Lee JS, Fridlyand J, Sahin A, Agarwal R, Joy C, Liu W, Stivers D, Baggerly K, Carey M, Lluch A, Monteagudo C, He X, Weigman V, Fan C, Palazzo J et al. (2009). Characterization of a naturally occurring breast cancer subset enriched in epithelial-to-mesenchymal transition and stem cell characteristics. Cancer Res 69: 4116–4124.
568C. Hennessy BT, Krishnamurthy S,

Giordano S, Buchholz TA, Kau SW, Duan Z, Valero V, Hortobagyi GN (2005). Squamous cell carcinoma of the breast. J Clin Oncol 23: 7827–7835.
569. Herbert M, Sandbank J, Liokumovich P, Yanai O, Pappo I, Karni T, Segal M (2002). Breast hamartomas: clinicopathological and immunohistochemical studies of 24 cases. Histopathology 41: 30–34.
570. Herbert M, Schvimer M, Zehavi S, Mendlovic S, Karni T, Pappo I, Sandbank J (2003). Breast hamartoma: fine-needle aspiration cytologic finding. Cancer 99: 255–258.
571. Herrington CS, Tarin D, Buley I, Athanasou N (1994). Osteosarcomatous differentiation in carcinoma of the breast: a case of 'metaplastic' carcinoma with osteoclasts and osteoclast-like giant cells. Histopathology 24: 282–285.
572. Herz H, Cooke B, Goldstein D (2000). Metastatic secretory breast cancer. Non-responsiveness to chemotherapy: case report and review of the literature. Ann Oncol 11: 1343–1347.
573. Heymann S, Delaloge S, Rahal A, Caron O, Frebourg T, Barreau L, Pachet C, Mathieu MC, Marsiglia H, Bourgier C (2010). Radio-induced malignancies after breast cancer postoperative radiotherapy in patients with Li-Fraumeni syndrome. Radiat.Oncol 5: 104. Abstract.
574. Hicks J, Krasnitz A, Lakshmi B, Navin NE, Riggs M, Leibu E, Esposito D, Alexander J, Troge J, Grubor V, Yoon S, Wigler M, Ye K, Borresen-Dale AL, Naume B, Schlicting E, Norton L, Hagerstrom T, Skoog L, Auer G et al. (2006). Novel patterns of genome rearrangement and their association with survival in breast cancer. Genome Res 16: 1465–1479.
575. Hill CB, Yeh IT (2005). Myoepithelial cell staining patterns of papillary breast lesions: from intraductal papillomas to invasive papillary carcinomas. Am J Clin Pathol 123: 36–44.
576. Hill RP, Miller FN, Jr (1954). Adenomas of the breast with case report of carcinomatous transformation in an adenoma. Cancer 7: 318–324.
577. Hilleren DJ, Andersson IT, Lindholm K, Linnell FS (1991). Invasive lobular carcinoma: mammographic findings in a 10-year experience. Radiology 178: 149–154.
578. Hilson JB, Schnitt SJ, Collins LC (2009). Phenotypic alterations in ductal carcinoma in situ-associated myoepithelial cells: biologic and diagnostic implications. Am J Surg Pathol 33: 227–232.
579. Hilson JB, Schnitt SJ, Collins LC (2010). Phenotypic alterations in myoepithelial cells associated with benign sclerosing lesions of the breast. Am J Surg Pathol 34: 896–900.
580. Hirokawa M, Sugihara K, Sai T, Monobe Y, Kudo H, Sano N, Sano T (2002). Secretory carcinoma of the breast: a tumour analogous to salivary gland acinic cell carcinoma? Histopathology 40: 223–229.
581. Hisada M, Garber JE, Fung CY, Fraumeni JF, Jr, Li FP (1998). Multiple primary cancers in families with Li-Fraumeni syndrome. J Natl Cancer Inst 90: 606–611.
582. Hisaoka M, Takamatsu Y, Hirano Y, Maeda H, Hamada T (2006). Sebaceous carcinoma of the breast: case report and review of the literature. Virchows Arch 449: 484–488.
582A. Hitchins MP, Ward RL (2009). Constitutional (germline) MLH1 epimutation as an aetiological mechanism for hereditary non-polyposis colorectal cancer. J Med Genet 46: 793–802.
583. Hitchins MP, Wong JJ, Suthers G, Suter CM, Martin DI, Hawkins NJ, Ward RL (2007). Inheritance of a cancer-associated MLH1 germ-line epimutation. N Engl J Med 356: 697–705.
584. Hittmair AP, Lininger RA, Tavassoli FA (1998). Ductal carcinoma in situ (DCIS) in the male breast: a morphologic study of 84 cases of pure DCIS and 30 cases of DCIS associated with invasive carcinoma—a preliminary report. Cancer 83: 2139–2149.
585. Hobert JA, Eng C (2009). PTEN hamartoma tumor syndrome: an overview. Genet Med 11: 687–694.
586. Hodi Z, Chakrabarti J, Lee AH, Ronan JE, Elston CW, Cheung KL, Robertson JF, Ellis IO (2007). The reliability of assessment of oestrogen receptor expression on needle core biopsy specimens of invasive carcinomas of the breast. J Clin Pathol 60: 299–302.
587. Holland R, Hendriks JH, Vebeek AL, Mravunac M, Schuurmans Stekhoven JH (1990). Extent, distribution, and mammographic/histological correlations of breast ductal carcinoma in situ. Lancet 335: 519–522.
588. Holland R, van Haelst UJ (1984). Mammary carcinoma with osteoclast-like giant cells. Additional observations on six cases. Cancer 53: 1963–1973.
589. Holmberg L, Garmo H, Granstrand B, Ringberg A, Arnesson LG, Sandelin K, Karlsson P, Anderson H, Emdin S (2008). Absolute risk reductions for local recurrence after postoperative radiotherapy after sector resection for ductal carcinoma in situ of the breast. J Clin Oncol 26: 1247–1252.
590. Holstege H, Horlings HM, Velds A, Langerod A, Borresen-Dale AL, Van de Vijver M, Nederlof PM, Jonkers J (2010). BRCA1-mutated and basal-like breast cancers have similar aCGH profiles and a high incidence of protein truncating TP53 mutations. BMC.Cancer 10: 654. Abstract.
591. Holstege H, Joosse SA, van Oostrom CT, Nederlof PM, de Vries A, Jonkers J (2009). High incidence of protein-truncating TP53 mutations in BRCA1-related breast cancer. Cancer Res 69: 3625–3633.
591A Honma N, Takubo K, Akiyama F, Sawabe M, Arai T, Younes M, Kasumi F, Sakamoto G (2005). Expression of GCDFP-15 and AR decreases in larger or node-positive apocrine carcinomas of the breast. Histopathology 47: 195–201.
592. Honrado E, Osorio A, Palacios J, Benitez J (2006). Pathology and gene expression of hereditary breast tumors associated with BRCA1, BRCA2 and CHEK2 gene mutations. Oncogene 25: 5837–5845.
593. Hooning MJ, Aleman BM, Hauptmann M, Baaijens MH, Klijn JG, Noyon R, Stovall M, van Leeuwen FE (2008). Roles of radiotherapy and chemotherapy in the development of contralateral breast cancer. J Clin Oncol 26: 5561–5568.
594. Hoorntje LE, Peeters PH, Mali WP, Borel Rinkes I (2003). Vacuum-assisted breast biopsy: a critical review. Eur J Cancer 39: 1676–1683.
595. Hoque MO, Prencipe M, Poeta ML, Barbano R, Valori VM, Copetti M, Gallo AP, Brait M, Maiello E, Apicella A, Rossiello R, Zito F, Stefania T, Paradiso A, Carella M, Dallapiccola B, Murgo R, Carosi I, Bisceglia M, Fazio VM et al. (2009). Changes in CpG islands promoter methylation patterns during ductal breast carcinoma progression. Cancer Epidemiol Biomarkers Prev 18: 2694–2700.
596. Horne CH, Reid IN, Milne GD (1976). Prognostic significance of inappropriate production of pregnancy proteins by breast cancers. Lancet 2: 279–282.
597. Hornick JL, Bosenberg MW, Mentzel T, McMenamin ME, Oliveira AM, Fletcher CD (2004). Pleomorphic liposarcoma: clinicopathologic analysis of 57 cases. Am J Surg Pathol 28: 1257–1267.
598. Hornychova H, Ryska A, Betlach J, Bohac R, Cizek T, Tomsova M, Obermannova R (2007). Mucoepidermoid carcinoma of the breast. Neoplasma 54: 168–172.
599. Hortobagyi GN, Ames FC, Buzdar AU, Kau SW, McNeese MD, Paulus D, Hug V, Holmes FA, Romsdahl MM, Fraschini G (1988). Management of stage III primary breast cancer with primary chemotherapy, surgery, and radiation therapy. Cancer 62: 2507–2516.
600. Houghton J, George WD, Cuzick J, Duggan C, Fentiman IS, Spittle M (2003). Radiotherapy and tamoxifen in women with completely excised ductal carcinoma in situ of the breast in the UK, Australia, and New Zealand: randomised controlled trial. Lancet 362: 95–102.
601. Howarth CB, Caces JN, Pratt CB (1980). Breast metastases in children with rhabdomyosarcoma. Cancer 46: 2520–2524.
602. Howe GR, Hirohata T, Hislop TG, Iscovich JM, Yuan JM, Katsouyanni K, Lubin F, Marubini E, Modan B, Rohan T (1990). Dietary factors and risk of breast cancer: combined analysis of 12 case-control studies. J Natl Cancer Inst 82: 561–569.
603. Howlett DC, Mason CH, Biswas S, Sangle PD, Rubin G, Allan SM (2003). Adenomyoepithelioma of the breast: spectrum of disease with associated imaging and pathology. AJR Am J Roentgenol 180: 799–803.
604. Hu M, Yao J, Carroll DK, Weremowicz S, Chen H, Carrasco D, Richardson A, Violette S, Nikolskaya T, Nikolsky Y, Bauerlein EL, Hahn WC, Gelman RS, Allred C, Bissell MJ, Schnitt S, Polyak K (2008). Regulation of in situ to invasive breast carcinoma transition. Cancer Cell 13: 394–406.
605. Huang CY, Sheen-Chen SM, Eng HL, Ko SF (2007). Adenomyoepithelioma of the breast. Tumori 93: 493–495.
606. Huang KT, Dobrovic A, Yan M, Karim RZ, Lee CS, Lakhani SR, Fox SB (2010). DNA methylation profiling of phyllodes and fibroadenoma tumours of the breast. Breast Cancer Res Treat 124: 555–565.
607. Huang Z, Hankinson SE, Colditz GA, Stampfer MJ, Hunter DJ, Manson JE, Hennekens CH, Rosner B, Speizer FE, Willett WC (1997). Dual effects of weight and weight gain on breast cancer risk. JAMA 278: 1407–1411.
608. Huen MS, Sy SM, Chen J (2010). BRCA1 and its toolbox for the maintenance of genome integrity. Nat Rev Mol Cell Biol 11: 138–148.
609. Hugh JC, Jackson FI, Hanson J, Poppema S (1990). Primary breast lymphoma. An immunohistologic study of 20 new cases. Cancer 66: 2602–2611.
609A. Hughes LL, Wang M, Page DL, Gray R, Solin LJ, Davidson NE, Lowen MA, Ingle JN, Recht A, Wood WC (2009). Local excision alone without irradiation for ductal carcinoma in situ of the breast: a trial of the Eastern Cooperative Oncology Group. J Clin Oncol 27: 5319–5324.
610. Huijts PE, van Dongen M, de Goeij MC, van Moolenbroek AJ, Blanken F, Vreeswijk MP, de Kruijf EM, Mesker WE, van Zwet EW, Tollenaar RA, Smit VT, van Asperen CJ, Devilee P (2011). Allele-specific regulation of FGFR2 expression is cell type-dependent and may increase breast cancer risk through a paracrine stimulus involving FGF10. Breast Cancer Res 13: R72
611. Hull MT, Warfel KA (1987). Mucinous breast carcinomas with abundant intracytoplasmic mucin and neuroendocrine features: light microscopic, immunohistochemical, and ultrastructural study. Ultrastruct Pathol 11: 29–38.
612. Hultborn R, Hanson C, Kopf I, Verbiene I, Warnhammar E, Weimarck A (1997). Prevalence of Klinefelter's syndrome in male breast cancer patients. Anticancer Res 17: 4293–4297.
613. Hungermann D, Buerger H, Oehlschlegel C, Herbst H, Boecker W (2005). Adenomyoepithelial tumours and myoepithelial carcinomas of the breast—a spectrum of monophasic and biphasic tumours dominated by immature myoepithelial cells. BMC.Cancer 5: 92. Abstract.
613A. Hungermann D, Schmidt H, Natrajan R, Tidow N, Poos K, Reis-Filho JS, Brandt B, Buerger H, Korsching E (2011). Influence of whole arm loss of chromosome 16q on gene expression patterns in oestrogen receptor-positive, invasive breast cancer. J Pathol 224: 517–528.
613B. Hunter DJ, Kraft P, Jacobs KB, Cox DG, Yeager M, Hankinson SE, Wacholder S, Wang Z, Welch R, Hutchinson A, Wang J, Yu K, Chatterjee N, Orr N, Willett WC, Colditz GA, Ziegler RG, Berg CD, Buys SS, McCarty CA et al. (2007). A genome-wide association study identifies alleles in FGFR2 associated with risk of sporadic postmenopausal breast cancer. Nat Genet 39: 870–874.
614. Hunter DJ, Willett WC (1993). Diet, body size, and breast cancer. Epidemiol Rev 15: 110–132.
615. Huo D, Melkonian S, Rathouz PJ, Khramtsov A, Olopade OI (2010). Concordance in histological and biological parameters between first and second primary breast cancers. Cancer 117: 907–915.
616. Huo L, Gilcrease MZ (2009). Fibroepithelial lesions of the breast with pleomorphic stromal giant cells: a clinicopathologic study of 4 cases and review of the literature. Ann Diagn Pathol 13: 226–232.
616A. Huvos AG, Lucas JC, Jr, Foote FW, Jr (1973). Metaplastic breast carcinoma. Rare form of mammary cancer. N Y State J Med 73: 1078–1082.
617. Hwang ES, Nyante SJ, Yi CY, Moore D, DeVries S, Korkola JE, Esserman LJ, Waldman FM (2004). Clonality of lobular carcinoma in situ and synchronous invasive lobular carcinoma. Cancer 100: 2562–2572.
618. IARC Working Group on the Evaluation of Carcinogenic Risks to Humans (2007). Combined estrogen-progestogen contraceptives and combined estrogen-progestogen menopausal therapy. IARC Monogr Eval Carcinog Risks Hum 91: 1–528.
619. Iaria G, Pisani F, De Luca L, Sforza D, Manuelli M, Perrone L, Bellini I, Angelico R, Tisone G (2010). Prospective study of switch from cyclosporine to tacrolimus for fibroadenomas of the breast in kidney transplantation. Transplant Proc 42: 1169–1170.
619A. Ichihara S, Fujimoto T, Hashimoto K, Moritani S, Hasegawa M, Yokoi T (2007). Double immunostaining with p63 and high-molecular-weight cytokeratins distinguishes borderline papillary lesions of the breast. Pathol Int 57: 126–132.

620. Imyanitov EN, Suspitsin EN, Grigoriev MY, Togo AV, Kuligina ES, Belogubova EV, Pozharisski KM, Turkevich EA, Rodriquez C, Cornelisse CJ, Hanson KP, Theillet C (2002). Concordance of allelic imbalance profiles in synchronous and metachronous bilateral breast carcinomas. Int J Cancer 100: 557–564.

621. Inaji H, Koyama H, Higashiyama M, Noguchi S, Yamamoto H, Ishikawa O, Omichi K, Iwanaga T, Wada A (1991). Immunohistochemical, ultrastructural and biochemical studies of an amylase-producing breast carcinoma. Virchows Arch A Pathol Anat Histopathol 419: 29–33.

622. International Agency for Research on Cancer (2002). Weight control and physical activity. IARC Handbooks of Cancer Prevention, Volume 6. IARC Press: Lyon.

623. Intra M, Rotmensz N, Viale G, Mariani L, Bonanni B, Mastropasqua MG, Galimberti V, Gennari R, Veronesi P, Colleoni M, Tousimis E, Galli A, Goldhirsch A, Veronesi U (2004). Clinicopathologic characteristics of 143 patients with synchronous bilateral invasive breast carcinomas treated in a single institution. Cancer 101: 905–912.

624. Iodice S, Barile M, Rotmensz N, Feroce I, Bonanni B, Radice P, Bernard L, Maisonneuve P, Gandini S (2010). Oral contraceptive use and breast or ovarian cancer risk in BRCA1/2 carriers: a meta-analysis. Eur J Cancer 46: 2275–2284.

625. Irvine T, Allen DS, Gillett C, Hamed H, Fentiman IS (2009). Prognosis of synchronous bilateral breast cancer. Br J Surg 96: 376–380.

626. Isaacson PG, Spencer J (1987). Malignant lymphoma of mucosa-associated lymphoid tissue. Histopathology 11: 445–462.

627. Iscovich J, Abdulrazik M, Cour C, Fischbein A, Pe'er J, Goldgar DE (2002). Prevalence of the BRCA2 6174 del T mutation in Israeli uveal melanoma patients. Int J Cancer 98: 42–44.

628. Itoh H, Miyajima Y, Kato N, Serizawa A, Machida T, Umemura S, Osamura RY (2010). Fine needle aspiration cytology of ductal adenoma of the breast with intracellular mucin: a report of three cases. Acta Cytol 54: 753–758.

629. Iwamoto T, Bianchini G, Booser D, Qi Y, Coutant C, Shiang CY, Santarpia L, Matsuoka J, Hortobagyi GN, Symmans WF, Holmes FA, O'Shaughnessy J, Hellerstedt B, Pippen J, Andre F, Simon R, Pusztai L (2011). Gene pathways associated with prognosis and chemotherapy sensitivity in molecular subtypes of breast cancer. J Natl Cancer Inst 103: 264–272.

630. Jackman RJ, Rodriguez-Soto J (2006). Breast microcalcifications: retrieval failure at prone stereotactic core and vacuum breast biopsy–frequency, causes, and outcome. Radiology 239: 61–70.

631. Jacobs TW, Byrne C, Colditz G, Connolly JL, Schnitt SJ (1999). Radial scars in benign breast-biopsy specimens and the risk of breast cancer. N Engl J Med 340: 430–436.

632. Jacobs TW, Chen YY, Guinee DG, Jr, Holden JA, Cha I, Bauermeister DE, Hashimoto B, Wolverton D, Hartzog G (2005). Fibroepithelial lesions with cellular stroma on breast core needle biopsy: are there predictors of outcome on surgical excision? Am J Clin Pathol 124: 342–354.

633. Jacobs TW, Pliss N, Kouria G, Schnitt SJ (2001). Carcinomas in situ of the breast with indeterminate features: role of E-cadherin staining in categorization. Am J Surg Pathol 25: 229–236.

634. Jacquemier J, Padovani L, Rabayrol L, Lakhani SR, Penault-Llorca F, Denoux Y, Fiche M, Figueiro P, Maisongrosse V, Ledoussal V, Martinez Penuela J, Udvarhely N, El Makdissi G, Ginestier C, Geneix J, Charafe-Jauffret E, Xerri L, Eisinger F, Birnbaum D, Sobol H (2005). Typical medullary breast carcinomas have a basal/myoepithelial phenotype. J Pathol 207: 260–268.

635. Jain RK, Mehta R, Dimitrov R, Larsson LG, Musto PM, Hodges KB, Ulbright TM, Hattab EM, Agaram N, Idrees MT, Badve S (2011). Atypical ductal hyperplasia: interobserver and intraobserver variability. Mod Pathol 24: 917–923.

636. Jain S, Fisher C, Smith P, Millis RR, Rubens RD (1993). Patterns of metastatic breast cancer in relation to histological type. Eur J Cancer 29A: 2155–2157.

637. James BA, Cranor ML, Rosen PP (1993). Carcinoma of the breast arising in microglandular adenosis. Am J Clin Pathol 100: 507–513.

638. James K, Bridger J, Anthony PP (1988). Breast tumour of pregnancy ('lactating' adenoma). J Pathol 156: 37–44.

639. James PA, Doherty R, Harris M, Mukesh BN, Milner A, Young MA, Scott C (2006). Optimal selection of individuals for BRCA mutation testing: a comparison of available methods. J Clin Oncol 24: 707–715.

640. Jamshed S, Farhan MI, Marshall MB, Nahabedian MY, Liu MC (2008). Fibromatosis of the breast after mammary prosthesis implantation. Clin Adv Hematol Oncol 6: 687–694.

641. Jansen L, Doting MH, Rutgers EJ, de Vries J, Olmos RA, Nieweg OE (2000). Clinical relevance of sentinel lymph nodes outside the axilla in patients with breast cancer. Br J Surg 87: 920–925.

642. Japaze H, Emina J, Diaz C, Schwam RJ, Gercovich N, Demonty G, Morgenfeld E, Rivarola E, Gil DE, Gercovich FG (2005). 'Pure' invasive apocrine carcinoma of the breast: a new clinicopathological entity? Breast 14: 3–10.

643. Jara-Lazaro AR, Akhilesh M, Thike AA, Lui PC, Tse GM, Tan PH (2010). Predictors of phyllodes tumours on core biopsy specimens of fibroepithelial neoplasms. Histopathology 57: 220–232.

644. Jara-Lazaro AR, Tan PH (2009). Molecular pathogenesis of progression and recurrence in breast phyllodes tumors. Am J Transl Res 1: 23–34.

645. Javid SH, Smith BL, Mayer E, Bellon J, Murphy CD, Lipsitz S, Golshan M (2009). Tubular carcinoma of the breast: results of a large contemporary series. Am J Surg 197: 674–677.

646. Jemal A, Siegel R, Ward E, Hao Y, Xu J, Thun MJ (2009). Cancer statistics, 2009. CA Cancer J Clin 59: 225–249.

647. Jemal A, Siegel R, Xu J, Ward E (2010). Cancer statistics, 2010. CA Cancer J Clin 60: 277–300.

648. Jensen RA, Page DL, Dupont WD, Rogers LW (1989). Invasive breast cancer risk in women with sclerosing adenosis. Cancer 64: 1977–1983.

649. Jensen UB, Sunde L, Timshel S, Halvarsson B, Nissen A, Bernstein I, Nilbert M (2010). Mismatch repair defective breast cancer in the hereditary nonpolyposis colorectal cancer syndrome. Breast Cancer Res Treat 120: 777–782.

650. Jeruss JS, Mittendorf EA, Tucker SL, Gonzalez-Angulo AM, Buchholz TA, Sahin AA, Cormier JN, Buzdar AU, Hortobagyi GN, Hunt KK (2008). Staging of breast cancer in the neoadjuvant setting. Cancer Res 68: 6477–6481.

651. Jeyaretna DS, Oriolowo A, Smith ME, Watkins RM (2007). Solitary neurofibroma in the male breast. World J Surg Oncol 5: 23. Abstract.

652. Jiao YF, Nakamura S, Oikawa T, Sugai T, Uesugi N (2001). Sebaceous gland metaplasia in intraductal papilloma of the breast. Virchows Arch 438: 505–508.

653. John BJ, Griffiths C, Ebbs SR (2007). Pleomorphic adenoma of the breast should be excised with a cuff of normal tissue. Breast J 13: 418–420.

654. Johnson NB, Collins LC (2009). Update on percutaneous needle biopsy of nonmalignant breast lesions. Adv Anat Pathol 16: 183–195.

655. Johnson RE, Murad MH (2009). Gynecomastia: pathophysiology, evaluation, and management. Mayo Clin Proc 84: 1010–1015.

656. Jones AM, Mitter R, Poulsom R, Gillett C, Hanby AM, Tomlinson IP, Sawyer EJ (2008). mRNA expression profiling of phyllodes tumours of the breast: identification of genes important in the development of borderline and malignant phyllodes tumours. J Pathol 216: 408–417.

657. Jones AM, Mitter R, Springall R, Graham T, Winter E, Gillett C, Hanby AM, Tomlinson IP, Sawyer EJ (2008). A comprehensive genetic profile of phyllodes tumours of the breast detects important mutations, intratumoral genetic heterogeneity and new genetic changes on recurrence. J Pathol 214: 533–544.

657A. Jones C, Damiani S, Wells D, Chaggar R, Lakhani SR, Eusebi V (2001). Molecular cytogenetic comparison of apocrine hyperplasia and apocrine carcinoma of the breast. Am J Pathol 158: 207–214.

658. Jones C, Merrett S, Thomas VA, Barker TH, Lakhani SR (2003). Comparative genomic hybridization analysis of bilateral hyperplasia of usual type of the breast. J Pathol 199: 152–156.

659. Jones C, Tooze R, Lakhani SR (2003). Malignant adenomyoepithelioma of the breast metastasizing to the liver. Virchows Arch 442: 504–506.

659A. Jones EL (1969). Primary squamous-cell carcinoma of breast with pseudosarcomatous stroma. J Pathol 97: 383–385.

660. Jones JL, Shaw JA, Pringle JH, Walker RA (2003). Primary breast myoepithelial cells exert an invasion-suppressor effect on breast cancer cells via paracrine down-regulation of MMP expression in fibroblasts and tumour cells. J Pathol 201: 562–572.

661. Jones KN, Glazebrook KN, Reynolds C (2010). Pseudoangiomatous stromal hyperplasia: imaging findings with pathologic and clinical correlation. AJR Am J Roentgenol 195: 1036–1042.

662. Jones MW, Norris HJ, Snyder RC (1989). Infiltrating syringomatous adenoma of the nipple. A clinical and pathological study of 11 cases. Am J Surg Pathol 13: 197–201.

662A. Jones MW, Norris HJ, Wargotz ES (1991). Hamartomas of the breast. Surg Gynecol Obstet 173: 54–56.

663. Jones MW, Tavassoli FA (1995). Coexistence of nipple duct adenoma and breast carcinoma: a clinicopathologic study of five cases and review of the literature. Mod Pathol 8: 633–636.

664. Jonsson G, Staaf J, Vallon-Christersson J, Ringner M, Holm K, Hegardt C, Gunnarsson H, Fagerholm R, Strand C, Agnarsson BA, Kilpivaara O, Luts L, Heikkila P, Aittomaki K, Blomqvist C, Loman N, Malmstrom P, Olsson H, Johannsson OT, Arason A et al. (2010). Genomic subtypes of breast cancer identified by array-comparative genomic hybridization display distinct molecular and clinical characteristics. Breast Cancer Res 12: R42

665. Joosse SA, Brandwijk KI, Devilee P, Wesseling J, Hogervorst FB, Verhoef S, Nederlof PM (2010). Prediction of BRCA2-association in hereditary breast carcinomas using array-CGH. Breast Cancer Res Treat

666. Joosse SA, Brandwijk KI, Mulder L, Wesseling J, Hannemann J, Nederlof PM (2011). Genomic signature of BRCA1 deficiency in sporadic basal-like breast tumors. Genes Chromosomes Cancer 50: 71–81.

667. Joosse SA, van Beers EH, Tielen IH, Horlings H, Peterse JL, Hoogerbrugge N, Ligtenberg MJ, Wessels LF, Axwijk P, Verhoef S, Hogervorst FB, Nederlof PM (2009). Prediction of BRCA1-association in hereditary non-BRCA1/2 breast carcinomas with array-CGH. Breast Cancer Res Treat 116: 479–489.

668. Jordan AC, Jaffer S, Mercer SE (2011). Massive nodular pseudoangiomatous stromal hyperplasia (PASH) of the breast arising simultaneously in the axilla and vulva. Int J Surg Pathol 19: 113–116.

668A. Joshi MG, Lee AK, Pedersen CA, Schnitt S, Camus MG, Hughes KS (1996). The role of immunocytochemical markers in the differential diagnosis of proliferative and neoplastic lesions of the breast. Mod Pathol 9: 57–62.

669. Jozefczyk MA, Rosen PP (1985). Vascular tumors of the breast. II. Perilobular hemangiomas and hemangiomas. Am J Surg Pathol 9: 491–503.

670. Julien M, Trojani M, Coindre JM (1994). [Myofibroblastoma of the breast. Report of 8 cases]. Ann Pathol 14: 143–147.

670A. Jung SY, Kim HY, Nam BH, Min SY, Lee SJ, Park C, Kwon Y, Kim EA, Ko KL, Shin KH, Lee KS, Park IH, Lee S, Kim SW, Kang HS, Ro J (2010). Worse prognosis of metaplastic breast cancer patients than other patients with triple-negative breast cancer. Breast Cancer Res Treat 120: 627–637.

671. Kabat GC, Cross AJ, Park Y, Schatzkin A, Hollenbeck AR, Rohan TE, Sinha R (2009). Meat intake and meat preparation in relation to risk of postmenopausal breast cancer in the NIH-AARP diet and health study. Int J Cancer 124: 2430–2435.

672. Kader HA, Jackson J, Mates D, Andersen S, Hayes M, Olivotto IA (2001). Tubular carcinoma of the breast: a population-based study of nodal metastases at presentation and of patterns of relapse. Breast J 7: 8–13.

673. Kahn R, Holtveg H, Nissen F, Holck S (2003). Are acinic cell carcinoma and microglandular carcinoma of the breast related lesions? Histopathology 42: 195–196.

674. Kalof AN, Tam D, Beatty B, Cooper K (2004). Immunostaining patterns of myoepithelial cells in breast lesions: a comparison of CD10 and smooth muscle myosin heavy chain. J Clin Pathol 57: 625–629.

675. Kambouchner M, Godmer P, Guillevin L, Raphael M, Droz D, Martin A (2003). Low grade marginal zone B cell lymphoma of the breast associated with localised amyloidosis and corpora amylacea in a woman with long standing primary Sjogren's syndrome. J Clin Pathol 56: 74–77.

676. Kamitani K, Kamitani T, Ono M,

Toyoshima S, Mitsuyama S (2011). Ultrasonographic findings of invasive micropapillary carcinoma of the breast: correlation between internal echogenicity and histological findings. Breast Cancer. In press.

676A. Kan Z, Jaiswal BS, Stinson J, Janakiraman V, Bhatt D, Stern HM, Yue P, Haverty PM, Bourgon R, Zheng J, Moorhead M, Chaudhuri S, Tomsho LP, Peters BA, Pujara K, Cordes S, Davis DP, Carlton VE, Yuan W, Li L et al. (2010). Diverse somatic mutation patterns and pathway alterations in human cancers. Nature 466: 869–873.

677. Kanaan N, Goffin E (2004). Multiple bilateral fibroadenomas of the breasts requiring mastectomy in a renal transplant patient. Clin Nephrol 61: 151–154.

678. Kanai Y, Oda T, Tsuda H, Ochiai A, Hirohashi S (1994). Point mutation of the E-cadherin gene in invasive lobular carcinoma of the breast. Jpn J Cancer Res 85: 1035–1039.

679. Karabagli P and Kilic H (2010). Primary pure signet cell carcinoma of the breast: a case report and review of the literature. Breast Cancer. In press.

679A. Karim RZ, Gerega SK, Yang YH, Spillane A, Carmalt H, Scolyer RA, Lee CS (2010). p16 and pRb immunohistochemical expression increases with increasing tumour grade in mammary phyllodes tumours. Histopathology 56: 868–875

679B. Kaufman MW, Marti JR, Gallager HS, Hoehn JL (1984). Carcinoma of the breast with pseudosarcomatous metaplasia. Cancer 53: 1908–1917.

680. Kaufmann O, Dietel M (2000). Expression of thyroid transcription factor-1 in pulmonary and extrapulmonary small cell carcinomas and other neuroendocrine carcinomas of various primary sites. Histopathology 36: 415–420.

681. Kazakov DV, Vanecek T, Belousova IE, Mukensnabl P, Kollertova D, Michal M (2007). Skin-type hidradenoma of the breast parenchyma with t(11;19) translocation: hidradenoma of the breast. Am J Dermatopathol 29: 457–461.

682. Kell MR, Burke JP, Barry M, Morrow M (2010). Outcome of axillary staging in early breast cancer: a meta-analysis. Breast Cancer Res Treat 120: 441–447.

683. Kennedy S, Merino MJ, Swain SM, Lippman ME (1990). The effects of hormonal and chemotherapy on tumoral and nonneoplastic breast tissue. Hum Pathol 21: 192–198.

684. Kerlikowske K, Barclay J, Grady D, Sickles EA, Ernster V (1997). Comparison of risk factors for ductal carcinoma in situ and invasive breast cancer. J Natl Cancer Inst 89: 76–82.

685. Kettritz U, Rotter K, Schreer I, Murauer M, Schulz-Wendtland R, Peter D, Heywang-Kobrunner SH (2004). Stereotactic vacuum-assisted breast biopsy in 2874 patients: a multicenter study. Cancer 100: 245–251.

686. Key T, Appleby P, Barnes I, Reeves G (2002). Endogenous sex hormones and breast cancer in postmenopausal women: reanalysis of nine prospective studies. J Natl Cancer Inst 94: 606–616.

686A. Khalifeh IM, Albarracin C, Diaz LK, Symmans FW, Edgerton ME, Hwang RF, Sneige N (2008). Clinical, histopathologic, and immunohistochemical features of microglandular adenosis and transition into in situ and invasive carcinoma. Am J Surg Pathol 32: 544–552.

687. Khanafshar E, Phillipson J, Schammel DP, Minobe L, Cymerman J, Weidner N (2005). Inflammatory myofibroblastic tumor of the breast. Ann Diagn Pathol 9: 123–129.

688. Khanna KK, Chenevix-Trench G (2004). ATM and genome maintenance: defining its role in breast cancer susceptibility. J Mammary Gland Biol Neoplasia 9: 247–262.

689. Kiaer H, Nielsen B, Paulsen S, Sorensen IM, Dyreborg U, Blichert-Toft M (1984). Adenomyoepithelial adenosis and low-grade malignant adenomyoepithelioma of the breast. Virchows Arch A Pathol Anat Histopathol 405: 55–67.

690. Kidwai N, Gong Y, Sun X, Deshpande CG, Yeldandi AV, Rao MS, Badve S (2004). Expression of androgen receptor and prostate-specific antigen in male breast carcinoma. Breast Cancer Res 6: R18–R23.

691. Kihara M, Yokomise H, Irie A, Kobayashi S, Kushida Y, Yamauchi A (2001). Malignant adenomyoepithelioma of the breast with lung metastases: report of a case. Surg Today 31: 899–903.

692. Kim BI (2010). Nanotribology and nanoindentation using advanced scanning probe techniques. Scanning 32: v–vi.

693. Kim MJ, Gong G, Joo HJ, Ahn SH, Ro JY (2005). Immunohistochemical and clinicopathologic characteristics of invasive ductal carcinoma of breast with micropapillary carcinoma component. Arch Pathol Lab Med 129: 1277–1282.

694. Kim SM, Kim HH, Shin HJ, Gong G, Ahn SH (2006). Cavernous haemangioma of the breast. Br J Radiol 79: e177–e180.

695. King MC, Marks JH, Mandell JB (2003). Breast and ovarian cancer risks due to inherited mutations in BRCA1 and BRCA2. Science 302: 643–646.

696. Kinkor Z (2002). [Myoepithelial carcinoma in adenomyoepithelioma of the breast (malignant adenomyoepithelioma)—case report]. Cesk Patol 38: 46–50.

697. Kinonen C, Gattuso P, Reddy VB (2010). Lupus mastitis: an uncommon complication of systemic or discoid lupus. Am J Surg Pathol 34: 901–906.

698. Kirova YM, Feuilhade F, Le Bourgeois JP (2002). Breast lipoma. Breast J 8: 117–118.

699. Klauber-DeMore N, Ollila DW, Moore DT, Livasy C, Calvo BF, Kim HJ, Dees EC, Sartor CI, Sawyer LR, Graham M, Carey LA (2006). Size of residual lymph node metastasis after neoadjuvant chemotherapy in locally advanced breast cancer patients is prognostic. Ann Surg Oncol 13: 685–691.

700. Kleer CG, Oberman HA (1998). Adenoid cystic carcinoma of the breast: value of histologic grading and proliferative activity. Am J Surg Pathol 22: 569–575.

701. Kleer CG, van Golen KL, Braun T, Merajver SD (2001). Persistent E-cadherin expression in inflammatory breast cancer. Mod Pathol 14: 458–464.

702. Kleer CG, Zhang Y, Pan Q, Merajver SD (2004). WISP3 (CCN6) is a secreted tumor-suppressor protein that modulates IGF signaling in inflammatory breast cancer. Neoplasia 6: 179–185.

703. Kleer CG, Zhang Y, Pan Q, van Golen KL, Wu ZF, Livant D, Merajver SD (2002). WISP3 is a novel tumor suppressor gene of inflammatory breast cancer. Oncogene 21: 3172–3180.

703A. Knauer M, Cardoso F, Wesseling J, Bedard PL, Linn SC, Rutgers EJ et al. (2010). Identification of a low-risk subgroup of HER-2-positive breast cancer by the 70-gene prognosis signature. Br J Cancer 103: 1788–1793.

703B. Kan Z, Jaiswal BS, Stinson J, Janakiraman V, Bhatt D, Stern HM, Yue P,

Haverty PM, Bourgon R, Zheng J, Moorhead M, Chaudhuri S, Tomsho LP, Peters BA, Pujara K, Cordes S, Davis DP, Carlton VE, Yuan W, Li L et al. (2010). Diverse somatic mutation patterns and pathway alterations in human cancers. Nature 466: 869–873.

704. Kocjan G, Bourgain C, Fassina A, Hagmar B, Herbert A, Kapila K, Kardum-Skelin I, Kloboves-Prevodnik V, Krishnamurthy S, Koutselini H, Majak B, Olszewski W, Onal B, Pohar-Marinsek Z, Shabalova I, Smith J, Tani E, Vielh P, Wiener H, Schenck U et al. (2008). The role of breast FNAC in diagnosis and clinical management: a survey of current practice. Cytopathology 19: 271–278.

705. Koenig C, Dadmanesh F, Bratthauer GL, Tavassoli FA (2000). Carcinoma arising in microglandular adenosis: an immunohistochemical analysis of 20 intraepithelial and invasive neoplasms. Int J Surg Pathol 8: 303–315.

706. Koerner F (2010). Papilloma and papillary carcinoma. Semin Diagn Pathol 27: 13–30.

707. Koker MM, Kleer CG (2004). p63 expression in breast cancer: a highly sensitive and specific marker of metaplastic carcinoma. Am J Surg Pathol 28: 1506–1512.

708. Kollias J, Elston CW, Ellis IO, Robertson JF, Blamey RW (1997). Early-onset breast cancer—histopathological and prognostic considerations. Br J Cancer 75: 1318–1323.

709. Kollmorgen DR, Varanasi JS, Edge SB, Carson WE, III (1998). Paget's disease of the breast: a 33-year experience. J Am Coll Surg 187: 171–177.

710. Kolodner RD, Hall NR, Lipford J, Kane MF, Morrison PT, Finan PJ, Burn J, Chapman P, Earabino C, Merchant E, . (1995). Structure of the human MLH1 locus and analysis of a large hereditary nonpolyposis colorectal carcinoma kindred for mlh1 mutations. Cancer Res 55: 242–248.

711. Kolodner RD, Hall NR, Lipford J, Kane MF, Rao MR, Morrison P, Wirth L, Finan PJ, Burn J, Chapman P (1994). Structure of the human MSH2 locus and analysis of two Muir-Torre kindreds for msh2 mutations. Genomics 24: 516–526.

712. Komaki K, Sakamoto G, Sugano H, Morimoto T, Monden Y (1988). Mucinous carcinoma of the breast in Japan. A prognostic analysis based on morphologic features. Cancer 61: 989–996.

713. Koninki K, Tanner M, Auvinen A, Isola J (2009). HER-2 positive breast cancer: decreasing proportion but stable incidence in Finnish population from 1982 to 2005. Breast Cancer Res. 11: R37. Abstract.

714. Koo JS, Jung W (2009). Xanthogranulomatous mastitis: clinicopathology and pathological implications. Pathol Int 59: 234–240.

715. Korde LA, Zujewski JA, Kamin L, Giordano S, Domchek S, Anderson WF, Bartlett JM, Gelmon K, Nahleh Z, Bergh J, Cutuli B, Pruneri G, Caskill-Stevens W, Gralow J, Hortobagyi G, Cardoso F (2010). Multidisciplinary meeting on male breast cancer: summary and research recommendations. J Clin Oncol 28: 2114–2122.

716. Korhonen T, Huhtala H, Holli K (2004). A comparison of the biological and clinical features of invasive lobular and ductal carcinomas of the breast. Breast Cancer Res Treat 85: 23–29.

717. Korkola JE, DeVries S, Fridlyand J, Hwang ES, Estep AL, Chen YY, Chew KL, Dairkee SH, Jensen RM, Waldman FM (2003). Differentiation of lobular versus ductal breast

carcinomas by expression microarray analysis. Cancer Res 63: 7167–7175.

718. Kothari AS, Beechey-Newman N, Hamed H, Fentiman IS, D'Arrigo C, Hanby AM, Ryder K (2002). Paget disease of the nipple: a multifocal manifestation of higher-risk disease. Cancer 95: 1–7.

719. Kovi J, Duong HD, Leffall LS, Jr (1981). High-grade mucoepidermoid carcinoma of the breast. Arch Pathol Lab Med 105: 612–614.

720. Koyama M, Kurotaki H, Yagihashi N, Aizawa S, Sugai M, Kamata Y, Oyama T, Yagihashi S (1997). Immunohistochemical assessment of proliferative activity in mammary adenomyoepithelioma. Histopathology 31: 134–139.

721. Krag DN, Anderson SJ, Julian TB, Brown AM, Harlow SP, Costantino JP, Ashikaga T, Weaver DL, Mamounas EP, Jalovec LM, Frazier TG, Noyes RD, Robidoux A, Scarth HM, Wolmark N (2010). Sentinel-lymph-node resection compared with conventional axillary-lymph-node dissection in clinically node-negative patients with breast cancer: overall survival findings from the NSABP B-32 randomised phase 3 trial. Lancet Oncol 11: 927–933.

722. Krausz T, Jenkins D, Grontoft O, Pollock DJ, Azzopardi JG (1989). Secretory carcinoma of the breast in adults: emphasis on late recurrence and metastasis. Histopathology 14: 25–36.

723. Krecke KN, Gisvold JJ (1993). Invasive lobular carcinoma of the breast: mammographic findings and extent of disease at diagnosis in 184 patients. AJR Am J Roentgenol 161: 957–960.

724. Kryvenko ON, Chitale DA, VanEgmond EM, Gupta NS, Schultz D, Lee MW (2011). Angiolipoma of the female breast: clinicomorphological correlation of 52 cases. Int J Surg Pathol 19: 35–43.

725. Kubota K, Ogawa Y, Nishioka A, Murata Y, Itoh S, Hamada N, Morio K, Maeda H, Tanaka Y (2008). Radiological imaging features of invasive micropapillary carcinoma of the breast and axillary lymph nodes. Oncol Rep 20: 1143–1147.

726. Kuerer HM, Newman LA, Buzdar AU, Hunt KK, Dhingra K, Buchholz TA, Binkley SM, Ames FC, Feig BW, Ross MI, Hortobagyi GN, Singletary SE (1998). Residual metastatic axillary lymph nodes following neoadjuvant chemotherapy predict disease-free survival in patients with locally advanced breast cancer. Am J Surg 176: 502–509.

727. Kuerer HM, Newman LA, Smith TL, Ames FC, Hunt KK, Dhingra K, Theriault RL, Singh G, Binkley SM, Sneige N, Buchholz TA, Ross MI, McNeese MD, Buzdar AU, Hortobagyi GN, Singletary SE (1999). Clinical course of breast cancer patients with complete pathologic primary tumor and axillary lymph node response to doxorubicin-based neoadjuvant chemotherapy. J Clin Oncol 17: 460–469.

728. Kuhl CK, Schrading S, Bieling HB, Wardelmann E, Leutner CC, Koenig R, Kuhn W, Schild HH (2007). MRI for diagnosis of pure ductal carcinoma in situ: a prospective observational study. Lancet 370: 485–492.

729. Kuijper A, Buerger H, Simon R, Schaefer KL, Croonen A, Boecker W, van der Wall E, van Diest PJ (2002). Analysis of the progression of fibroepithelial tumours of the breast by PCR-based clonality assay. J Pathol 197: 575–581.

730. Kuijper A, Mommers EC, van der Wall E, van Diest PJ (2001). Histopathology of

fibroadenoma of the breast. Am J Clin Pathol 115: 736–742.
730A. Kumar R, Neilsen PM, Crawford J, McKirdy R, Lee J, Powell JA, Saif Z, Martin JM, Lombaerts M, Cornelisse CJ, Cleton-Jansen AM, Callen DF (2005). FBXO31 is the chromosome 16q24.3 senescence gene, a candidate breast tumor suppressor, and a component of an SCF complex. Cancer Res 65: 11304–11313.
731. Kurebayashi J, Izuo M, Ishida T, Kurosumi M, Kawai T (1988). Two cases of lipid-secreting carcinoma of the breast: case reports with an electron microscopic study. Jpn J Clin Oncol 18: 249–254.
732. Kurian AW, McClure LA, John EM, Horn-Ross PL, Ford JM, Clarke CA (2009). Second primary breast cancer occurrence according to hormone receptor status. J Natl Cancer Inst 101: 1058–1065.
733. Kuroda H, Sakamoto G, Ohnisi K, Itoyama S (2004). Overexpression of Her2/neu, estrogen and progesterone receptors in invasive micropapillary carcinoma of the breast. Breast Cancer 11: 301–306.
734. Kuroda H, Tamaru J, Sakamoto G, Ohnisi K, Itoyama S (2005). Immunophenotype of lymphocytic infiltration in medullary carcinoma of the breast. Virchows Arch 446: 10–14.
735. Kurokawa K, Mouri Y, Asano A, Kamei K, Iwata Y, Isogai M, Saga S, Ichihara S (2009). Pleomorphic carcinoma with osteoclastic giant cells of the breast: immunohistochemical differentiation between coexisting neoplastic and reactive giant cells. Pathol Int 59: 91–97.
736. La Vecchia C, Parazzini F, Franceschi S, Decarli A (1985). Risk factors for benign breast disease and their relation with breast cancer risk. Pooled information from epidemiologic studies. Tumori 71: 167–178.
737. Lack EE, Worsham GF, Callihan MD, Crawford BE, Klappenbach S, Rowden G, Chun B (1980). Granular cell tumor: a clinicopathologic study of 110 patients. J Surg Oncol 13: 301–316.
738. Lacroix-Triki M, Geyer FC, Lambros MB, Savage K, Ellis IO, Lee AH, Reis-Filho JS (2010). Beta-catenin/Wnt signalling pathway in fibromatosis, metaplastic carcinomas and phyllodes tumours of the breast. Mod Pathol 23: 1438–1448.
739. Lacroix-Triki M, Suarez PH, Mackay A, Lambros MB, Natrajan R, Savage K, Geyer FC, Weigelt B, Ashworth A, Reis-Filho JS (2010). Mucinous carcinoma of the breast is genomically distinct from invasive ductal carcinomas of no special type. J Pathol 222: 282–298.
740. Lae M, Freneaux P, Sastre-Garau X, Chouchane O, Sigal-Zafrani B, Vincent-Salomon A (2009). Secretory breast carcinomas with ETV6-NTRK3 fusion gene belong to the basal-like carcinoma spectrum. Mod Pathol 22: 291–298.
741. Lae M, Vincent-Salomon A, Savignoni A, Huon I, Freneaux P, Sigal-Zafrani B, Aurias A, Sastre-Garau X, Couturier J (2007). Phyllodes tumors of the breast segregate in two groups according to genetic criteria. Mod Pathol 20: 435–444.
742. Lakhani SR (1999). The transition from hyperplasia to invasive carcinoma of the breast. J Pathol 187: 272–278.
743. Lakhani SR, Chaggar R, Davies S, Jones C, Collins N, Odel C, Stratton MR, O'Hare MJ (1999). Genetic alterations in 'normal' luminal and myoepithelial cells of the breast. J Pathol 189: 496–503.
744. Lakhani SR, Collins N, Sloane JP, Stratton MR (1995). Loss of heterozygosity in lobular carcinoma in situ of the breast. Clin Mol Pathol 48: M74–M78.
745. Lakhani SR, Collins N, Stratton MR, Sloane JP (1995). Atypical ductal hyperplasia of the breast: clonal proliferation with loss of heterozygosity on chromosomes 16q and 17p. J Clin Pathol 48: 611–615.
746. Lakhani SR, Gusterson BA, Jacquemier J, Sloane JP, Anderson TJ, Van de Vijver, MJ, Venter D, Freeman A, Antoniou A, McGuffog L, Smyth E, Steel CM, Haites N, Scott RJ, Goldgar D, Neuhausen S, Daly PA, Ormiston W, McManus R, Scherneck S et al. (2000). The pathology of familial breast cancer: histological features of cancers in families not attributable to mutations in BRCA1 or BRCA2. Clin Cancer Res 6: 782–789.
747. Lakhani SR, Jacquemier J, Sloane JP, Gusterson BA, Anderson TJ, Van de Vijver M, Farid LM, Venter D, Antoniou A, Storfer-Isser A, Smyth E, Steel CM, Haites N, Scott RJ, Goldgar D, Neuhausen S, Daly PA, Ormiston W, McManus R, Scherneck S et al. (1998). Multifactorial analysis of differences between sporadic breast cancers and cancers involving BRCA1 and BRCA2 mutations. J Natl Cancer Inst 90: 1138–1145.
748. Lakhani SR, O'Hare MJ (2001). The mammary myoepithelial cell—Cinderella or ugly sister? Breast Cancer Res 3: 1–4.
749. Lakhani SR, O'Hare MJ, Monaghan P, Winehouse J, Gazet JC, Sloane JP (1995). Malignant myoepithelioma (myoepithelial carcinoma) of the breast: a detailed cytokeratin study. J Clin Pathol 48: 164–167.
750. Lakhani SR, Reis-Filho JS, Fulford L, Penault-Llorca F, van der Vijver M, Parry S, Bishop T, Benitez J, Rivas C, Bignon YJ, Chang-Claude J, Hamann U, Cornelisse CJ, Devilee P, Beckmann MW, Nestle-Kramling C, Daly PA, Haites N, Varley J, Lalloo F et al. (2005). Prediction of BRCA1 status in patients with breast cancer using estrogen receptor and basal phenotype. Clin Cancer Res 11: 5175–5180.
751. Lakhani SR, Slack DN, Hamoudi RA, Collins N, Stratton MR, Sloane JP (1996). Detection of allelic imbalance indicates that a proportion of mammary hyperplasia of usual type are clonal, neoplastic proliferations. Lab Invest 74: 129–135.
752. Lakhani SR, Van de Vijver MJ, Jacquemier J, Anderson TJ, Osin PP, McGuffog L, Easton DF (2002). The pathology of familial breast cancer: predictive value of immunohistochemical markers estrogen receptor, progesterone receptor, HER-2, and p53 in patients with mutations in BRCA1 and BRCA2. J Clin Oncol 20: 2310–2318.
753. Lalloo F, Varley J, Ellis D, Moran A, O'Dair L, Pharoah P, Evans DG (2003). Prediction of pathogenic mutations in patients with early-onset breast cancer by family history. Lancet 361: 1101–1102.
754. Lalloo F, Varley J, Moran A, Ellis D, O'Dair L, Pharoah P, Antoniou A, Hartley R, Shenton A, Seal S, Bulman B, Howell A, Evans DG (2006). BRCA1, BRCA2 and TP53 mutations in very early-onset breast cancer with associated risks to relatives. Eur J Cancer 42: 1143–1150.
755. Lammens CR, Aaronson NK, Wagner A, Sijmons RH, Ausems MG, Vriends AH, Ruijs MW, van Os TA, Spruijt L, Gomez Garcia EB, Kluijt I, Nagtegaal T, Verhoef S, Bleiker EM (2010). Genetic testing in Li-Fraumeni syndrome: uptake and psychosocial consequences. J Clin Oncol 28: 3008–3014.
756. Lammie GA, Millis RR (1989). Ductal adenoma of the breast—a review of fifteen cases. Hum Pathol 20: 903–908.
757. Lamovec J, Bracko M (1991). Metastatic pattern of infiltrating lobular carcinoma of the breast: an autopsy study. J Surg Oncol 48: 28–33.
758. Lamovec J, Us-Krasovec M, Zidar A, Kljun A (1989). Adenoid cystic carcinoma of the breast: a histologic, cytologic, and immunohistochemical study. Semin Diagn Pathol 6: 153–164.
759. Lanng C, Eriksen BO, Hoffmann J (2004). Lipoma of the breast: a diagnostic dilemma. Breast 13: 408–411.
760. Lapey JD (1977). Lipid-rich mammary carcinoma — diagnosis by cytology. Case report. Acta Cytol 21: 120–122.
761. Lazard D, Sastre X, Frid MG, Glukhova MA, Thiery JP, Koteliansky VE (1993). Expression of smooth muscle-specific proteins in myoepithelium and stromal myofibroblasts of normal and malignant human breast tissue. Proc Natl Acad Sci U S A 90: 999–1003.
762. Le Calvez-Kelm F, Lesueur F, Damiola F, Vallee M, Voegele C, Babikyan D, Durand G, Forey N, McKay-Chopin S, Robinot N, Nguyen-Dumont T, Thomas A, Byrnes GB, Hopper JL, Southey MC, Andrulis IL, John EM, Tavtigian SV (18-1-2011). Rare, evolutionarily unlikely missense substitutions in CHEK2 contribute to breast cancer susceptibility: results from a breast cancer family registry case-control mutation-screening study. Breast Cancer Res. 13: R6. Abstract.
763. Le BH, Boyer PJ, Lewis JE, Kapadia SB (2004). Granular cell tumor: immunohistochemical assessment of inhibin-alpha, protein gene product 9.5, S100 protein, CD68, and Ki-67 proliferative index with clinical correlation. Arch Pathol Lab Med 128: 771–775.
764. Le GM, Ollivier L, Asselain B, Meunier M, Laurent M, Vielh P, Neuenschwander S (1992). Mammographic features of 455 invasive lobular carcinomas. Radiology 185: 705–708.
765. Le ML, Kolonel LN, Earle ME, Mi MP (1988). Body size at different periods of life and breast cancer risk. Am J Epidemiol 128: 137–152.
766. Leach FS, Nicolaides NC, Papadopoulos N, Liu B, Jen J, Parsons R, Peltomaki P, Sistonen P, Aaltonen LA, Nystrom-Lahti M (1993). Mutations of a mutS homolog in hereditary nonpolyposis colorectal cancer. Cell 75: 1215–1225.
767. Leal C, Costa I, Fonseca D, Lopes P, Bento MJ, Lopes C (1998). Intracystic (encysted) papillary carcinoma of the breast: a clinical, pathological, and immunohistochemical study. Hum Pathol 29: 1097–1104.
768. Leal C, Henrique R, Monteiro P, Lopes C, Bento MJ, De Sousa CP, Lopes P, Olson S, Silva MD, Page DL (2001). Apocrine ductal carcinoma in situ of the breast: histologic classification and expression of biologic markers. Hum Pathol 32: 487–493.
769. Lee AH (2007). The histological diagnosis of metastases to the breast from extramammary malignancies. J Clin Pathol 60: 1333–1341.
770. Lee AH (2008). Recent developments in the histological diagnosis of spindle cell carcinoma, fibromatosis and phyllodes tumour of the breast. Histopathology 52: 45–57.
771. Lee AH, Hodi Z, Ellis IO, Elston CW (2007). Histological features useful in the distinction of phyllodes tumour and fibroadenoma on needle core biopsy of the breast. Histopathology 51: 336–344.
772. Lee AH, Pinder SE, Macmillan RD, Mitchell M, Ellis IO, Elston CW, Blamey RW (2006). Prognostic value of lymphovascular invasion in women with lymph node negative invasive breast carcinoma. Eur J Cancer 42: 357–362.
773. Lee E, Ma H, Kean-Cowdin R, Van Den Berg D, Bernstein L, Henderson BE, Ursin G (2008). Effect of reproductive factors and oral contraceptives on breast cancer risk in BRCA1/2 mutation carriers and noncarriers: results from a population-based study. Cancer Epidemiol Biomarkers Prev 17: 3170–3178.
774. Lee EK, Kook SH, Kwag HJ, Park YL, Bae WG (2006). Schwannoma of the breast showing massive exophytic growth: a case report. Breast 15: 562–566.
775. Lee JO, Yang H, Georgescu MM, Di CA, Maehama T, Shi Y, Dixon JE, Pandolfi P, Pavletich NP (1999). Crystal structure of the PTEN tumor suppressor: implications for its phosphoinositide phosphatase activity and membrane association. Cell 99: 323–334.
776. Lee SH, Park JM, Kook SH, Han BK, Moon WK (2000). Metastatic tumors to the breast: mammographic and ultrasonographic findings. J Ultrasound Med 19: 257–262.
777. Lee SK, Kim WW, Kim SH, Hur SM, Kim S, Choi JH, Cho EY, Han SY, Hahn BK, Choe JH, Kim JH, Kim JS, Lee JE, Nam SJ, Yang JH (2010). Characteristics of metastasis in the breast from extramammary malignancies. J Surg Oncol 101: 137–140.
778. Lefkowitz M, Lefkowitz W, Wargotz ES (1994). Intraductal (intracystic) papillary carcinoma of the breast and its variants: a clinicopathological study of 77 cases. Hum Pathol 25: 802–809.
779. Leibl S, Regitnig P, Moinfar F (2007). Flat epithelial atypia (DIN 1a, atypical columnar change): an underdiagnosed entity very frequently coexisting with lobular neoplasia. Histopathology 50: 859–865.
780. Leikola J, Heikkila P, von Smitten K, Leidenius M (2006). The prevalence of axillary lymph-node metastases in patients with pure tubular carcinoma of the breast and sentinel node biopsy. Eur J Surg Oncol 32: 488–491.
781. Lempiainen H, Halazonetis TD (2009). Emerging common themes in regulation of PIKKs and PI3Ks. EMBO J 28: 3067–3073.
782. Leonard GD, Swain SM (2004). Ductal carcinoma in situ, complexities and challenges. J Natl Cancer Inst 96: 906–920.
783. Leong AS, Williams JA (1985). Mucoepidermoid carcinoma of the breast: high grade variant. Pathology 17: 516–521.
784. Lerwill MF (2004). Current practical applications of diagnostic immunohistochemistry in breast pathology. Am J Surg Pathol 28: 1076–1091.
785. Lesser ML, Rosen PP, Kinne DW (1982). Multicentricity and bilaterality in invasive breast carcinoma. Surgery 91: 234–240.
785A. Lester SC, Bose S, Chen YY, Connolly JL, de Baca ME, Fitzgibbons PL, Hayes DF, Kleer C, O'Malley FP, Page DL, Smith BL, Weaver DL, Winer E (2009). Protocol for the examination of specimens from patients with ductal carcinoma in situ of the breast. Arch Pathol Lab Med 133: 15–25.
786. Levrero M, De Laurenzi V, Costanzo A, Gong J, Wang JY, Melino G (2000). The p53/p63/p73 family of transcription factors: overlapping and distinct functions. J Cell Sci 113 (Pt 10): 1661–1670.

787. Lewis JT, Hartmann LC, Vierkant RA, Maloney SD, Shane Pankratz V, Allers TM, Frost MH, Visscher DW (2006). An analysis of breast cancer risk in women with single, multiple, and atypical papilloma. Am J Surg Pathol 30: 665–672.
788. Li CI, Anderson BO, Daling JR, Moe RE (2002). Changing incidence of lobular carcinoma in situ of the breast. Breast Cancer Res Treat 75: 259–268.
789. Li CI, Anderson BO, Daling JR, Moe RE (2003). Trends in incidence rates of invasive lobular and ductal breast carcinoma. JAMA 289: 1421–1424.
790. Li CI, Anderson BO, Porter P, Holt SK, Daling JR, Moe RE (2000). Changing incidence rate of invasive lobular breast carcinoma among older women. Cancer 88: 2561–2569.
791. Li CI, Chlebowski RT, Freiberg M, Johnson KC, Kuller L, Lane D, Lessin L, O'Sullivan MJ, Wactawski-Wende J, Yasmeen S, Prentice R (2010). Alcohol consumption and risk of postmenopausal breast cancer by subtype: the women's health initiative observational study. J Natl Cancer Inst 102: 1422–1431.
792. Li CI, Daling JR, Malone KE (2005). Age-specific incidence rates of in situ breast carcinomas by histologic type, 1980 to 2001. Cancer Epidemiol Biomarkers Prev 14: 1008–1011.
793. Li CI, Daling JR, Malone KE, Bernstein L, Marchbanks PA, Liff JM, Strom BL, Simon MS, Press MF, McDonald JA, Ursin G, Burkman RT, Deapen D, Spirtas R (2006). Relationship between established breast cancer risk factors and risk of seven different histologic types of invasive breast cancer. Cancer Epidemiol Biomarkers Prev 15: 946–954.
794. Li CI, Malone KE, Daling JR, Potter JD, Bernstein L, Marchbanks PA, Strom BL, Simon MS, Press MF, Ursin G, Burkman RT, Folger SG, Norman S, McDonald JA, Spirtas R (2008). Timing of menarche and first full-term birth in relation to breast cancer risk. Am J Epidemiol 167: 230–239.
795. Li CI, Uribe DJ, Daling JR (2005). Clinical characteristics of different histologic types of breast cancer. Br J Cancer 93: 1046–1052.
796. Li CI, Weiss NS, Stanford JL, Daling JR (2000). Hormone replacement therapy in relation to risk of lobular and ductal breast carcinoma in middle-aged women. Cancer 88: 2570–2577.
797. Li DM, Sun H (1997). TEP1, encoded by a candidate tumor suppressor locus, is a novel protein tyrosine phosphatase regulated by transforming growth factor beta. Cancer Res 57: 2124–2129.
798. Li FP, Fraumeni JF, Jr, Mulvihill JJ, Blattner WA, Dreyfus MG, Tucker MA, Miller RW (1988). A cancer family syndrome in twenty-four kindreds. Cancer Res 48: 5358–5362.
799. Li J, Yen C, Liaw D, Podsypanina K, Bose S, Wang SI, Puc J, Miliaresis C, Rodgers L, McCombie R, Bigner SH, Giovanella BC, Ittmann M, Tycko B, Hibshoosh H, Wigler MH, Parsons R (1997). PTEN, a putative protein tyrosine phosphatase gene mutated in human brain, breast, and prostate cancer. Science 275: 1943–1947.
800. Li M, Cordon-Cardo C, Gerald WL, Rosai J (1996). Desmoid fibromatosis is a clonal process. Hum Pathol 27: 939–943.
801. Li S, Lee AK (2009). Silicone implant and primary breast ALK1-negative anaplastic large cell lymphoma, fact or fiction? Int J Clin Exp Pathol 3: 117–127.
802. Li YS, Kaneko M, Amatya VJ, Takeshima Y, Arihiro K, Inai K (2006). Expression of vascular endothelial growth factor-C and its receptor in invasive micropapillary carcinoma of the breast. Pathol Int 56: 256–261.
803. Lian D, Cheah E, Tan PH, Thng CH, Tan SM (2007). Phyllodes tumour with intraductal growth: a rare cause of nipple discharge. Histopathology 50: 666–669.
804. Liaw D, Marsh DJ, Li J, Dahia PL, Wang SI, Zheng Z, Bose S, Call KM, Tsou HC, Peacocke M, Eng C, Parsons R (1997). Germline mutations of the PTEN gene in Cowden disease, an inherited breast and thyroid cancer syndrome. Nat Genet 16: 64–67.
805. Liberman L (2000). Centennial dissertation. Percutaneous imaging-guided core breast biopsy: state of the art at the millennium. AJR Am J Roentgenol 174: 1191–1199.
806. Liberman L, Giess CS, Dershaw DD, Louie DC, Deutch BM (1994). Non-Hodgkin lymphoma of the breast: imaging characteristics and correlation with histopathologic findings. Radiology 192: 157–160.
806A. Lien HC, Hsiao YH, Lin YS, Yao YT, Juan HF, Kuo WH, Hung MC, Chang KJ, Hsieh FJ (2007). Molecular signatures of metaplastic carcinoma of the breast by large-scale transcriptional profiling: identification of genes potentially related to epithelial-mesenchymal transition. Oncogene 26: 7859–7871.
806B. Lien HC, Lin CW, Mao TL, Kuo SH, Hsiao CH, Huang CS (2004). p53 overexpression and mutation in metaplastic carcinoma of the breast: genetic evidence for a monoclonal origin of both the carcinomatous and the heterogeneous sarcomatous components. J Pathol 204: 131–139.
807. Ligtenberg MJ, Kuiper RP, Chan TL, Goossens M, Hebeda KM, Voorendt M, Lee TY, Bodmer D, Hoenselaar E, Hendriks-Cornelissen SJ, Tsui WY, Kong CK, Brunner HG, van Kessel AG, Yuen ST, van Krieken JH, Leung SY, Hoogerbrugge N (2009). Heritable somatic methylation and inactivation of MSH2 in families with Lynch syndrome due to deletion of the 3' exons of TACSTD1. Nat Genet 41: 112–117.
808. Lim YT (1991). Cardiac magnetic resonance imaging. Singapore Med J 32: 296–298.
809. Lim-Co RY, Gisser SD (1978). Unusual variant of lipid-rich mammary carcinoma. Arch Pathol Lab Med 102: 193–195.
810. Limacher JM, Frebourg T, Natarajan-Ame S, Bergerat JP (2001). Two metachronous tumors in the radiotherapy fields of a patient with Li-Fraumeni syndrome. Int J Cancer 96: 238–242.
811. Linardic CM (2008). PAX3-FOXO1 fusion gene in rhabdomyosarcoma. Cancer Lett 270: 10–18.
812. Linda A, Machin P, Bazzocchi M, Zuiani C (2008). Painful schwannoma of the breast completely removed by a vacuum-assisted device with symptom resolution. Breast J 14: 496–497.
813. Lindblom A, Tannergard P, Werelius B, Nordenskjold M (1993). Genetic mapping of a second locus predisposing to hereditary non-polyposis colon cancer. Nat Genet 5: 279–282.
814. Linell F, Ljungberg O, Andersson I (1980). Breast carcinoma. Aspects of early stages, progression and related problems. Acta Pathol Microbiol Scand Suppl 1–233.
815. Lininger RA, Park WS, Man YG, Pham T, MacGrogan G, Zhuang Z, Tavassoli FA (1998). LOH at 16p13 is a novel chromosomal alteration detected in benign and malignant microdissected papillary neoplasms of the breast. Hum Pathol 29: 1113–1118.
816. Lipkin SM, Wang V, Jacoby R, Banerjee-Basu S, Baxevanis AD, Lynch HT, Elliott RM, Collins FS (2000). MLH3: a DNA mismatch repair gene associated with mammalian microsatellite instability. Nat Genet 24: 27–35.
817. Liu B, Nicolaides NC, Markowitz S, Willson JK, Parsons RE, Jen J, Papadopolous N, Peltomaki P, de la Chapelle A, Hamilton SR (1995). Mismatch repair gene defects in sporadic colorectal cancers with microsatellite instability. Nat Genet 9: 48–55.
817A. Liu B, Parsons R, Papadopoulos N, Nicolaides NC, Lynch HT, Watson P, Jass JR, Dunlop M, Wyllie A, Peltomaki P, de la CA, Hamilton SR, Vogelstein B, Kinzler KW (1996). Analysis of mismatch repair genes in hereditary non-polyposis colorectal cancer patients. Nat Med 2: 169–174.
818. Liu B, Parsons RE, Hamilton SR, Petersen GM, Lynch HT, Watson P, Markowitz S, Willson JK, Green J, de la Chapelle A (1994). hMSH2 mutations in hereditary non-polyposis colorectal cancer kindreds. Cancer Res 54: 4590–4594.
819. Liu F, Lang R, Wei J, Fan Y, Cui L, Gu F, Guo X, Pringle GA, Zhang X, Fu L (2009). Increased expression of SDF-1/CXCR4 is associated with lymph node metastasis of invasive micropapillary carcinoma of the breast. Histopathology 54: 741–750.
820. Liu GF, Yang Q, Haffty BG, Moran MS (2009). Clinical-pathologic features and long-term outcomes of tubular carcinoma of the breast compared with invasive ductal carcinoma treated with breast conservation therapy. Int J Radiat Oncol Biol Phys 75: 1304–1308.
821. Liu H, Tan H, Cheng Y, Zhang X, Gu Y, Peng W (2010). Imaging findings in mucinous breast carcinoma and correlating factors. Eur J Radiol 80: 706–712.
822. Lobo GP, Waite KA, Planchon SM, Romigh T, Houghton JA, Eng C (2008). ATP modulates PTEN subcellular localization in multiple cancer cell lines. Hum Mol Genet 17: 2877–2885.
823. Lobo GP, Waite KA, Planchon SM, Romigh T, Nassif NT, Eng C (2009). Germline and somatic cancer-associated mutations in the ATP-binding motifs of PTEN influence its subcellular localization and tumor suppressive function. Hum Mol Genet 18: 2851–2862.
824. Lomoschitz FM, Helbich TH, Rudas M, Pfarl G, Linnau KF, Stadler A, Jackman RJ (2004). Stereotactic 11-gauge vacuum-assisted breast biopsy: influence of number of specimens on diagnostic accuracy. Radiology 232: 897–903.
825. London SJ, Connolly JL, Schnitt SJ, Colditz GA (1992). A prospective study of benign breast disease and the risk of breast cancer. JAMA 267: 941–944.
826. Longy M, Lacombe D (1996). Cowden disease. Report of a family and review. Ann Genet 39: 35–42.
827. Loo LW, Grove DI, Williams EM, Neal CL, Cousens LA, Schubert EL, Holcomb IN, Massa HF, Glogovac J, Li CI, Malone KE, Daling JR, Delrow JJ, Trask BJ, Hsu L, Porter PL (2004). Array comparative genomic hybridization analysis of genomic alterations in breast cancer subtypes. Cancer Res 64: 8541–8549.
828. Loof-Johanson M, Brudin L, Sundquist M, Thorstenson S, Rudebeck CE (2010). Breastfeeding and prognostic markers in breast cancer. Breast 20: 170–175.
829. Loose JH, Patchefsky AS, Hollander IJ, Lavin LS, Cooper HS, Katz SM (1992). Adenomyoepithelioma of the breast. A spectrum of biologic behavior. Am J Surg Pathol 16: 868–876.
830. Lopez-Garcia MA, Geyer FC, Lacroix-Triki M, Marchio C, Reis-Filho JS (2010). Breast cancer precursors revisited: molecular features and progression pathways. Histopathology 57: 171–192.
831. Lopez-Garcia MA, Geyer FC, Natrajan R, Kreike B, Mackay A, Grigoriadis A, Reis-Filho JS, Weigelt B (2010). Transcriptomic analysis of tubular carcinomas of the breast reveals similarities and differences with molecular subtype-matched ductal and lobular carcinomas. J Pathol 222: 64–75.
832. Louwman MW, Vriezen M, van Beek MW, Nolthenius-Puylaert MC, van der Sangen MJ, Roumen RM, Kiemeney LA, Coebergh JW (2007). Uncommon breast tumors in perspective: incidence, treatment and survival in the Netherlands. Int J Cancer 121: 127–135.
833. Loveday C, Turnbull C, Ramsay E, Hughes D, Ruark E, Frankum JR, Bowden G, Kalmyrzaev B, Warren-Perry M, Snape K, Adlard JW, Barwell J, Berg J, Brady AF, Brewer C, Brice G, Chapman C, Cook J, Davidson R, Donaldson A et al. (2011). Germline mutations in RAD51D confer susceptibility to ovarian cancer. Nat Genet 43: 879–882.
834. Lu X, Lu X, Wang ZC, Iglehart JD, Zhang X, Richardson AL (2008). Predicting features of breast cancer with gene expression patterns. Breast Cancer Res Treat 108: 191–201.
835. Lu YJ, Osin P, Lakhani SR, Di PS, Gusterson BA, Shipley JM (1998). Comparative genomic hybridization analysis of lobular carcinoma in situ and atypical lobular hyperplasia and potential roles for gains and losses of genetic material in breast neoplasia. Cancer Res 58: 4721–4727.
836. Lucas FV, Perez-Mesa C (1978). Inflammatory carcinoma of the breast. Cancer 41: 1595–1605.
836A. Luini A, Aguilar M, Gatti G, Fasani R, Botteri E, Brito JA, Maisonneuve P, Vento AR, Viale G (2007). Metaplastic carcinoma of the breast, an unusual disease with worse prognosis: the experience of the European Institute of Oncology and review of the literature. Breast Cancer Res Treat 101: 349–353.
837. Luna-More S, Casquero S, Perez-Mellado A, Rius F, Weill B, Gornemann I (2000). Importance of estrogen receptors for the behavior of invasive micropapillary carcinoma of the breast. Review of 68 cases with follow-up of 54. Pathol Res Pract 196: 35–39.
838. Luna-More S, de los SF, Breton JJ, Canadas MA (1996). Estrogen and progesterone receptors, c-erbB-2, p53, and Bcl-2 in thirty-three invasive micropapillary breast carcinomas. Pathol Res Pract 192: 27–32.
838A. Lusa L, McShane LM, Reid JF, de Cecco L, Ambrogi F, Biganzoli E et al. (2007). Challenges in projecting clustering results across gene expression-profiling datasets. J Natl Cancer Inst 99: 1715–1723.
839. Lyman GH, Giuliano AE, Somerfield MR, Benson AB, III, Bodurka DC, Burstein HJ, Cochran AJ, Cody HS, III, Edge SB, Galper S, Hayman JA, Kim TY, Perkins CL, Podoloff DA, Sivasubramaniam VH, Turner RR, Wahl R, Weaver DL, Wolff AC, Winer EP (2005). American Society of Clinical Oncology guide-

line recommendations for sentinel lymph node biopsy in early-stage breast cancer. J Clin Oncol 23: 7703–7720.

840. Ma CX, Sanchez CG, Ellis MJ (2009). Predicting endocrine therapy responsiveness in breast cancer. Oncology (Williston Park) 23: 133–142.

841. Ma H, Wang Y, Sullivan-Halley J, Weiss L, Marchbanks PA, Spirtas R, Ursin G, Burkman RT, Simon MS, Malone KE, Strom BL, McDonald JA, Press MF, Bernstein L (2010). Use of four biomarkers to evaluate the risk of breast cancer subtypes in the women's contraceptive and reproductive experiences study. Cancer Res 70: 575–587.

842. Ma XJ, Dahiya S, Richardson E, Erlander M, Sgroi DC (2009). Gene expression profiling of the tumor microenvironment during breast cancer progression. Breast Cancer Res 11: R7

843. Ma XJ, Hilsenbeck SG, Wang W, Ding L, Sgroi DC, Bender RA, Osborne CK, Allred DC, Erlander MG (2006). The HOXB13:IL17BR expression index is a prognostic factor in early-stage breast cancer. J Clin Oncol 24: 4611–4619.

844. Ma XJ, Salunga R, Tuggle JT, Gaudet J, Enright E, McQuary P, Payette T, Pistone M, Stecker K, Zhang BM, Zhou YX, Varnholt H, Smith B, Gadd M, Chatfield E, Kessler J, Baer TM, Erlander MG, Sgroi DC (2003). Gene expression profiles of human breast cancer progression. Proc Natl Acad Sci U S A 100: 5974–5979.

845. Ma XJ, Salunga R, Tuggle JT, Gaudet J, Enright E, McQuary P, Payette T, Pistone M, Stecker K, Zhang BM, Zhou YX, Varnholt H, Smith B, Gadd M, Chatfield E, Kessler J, Baer TM, Erlander MG, Sgroi DC (2003). Gene expression profiles of human breast cancer progression. Proc Natl Acad Sci U S A 100: 5974–5979.

846. Ma XJ, Wang Z, Ryan PD, Isakoff SJ, Barmettler A, Fuller A, Muir B, Mohapatra G, Salunga R, Tuggle JT, Tran Y, Tran D, Tassin A, Amon P, Wang W, Wang W, Enright E, Stecker K, Estepa-Sabal E, Smith B et al. (2004). A two-gene expression ratio predicts clinical outcome in breast cancer patients treated with tamoxifen. Cancer Cell 5: 607–616.

846A. MacDonald HR, Silverstein MJ, Mabry H, Moorthy B, Ye W, Epstein MS, Holmes D, Silberman H, Lagios M (2005). Local control in ductal carcinoma in situ treated by excision alone: incremental benefit of larger margins. Am J Surg 190: 521–525.

847. MacGrogan G, Moinfar F, Raju U (2003). Intraductal papillary neoplasms. In: Pathology and genetics of tumours of the breast and female genital organs.Tavassoli FE, Devilee P, eds. WHO Classification of Tumours, 3rd edition. IARCPress: Lyon: pp 76–80.

848. MacGrogan G, Tavassoli FA (2003). Central atypical papillomas of the breast: a clinicopathological study of 119 cases. Virchows Arch 443: 609–617.

849. Machiavelli MR, Romero AO, Perez JE, Lacava JA, Dominguez ME, Rodriguez R, Barbieri MR, Romero Acuna LA, Romero Acuna JM, Langhi MJ, Amato S, Ortiz EH, Vallejo CT, Leone BA (1998). Prognostic significance of pathological response of primary tumor and metastatic axillary lymph nodes after neoadjuvant chemotherapy for locally advanced breast carcinoma. Cancer J Sci Am 4: 125–131.

849A, Mackay A, Weigelt B, Grigoriadis A,

Kreike B, Natrajan R, A'Hern R, Tan DS, Dowsett M, Ashworth A, Reis-Filho JS (2011). Microarray-based class discovery for molecular classification of breast cancer: analysis of inter-observer agreement. J Natl Cancer Inst 103: 662–673.

850. MacKenzie TA, Titus-Ernstoff L, Vacek PM, Geller B, Weiss JE, Goodrich ME, Carney PA (2007). Breast density in relation to risk of ductal carcinoma in situ of the breast in women undergoing screening mammography. Cancer Causes Control 18: 939–945.

851. Maehama T, Dixon JE (1998). The tumor suppressor, PTEN/MMAC1, dephosphorylates the lipid second messenger, phosphatidylinositol 3,4,5-trisphosphate. J Biol Chem 273: 13375–13378.

852. Magrath IT (1991). African Burkitt's lymphoma. History, biology, clinical features, and treatment. Am J Pediatr Hematol Oncol 13: 222–246.

853. Magro G (2008). Mammary myofibroblastoma: a tumor with a wide morphologic spectrum. Arch Pathol Lab Med 132: 1813–1820.

854. Magro G (2009). Epithelioid-cell myofibroblastoma of the breast: expanding the morphologic spectrum. Am J Surg Pathol 33: 1085–1092.

855. Magro G, Bisceglia M, Michal M, Eusebi V (2002). Spindle cell lipoma-like tumor, solitary fibrous tumor and myofibroblastoma of the breast: a clinico-pathological analysis of 13 cases in favor of a unifying histogenetic concept. Virchows Arch 440: 249–260.

856. Magro G, Gangemi P, Greco P (2008). Deciduoid-like myofibroblastoma of the breast: a potential pitfall of malignancy. Histopathology 52: 652–654.

857. Magro G, Gurrera A, Bisceglia M (2003). H-caldesmon expression in myofibroblastoma of the breast: evidence supporting the distinction from leiomyoma. Histopathology 42: 233–238.

858. Magro G, Michal M, Vasquez E, Bisceglia M (2000). Lipomatous myofibroblastoma: a potential diagnostic pitfall in the spectrum of the spindle cell lesions of the breast. Virchows Arch 437: 540–544.

858A. Magro G, Righi A, Casorzo L, Torrisi A, Salvatorelli L, Kacerovska D, Michal M (2012). Mammary and vaginal myofibroblastoma are genetically related lesions: FISH analysis showing deletion of 13q14 region. Hum Pathol. In press.

859. Maitra A, Tavassoli FA, bores-Saavedra J, Behrens C, Wistuba II, Bryant D, Weinberg AG, Rogers BB, Saboorian MH, Gazdar AF (1999). Molecular abnormalities associated with secretory carcinomas of the breast. Hum Pathol 30: 1435–1440.

860. Malkin D (2011). Li-Fraumeni syndrome. Genes Cancer 2: 475–484.

861. Malkin D, Li FP, Strong LC, Fraumeni JF, Jr, Nelson CE, Kim DH, Kassel J, Gryka MA, Bischoff FZ, Tainsky MA (1990). Germ line p53 mutations in a familial syndrome of breast cancer, sarcomas, and other neoplasms. Science 250: 1233–1238.

862. Malone KE, Begg CB, Haile RW, Borg A, Concannon P, Tellhed L, Xue S, Teraoka S, Bernstein L, Capanu M, Reiner AS, Riedel ER, Thomas DC, Mellemkjaer L, Lynch CF, Boice JD, Jr, Anton-Culver H, Bernstein JL (2010). Population-based study of the risk of second primary contralateral breast cancer associated with carrying a mutation in BRCA1 or BRCA2. J Clin Oncol 28: 2404–2410.

863. Maluf HM, Koerner FC (1995). Solid

papillary carcinoma of the breast. A form of intraductal carcinoma with endocrine differentiation frequently associated with mucinous carcinoma. Am J Surg Pathol 19: 1237–1244.

864. Mambo NC, Burke JS, Butler JJ (1977). Primary malignant lymphomas of the breast. Cancer 39: 2033–2040.

865. Man S, Ellis IO, Sibbering M, Blamey RW, Brook JD (1996). High levels of allele loss at the FHIT and ATM genes in non-comedo ductal carcinoma in situ and grade I tubular invasive breast cancers. Cancer Res 56: 5484–5489.

866. Manavi M, Hudelist G, Schatten C, Battistutti WB, Pischinger KI, Czerwenka KF (2002). Characteristics of clear cells and Toker cells in the epidermis of underlying nipple duct adenoma. Anticancer Res 22: 3691–3700.

867. Mandrell J, Mehta S, McClure S (2010). Atypical vascular lesion of the breast. J Am Acad Dermatol 63: 337–340.

868. Manie E, Vincent-Salomon A, Lehmann-Che J, Pierron G, Turpin E, Warcoin M, Gruel N, Lebigot I, Sastre-Garau X, Lidereau R, Remenieras A, Feunteun J, Delattre O, de The H, Stoppa-Lyonnet D, Stern MH (2009). High frequency of TP53 mutation in BRCA1 and sporadic basal-like carcinomas but not in BRCA1 luminal breast tumors. Cancer Res 69: 663–671.

869. Manner J, Radlwimmer B, Hohenberger P, Mossinger K, Kuffer S, Sauer C, Belharazem D, Zettl A, Coindre JM, Hallermann C, Hartmann JT, Katenkamp D, Katenkamp K, Schoffski P, Sciot R, Wozniak A, Lichter P, Marx A, Strobel P (2010). MYC high level gene amplification is a distinctive feature of angiosarcomas after irradiation or chronic lymphedema. Am J Pathol 176: 34–39.

870. Mansel RE, Webster DJT, Sweetland HM, eds (2009). Hughes, Mansel & Webster's benign disorders and diseases of the breast, 3rd edition. Saunders-Elsevier

871. Mansouri H, Jalil A, Chouhou L, Benjaafar N, Souadka A, El GB (2000). A rare case of angiosarcoma of the breast in a man: case report. Eur J Gynaecol Oncol 21: 603–604.

872. Marcel V, Palmero EI, Falagan-Lotsch P, Martel-Planche G, Ashton-Prolla P, Olivier M, Brentani RR, Hainaut P, Achatz MI (2009). TP53 PIN3 and MDM2 SNP309 polymorphisms as genetic modifiers in the Li-Fraumeni syndrome: impact on age at first diagnosis. J Med Genet 46: 766–772.

873. Marchbanks PA, McDonald JA, Wilson HG, Folger SG, Mandel MG, Daling JR, Bernstein L, Malone KE, Ursin G, Strom BL, Norman SA, Wingo PA, Burkman RT, Berlin JA, Simon MS, Spirtas R, Weiss LK (2002). Oral contraceptives and the risk of breast cancer. N Engl J Med 346: 2025–2032.

874. Marchese C, Montera M, Torrini M, Goldoni F, Mareni C, Forni M, Locatelli L (2003). Granular cell tumor in a PHTS patient with a novel germline PTEN mutation. Am J Med Genet A 120A: 286–288.

875. Marchio C, Iravani M, Natrajan R, Lambros MB, Geyer FC, Savage K, Parry S, Tamber N, Fenwick K, Mackay A, Schmitt FC, Bussolati G, Ellis I, Ashworth A, Sapino A, Reis-Filho JS (2009). Mixed micropapillary-ductal carcinomas of the breast: a genomic and immunohistochemical analysis of morphologically distinct components. J Pathol 218: 301–315.

876. Marchio C, Iravani M, Natrajan R, Lambros MB, Savage K, Tamber N, Fenwick K,

Mackay A, Senetta R, Di PS, Schmitt FC, Bussolati G, Ellis LO, Ashworth A, Sapino A, Reis-Filho JS (2008). Genomic and immunophenotypical characterization of pure micropapillary carcinomas of the breast. J Pathol 215: 398–410.

877. Marchio C, Weigelt B, Reis-Filho JS (2010). Adenoid cystic carcinomas of the breast and salivary glands (or 'The strange case of Dr Jekyll and Mr Hyde' of exocrine gland carcinomas). J Clin Pathol 63: 220–228.

878. Marcus JN, Watson P, Page DL, Narod SA, Lenoir GM, Tonin P, Linder-Stephenson L, Salerno G, Conway TA, Lynch HT (1996). Hereditary breast cancer: pathobiology, prognosis, and BRCA1 and BRCA2 gene linkage. Cancer 77: 697–709.

879. Marsh DJ, Coulon V, Lunetta KL, Rocca-Serra P, Dahia PL, Zheng Z, Liaw D, Caron S, Duboue B, Lin AY, Richardson AL, Bonnetblanc JM, Bressieux JM, Cabarrot-Moreau A, Chompret A, Demange L, Eeles RA, Yahanda AM, Fearon ER, Fricker JP et al. (1998). Mutation spectrum and genotype-phenotype analyses in Cowden disease and Bannayan-Zonana syndrome, two hamartoma syndromes with germline PTEN mutation. Hum Mol Genet 7: 507–515.

880. Marsh DJ, Dahia PL, Zheng Z, Liaw D, Parsons R, Gorlin RJ, Eng C (1997). Germline mutations in PTEN are present in Bannayan-Zonana syndrome. Nat Genet 16: 333–334.

881. Marshall LM, Hunter DJ, Connolly JL, Schnitt SJ, Byrne C, London SJ, Colditz GA (1997). Risk of breast cancer associated with atypical hyperplasia of lobular and ductal types. Cancer Epidemiol Biomarkers Prev 6: 297–301.

882. Martin RW, III, Neldner KH, Boyd AS, Coates PW (1990). Multiple cutaneous granular cell tumors and neurofibromatosis in childhood. A case report and review of the literature. Arch Dermatol 126: 1051–1056.

883. Martinelli G, Ryan G, Seymour JF, Nassi L, Steffanoni S, Alietti A, Calabrese L, Pruneri G, Santoro L, Kuper-Hommel M, Tsang R, Zinzani PL, Taghian A, Zucca E, Cavalli F (2009). Primary follicular and marginal-zone lymphoma of the breast: clinical features, prognostic factors and outcome: a study by the International Extranodal Lymphoma Study Group. Ann Oncol 20: 1993–1999.

884. Martinez SR, Beal SH, Canter RJ, Chen SL, Khatri VP, Bold RJ (2010). Medullary carcinoma of the breast: a population-based perspective. Med Oncol. 28:738-744..

885. Martinez V, Azzopardi JG (1979). Invasive lobular carcinoma of the breast: incidence and variants. Histopathology 3: 467–488.

886. Marty B, Maire V, Gravier E, Rigaill G, Vincent-Salomon A, Kappler M, Lebigot I, Djelti F, Tourdes A, Gestraud P, Hupe P, Barillot E, Cruzalegui F, Tucker GC, Stern MH, Thiery JP, Hickman JA, Dubois T (2008). Frequent PTEN genomic alterations and activated phosphatidylinositol 3-kinase pathway in basal-like breast cancer cells. Breast Cancer Res 10: R101

887. Marucci G, Betts CM, Golouh R, Peterse JL, Foschini MP, Eusebi V (2002). Toker cells are probably precursors of Paget cell carcinoma: a morphological and ultrastructural description. Virchows Arch 441: 117–123.

888. Maruti SS, Willett WC, Feskanich D, Rosner B, Colditz GA (2008). A prospective study of age-specific physical activity and premenopausal breast cancer. J Natl Cancer Inst 100: 728–737.

889. Marzullo F, Zito FA, Marzullo A, Labriola A, Schittulli F, Gargano G, De Girolamo R, Colonna F (1996). Infiltrating cribriform carcinoma of the breast. A clinico-pathologic and immunohistochemical study of 5 cases. Eur J Gynaecol Oncol 17: 228–231.

890. Mastracci TL, Shadeo A, Colby SM, Tuck AB, O'Malley FP, Bull SB, Lam WL, Andrulis IL (2006). Genomic alterations in lobular neoplasia: a microarray comparative genomic hybridization signature for early neoplastic proliferationin the breast. Genes Chromosomes Cancer 45: 1007–1017.

891. Mastracci TL, Tjan S, Bane AL, O'Malley FP, Andrulis IL (2005). E-cadherin alterations in atypical lobular hyperplasia and lobular carcinoma in situ of the breast. Mod Pathol 18: 741–751.

892. Mastropasqua MG, Maiorano E, Pruneri G, Orvieto E, Mazzarol G, Vento AR, Viale G (2005). Immunoreactivity for c-kit and p63 as an adjunct in the diagnosis of adenoid cystic carcinoma of the breast. Mod Pathol 18: 1277–1282.

893. Mattia AR, Ferry JA, Harris NL (1993). Breast lymphoma. A B-cell spectrum including the low grade B-cell lymphoma of mucosa associated lymphoid tissue. Am J Surg Pathol 17: 574–587.

894. Mazzella FM, Sieber SC, Braza F (1995). Ductal carcinoma of male breast with prominent lipid-rich component. Pathology 27: 280–283.

895. McCague A, Davis JV (2010). Giant fibroadenoma in a 22 year old patient: case report and literature review. Breast Dis 31: 49–52.

896. McCarthy NJ, Yang X, Linnoila IR, Merino MJ, Hewitt SM, Parr AL, Paik S, Steinberg SM, Hartmann DP, Mourali N, Levine PH, Swain SM (2002). Microvessel density, expression of estrogen receptor alpha, MIB-1, p53, and c-erbB-2 in inflammatory breast cancer. Clin Cancer Res 8: 3857–3862.

897. McClenathan JH, de la Roza G (2002). Adenoid cystic breast cancer. Am J Surg 183: 646–649.

898. McDivitt RW, Boyce W, Gersell D (1982). Tubular carcinoma of the breast. Clinical and pathological observations concerning 135 cases. Am J Surg Pathol 6: 401–411.

899. McDivitt RW, Stewart FW (1966). Breast carcinoma in children. JAMA 195: 388–390.

900. McIntosh IH, Hooper AA, Millis RR, Greening WP (1976). Metastatic carcinoma within the breast. Clin Oncol 2: 393–401.

901. McKinnon PJ (2004). ATM and ataxia telangiectasia. EMBO Rep 5: 772–776.

902. McKusick VA (1998). Mendelian inheritance in man. Catalogs of human genes and genetic disorders. 12th edition. Johns Hopkins University Press: Baltimore.

903. McLaren BK, Smith J, Schuyler PA, Dupont WD, Page DL (2005). Adenomyoepithelioma: clinical, histologic, and immunohistologic evaluation of a series of related lesions. Am J Surg Pathol 29: 1294–1299.

904. McLaughlin ER, Morris R, Weiss SW, Arbiser JL (2001). Diffuse dermal angiomatosis of the breast: response to isotretinoin. J Am Acad Dermatol 45: 462–465.

905. McLaughlin JR, Risch HA, Lubinski J, Moller P, Ghadirian P, Lynch H, Karlan B, Fishman D, Rosen B, Neuhausen SL, Offit K, Kauff N, Domchek S, Tung N, Friedman E, Foulkes W, Sun P, Narod SA (2007). Reproductive risk factors for ovarian cancer in carriers of BRCA1 or BRCA2 mutations: a case-control study. Lancet Oncol 8: 26–34.

906. McMenamin ME, DeSchryver K, Fletcher CD (2000). Fibrous lesions of the breast: a review. Int J Surg Pathol 8: 99–108.

907. Medina-Franco H, Gamboa-Dominguez A, de La Medina AR (2003). Malignant peripheral nerve sheath tumor of the breast. Breast J 9: 332.

908. Meijers-Heijboer H, van den Ouweland A, Klijn J, Wasielewski M, de Snoo A, Oldenburg R, Hollestelle A, Houben M, Crepin E, van Veghel-Plandsoen M, Elstrodt F, van Duijn C, Bartels C, Meijers C, Schutte M, McGuffog L, Thompson D, Easton D, Sodha N, Seal S et al. (2002). Low-penetrance susceptibility to breast cancer due to CHEK2(*)1100delC in noncarriers of BRCA1 or BRCA2 mutations. Nat Genet 31: 55–59.

909. Meindl A, Hellebrand H, Wiek C, Erven V, Wappenschmidt B, Niederacher D, Freund M, Lichtner P, Hartmann L, Schaal H, Ramser J, Honisch E, Kubisch C, Wichmann HE, Kast K, Deissler H, Engel C, Muller-Myhsok B, Neveling K, Kiechle M et al. (2010). Germline mutations in breast and ovarian cancer pedigrees establish RAD51C as a human cancer susceptibility gene. Nat Genet 42: 410–414.

910. Melchor L, Alvarez S, Honrado E, Palacios J, Barroso A, Diez O, Osorio A, Benitez J (2005). The accumulation of specific amplifications characterizes two different genomic pathways of evolution of familial breast tumors. Clin Cancer Res 11: 8577–8584.

911. Melchor L, Honrado E, Garcia MJ, Alvarez S, Palacios J, Osorio A, Nathanson KL, Benitez J (2008). Distinct genomic aberration patterns are found in familial breast cancer associated with different immunohistochemical subtypes. Oncogene 27: 3165–3175.

912. Melchor L, Honrado E, Huang J, Alvarez S, Naylor TL, Garcia MJ, Osorio A, Blesa D, Stratton MR, Weber BL, Cigudosa JC, Rahman N, Nathanson KL, Benitez J (2007). Estrogen receptor status could modulate the genomic pattern in familial and sporadic breast cancer. Clin Cancer Res 13: 7305–7313.

913. Mentzel T, Fletcher CD (1995). Lipomatous tumours of soft tissues: an update. Virchows Arch 427: 353–363.

914. Mercado CL, Toth HK, Axelrod D, Cangiarella J (2007). Fine-needle aspiration biopsy of benign adenomyoepithelioma of the breast: radiologic and pathologic correlation in four cases. Diagn Cytopathol 35: 690–694.

915. Merino MJ, LiVolsi VA (1981). Signet ring carcinoma of the female breast: a clinicopathologic analysis of 24 cases. Cancer 48: 1830–1837.

916. Mery CM, George S, Bertagnolli MM, Raut CP (2009). Secondary sarcomas after radiotherapy for breast cancer: sustained risk and poor survival. Cancer 115: 4055–4063.

917. Mesurolle B, Sygal V, Lalonde L, Lisbona A, Dufresne MP, Gagnon JH, Kao E (2008). Sonographic and mammographic appearances of breast hemangioma. AJR Am J Roentgenol 191: W17–W22.

918. Meyer KB, Maia AT, O'Reilly M, Teschendorff AE, Chin SF, Caldas C, Ponder BA (2008). Allele-specific up-regulation of FGFR2 increases susceptibility to breast cancer. PLoS Biol 6: e108

919. Mezzabotta M, Riccardi S, Bonvini S, Declich P, Tavani E, Morandi E (2009). Giant nodular pseudoangiomatous stromal hyperplasia (PASH) of the breast presenting as a rapidly growing tumour. Chir Ital 61: 369–373.

920. Michaelson JS, Silverstein M, Sgroi D, Cheongsiatmoy JA, Taghian A, Powell S, Hughes K, Comegno A, Tanabe KK, Smith B (2003). The effect of tumor size and lymph node status on breast carcinoma lethality. Cancer 98: 2133–2143.

921. Michal M, Baumruk L, Burger J, Manhalova M (1994). Adenomyoepithelioma of the breast with undifferentiated carcinoma component. Histopathology 24: 274–276.

921A. Michal M, Skalova A (1990). Collagenous spherulosis. A comment on its histogenesis. Pathol Res Pract 186: 365–370.

922. Middleton LP, Palacios DM, Bryant BR, Krebs P, Otis CN, Merino MJ (2000). Pleomorphic lobular carcinoma: morphology, immunohistochemistry, and molecular analysis. Am J Surg Pathol 24: 1650–1656.

923. Middleton LP, Tressera F, Sobel ME, Bryant BR, Alburquerque A, Grases P, Merino MJ (1999). Infiltrating micropapillary carcinoma of the breast. Mod Pathol 12: 499–504.

924. Miettinen M (1988). Immunoreactivity for cytokeratin and epithelial membrane antigen in leiomyosarcoma. Arch Pathol Lab Med 112: 637–640.

925. Miki Y, Swensen J, Shattuck-Eidens D, Futreal PA, Harshman K, Tavtigian S, Liu Q, Cochran C, Bennett LM, Ding W (1994). A strong candidate for the breast and ovarian cancer susceptibility gene BRCA1. Science 266: 66–71.

925A. Milne RL, Goode EL, Garcia-Closas M, Couch FJ, Severi G, Hein R, Fredericksen Z, Malats N, Zamora MP, Perez JI, Benitez J, Dork T, Schurmann P, Karstens JH, Hillemanns P, Cox A, Brock IW, Elliot G, Cross SS, Seal S et al. (2011). Confirmation of 5p12 as a susceptibility locus for progesterone-receptor-positive, lower grade breast cancer. Cancer Epidemiol Biomarkers Prev 20: 2222–2231.

926. Miranda RN, Lin L, Talwalkar SS, Manning JT, Medeiros LJ (2009). Anaplastic large cell lymphoma involving the breast: a clinicopathologic study of 6 cases and review of the literature. Arch Pathol Lab Med 133: 1383–1390.

927. Missmer SA, Eliassen AH, Barbieri RL, Hankinson SE (2004). Endogenous estrogen, androgen, and progesterone concentrations and breast cancer risk among postmenopausal women. J Natl Cancer Inst 96: 1856–1865.

928. Mitnick JS, Gianutsos R, Pollack AH, Susman M, Baskin BL, Ko WD, Pressman PI, Feiner HD, Roses DF (1999). Tubular carcinoma of the breast: sensitivity of diagnostic techniques and correlation with histopathology. AJR Am J Roentgenol 172: 319–323.

929. Mohammed RA, Ellis IO, Lee AH, Martin SG (2009). Vascular invasion in breast cancer; an overview of recent prognostic developments and molecular pathophysiological mechanisms. Histopathology 55: 1–9.

930. Mohammed RA, Martin SG, Gill MS, Green AR, Paish EC, Ellis IO (2007). Improved methods of detection of lymphovascular invasion demonstrate that it is the predominant method of vascular invasion in breast cancer and has important clinical consequences. Am J Surg Pathol 31: 1825–1833.

931. Mohammed RA, Martin SG, Mahmmod AM, Macmillan RD, Green AR, Paish EC, Ellis IO (2011). Objective assessment of lymphatic and blood vascular invasion in lymph node-negative breast carcinoma: findings from a large case series with long-term follow-up. J Pathol 223: 358–365.

932. Mohsin SK, Weiss H, Havighurst T, Clark GM, Berardo M, Roanh ID, To TV, Qian Z, Love RR, Allred DC (2004). Progesterone receptor by immunohistochemistry and clinical outcome in breast cancer: a validation study. Mod Pathol 17: 1545–1554.

933. Moinfar F (2010). Flat ductal intraepithelial neoplasia of the breast: evolution of Azzopardi's «clinging» concept. Semin Diagn Pathol 27: 37–48.

934. Moinfar F, Man YG, Arnould L, Bratthauer GL, Ratschek M, Tavassoli FA (2000). Concurrent and independent genetic alterations in the stromal and epithelial cells of mammary carcinoma: implications for tumorigenesis. Cancer Res 60: 2562–2566.

935. Moinfar F, Man YG, Bratthauer GL, Ratschek M, Tavassoli FA (2000). Genetic abnormalities in mammary ductal intraepithelial neoplasia-flat type («clinging ductal carcinoma in situ»): a simulator of normal mammary epithelium. Cancer 88: 2072–2081.

936. Moinfar F, Man YG, Lininger RA, Bodian C, Tavassoli FA (1999). Use of keratin 35betaE12 as an adjunct in the diagnosis of mammary intraepithelial neoplasia-ductal type—benign and malignant intraductal proliferations. Am J Surg Pathol 23: 1048–1058.

937. Mokbel K (2001). Grading of infiltrating lobular carcinoma. Eur J Surg Oncol 27: 609–610.

938. Moll R, Mitze M, Frixen UH, Birchmeier W (1993). Differential loss of E-cadherin expression in infiltrating ductal and lobular breast carcinomas. Am J Pathol 143: 1731–1742.

939. Moll UM, Chumas J (1997). Morphologic effects of neoadjuvant chemotherapy in locally advanced breast cancer. Pathol Res Pract 193: 187–196.

940. Molland JG, Donnellan M, Janu NC, Carmalt HL, Kennedy CW, Gillett DJ (2004). Infiltrating lobular carcinoma—a comparison of diagnosis, management and outcome with infiltrating duct carcinoma. Breast 13: 389–396.

941. Mollerstrom E, Delle U, Danielsson A, Parris T, Olsson B, Karlsson P, Helou K (2010). High-resolution genomic profiling to predict 10-year overall survival in node-negative breast cancer. Cancer Genet Cytogenet 198: 79–89.

942. Montgomery EA, Meis JM (1991). Nodular fasciitis. Its morphologic spectrum and immunohistochemical profile. Am J Surg Pathol 15: 942–948.

943. Monti P, Ciribilli Y, Jordan J, Menichini P, Umbach DM, Resnick MA, Luzzatto L, Inga A, Fronza G (2007). Transcriptional functionality of germ line p53 mutants influences cancer phenotype. Clin Cancer Res 13: 3789–3795.

944. Monticciolo DL (2005). Histologic grading at breast core needle biopsy: comparison with results from the excised breast specimen. Breast J 11: 9–14.

944A. Mook S, Schmidt MK, Viale G, Pruneri G, Eekhout I, Floore A et al. (2009). The 70-gene prognosis-signature predicts disease outcome in breast cancer patients with 1-3 positive lymph nodes in an independent validation study. Breast Cancer Res Treat 116: 295–302.

944B. Mooney EE, Kayani N, Tavassoli FA (1999). Spherulosis of the breast. A spectrum of municous and collagenous lesions. Arch Pathol Lab Med 123: 626–630.

945. Morak M, Schackert HK, Rahner N, Betz B, Ebert M, Walldorf C, Royer-Pokora B, Schulmann K, von Knebel-Doeberitz M, Dietmaier W, Keller G, Kerker B, Leitner G, Holinski-Feder E (2008). Further evidence for heritability of an epimutation in one of 12 cases with MLH1 promoter methylation in blood cells

clinically displaying HNPCC. Eur J Hum Genet 16: 804–811.
946. Morandi L, Pession A, Marucci GL, Foschini MP, Pruneri G, Viale G, Eusebi V (2003). Intraepidermal cells of Paget's carcinoma of the breast can be genetically different from those of the underlying carcinoma. Hum Pathol 34: 1321–1330.
947. Moritani S, Ichihara S, Hasegawa M, Endo T, Oiwa M, Shiraiwa M, Nishida C, Morita T, Sato Y, Hayashi T, Kato A (2011). Intracytoplasmic lipid accumulation in apocrine carcinoma of the breast evaluated with adipophilin immunoreactivity: a possible link between apocrine carcinoma and lipid-rich carcinoma. Am J Surg Pathol 35: 861–867.
947A. Moritani S, Ichihara S, Hasegawa M, Endo T, Oiwa M, Shiraiwa M, Nishida C, Morita T, Sato Y, Hayashi T, Kato A, Aoyama H, Yoshikawa K (2011). Topographical, morphological and immunohistochemical characteristics of carcinoma in situ of the breast involving sclerosing adenosis. Two distinct topographical patterns and histological types of carcinoma in situ. Histopathology 58: 835–846.
948. Moritani S, Ichihara S, Kushima R, Okabe H, Bamba M, Kobayashi TK, Hattori T (2007). Myoepithelial cells in solid variant of intraductal papillary carcinoma of the breast: a potential diagnostic pitfall and a proposal of an immunohistochemical panel in the differential diagnosis with intraductal papilloma with usual ductal hyperplasia. Virchows Arch 450: 539–547.
949. Moross T, Lang AP, Mahoney L (1983). Tubular adenoma of breast. Arch Pathol Lab Med 107: 84–86.
950. Morrow M, Berger D, Thelmo W (1988). Diffuse cystic angiomatosis of the breast. Cancer 62: 2392–2396.
951. Mouchawar J, Korch C, Byers T, Pitts TM, Li E, McCredie MR, Giles GG, Hopper JL, Southey MC (2010). Population-based estimate of the contribution of TP53 mutations to subgroups of early-onset breast cancer: Australian Breast Cancer Family Study. Cancer Res 70: 4795–4800.
951A. Moulder S, Moroney J, Helgason T, Wheler J, Booser D, Albarracin C, Morrow PK, Koenig K, Kurzrock R (2011). Responses to liposomal Doxorubicin, bevacizumab, and temsirolimus in metaplastic carcinoma of the breast: biologic rationale and implications for stem-cell research in breast cancer. J Clin Oncol 29: e572–e575.
952. Moy L, Slanetz PJ, Moore R, Satija S, Yeh ED, McCarthy KA, Hall D, Staffa M, Rafferty EA, Halpern E, Kopans DB (2002). Specificity of mammography and US in the evaluation of a palpable abnormality: retrospective review. Radiology 225: 176–181.
953. Muller A, Edmonston TB, Corao DA, Rose DG, Palazzo JP, Becker H, Fry RD, Rueschoff J, Fishel R (2002). Exclusion of breast cancer as an integral tumor of hereditary nonpolyposis colorectal cancer. Cancer Res 62: 1014–1019.
954. Mulligan AM, O'Malley FP (2007). Metastatic potential of encapsulated (intracystic) papillary carcinoma of the breast: a report of 2 cases with axillary lymph node micrometastases. Int J Surg Pathol 15: 143–147.
955. Mulligan AM, O'Malley FP (2007). Papillary lesions of the breast: a review. Adv Anat Pathol 14: 108–119.
956. Murakami A, Kawachi K, Sasaki T, Ishikawa T, Nagashima Y, Nozawa A (2009). Sebaceous carcinoma of the breast. Pathol Int 59: 188–192.
957. Murat A, Kansiz F, Kabakus N, Kazez A, Ozercan R (2004). Neurofibroma of the breast in a boy with neurofibromatosis type 1. Clin Imaging 28: 415–417.
958. Nadelman CM, Leslie KO, Fishbein MC (2006). «Benign,» metastasizing adenomyoepithelioma of the breast: a report of 2 cases. Arch Pathol Lab Med 130: 1349–1353.
959. Nagi C, Bleiweiss I, Jaffer S (2005). Epithelial displacement in breast lesions: a papillary phenomenon. Arch Pathol Lab Med 129: 1465–1469.
960. Narita T, Matsuda K (1995). Pleomorphic adenoma of the breast: case report and review of the literature. Pathol Int 45: 441–447.
961. Narod SA, Dube MP, Klijn J, Lubinski J, Lynch HT, Ghadirian P, Provencher D, Heimdal K, Moller P, Robson M, Offit K, Isaacs C, Weber B, Friedman E, Gershoni-Baruch R, Rennert G, Pasini B, Wagner T, Daly M, Garber JE et al. (2002). Oral contraceptives and the risk of breast cancer in BRCA1 and BRCA2 mutation carriers. J Natl Cancer Inst 94: 1773–1779.
962. Narod SA, Sun P, Risch HA (2001). Ovarian cancer, oral contraceptives, and BRCA mutations. N Engl J Med 345: 1706–1707.
963. Narula HS, Carlson HE (2007). Gynecomastia. Endocrinol Metab Clin North Am 36: 497–519.
964. Nascimento AF, Raut CP, Fletcher CD (2008). Primary angiosarcoma of the breast: clinicopathologic analysis of 49 cases, suggesting that grade is not prognostic. Am J Surg Pathol 32: 1896–1904.
965. Nascimento AG, Karas M, Rosen PP, Caron AG (1979). Leiomyoma of the nipple. Am J Surg Pathol 3: 151–154.
966. Nassar A (2010). Core needle biopsy versus fine needle aspiration biopsy in breast. A historical perspective and opportunities in the modern era. Diagn Cytopathol 39: 380–388.
967. Nassar H (2004). Carcinomas with micropapillary morphology: clinical significance and current concepts. Adv Anat Pathol 11: 297–303.
968. Nassar H, Elieff MP, Kronz JD, Argani P (2010). Pseudoangiomatous stromal hyperplasia (PASH) of the breast with foci of morphologic malignancy: a case of PASH with malignant transformation? Int J Surg Pathol 18: 564–569.
969. Nassar H, Qureshi H, Adsay NV, Visscher D (2006). Clinicopathologic analysis of solid papillary carcinoma of the breast and associated invasive carcinomas. Am J Surg Pathol 30: 501–507.
970. Natrajan R, Lambros MB, Geyer FC, Marchio C, Tan DS, Vatcheva R, Shiu KK, Hungermann D, Rodriguez-Pinilla SM, Palacios J, Ashworth A, Buerger H, Reis-Filho JS (2009). Loss of 16q in high grade breast cancer is associated with estrogen receptor status: Evidence for progression in tumors with a luminal phenotype? Genes Chromosomes Cancer 48: 351–365.
970A. Natrajan R, Lambros MB, Rodriguez-Pinilla SM, Moreno-Bueno G, Tan DS, Marchio C, Vatcheva R, Rayter S, Mahler-Araujo B, Fulford LG, Hungermann D, Mackay A, Grigoriadis A, Fenwick K, Tamber N, Hardisson D, Tutt A, Palacios J, Lord CJ, Buerger H et al. (2009). Tiling path genomic profiling of grade 3 invasive ductal breast cancers. Clin Cancer Res 15: 2711–2722.
970B. Natrajan R, Weigelt B, Mackay A, Geyer FC, Grigoriadis A, Tan DS, Jones C, Lord CJ, Vatcheva R, Rodriguez-Pinilla SM, Palacios J, Ashworth A, Reis-Filho JS (2010). An integrative genomic and transcriptomic analysis reveals molecular pathways and networks regulated by copy number aberrations in basal-like, HER2 and luminal cancers. Breast Cancer Res Treat 121: 575–589.
970C. Navin N, Kendall J, Troge J, Andrews P, Rodgers L, McIndoo J, Cook K, Stepansky A, Levy D, Esposito D, Muthuswamy L, Krasnitz A, McCombie WR, Hicks J, Wigler M (2011). Tumour evolution inferred by single-cell sequencing. Nature 472: 90–94.
971. Nayar R, Zhuang Z, Merino MJ, Silverberg SG (1997). Loss of heterozygosity on chromosome 11q13 in lobular lesions of the breast using tissue microdissection and polymerase chain reaction. Hum Pathol 28: 277–282.
972. Nelen MR, Kremer H, Konings IB, Schoute F, van Essen AJ, Koch R, Woods CG, Fryns JP, Hamel B, Hoefsloot LH, Peeters EA, Padberg GW (1999). Novel PTEN mutations in patients with Cowden disease: absence of clear genotype-phenotype correlations. Eur J Hum Genet 7: 267–273.
973. Nelen MR, Padberg GW, Peeters EA, Lin AY, van den Helm B, Frants RR, Coulon V, Goldstein AM, van Reen MM, Easton DF, Eeles RA, Hodgsen S, Mulvihill JJ, Murday VA, Tucker MA, Mariman EC, Starink TM, Ponder BA, Ropers HH, Kremer H et al. (1996). Localization of the gene for Cowden disease to chromosome 10q22-23. Nat Genet 13: 114–116.
974. Nelen MR, van Staveren WC, Peeters EA, Hassel MB, Gorlin RJ, Hamm H, Lindboe CF, Fryns JP, Sijmons RH, Woods DG, Mariman EC, Padberg GW, Kremer H (1997). Germline mutations in the PTEN/MMAC1 gene in patients with Cowden disease. Hum Mol Genet 6: 1383–1387.
975. Nemoto T, Castillo N, Tsukada Y, Koul A, Eckhert KH, Jr, Bauer RL (1998). Lobular carcinoma in situ with microinvasion. J Surg Oncol 67: 41–46.
976. Nemoto T, Vana J, Bedwani RN, Baker HW, McGregor FH, Murphy GP (1980). Management and survival of female breast cancer: results of a national survey by the American College of Surgeons. Cancer 45: 2917–2924.
977. Nesland JM, Holm R, Johannessen JV (1985). Ultrastructural and immunohistochemical features of lobular carcinoma of the breast. J Pathol 145: 39–52.
978. Neuman HB, Brogi E, Ebrahim A, Brennan MF, Van Zee KJ (2008). Desmoid tumors (fibromatoses) of the breast: a 25-year experience. Ann Surg Oncol 15: 274–280.
979. Neves Cde O, Soares AB, Costa AF, de Araujo V, Furuse C, Juliano PB, Altemani A (2010). CD10 (neutral endopeptidase) expression in myoepithelial cells of salivary neoplasms. Appl Immunohistochem Mol Morphol 18: 172–178.
980. Neville BW, Damm DD, Allen C, Bouquot JE (2008). Oral and maxillofacial pathology, 3rd edition. Saunders: Philadelphia.
981. Newcomb PA, Trentham-Dietz A, Hampton JM, Egan KM, Titus-Ernstoff L, Warren AS, Greenberg ER, Willett WC MD (2010). Late age at first full term birth is strongly associated with lobular breast cancer. Cancer. 117:1946-1956.
982. Newman B, Austin MA, Lee M, King MC (1988). Inheritance of human breast cancer: evidence for autosomal dominant transmission in high-risk families. Proc Natl Acad Sci U S A 85: 3044–3048.
983. Newman PL, Fletcher CD (1991). Smooth muscle tumours of the external genitalia: clinicopathological analysis of a series. Histopathology 18: 523–529.
984. Newman W (1966). Lobular carcinoma of the female breast. Report of 73 cases. Ann Surg 164: 305–314.
985. Ng TL, Gown AM, Barry TS, Cheang MC, Chan AK, Turbin DA, Hsu FD, West RB, Nielsen TO (2005). Nuclear beta-catenin in mesenchymal tumors. Mod Pathol 18: 68–74.
986. Ng WK (2001). Fine needle aspiration cytology of invasive cribriform carcinoma of the breast with osteoclastlike giant cells: a case report. Acta Cytol 45: 593–598.
987. Nga ME, Lim KH, Tan EY, Chan P, Tan SY, Walford N (2008). Malignant adenomyoepithelial tumor of the breast: multi-immunolabeling technique and detailed immunophenotypic study. Appl Immunohistochem Mol Morphol 16: 100–104.
988. Nguyen CV, Albarracin CT, Whitman GJ, Lopez A, Sneige N (2010). Atypical ductal hyperplasia in directional vacuum-assisted biopsy of breast microcalcifications: considerations for surgical excision. Ann Surg Oncol 18: 752–761.
989. Nguyen CV, Falcon-Escobedo R, Hunt KK, Nayeemuddin KM, Lester TR, Harrell RK, Bassett RL, Jr, Gilcrease MZ (2010). Pleomorphic ductal carcinoma of the breast: predictors of decreased overall survival. Am J Surg Pathol 34: 486–493.
990. NHS Cancer Screening Programmes (2010). NHS breast screening programme & association of breast surgery at BASO. An audit of screen-detected breast cancers for the year of screening April 2008 to March 2009. West Midlands Cancer Intelligence Unit
991. Ni Y, Zbuk KM, Sadler T, Patocs A, Lobo G, Edelman E, Platzer P, Orloff MS, Waite KA, Eng C (2008). Germline mutations and variants in the succinate dehydrogenase genes in Cowden and Cowden-like syndromes. Am J Hum Genet 83: 261–268.
992. Nicolaides NC, Carter KC, Shell BK, Papadopoulos N, Vogelstein B, Kinzler KW (1995). Genomic organization of the human PMS2 gene family. Genomics 30: 195–206.
993. Nicolaides NC, Palombo F, Kinzler KW, Vogelstein B, Jiricny J (1996). Molecular cloning of the N-terminus of GTBP. Genomics 31: 395–397.
994. Nicolaides NC, Papadopoulos N, Liu B, Wei YF, Carter KC, Ruben SM, Rosen CA, Haseltine WA, Fleischmann RD, Fraser CM (1994). Mutations of two PMS homologues in hereditary nonpolyposis colon cancer. Nature 371: 75–80.
995. Nicolas MM, Wu Y, Middleton LP, Gilcrease MZ (2007). Loss of myoepithelium is variable in solid papillary carcinoma of the breast. Histopathology 51: 657–665.
996. Nielsen M, Andersen JA, Henriksen FW, Kristensen PB, Lorentzen M, Ravn V, Schiodt T, Thorborg JV, Ornvold K (1981). Metastases to the breast from extramammary carcinomas. Acta Pathol Microbiol Scand A 89: 251–256.
997. Nielsen TO, Hsu FD, Jensen K, Cheang M, Karaca G, Hu Z, Hernandez-Boussard T, Livasy C, Cowan D, Dressler L, Akslen LA, Ragaz J, Gown AM, Gilks CB, van de Rijn M, Perou CM (2004). Immunohistochemical and clinical characterization of the basal-like subtype of invasive breast carcinoma. Clin Cancer Res 10: 5367–5374.
997A. Nielsen TO, Parker JS, Leung S, Voduc D, Ebbert M, Vickery T et al. (2010). A compar-

ison of PAM50 intrinsic subtyping with immunohistochemistry and clinical prognostic factors in tamoxifen-treated estrogen receptor-positive breast cancer. Clin Cancer Res 16: 5222–5232.

998. Niemeier LA, Dabbs DJ, Beriwal S, Striebel JM, Bhargava R (2010). Androgen receptor in breast cancer: expression in estrogen receptor-positive tumors and in estrogen receptor-negative tumors with apocrine differentiation. Mod Pathol 23: 205–212.

999. Nigro DM, Organ CH, Jr (1976). Fibroadenoma of the female breast. Some epidemiologic surprises. Postgrad Med 59: 113–117.

1000. NIH Consensus Development Conference (1997). The uniform approach to breast fine-needle aspiration biopsy. NIH Consensus Development Conference. Am J Surg 174: 371–385.

1001. Nikolsky Y, Sviridov E, Yao J, Dosymbekov D, Ustyansky V, Kaznacheev V, Dezso Z, Mulvey L, Macconaill LE, Winckler W, Serebryiskaya T, Nikolskaya T, Polyak K (2008). Genome-wide functional synergy between amplified and mutated genes in human breast cancer. Cancer Res 68: 9532–9540.

1002. Nishimori H, Sasaki M, Hirata K, Zembutsu H, Yasoshima T, Fukui R, Kobayashi K (2000). Tubular adenoma of the breast in a 73-year-old woman. Breast Cancer 7: 169–172.

1003. Nishimura R, Ohsumi S, Teramoto N, Yamakawa T, Saeki T, Takashima S (2005). Invasive cribriform carcinoma with extensive microcalcifications in the male breast. Breast Cancer 12: 145–148.

1004. Nishizaki T, Chew K, Chu L, Isola J, Kallioniemi A, Weidner N, Waldman FM (1997). Genetic alterations in lobular breast cancer by comparative genomic hybridization. Int J Cancer 74: 513–517.

1005. Nobukawa B, Fujii H, Hirai S, Kumasaka T, Shimizu H, Matsumoto T, Suda K, Futagawa S (1999). Breast carcinoma diverging to aberrant melanocytic differentiation: a case report with histopathologic and loss of heterozygosity analyses. Am J Surg Pathol 23: 1280–1287.

1006. Noel JC, Simon P, Aguilar SF (2006). Malignant myoepithelioma arising in cystic adenomyoepithelioma. Breast J 12: 386.

1007. Nofech-Mozes S, Hanna W (2009). Toker cells revisited. Breast J 15: 394–398.

1008. Noguchi S, Motomura K, Inaji H, Imaoka S, Koyama H (1994). Clonal analysis of solitary intraductal papilloma of the breast by means of polymerase chain reaction. Am J Pathol 144: 1320–1325.

1009. Noguchi S, Yokouchi H, Aihara T, Motomura K, Inaji H, Imaoka S, Koyama H (1995). Progression of fibroadenoma to phyllodes tumor demonstrated by clonal analysis. Cancer 76: 1779–1785.

1010. Nomura K, Fukunaga M, Uchida K, Aizawa S (1996). Adenomyoepithelioma of the breast with exaggerated proliferation of epithelial cells: report of a case. Pathol Int 46: 1011–1014.

1011. Nonaka D, Rosai J, Spagnolo D, Fiaccavento S, Bisceglia M (2004). Cylindroma of the breast of skin adnexal type: a study of 4 cases. Am J Surg Pathol 28: 1070–1075.

1012. Norris HJ, Taylor HB (1965). Prognosis of mucinous (gelatinous) carcinoma of the breast. Cancer 18: 879–885.

1013. Nystrom-Lahti M, Wu Y, Moisio AL, Hofstra RM, Osinga J, Mecklin JP, Jarvinen HJ, Leisti J, Buys CH, de la Chapelle A, Peltomaki P (1996). DNA mismatch repair gene mutations

in 55 kindreds with verified or putative hereditary non-polyposis colorectal cancer. Hum Mol Genet 5: 763–769.

1014. O'Connell FP, Wang HH, Odze RD (2005). Utility of immunohistochemistry in distinguishing primary adenocarcinomas from metastatic breast carcinomas in the gastrointestinal tract. Arch Pathol Lab Med 129: 338–347.

1015. O'Connell P, Pekkel V, Fuqua SA, Osborne CK, Clark GM, Allred DC (1998). Analysis of loss of heterozygosity in 399 premalignant breast lesions at 15 genetic loci. J Natl Cancer Inst 90: 697–703.

1016. O'Connor IF, Shembekar MV, Shousha S (1998). Breast carcinoma developing in patients on hormone replacement therapy: a histological and immunohistological study. J Clin Pathol 51: 935–938.

1017. O'Hara MF, Page DL (1985). Adenomas of the breast and ectopic breast under lactational influences. Hum Pathol 16: 707–712.

1018. O'Malley FP (2010). Lobular neoplasia: morphology, biological potential and management in core biopsies. Mod Pathol 23 Suppl 2: S14–S25.

1019. Oberman HA (1980). Secretory carcinoma of the breast in adults. Am J Surg Pathol 4: 465–470.

1019A. Oberman HA (1987). Metaplastic carcinoma of the breast. A clinicopathologic study of 29 patients. Am J Surg Pathol 11: 918–929.

1020. Oberman HA (1989). Hamartomas and hamartoma variants of the breast. Semin Diagn Pathol 6: 135–145.

1021. Oberman HA, Fidler WJ, Jr (1979). Tubular carcinoma of the breast. Am J Surg Pathol 3: 387–395.

1022. Ognjanovic S, Oliver M, Bergemann TL, Hainaut P (2011). Sarcomas in TP53 germline mutation carriers: A review of the IARC TP53 database. Cancer. 118:1387-1396.

1023. Ogston KN, Miller ID, Payne S, Hutcheon AW, Sarkar TK, Smith I, Schofield A, Heys SD (2003). A new histological grading system to assess response of breast cancers to primary chemotherapy: prognostic significance and survival. Breast 12: 320–327.

1024. Oh DS, Troester MA, Usary J, Hu Z, He X, Fan C, Wu J, Carey LA, Perou CM (2006). Estrogen-regulated genes predict survival in hormone receptor-positive breast cancers. J Clin Oncol 24: 1656–1664.

1025. Ohi Y, Umekita Y, Rai Y, Kukita T, Sagara Y, Sagara Y, Takahama T, Andou M, Sagara Y, Yoshida A, Yoshida H (2007). Clear cell hidradenoma of the breast: a case report with review of the literature. Breast Cancer 14: 307–311.

1026. Ohta M, Mori M, Kawada T, Maegawa H, Yamamoto S, Imamura Y (2010). Collagenous spherulosis associated with adenomyoepithelioma of the breast: a case report. Acta Cytol 54: 314–318.

1027. Ohtake T, Abe R, Kimijima I, Fukushima T, Tsuchiya A, Hoshi K, Wakasa H (1995). Intraductal extension of primary invasive breast carcinoma treated by breast-conservative surgery. Computer graphic three-dimensional reconstruction of the mammary duct-lobular systems. Cancer 76: 32–45.

1028. Ohuchi N (1999). Breast-conserving surgery for invasive cancer: a principle based on segmental anatomy. Tohoku J Exp Med 188: 103–118.

1029. Ohuchi N, Abe R, Kasai M (1984). Possible cancerous change of intraductal papillomas of the breast. A 3-D reconstruction study of 25 cases. Cancer 54: 605–611.

1030. Ohuchi N, Abe R, Takahashi T, Tezuka F (1984). Origin and extension of intraductal papillomas of the breast: a three-dimensional reconstruction study. Breast Cancer Res Treat 4: 117–128.

1031. Ohuchi N, Furuta A, Mori S (1994). Management of ductal carcinoma in situ with nipple discharge. Intraductal spreading of carcinoma is an unfavorable pathologic factor for breast-conserving surgery. Cancer 74: 1294–1302.

1032. Oka H, Shiozaki H, Kobayashi K, Inoue M, Tahara H, Kobayashi T, Takatsuka Y, Matsuyoshi N, Hirano S, Takeichi M, . (1993). Expression of E-cadherin cell adhesion molecules in human breast cancer tissues and its relationship to metastasis. Cancer Res 53: 1696–1701.

1033. Okada K, Suzuki Y, Saito Y, Umemura S, Tokuda Y (2006). Two cases of ductal adenoma of the breast. Breast Cancer 13: 354–359.

1034. Olivier M, Goldgar DE, Sodha N, Ohgaki H, Kleihues P, Hainaut P, Eeles RA (2003). Li-Fraumeni and related syndromes: correlation between tumor type, family structure, and TP53 genotype. Cancer Res 63: 6643–6650.

1035. Olivier M, Hollstein M, Hainaut P (2010). TP53 mutations in human cancers: origins, consequences, and clinical use. Cold Spring Harb Perspect Biol 2: a001008.

1036. Olsen JH, Hahnemann JM, Borresen-Dale AL, Brondum-Nielsen K, Hammarstrom L, Kleinerman R, Kaariainen H, Lonnqvist T, Sankila R, Seersholm N, Tretli S, Yuen J, Boice JD, Jr, Tucker M (2001). Cancer in patients with ataxia-telangiectasia and in their relatives in the Nordic countries. J Natl Cancer Inst 93: 121–127.

1037. Olsen JH, Hahnemann JM, Borresen-Dale AL, Tretli S, Kleinerman R, Sankila R, Hammarstrom L, Robsahm TE, Kaariainen H, Bregard A, Brondum-Nielsen K, Yuen J, Tucker M (2005). Breast and other cancers in 1445 blood relatives of 75 Nordic patients with ataxia telangiectasia. Br J Cancer 93: 260–265.

1038. Oo KZ, Xiao PQ (2009). Infiltrating syringomatous adenoma of the nipple: clinical presentation and literature review. Arch Pathol Lab Med 133: 1487–1489.

1039. Orban TI, Olah E (2003). Emerging roles of BRCA1 alternative splicing. Mol Pathol 56: 191–197.

1040. Organ CH, Jr, Organ BC (1983). Fibroadenoma of the female breast: a critical clinical assessment. J Natl Med Assoc 75: 701–704.

1041. Orlando L, Renne G, Rocca A, Curigliano G, Colleoni M, Severi G, Peruzzotti G, Cinieri S, Viale G, Sanna G, Goldhirsch A (2005). Are all high-grade breast cancers with no steroid receptor hormone expression alike? The special case of the medullary phenotype. Ann Oncol 16: 1094–1099.

1042. Orloff MS, Eng C (2008). Genetic and phenotypic heterogeneity in the PTEN hamartoma tumour syndrome. Oncogene 27: 5387–5397.

1043. Orvieto E, Maiorano E, Bottiglieri L, Maisonneuve P, Rotmensz N, Galimberti V, Luini A, Brenelli F, Gatti G, Viale G (2008). Clinicopathologic characteristics of invasive lobular carcinoma of the breast: results of an analysis of 530 cases from a single institution. Cancer 113: 1511–1520.

1044. Osin P, Lu YJ, Stone J, Crook T, Houlston RS, Gasco M, Gusterson BA, Shipley J (2003). Distinct genetic and epigenetic

changes in medullary breast cancer. Int J Surg Pathol 11: 153–158.

1045. Otsuki Y, Yamada M, Shimizu S, Suwa K, Yoshida M, Tanioka F, Ogawa H, Nasuno H, Serizawa A, Kobayashi H (2007). Solid-papillary carcinoma of the breast: clinicopathological study of 20 cases. Pathol Int 57: 421–429.

1046. Otterbach F, Bankfalvi A, Bergner S, Decker T, Krech R, Boecker W (2000). Cytokeratin 5/6 immunohistochemistry assists the differential diagnosis of atypical proliferations of the breast. Histopathology 37: 232–240.

1047. Ottini L, Masala G, D'Amico C, Mancini B, Saieva C, Aceto G, Gestri D, Vezzosi V, Falchetti M, De Marco M, Paglierani M, Cama A, Bianchi S, Mariani-Costantini R, Palli D (2003). BRCA1 and BRCA2 mutation status and tumor characteristics in male breast cancer: a population-based study in Italy. Cancer Res 63: 342–347.

1048. Ottini L, Rizzolo P, Zanna I, Falchetti M, Masala G, Ceccarelli K, Vezzosi V, Gulino A, Giannini G, Bianchi S, Sera F, Palli D (2009). BRCA1/BRCA2 mutation status and clinical-pathologic features of 108 male breast cancer cases from Tuscany: a population-based study in central Italy. Breast Cancer Res Treat 116: 577–586.

1049. Ou J, Niessen RC, Vonk J, Westers H, Hofstra RM, Sijmons RH (2008). A database to support the interpretation of human mismatch repair gene variants. Hum Mutat 29: 1337–1341.

1050. Ozmen V, Unal ES, Muslumanoglu ME, Igci A, Canbay E, Ozcinar B, Mudun A, Tunaci M, Tuzlali S, Kecer M (2010). Axillary sentinel node biopsy after neoadjuvant chemotherapy. Eur J Surg Oncol 36: 23–29.

1050A. Padilla-Rodriguez AL (2011). Pure hibernoma of the breast: insights about its origins. Ann Diagn Pathol. In press.

1051. Padmore RF, Lara JF, Ackerman DJ, Gales T, Sigurdson ER, Ehya H, Cooper HS, Patchefsky AS (1996). Primary combined malignant melanoma and ductal carcinoma of the breast. A report of two cases. Cancer 78: 2515–2525.

1052. Page DL, Anderson TJ, Sakamoto G (198). Infiltrating carcinoma: major histological types. WB Saunders: London.

1053. Page DL, Dixon JM, Anderson TJ, Lee D, Stewart HJ (1983). Invasive cribriform carcinoma of the breast. Histopathology 7: 525–536.

1054. Page DL, Dupont WD (1990). Anatomic markers of human premalignancy and risk of breast cancer. Cancer 66: 1326–1335.

1055. Page DL, Dupont WD, Rogers LW, Rados MS (1985). Atypical hyperplastic lesions of the female breast. A long-term follow-up study. Cancer 55: 2698–2708.

1056. Page DL, Kidd TE, Jr, Dupont WD, Simpson JF, Rogers LW (1991). Lobular neoplasia of the breast: higher risk for subsequent invasive cancer predicted by more extensive disease. Hum Pathol 22: 1232–1239.

1057. Page DL, Salhany KE, Jensen RA, Dupont WD (1996). Subsequent breast carcinoma risk after biopsy with atypia in a breast papilloma. Cancer 78: 258–266.

1058. Page DL, Schuyler PA, Dupont WD, Jensen RA, Plummer WD, Jr, Simpson JF (2003). Atypical lobular hyperplasia as a unilateral predictor of breast cancer risk: a retrospective cohort study. Lancet 361: 125–129.

1059. Paik S, Shak S, Tang G, Kim C, Baker J, Cronin M, Baehner FL, Walker MG, Watson D, Park T, Hiller W, Fisher ER, Wickerham DL,

Bryant J, Wolmark N (2004). A multigene assay to predict recurrence of tamoxifen-treated, node-negative breast cancer. N Engl J Med 351: 2817–2826.

1059A. Paik S, Tang G, Shak S, Kim C, Baker J, Kim W et al. (2006). Gene expression and benefit of chemotherapy in women with node-negative, estrogen receptor-positive breast cancer. J Clin Oncol 24: 3726–3734.

1060. Palacios J, Benito N, Pizarro A, Suarez A, Espada J, Cano A, Gamallo C (1995). Anomalous expression of P-cadherin in breast carcinoma. Correlation with E-cadherin expression and pathological features. Am J Pathol 146: 605–612.

1061. Palacios J, Honrado E, Osorio A, Cazorla A, Sarrio D, Barroso A, Rodriguez S, Cigudosa JC, Diez O, Alonso C, Lerma E, Sanchez L, Rivas C, Benitez J (2003). Immunohistochemical characteristics defined by tissue microarray of hereditary breast cancer not attributable to BRCA1 or BRCA2 mutations: differences from breast carcinomas arising in BRCA1 and BRCA2 mutation carriers. Clin Cancer Res 9: 3606–3614.

1062. Palacios J, Sarrio D, Garcia-Macias MC, Bryant B, Sobel ME, Merino MJ (2003). Frequent E-cadherin gene inactivation by loss of heterozygosity in pleomorphic lobular carcinoma of the breast. Mod Pathol 16: 674–678.

1063. Palau F and Espinos C (2006). Autosomal recessive cerebellar ataxias. Orphanet J Rare Dis 1: 47.

1064. Palazzo JP, Hyslop T (1998). Hyperplastic ductal and lobular lesions and carcinomas in situ of the breast: reproducibility of current diagnostic criteria among community- and academic-based pathologists. Breast J 4: 230–237.

1065. Palli D, Galli M, Bianchi S, Bussolati G, Di PS, Eusebi V, Gambacorta M, Rosselli Del TM (1996). Reproducibility of histological diagnosis of breast lesions: results of a panel in Italy. Eur J Cancer 32A: 603–607.

1066. Pallis L, Wilking N, Cedermark B, Rutqvist LE, Skoog L (1992). Receptors for estrogen and progesterone in breast carcinoma in situ. Anticancer Res 12: 2113–2115.

1067. Palmero EI, Achatz MI, Ashton-Prolla P, Olivier M, Hainaut P (2010). Tumor protein 53 mutations and inherited cancer: beyond Li-Fraumeni syndrome. Curr Opin Oncol 22: 64–69.

1068. Palombo F, Gallinari P, Iaccarino I, Lettieri T, Hughes M, D'Arrigo A, Truong O, Hsuan JJ, Jiricny J (1995). GTBP, a 160-kilo-dalton protein essential for mismatch-binding activity in human cells. Science 268: 1912–1914.

1069. Papachristou DJ, Palekar A, Surti U, Cieply K, McGough RL, Rao UN (2009). Malignant granular cell tumor of the ulnar nerve with novel cytogenetic and molecular genetic findings. Cancer Genet Cytogenet 191: 46–50.

1070. Papachristou DN, Kinne D, Ashikari R, Fortner JG (1979). Melanoma of the nipple and areola. Br J Surg 66: 287–288.

1071. Papadatos G, Rangan AM, Psarianos T, Ung O, Taylor R, Boyages J (2001). Probability of axillary node involvement in patients with tubular carcinoma of the breast. Br J Surg 88: 860–864.

1072. Papadopoulos N, Nicolaides NC, Wei YF, Ruben SM, Carter KC, Rosen CA, Haseltine WA, Fleischmann RD, Fraser CM, Adams MD (1994). Mutation of a mutL homolog in hereditary colon cancer. Science 263: 1625–1629.

1073. Park S, Koo J, Park HS, Kim JH, Choi SY, Lee JH, Park BW, Lee KS (2010). Expression of androgen receptors in primary breast cancer. Ann Oncol 21: 488–492.

1073A. Parker JS, Mullins M, Cheang MC, Leung S, Voduc D, Vickery T et al. (2009). Supervised risk predictor of breast cancer based on intrinsic subtypes. J Clin Oncol 27: 1160–1167.

1074. Parmigiani G, Berry D, Aguilar O (1998). Determining carrier probabilities for breast cancer-susceptibility genes BRCA1 and BRCA2. Am J Hum Genet 62: 145–158.

1075. Pasquale-Styles MA, Milikowski C (2003). Three-millimeter apocrine adenoma in a man: a case report and review of the literature. Arch Pathol Lab Med 127: 1498–1500.

1076. Paterakos M, Watkin WG, Edgerton SM, Moore DH, Thor AD (1999). Invasive micropapillary carcinoma of the breast: a prognostic study. Hum Pathol 30: 1459–1463.

1077. Patey DH, Scarff RW (1928). The position of histology in the prognosis of carcinoma of the breast. Lancet 1: 801–804.

1078. Patnick J, ed. (2010). NHS breast screening programme. Annual review 2010. Overcoming barriers. NHS Cancer Screening Programmes: Sheffield.

1079. Patton KT, Deyrup AT, Weiss SW (2008). Atypical vascular lesions after surgery and radiation of the breast: a clinicopathologic study of 32 cases analyzing histologic heterogeneity and association with angiosarcoma. Am J Surg Pathol 32: 943–950.

1080. Paulus DD (1990). Lymphoma of the breast. Radiol Clin North Am 28: 833–840.

1081. Pauwels P, Sciot R, Croiset F, Rutten H, Van den Berghe H, Dal CP (2000). Myofibroblastoma of the breast: genetic link with spindle cell lipoma. J Pathol 191: 282–285.

1082. Pedersen L, Holck S, Mouridsen HT, Schodt T, Zedeler K (1999). Prognostic comparison of three classifications for medullary carcinoma of the breast. Histopathology 34: 175–178.

1083. Peintinger F, Leibl S, Reitsamer R, Moinfar F (2004). Primary acinic cell carcinoma of the breast: a case report with long-term follow-up and review of the literature. Histopathology 45: 645–648.

1084. Peiro G, Bornstein BA, Connolly JL, Gelman R, Hetelekidis S, Nixon AJ, Recht A, Silver B, Harris JR, Schnitt SJ (2000). The influence of infiltrating lobular carcinoma on the outcome of patients treated with breast-conserving surgery and radiation therapy. Breast Cancer Res Treat 59: 49–54.

1085. Peltomaki P, Aaltonen LA, Sistonen P, Pylkkanen L, Mecklin JP, Jarvinen H, Green JS, Jass JR, Weber JL, Leach FS (1993). Genetic mapping of a locus predisposing to human colorectal cancer. Science 260: 810–812.

1086. Peltomaki P, Vasen H (2004). Mutations associated with HNPCC predisposition — Update of ICG-HNPCC/INSiGHT mutation database. Dis Markers 20: 269–276.

1087. Pelttari LM, Heikkinen T, Thompson D, Kallioniemi A, Schleutker J, Holli K, Blomqvist C, Aittomaki K, Butzow R, Nevanlinna H (2011). RAD51C is a susceptibility gene for ovarian cancer. Hum Mol Genet 20: 3278–3288.

1087A. Penault-Llorca F, Bilous M, Dowsett M, Hanna W, Osamura RY, Ruschoff J, Van de Vijver M, (2009). Emerging technologies for assessing HER2 amplification. Am J Clin Pathol 132: 539–548.

1088. Penner CG, Murphy LC, Huzel NJ,

Yamada EW (1991). Antigenic reactivity of ribosomal protein S6 and the calcium-binding ATPase inhibitor protein of mammalian mitochondria. Mol Cell Biochem 108: 57–66.

1089. Pereira H, Pinder SE, Sibbering DM, Galea MH, Elston CW, Blamey RW, Robertson JF, Ellis IO (1995). Pathological prognostic factors in breast cancer. IV: Should you be a typer or a grader? A comparative study of two histological prognostic features in operable breast carcinoma. Histopathology 27: 219–226.

1089A. Perou CM, Parker JS, Prat A, Ellis MJ, Bernard PS (2010). Clinical implementation of the intrinsic subtypes of breast cancer. Lancet Oncol 11: 718–719.

1090. Perou CM, Sorlie T, Eisen MB, van de Rijn M, Jeffrey SS, Rees CA, Pollack JR, Ross DT, Johnsen H, Akslen LA, Fluge O, Pergamenschikov A, Williams C, Zhu SX, Lonning PE, Borresen-Dale AL, Brown PO, Botstein D (2000). Molecular portraits of human breast tumours. Nature 406: 747–752.

1091. Perry N, Broeders M, de Wolf C, Tornberg S, Holland R, von Karsa L (2008). European guidelines for quality assurance in breast cancer screening and diagnosis. Fourth edition—summary document. Ann Oncol 19: 614–622.

1092. Persson M, Andren Y, Mark J, Horlings HM, Persson F, Stenman G (2009). Recurrent fusion of MYB and NFIB transcription factor genes in carcinomas of the breast and head and neck. Proc Natl Acad Sci U S A 106: 18740–18744.

1093. Perzin KH, Lattes R (1972). Papillary adenoma of the nipple (florid papillomatosis, adenoma, adenomatosis). A clinicopathologic study. Cancer 29: 996–1009.

1094. Pestalozzi BC, Zahrieh D, Mallon E, Gusterson BA, Price KN, Gelber RD, Holmberg SB, Lindtner J, Snyder R, Thurlimann B, Murray E, Viale G, Castiglione-Gertsch M, Coates AS, Goldhirsch A (2008). Distinct clinical and prognostic features of infiltrating lobular carcinoma of the breast: combined results of 15 International Breast Cancer Study Group clinical trials. J Clin Oncol 26: 3006–3014.

1095. Peters GN, Wolff M (1983). Adenoid cystic carcinoma of the breast. Report of 11 new cases: review of the literature and discussion of biological behavior. Cancer 52: 680–686.

1096. Peters GN, Wolff M, Haagensen CD (1981). Tubular carcinoma of the breast. Clinical pathologic correlations based on 100 cases. Ann Surg 193: 138–149.

1097. Petitjean A, Mathe E, Kato S, Ishioka C, Tavtigian SV, Hainaut P, Olivier M (2007). Impact of mutant p53 functional properties on TP53 mutation patterns and tumor phenotype: lessons from recent developments in the IARC TP53 database (R15, November 2010). Hum Mutat 28: 622–629.

1098. Pettigrew CA, French JD, Saunus JM, Edwards SL, Sauer AV, Smart CE, Lundstrom T, Wiesner C, Spurdle AB, Rothnagel JA, Brown MA (2010). Identification and functional analysis of novel BRCA1 transcripts, including mouse Brca1-Iris and human pseudo-BRCA1. Breast Cancer Res Treat 119: 239–247.

1099. Pettinato G, Manivel CJ, Panico L, Sparano L, Petrella G (2004). Invasive micropapillary carcinoma of the breast: clinicopathologic study of 62 cases of a poorly recognized variant with highly aggressive behavior. Am J Clin Pathol 121: 857–866.

1100. Pettinato G, Manivel JC, Kelly DR, Wold LE, Dehner LP (1989). Lesions of the breast in

children exclusive of typical fibroadenoma and gynecomastia. A clinicopathologic study of 113 cases. Pathol Annu 24 Pt 2: 296–328.

1100A. Pezzi CM, Patel-Parekh L, Cole K, Franko J, Klimberg VS, Bland K (2007). Characteristics and treatment of metaplastic breast cancer: analysis of 892 cases from the National Cancer Data Base. Ann Surg Oncol 14: 166–173.

1101. Pharoah PD, Antoniou AC, Easton DF, Ponder BA (2008). Polygenes, risk prediction, and targeted prevention of breast cancer. N Engl J Med 358: 2796–2803.

1102. Pharoah PD, Tyrer J, Dunning AM, Easton DF, Ponder BA (16-3-2007). Association between common variation in 120 candidate genes and breast cancer risk. PLoS.Genet. 3: e42. Abstract.

1103. Phillipson J, Ostrzega N (1994). Fine needle aspiration of invasive cribriform carcinoma with benign osteoclast-like giant cells of histiocytic origin. A case report. Acta Cytol 38: 479–482.

1104. Pia-Foschini M, Reis-Filho JS, Eusebi V, Lakhani SR (2003). Salivary gland-like tumours of the breast: surgical and molecular pathology. J Clin Pathol 56: 497–506.

1105. Pierga JY, Mouret E, Laurence V, Dieras V, Savigioni A, Beuzeboc P, Dorval T, Palangie T, Jouve M, Pouillart P (2003). Prognostic factors for survival after neoadjuvant chemotherapy in operable breast cancer. the role of clinical response. Eur J Cancer 39: 1089–1096.

1106. Pina L, Apesteguia L, Cojo R, Cojo F, Arias-Camison I, Rezola R, De Miguel C (1997). Myofibroblastoma of male breast: report of three cases and review of the literature. Eur Radiol 7: 931–934.

1107. Pinder SE, Duggan C, Ellis IO, Cuzick J, Forbes JF, Bishop H, Fentiman IS, George WD (2010). A new pathological system for grading DCIS with improved prediction of local recurrence: results from the UKCCCR/ANZ DCIS trial. Br J Cancer 103: 94–100.

1108. Pinder SE, Ellis IO, Galea M, O'Rouke S, Blamey RW, Elston CW (1994). Pathological prognostic factors in breast cancer. III. Vascular invasion: relationship with recurrence and survival in a large study with long-term follow-up. Histopathology 24: 41–47.

1109. Pinder SE, Provenzano E, Earl H, Ellis IO (2007). Laboratory handling and histology reporting of breast specimens from patients who have received neoadjuvant chemotherapy. Histopathology 50: 409–417.

1110. Pinder SE, Reis-Filho JS (2007). Non-operative breast pathology: columnar cell lesions. J Clin Pathol 60: 1307–1312.

1111. Pinilla SM, Honrado E, Hardisson D, Benitez J, Palacios J (2006). Caveolin-1 expression is associated with a basal-like phenotype in sporadic and hereditary breast cancer. Breast Cancer Res Treat 99: 85–90.

1111A. Pitts WC, Rojas VA, Gaffey MJ, Rouse RV, Esteban J, Frierson HF, Kempson RL, Weiss LM (1991). Carcinomas with metaplasia and sarcomas of the breast. Am J Clin Pathol 95: 623–632.

1112. Planchon SM, Waite KA, Eng C (2008). The nuclear affairs of PTEN. J Cell Sci 121: 249–253.

1113. Pluquet O, Hainaut P (2001). Genotoxic and non-genotoxic pathways of p53 induction. Cancer Lett 174: 1–15.

1113A. Podetta M, D'Ambrosio G, Ferrari A, Sgarella A, Dal BB, Fossati GS, Zonta S, Silini E, Dionigi P (2009). Low-grade fibromatosis-

like spindle cell metaplastic carcinoma: a basal-like tumor with a favorable clinical outcome. Report of two cases. Tumori 95: 264–267.
1114. Polednak AP (2003). Bilateral synchronous breast cancer: a population-based study of characteristics, method of detection, and survival. Surgery 133: 383–389.
1115. Polyak K (2010). Molecular markers for the diagnosis and management of ductal carcinoma in situ. J Natl Cancer Inst Monogr 2010: 210–213.
1116. Popnikolov NK, Ayala AG, Graves K, Gatalica Z (2003). Benign myoepithelial tumors of the breast have immunophenotypic characteristics similar to metaplastic matrix-producing and spindle cell carcinomas. Am J Clin Pathol 120: 161–167.
1117. Porter PL, Garcia R, Moe R, Corwin DJ, Gown AM (1991). C-erbB-2 oncogene protein in in situ and invasive lobular breast neoplasia. Cancer 68: 331–334.
1118. Powell CM, Cranor ML, Rosen PP (1995). Pseudoangiomatous stromal hyperplasia (PASH). A mammary stromal tumor with myofibroblastic differentiation. Am J Surg Pathol 19: 270–277.
1119. Powell CM, Rosen PP (1994). Adipose differentiation in cystosarcoma phyllodes. A study of 14 cases. Am J Surg Pathol 18: 720–727.
1120. Prasad ML, Osborne MP, Giri DD, Hoda SA (2000). Microinvasive carcinoma (T1mic) of the breast: clinicopathologic profile of 21 cases. Am J Surg Pathol 24: 422–428.
1121. Prasad SN, Houserkova D, Svach I, Zlamalova N, Kucerova L, Cwiertka K (2008). Pseudoangiomatous stromal hyperplasia of breast: a case report. Biomed Pap Med Fac Univ Palacky Olomouc Czech Repub 152: 117–120.
1122. Prat A, Parker JS, Karginova O, Fan C, Livasy C, Herschkowitz JI, He X, Perou CM (2010). Phenotypic and molecular characterization of the claudin-low intrinsic subtype of breast cancer. Breast Cancer Res 12: R68.
1123. Prat A, Perou CM (2011). Deconstructing the molecular portraits of breast cancer. Mol Oncol 5: 5–23.
1124. Prescott RJ, Eyden BP, Reeve NL (1992). Sebaceous differentiation in a breast carcinoma with ductal, myoepithelial and squamous elements. Histopathology 21: 181–184.
1125. Pugliese M, Stempel M, Patil S, Hsu M, Ho A, Traina T, Morrow M, Cody H, III, Gemignani ML (2010). The clinical impact and outcomes of immunohistochemistry-only metastasis in breast cancer. Am J Surg 200: 368–373.
1126. Pugliese MS, Stempel MM, Cody HS, III, Morrow M, Gemignani ML (2009). Surgical management of the axilla: do intramammary nodes matter? Am J Surg 198: 532–537.
1126A. Pusztai L, Mazouni C, Anderson K, Wu Y, Symmans WF (2006). Molecular classification of breast cancer: limitations and potential. Oncologist 11: 868–877.
1127. Quenneville LA, Phillips KA, Ozcelik H, Parkes RK, Knight JA, Goodwin PJ, Andrulis IL, O'Malley FP (2002). HER-2/neu status and tumor morphology of invasive breast carcinomas in Ashkenazi women with known BRCA1 mutation status in the Ontario Familial Breast Cancer Registry. Cancer 95: 2068–2075.
1128. Quincey C, Raitt N, Bell J, Ellis IO (1991). Intracytoplasmic lumina—a useful diagnostic feature of adenocarcinomas. Histopathology 19: 83–87.
1129. Rabban JT, Koerner FC, Lerwill MF (2006). Solid papillary ductal carcinoma in situ versus usual ductal hyperplasia in the breast: a potentially difficult distinction resolved by cytokeratin 5/6. Hum Pathol 37: 787–793.
1130. Radhi JM (2000). Immunohistochemical analysis of pleomorphic lobular carcinoma: higher expression of p53 and chromogranin and lower expression of ER and PgR. Histopathology 36: 156–160.
1131. Ragazzi M, de Biase D., Betts CM, Farnedi A, Ramadan SS, Tallini G, Reis-Filho JS, Eusebi V (2011). Oncocytic carcinoma of the breast: frequency, morphology and follow-up. Hum Pathol 42: 166–175.
1132. Rahman N, Seal S, Thompson D, Kelly P, Renwick A, Elliott A, Reid S, Spanova K, Barfoot R, Chagtai T, Jayatilake H, McGuffog L, Hanks S, Evans DG, Eccles D, Easton DF, Stratton MR (2007). PALB2, which encodes a BRCA2-interacting protein, is a breast cancer susceptibility gene. Nat Genet 39: 165–167.
1133. Rajan JV, Wang M, Marquis ST, Chodosh LA (1996). Brca2 is coordinately regulated with Brca1 during proliferation and differentiation in mammary epithelial cells. Proc Natl Acad Sci U S A 93: 13078–13083.
1134. Raju GC, O'Reilly AP (1987). Immunohistochemical study of granular cell tumour. Pathology 19: 402–406.
1135. Rakha EA, Aleskandarany M, El-Sayed ME, Blamey RW, Elston CW, Ellis IO, Lee AH (2009). The prognostic significance of inflammation and medullary histological type in invasive carcinoma of the breast. Eur J Cancer 45: 1780–1787.
1135A. Rakha EA, Armour JA, Pinder SE, Paish CE, Ellis IO (2005). High-resolution analysis of 16q22.1 in breast carcinoma using DNA amplifiable probes (multiplex amplifiable probe hybridization technique) and immunohistochemistry. Int J Cancer 114: 720–729.
1136. Rakha EA, El-Sayed ME, Lee AH, Elston CW, Grainge MJ, Hodi Z, Blamey RW, Ellis IO (2008). Prognostic significance of Nottingham histologic grade in invasive breast carcinoma. J Clin Oncol 26: 3153–3158.
1137. Rakha EA, El-Sayed ME, Menon S, Green AR, Lee AH, Ellis IO (2008). Histologic grading is an independent prognostic factor in invasive lobular carcinoma of the breast. Breast Cancer Res Treat 111: 121–127.
1138. Rakha EA, El-Sayed ME, Powe DG, Green AR, Habashy H, Grainge MJ, Robertson JF, Blamey R, Gee J, Nicholson RI, Lee AH, Ellis IO (2008). Invasive lobular carcinoma of the breast: response to hormonal therapy and outcomes. Eur J Cancer 44: 73–83.
1139. Rakha EA, El-Sayed ME, Reed J, Lee AH, Evans AJ, Ellis IO (2009). Screen-detected breast lesions with malignant needle core biopsy diagnoses and no malignancy identified in subsequent surgical excision specimens (potential false-positive diagnosis). Eur J Cancer 45: 1162–1167.
1140. Rakha EA, Gandhi N, Climent F, van Deurzen CH, Haider SA, Dunk L, Lee AH, Macmillan D, Ellis IO (2011). Encapsulated papillary carcinoma of the breast: an invasive tumor with excellent prognosis. Am J Surg Pathol 35: 1093–1103.
1141. Rakha EA, Lee AH, Evans AJ, Menon S, Assad NY, Hodi Z, Macmillan D, Blamey RW, Ellis IO (2010). Tubular carcinoma of the breast: further evidence to support its excellent prognosis. J Clin Oncol 28: 99–104.
1142. Rakha EA, Lee AH, Jenkins JA, Murphy AE, Hamilton LJ, Ellis IO (2010). Characterisation and outcome of breast needle core biopsy diagnoses of lesions of uncertain malignant potential (B3) in abnormalities detected by mammographic screening. Int J Cancer 129: 1417–1424.
1143. Rakha EA, Lee AH, Reed J, Murphy A, El-Sayed M, Burrell H, Evans AJ, Ellis IO (2010). Screen-detected malignant breast lesions diagnosed following benign (B2) or normal (B1) needle core biopsy diagnoses. Eur J Cancer 46: 1835–1840.
1144. Rakha EA, Patel A, Powe DG, Benhasouna A, Green AR, Lambros MB, Reis-Filho JS, Ellis IO (2010). Clinical and biological significance of E-cadherin protein expression in invasive lobular carcinoma of the breast. Am J Surg Pathol 34: 1472–1479.
1145. Rakha EA, Putti TC, Abd El-Rehim DM, Paish C, Green AR, Powe DG, Lee AH, Robertson JF, Ellis IO (2006). Morphological and immunophenotypic analysis of breast carcinomas with basal and myoepithelial differentiation. J Pathol 208: 495–506.
1146. Rakha EA, Reis-Filho JS, Baehner F, Dabbs DJ, Decker T, Eusebi V, Fox SB, Ichihara S, Jacquemier J, Lakhani SR, Palacios J, Richardson AL, Schnitt SJ, Schmitt FC, Tan PH, Tse GM, Badve S, Ellis IO (2010). Breast cancer prognostic classification in the molecular era: the role of histological grade. Breast Cancer Res 12: 207
1147. Rakha EA, Reis-Filho JS, Ellis IO (2008). Basal-like breast cancer: a critical review. J Clin Oncol 26: 2568–2581.
1148. Ramachandra S, Machin L, Ashley S, Monaghan P, Gusterson BA (1990). Immunohistochemical distribution of c-erbB-2 in in situ breast carcinoma—a detailed morphological analysis. J Pathol 161: 7–14.
1149. Ramaswamy PV, Storm CA, Filiano JJ, Dinulos JG (2010). Multiple granular cell tumors in a child with Noonan syndrome. Pediatr Dermatol 27: 209–211.
1150. Ramljak V, Sarcevic B, Vrdoljak DV, Kelcec IB, Agai M, Ostovic KT (2010). Fine needle aspiration cytology in diagnosing rare breast carcinoma—two case reports. Coll Antropol 34: 201–205.
1151. Rammeh-Rommani S, Mrad K, Dhouib R, Sassi S, Driss M, Khattech R, Ben RK (2000). [Adenomyoepithelioma of the breast: two cases]. Ann Pathol 20: 365–368.
1152. Ramos CV, TAYLOR HB (1974). Lipid-rich carcinoma of the breast. A clinicopathologic analysis of 13 examples. Cancer 33: 812–819.
1153. Rao P, Shousha S (2010). Male nipple adenoma with DCIS followed 9 years later by invasive carcinoma. Breast J 16: 317–318.
1154. Rao VK, Weiss SW (1992). Angiomatosis of soft tissue. An analysis of the histologic features and clinical outcome in 51 cases. Am J Surg Pathol 16: 764–771.
1155. Rasbridge SA, Gillett CE, Sampson SA, Walsh FS, Millis RR (1993). Epithelial (E-) and placental (P-) cadherin cell adhesion molecule expression in breast carcinoma. J Pathol 169: 245–250.
1156. Rasbridge SA, Millis RR (1998). Adenomyoepithelioma of the breast with malignant features. Virchows Arch 432: 123–130.
1157. Rasmussen BB, Rose C, Thorpe SM, Andersen KW, Hou-Jensen K (1985). Argyrophilic cells in 202 human mucinous breast carcinomas. Relation to histopathologic and clinical factors. Am.J.Clin.Pathol. 84: 737. Abstract.
1158. Ravdin PM, Siminoff LA, Davis GJ, Mercer MB, Hewlett J, Gerson N, Parker HL (2001). Computer program to assist in making decisions about adjuvant therapy for women with early breast cancer. J Clin Oncol 19: 980–991.
1159. Rawal A, Finn WG, Schnitzer B, Valdez R (2007). Site-specific morphologic differences in extranodal marginal zone B-cell lymphomas. Arch Pathol Lab Med 131: 1673–1678.
1160. Reardon W, Zhou XP, Eng C (2001). A novel germline mutation of the PTEN gene in a patient with macrocephaly, ventricular dilatation, and features of VATER association. J Med Genet 38: 820–823.
1161. Recine MA, Deavers MT, Middleton LP, Silva EG, Malpica A (2004). Serous carcinoma of the ovary and peritoneum with metastases to the breast and axillary lymph nodes: a potential pitfall. Am J Surg Pathol 28: 1646–1651.
1162. Reeves GK, Beral V, Green J, Gathani T, Bull D (2006). Hormonal therapy for menopause and breast-cancer risk by histological type: a cohort study and meta-analysis. Lancet Oncol 7: 910–918.
1163. Reeves GK, Pirie K, Green J, Bull D, Beral V (2009). Reproductive factors and specific histological types of breast cancer: prospective study and meta-analysis. Br J Cancer 100: 538–544.
1164. Regitnig P, Ploner F, Maderbacher M, Lax SF (2004). Bilateral carcinomas of the breast with local recurrence: analysis of genetic relationship of the tumors. Mod Pathol 17: 597–602.
1165. Reis-Filho JS, Fulford LG, Crebassa B, Carpentier S, Lakhani SR (2004). Collagenous spherulosis in an adenomyoepithelioma of the breast. J Clin Pathol 57: 83–86.
1166. Reis-Filho JS, Fulford LG, Lakhani SR, Schmitt FC (2003). Pathologic quiz case: a 62-year-old woman with a 4.5-cm nodule in the right breast. Lipid-rich breast carcinoma. Arch Pathol Lab Med 127: e396–e398.
1167. Reis-Filho JS, Lakhani SR (2003). The diagnosis and management of pre-invasive breast disease: genetic alterations in pre-invasive lesions. Breast Cancer Res 5: 313–319.
1168. Reis-Filho JS, Milanezi F, Amendoeira I, Albergaria A, Schmitt FC (2003). Distribution of p63, a novel myoepithelial marker, in fine-needle aspiration biopsies of the breast: an analysis of 82 samples. Cancer 99: 172–179.
1168A. Reis-Filho JS, Milanezi F, Carvalho S, Simpson PT, Steele D, Savage K, Lambros MB, Pereira EM, Nesland JM, Lakhani SR, Schmitt FC (2005). Metaplastic breast carcinomas exhibit EGFR, but not HER2, gene amplification and overexpression: immunohistochemical and chromogenic in situ hybridization analysis. Breast Cancer Res 7: R1028–R1035.
1168B. Reis-Filho JS, Milanezi F, Paredes J, Silva P, Pereira EM, Maeda SA, de Carvalho LV, Schmitt FC (2003). Novel and classic myoepithelial/stem cell markers in metaplastic carcinomas of the breast. Appl Immunohistochem Mol Morphol 11: 1–8.
1169. Reis-Filho JS, Milanezi F, Silva P, Schmitt FC (2001). Maspin expression in myoepithelial tumors of the breast. Pathol Res Pract 197: 817–821.
1169A. Reis-Filho JS, Milanezi F, Steele D, Savage K, Simpson PT, Nesland JM, Pereira EM, Lakhani SR, Schmitt FC (2006). Metaplastic breast carcinomas are basal-like tumours. Histopathology 49: 10–21.
1170. Reis-Filho JS, Natrajan R, Vatcheva R, Lambros MB, Marchio C, Mahler-Araujo B, Paish C, Hodi Z, Eusebi V, Ellis IO (2008). Is acinic cell carcinoma a variant of secretory car-

cinoma? A FISH study using ETV6 'split apart' probes. Histopathology 52: 840–846.

1170A. Reis-Filho JS, Pinheiro C, Lambros MB, Milanezi F, Carvalho S, Savage K, Simpson PT, Jones C, Swift S, Mackay A, Reis RM, Hornick JL, Pereira EM, Baltazar F, Fletcher CD, Ashworth A, Lakhani SR, Schmitt FC (2006). EGFR amplification and lack of activating mutations in metaplastic breast carcinomas. J Pathol 209: 445–453.

1171. Reis-Filho JS, Schmitt FC (2002). Taking advantage of basic research: p63 is a reliable myoepithelial and stem cell marker. Adv Anat Pathol 9: 280–289.

1171A. Reis-Filho JS, Schmitt FC (2003). p63 expression in sarcomatoid/metaplastic carcinomas of the breast. Histopathology 42: 94–95.

1172. Reis-Filho JS, Simpson PT, Jones C, Steele D, Mackay A, Iravani M, Fenwick K, Valgeirsson H, Lambros M, Ashworth A, Palacios J, Schmitt F, Lakhani SR (2005). Pleomorphic lobular carcinoma of the breast: role of comprehensive molecular pathology in characterization of an entity. J Pathol 207: 1–13.

1173. Reis-Filho JS, Simpson PT, Turner NC, Lambros MB, Jones C, Mackay A, Grigoriadis A, Sarrio D, Savage K, Dexter T, Iravani M, Fenwick K, Weber B, Hardisson D, Schmitt FC, Palacios J, Lakhani SR, Ashworth A (2006). FGFR1 emerges as a potential therapeutic target for lobular breast carcinomas. Clin Cancer Res 12: 6652–6662.

1173A. Reis-Filho JS, Weigelt B, Fumagalli D, Sotiriou C (2010). Molecular profiling: moving away from tumor philately. Sci Transl Med 2: 47ps43.

1173B. Rekhi B, Shet TM, Badwe RA, Chinoy RF (2007). Fibromatosis-like carcinoma-an unusual phenotype of a metaplastic breast tumor associated with a micropapilloma. World J Surg Oncol 5: 24

1174. Renehan AG, Harvie M, Howell A (2006). Insulin-like growth factor (IGF)-I, IGF binding protein-3, and breast cancer risk: eight years on. Endocr Relat Cancer 13: 273–278.

1175. Renwick A, Thompson D, Seal S, Kelly P, Chagtai T, Ahmed M, North B, Jayatilake H, Barfoot R, Spanova K, McGuffog L, Evans DG, Eccles D, Easton DF, Stratton MR, Rahman N (2006). ATM mutations that cause ataxia-telangiectasia are breast cancer susceptibility alleles. Nat Genet 38: 873–875.

1176. Requena L, Kutzner H, Mentzel T, Duran R, Rodriguez-Peralto JL (2002). Benign vascular proliferations in irradiated skin. Am J Surg Pathol 26: 328–337.

1176A. Resetkova E, Albarracin C, Sneige N (2006). Collagenous spherulosis of breast: morphologic study of 59 cases and review of the literature. Am J Surg Pathol 30: 20–27.

1177. Resetkova E, Flanders DJ, Rosen PP (2003). Ten-year follow-up of mammary carcinoma arising in microglandular adenosis treated with breast conservation. Arch Pathol Lab Med 127: 77–80.

1177A. Reyal F, van Vliet MH, Armstrong NJ, Horlings HM, de Visser KE, Kok M et al. (2008). A comprehensive analysis of prognostic signatures reveals the high predictive capacity of the proliferation, immune response and RNA splicing modules in breast cancer. Breast Cancer Res 10: R93,

1178. Rhodes DR, Yu J, Shanker K, Deshpande N, Varambally R, Ghosh D, Barrette T, Pandey A, Chinnaiyan AM (2004). Large-scale meta-analysis of cancer microarray data identifies common transcriptional profiles

of neoplastic transformation and progression. Proc Natl Acad Sci U S A 101: 9309–9314.

1179. Ribeiro RC, Saltz R, Espana Quintera LF (2008). Breast reconstruction with parenchymal cross after giant lipoma removal. Aesthetic Plast Surg 32: 695–697.

1180. Ribrag V, Bibeau F, El Weshi A, Frayfer J, Fadel C, Cebotaru C, Laribi K, Fenaux P (2001). Primary breast lymphoma: a report of 20 cases. Br J Haematol 115: 253–256.

1181. Rich-Edwards JW, Goldman MB, Willett WC, Hunter DJ, Stampfer MJ, Colditz GA, Manson JE (1994). Adolescent body mass index and infertility caused by ovulatory disorder. Am J Obstet Gynecol 171: 171–177.

1182. Richardson AL, Wang ZC, De Nicolo A, Lu X, Brown M, Miron A, Liao X, Iglehart JD, Livingston DM, Ganesan S (2006). X chromosomal abnormalities in basal-like human breast cancer. Cancer Cell 9: 121–132.

1183. Rickert CH, Paulus W (2002). Genetic characterisation of granular cell tumours. Acta Neuropathol 103: 309–312.

1184. Ridolfi RL, Rosen PP, Port A, Kinne D, Mike V (1977). Medullary carcinoma of the breast: a clinicopathologic study with 10 year follow-up. Cancer 40: 1365–1385.

1185. Riegert-Johnson DL, Gleeson FC, Roberts M, Tholen K, Youngborg L, Bullock M, Boardman LA (2010). Cancer and Lhermitte-Duclos disease are common in Cowden syndrome patients. Hered.Cancer Clin.Pract. 8: 6. Abstract.

1186. Riener MO, Nikolopoulos E, Herr A, Wild PJ, Hausmann M, Wiech T, Orlowska-Volk M, Lassmann S, Walch A, Werner M (2008). Microarray comparative genomic hybridization analysis of tubular breast carcinoma shows recurrent loss of the CDH13 locus on 16q. Hum Pathol 39: 1621–1629.

1187. Righi L, Sapino A, Marchio C, Papotti M, Bussolati G (2010). Neuroendocrine differentiation in breast cancer: established facts and unresolved problems. Semin Diagn Pathol 27: 69–76.

1188. Risch HA, McLaughlin JR, Cole DE, Rosen B, Bradley L, Fan I, Tang J, Li S, Zhang S, Shaw PA, Narod SA (2006). Population BRCA1 and BRCA2 mutation frequencies and cancer penetrances: a kin-cohort study in Ontario, Canada. J Natl Cancer Inst 98: 1694–1706.

1189. Rissanen T, Tikkakoski T, Autio AL, paja-Sarkkinen M (1998). Ultrasonography of invasive lobular breast carcinoma. Acta Radiol 39: 285–291.

1190. Ro JY, Silva EG, Gallager HS (1987). Adenoid cystic carcinoma of the breast. Hum Pathol 18: 1276–1281.

1191. Roa BB, Boyd AA, Volcik K, Richards CS (1996). Ashkenazi Jewish population frequencies for common mutations in BRCA1 and BRCA2. Nat Genet 14: 185–187.

1192. Robertson FM, Bondy M, Yang W, Yamauchi H, Wiggins S, Kamrudin S, Krishnamurthy S, Le-Petross H, Bidaut L, Player AN, Barsky SH, Woodward WA, Buchholz T, Lucci A, Ueno N, Cristofanilli M (2010). Inflammatory breast cancer: the disease, the biology, the treatment. CA Cancer J Clin 60: 351–375.

1192A. Robertson FM, Petricoin EF, Chu K, Jin J, Circo R, Fernandez SV, Alpaugh PK, Zook M, Sun G, Wulfkuhle J, Liotta LA, Ye Z, Krishnamurthy S, Luo AZ, Lui H, Wright MC, Woodward WA, Barsky SH, Cristofanilli M (2011). Amplification of anaplastic lymphoma kinase (ALK) as a common genetic alteration in

inflammatory breast cancer. San Antonio Breast Cancer Symposium 2011, P3-01-18 . Abstract.

1193. Roden AC, Macon WR, Keeney GL, Myers JL, Feldman AL, Dogan A (2008). Seroma-associated primary anaplastic large-cell lymphoma adjacent to breast implants: an indolent T-cell lymphoproliferative disorder. Mod Pathol 21: 455–463.

1194. Rodriguez-Pinilla SM, Rodriguez-Gil Y, Moreno-Bueno G, Sarrio D, Martin-Guijarro MC, Hernandez L, Palacios J (2007). Sporadic invasive breast carcinomas with medullary features display a basal-like phenotype: an immunohistochemical and gene amplification study. Am J Surg Pathol 31: 501–508.

1195. Rody A, Holtrich U, Pusztai L, Liedtke C, Gaetje R, Ruckhaeberle E, Solbach C, Hanker L, Ahr A, Metzler D, Engels K, Karn T, Kaufmann M (2009). T-cell metagene predicts a favorable prognosis in estrogen receptor-negative and HER2-positive breast cancers. Breast Cancer Res 11: R15

1196. Rogers DA, Lobe TE, Rao BN, Fleming ID, Schropp KP, Pratt AS, Pappo AS (1994). Breast malignancy in children. J Pediatr Surg 29: 48–51.

1197. Rohen C, Caselitz J, Stern C, Wanschura S, Schoenmakers EF, Van de Ven WJ, Bartnitzke S, Bullerdiek J (1995). A hamartoma of the breast with an aberration of 12q mapped to the MAR region by fluorescence in situ hybridization. Cancer Genet Cytogenet 84: 82–84.

1198. Roncaroli F, Lamovec J, Zidar A, Eusebi V (1996). Acinic cell-like carcinoma of the breast. Virchows Arch 429: 69–74.

1199. Rosai J (1991). Borderline epithelial lesions of the breast. Am J Surg Pathol 15: 209–221.

1200. Rosen PP (1989). Adenoid cystic carcinoma of the breast. A morphologically heterogeneous neoplasm. Pathol Annu 24: 237–254.

1201. Rosen PP (1983). Microglandular adenosis. A benign lesion simulating invasive mammary carcinoma. Am J Surg Pathol 7: 137–144.

1202. Rosen PP (1983). Syringomatous adenoma of the nipple. Am J Surg Pathol 7: 739–745.

1203. Rosen PP (1983). Tumor emboli in intramammary lymphatics in breast carcinoma: pathologic criteria for diagnosis and clinical significance. Pathol Annu 18 Pt 2: 215–232.

1204. Rosen PP (1985). Vascular tumors of the breast. III. Angiomatosis. Am J Surg Pathol 9: 652–658.

1205. Rosen PP (1985). Vascular tumors of the breast. V. Nonparenchymal hemangiomas of mammary subcutaneous tissues. Am J Surg Pathol 9: 723–729.

1206. Rosen PP (1987). Adenomyoepithelioma of the breast. Hum Pathol 18: 1232–1237.

1207. Rosen PP (1997). Mammary carcinoma with osteoclast-like giant cells. In: Rosen's breast pathology.Rosen PP, ed. Lippincott-Raven: Philadelphia/New York: pp 449–456.

1208. Rosen PP (2001). Myoepithelial neoplasms. In: Rosen's breast pathology, 2nd edition.Rosen PP, ed. Lippincott Williams & Wilkins: Philadelphia: pp 121–138.

1209. Rosen PP (2008). Angiomas and other benign vascular lesions of the breast. In: Rosen's breast pathology, 3rd edition.Rosen PP, ed. Wolters Kluwer, Lippincott Williams & Williams: Philadelphia: pp 872–890.

1210. Rosen PP (2008). Benign mesenchymal

neoplasms. In: Rosen's breast pathology, 3rd edition.Rosen PP, ed. Wolters Kluwer, Lippincott Williams & Williams: Philadelphia: pp 829–901.

1211. Rosen PP (2008). Myoepithelial neoplasms. In: Rosen's breast pathology, 3rd edition.Rosen PP, ed. Wolters Kluwer, Lippincott Williams & Williams: Philadelphia: pp

1212. Rosen PP, Caicco JA (1986). Florid papillomatosis of the nipple. A study of 51 patients, including nine with mammary carcinoma. Am J Surg Pathol 10: 87–101.

1213. Rosen PP, Cranor ML (1991). Secretory carcinoma of the breast. Arch Pathol Lab Med 115: 141–144.

1214. Rosen PP, ed. (2001). Rosen's breast pathology. 2nd ed Edition. Lippincott Williams & Wilkins: Philadelphia.

1215. Rosen PP, ed. (2008). Rosen's Breast Pathology, 3rd edition. Wolters Kluwer, Lippincott Williams & Williams: Philadelphia.

1215A. Rosen PP, Ernsberger D (1987). Low-grade adenosquamous carcinoma. A variant of metaplastic mammary carcinoma. Am J Surg Pathol 11: 351–358.

1216. Rosen PP, Ernsberger D (1989). Mammary fibromatosis. A benign spindle-cell tumor with significant risk for local recurrence. Cancer 63: 1363–1369.

1217. Rosen PP, Jozefczyk MA, Boram LH (1985). Vascular tumors of the breast. IV. The venous hemangioma. Am J Surg Pathol 9: 659–665.

1218. Rosen PP, Kimmel M, Ernsberger D (1988). Mammary angiosarcoma. The prognostic significance of tumor differentiation. Cancer 62: 2145–2151.

1219. Rosen PP, Kosloff C, Lieberman PH, Adair F, Braun DW, Jr (1978). Lobular carcinoma in situ of the breast. Detailed analysis of 99 patients with average follow-up of 24 years. Am J Surg Pathol 2: 225–251.

1220. Rosen PP, Oberman HA, eds (1993). Tumors of the mammary gland. Atlas of tumor pathology. Third series, fasc. 7. Armed Forces Institute of Pathology: Washington, D.C.

1221. Rosen PP, Senie R, Schottenfeld D, Ashikari R (1979). Noninvasive breast carcinoma: frequency of unsuspected invasion and implications for treatment. Ann Surg 189: 377–382.

1221A. Rosenblum MK, Purrazzella R, Rosen PP (1986). Is microglandular adenosis a precancerous disease? A study of carcinoma arising therein. Am J Surg Pathol 10: 237–245.

1222. Rosner B, Colditz GA, Willett WC (1994). Reproductive risk factors in a prospective study of breast cancer: the Nurses' Health Study. Am J Epidemiol 139: 819–835.

1223. Ross JS (2009). Multigene classifiers, prognostic factors, and predictors of breast cancer clinical outcome. Adv Anat Pathol 16: 204–215.

1224. Rosso R, Scelsi M, Carnevali L (2000). Granular cell traumatic neuroma: a lesion occurring in mastectomy scars. Arch Pathol Lab Med 124: 709–711.

1225. Rossouw JE, Anderson GL, Prentice RL, LaCroix AZ, Kooperberg C, Stefanick ML, Jackson RD, Beresford SA, Howard BV, Johnson KC, Kotchen JM, Ockene J (2002). Risks and benefits of estrogen plus progestin in healthy postmenopausal women: principal results From the Women's Health Initiative randomized controlled trial. JAMA 288: 321–333.

1226. Rouzier R, Extra JM, Klijanienko J, Falcou MC, Asselain B, Vincent-Salomon A, Vielh P, Bourstyn E (2002). Incidence and prog-

nostic significance of complete axillary downstaging after primary chemotherapy in breast cancer patients with T1 to T3 tumors and cytologically proven axillary metastatic lymph nodes. J Clin Oncol 20: 1304–1310.
1227. Rouzier R, Pusztai L, Garbay JR, Delaloge S, Hunt KK, Hortobagyi GN, Berry D, Kuerer HM (2006). Development and validation of nomograms for predicting residual tumor size and the probability of successful conservative surgery with neoadjuvant chemotherapy for breast cancer. Cancer 107: 1459–1466.
1228. Rovera F, Ferrari A, Carcano G, Dionigi G, Cinquepalmi L, Boni L, Diurni M, Dionigi R (2006). Tubular adenoma of the breast in an 84-year-old woman: report of a case simulating breast cancer. Breast J 12: 257–259.
1229. Roylance R, Gorman P, Hanby A, Tomlinson I (2002). Allelic imbalance analysis of chromosome 16q shows that grade I and grade III invasive ductal breast cancers follow different genetic pathways. J Pathol 196: 32–36.
1230. Roylance R, Gorman P, Harris W, Liebmann R, Barnes D, Hanby A, Sheer D (1999). Comparative genomic hybridization of breast tumors stratified by histological grade reveals new insights into the biological progression of breast cancer. Cancer Res 59: 1433–1436.
1231. Rozan S, Vincent-Salomon A, Zafrani B, Validire P, De CP, Bernoux A, Nieruchalski M, Fourquet A, Clough K, Dieras V, Pouillart P, Sastre-Garau X (1998). No significant predictive value of c-erbB-2 or p53 expression regarding sensitivity to primary chemotherapy or radiotherapy in breast cancer. Int J Cancer 79: 27–33.
1232. Rubin BP, Dal CP (2001). The genetics of lipomatous tumors. Semin Diagn Pathol 18: 286–293.
1233. Rubin E, Visscher DW, Alexander RW, Urist MM, Maddox WA (1988). Proliferative disease and atypia in biopsies performed for nonpalpable lesions detected mammographically. Cancer 61: 2077–2082.
1234. Rudas M, Neumayer R, Gnant MF, Mittelbock M, Jakesz R, Reiner A (1997). p53 protein expression, cell proliferation and steroid hormone receptors in ductal and lobular in situ carcinomas of the breast. Eur J Cancer 33: 39–44.
1235. Rudloff U, Jacks LM, Goldberg JI, Wynveen CA, Brogi E, Patil S, Van Zee KJ (2010). Nomogram for predicting the risk of local recurrence after breast-conserving surgery for ductal carcinoma in situ. J Clin Oncol 28: 3762–3769.
1236. Rudlowski C, Friedrichs N, Faridi A, Fuzesi L, Moll R, Bastert G, Rath W, Buttner R (2004). Her-2/neu gene amplification and protein expression in primary male breast cancer. Breast Cancer Res Treat 84: 215–223.
1237. Ruffolo EF, Koerner FC, Maluf HM (1997). Metaplastic carcinoma of the breast with melanocytic differentiation. Mod Pathol 10: 592–596.
1238. Ruijs MW, Broeks A, Menko FH, Ausems MG, Wagner A, Oldenburg R, Meijers-Heijboer H, Van't Veer LJ, Verhoef S (2009). The contribution of CHEK2 to the TP53-negative Li-Fraumeni phenotype. Hered Cancer Clin Pract 7: 4
1239. Ruijs MW, Verhoef S, Rookus MA, Pruntel R, van der Hout AH, Hogervorst FB, Kluijt I, Sijmons RH, Aalfs CM, Wagner A, Ausems MG, Hoogerbrugge N, van Asperen CJ, Gomez Garcia EB, Meijers-Heijboer H, Ten Kate LP, Menko FH, van 't Veer LJ (2010). TP53 germline mutation testing in 180 families suspected of Li-Fraumeni syndrome: mutation detection rate and relative frequency of cancers in different familial phenotypes. J Med Genet 47: 421–428.
1240. Ruijs MW, Verhoef S, Rookus MA, Pruntel R, van der Hout AH, Hogervorst FB, Kluijt I, Sijmons RH, Aalfs CM, Wagner A, Ausems MG, Hoogerbrugge N, van Asperen CJ, Gomez Garcia EB, Meijers-Heijboer H, Ten Kate LP, Menko FH, van't Veer LJ (2010). TP53 germline mutation testing in 180 families suspected of Li-Fraumeni syndrome: mutation detection rate and relative frequency of cancers in different familial phenotypes. J Med Genet 47: 421–428.
1241. Ruiz-Delgado ML, Lopez-Ruiz JA, Eizaguirre B, Saiz A, Astigarraga E, Fernandez-Temprano Z (2007). Benign adenomyoepithelioma of the breast: imaging findings mimicking malignancy and histopathological features. Acta Radiol 48: 27–29.
1242. Runswick SK, O'Hare MJ, Jones L, Streuli CH, Garrod DR (2001). Desmosomal adhesion regulates epithelial morphogenesis and cell positioning. Nat Cell Biol 3: 823–830.
1242A. Russnes HG, Vollan HK, Lingjaerde OC, Krasnitz A, Lundin P, Naume B, Sorlie T, Borgen E, Rye IH, Langerod A, Chin SF, Teschendorff AE, Stephens PJ, Maner S, Schlichting E, Baumbusch LO, Karesen R, Stratton MP, Wigler M, Caldas C et al. (2010). Genomic architecture characterizes tumor progression paths and fate in breast cancer patients. Sci Transl Med 2: 38ra47.
1243. Ryan G, Martinelli G, Kuper-Hommel M, Tsang R, Pruneri G, Yuen K, Roos D, Lennard A, Devizzi L, Crabb S, Hossfeld D, Pratt G, Dell'Olio M, Choo SP, Bociek RG, Radford J, Lade S, Gianni AM, Zucca E, Cavalli F et al. (2008). Primary diffuse large B-cell lymphoma of the breast: prognostic factors and outcomes of a study by the International Extranodal Lymphoma Study Group. Ann Oncol 19: 233–241.
1244. Ryu EM, Whang IY, Chang ED (2010). Rapidly growing bilateral pseudoangiomatous stromal hyperplasia of the breast. Korean J Radiol 11: 355–358.
1245. Saal LH, Gruvberger-Saal SK, Persson C, Lovgren K, Jumppanen M, Staaf J, Jonsson G, Pires MM, Maurer M, Holm K, Koujak S, Subramaniyam S, Vallon-Christersson J, Olsson H, Su T, Memeo L, Ludwig T, Ethier SP, Krogh M, Szabolcs M et al. (2008). Recurrent gross mutations of the PTEN tumor suppressor gene in breast cancers with deficient DSB repair. Nat Genet 40: 102–107.
1246. Sabate JM, Gomez A, Torrubia S, Blancas C, Sanchez G, Alonso MC, Lerma E (2006). Evaluation of breast involvement in relation to Cowden syndrome: a radiological and clinicopathological study of patients with PTEN germ-line mutations. Eur Radiol 16: 702–706.
1247. Sabatier R, Finetti P, Cervera N, Lambaudie E, Esterni B, Mamessier E, Tallet A, Chabannon C, Extra JM, Jacquemier J, Viens P, Birnbaum D, Bertucci F (2010). A gene expression signature identifies two prognostic subgroups of basal breast cancer. Breast Cancer Res Treat 126: 407–420.
1248. Saglam A, Can B (2005). Coexistence of lactating adenoma and invasive ductal adenocarcinoma of the breast in a pregnant woman. J Clin Pathol 58: 87–89.
1249. Sahlin P, Windh P, Lauritzen C, Emanuelsson M, Gronberg H, Stenman G (2007). Women with Saethre-Chotzen syndrome are at increased risk of breast cancer. Genes Chromosomes Cancer 46: 656–660.
1250. Saigo PE, Rosen PP (1981). Mammary carcinoma with «choriocarcinomatous» features. Am J Surg Pathol 5: 773–778.
1251. Salmon A, Amikam D, Sodha N, Davidson S, Basel-Vanagaite L, Eeles RA, Abeliovich D, Peretz T (2007). Rapid development of post-radiotherapy sarcoma and breast cancer in a patient with a novel germline 'denovo' TP53 mutation. Clin Oncol (R Coll Radiol) 19: 490–493.
1252. Salto-Tellez M, Putti TC, Lee CK, Chiu LL, Koay ES (2005). Adenomyoepithelioma of the breast: description of allelic imbalance and microsatellite instability. Histopathology 46: 230–231.
1253. Saltzstein SL (1974). Clinically occult inflammatory carcinoma of the breast. Cancer 34: 382–388.
1254. Sanders ME, Page DL, Simpson JF, Schuyler PA, Dale PW, Dupont WD (2006). Interdependence of radial scar and proliferative disease with respect to invasive breast carcinoma risk in patients with benign breast biopsies. Cancer 106: 1453–1461.
1254A. Sanders ME, Schuyler PA, Dupont WD, Page DL (2005). The natural history of low-grade ductal carcinoma in situ of the breast in women treated by biopsy only revealed over 30 years of long-term follow-up. Cancer 103: 2481–2484.
1255. Sano M, Kikuchi K, Zhao C, Kobayashi M, Nakanishi Y, Nemoto N (2004). Osteoclastogenesis in human breast carcinoma. Virchows Arch 444: 470–472.
1256. Santisteban M, Reynolds C, Barr Fritcher EG, Frost MH, Vierkant RA, Anderson SS, Degnim AC, Visscher DW, Pankratz VS, Hartmann LC (2010). Ki67: a time-varying biomarker of risk of breast cancer in atypical hyperplasia. Breast Cancer Res Treat 121: 431–437.
1257. Saout L, Leduc M, Suy-Beng PT, Meignie P (1985). [A new case of cribriform breast carcinoma associated with histiocytic giant cell reaction]. Arch Anat Cytol Pathol 33: 58–61.
1258. Sapino A, Frigerio A, Peterse JL, Arisio R, Coluccia C, Bussolati G (2000). Mammographically detected in situ lobular carcinomas of the breast. Virchows Arch 436: 421–430.
1259. Sapino A, Righi L, Cassoni P, Papotti M, Gugliotta P, Bussolati G (2001). Expression of apocrine differentiation markers in neuroendocrine breast carcinomas of aged women. Mod Pathol 14: 768–776.
1260. Sapino A, Righi L, Cassoni P, Papotti M, Pietribiasi F, Bussolati G (2000). Expression of the neuroendocrine phenotype in carcinomas of the breast. Semin Diagn Pathol 17: 127–137.
1261. Sarnaik AA, Meade T, King J, Acs G, Hoover S, Cox CE, Carter WB, Laronga C (2010). Adenoid cystic carcinoma of the breast: a review of a single institution's experience. Breast J 16: 208–210.
1262. Sarrio D, Perez-Mies B, Hardisson D, Moreno-Bueno G, Suarez A, Cano A, Martin-Perez J, Gamallo C, Palacios J (2004). Cytoplasmic localization of p120ctn and E-cadherin loss characterize lobular breast carcinoma from preinvasive to metastatic lesions. Oncogene 23: 3272–3283.
1263. Sashiyama H, Abe Y, Miyazawa Y, Nagashima T, Hasegawa M, Okuyama K, Kuwahara T, Takagi T (1999). Primary non-Hodgkin's lymphoma of the male breast: a case report. Breast Cancer 6: 55–58.
1264. Sastre-Garau X, Jouve M, Asselain B, Vincent-Salomon A, Beuzeboc P, Dorval T, Durand JC, Fourquet A, Pouillart P (1996). Infiltrating lobular carcinoma of the breast. Clinicopathologic analysis of 975 cases with reference to data on conservative therapy and metastatic patterns. Cancer 77: 113–120.
1265. Satake N, Durham JH, Brodsky WA (1981). Reversal of the luminal acidification current by a phosphodiesterase inhibitor in the turtle bladder: evidence for active electrogenic biocarbonate secretion. Prog Clin Biol Res 73: 13–24.
1266. Sataloff DM, Mason BA, Prestipino AJ, Seinige UL, Lieber CP, Baloch Z (1995). Pathologic response to induction chemotherapy in locally advanced carcinoma of the breast: a determinant of outcome. J Am Coll Surg 180: 297–306.
1267. Sau P, Solis J, Lupton GP, James WD (1989). Pigmented breast carcinoma. A clinical and histopathologic simulator of malignant melanoma. Arch Dermatol 125: 536–539.
1268. Sauer T (2010). Fine-needle aspiration cytology of extra mammary metastatic lesions in the breast: A retrospective study of 36 cases diagnosed during 18 years. Cytojournal. 7: 10.
1268A. Saul S (2010). Prone to error: earliest steps to find cancer. New York Times July 19: A1 (http://www.nytimes.com/2010/07/20/health/20cancer.html?pagewanted=all).
1269. Savitsky K, Bar-Shira A, Gilad S, Rotman G, Ziv Y, Vanagaite L, Tagle DA, Smith S, Uziel T, Sfez S, Ashkenazi M, Pecker I, Frydman M, Harnik R, Patanjali SR, Simmons A, Clines GA, Sartiel A, Gatti RA, Chessa L et al. (1995). A single ataxia telangiectasia gene with a product similar to PI-3 kinase. Science 268: 1749–1753.
1270. Sawyer EJ, Hanby AM, Rowan AJ, Gillett CE, Thomas RE, Poulsom R, Lakhani SR, Ellis IO, Ellis P, Tomlinson IP (2002). The Wnt pathway, epithelial-stromal interactions, and malignant progression in phyllodes tumours. J Pathol 196: 437–444.
1271. Sawyer EJ, Poulsom R, Hunt FT, Jeffery R, Elia G, Ellis IO, Ellis P, Tomlinson IP, Hanby AM (2003). Malignant phyllodes tumours show stromal overexpression of c-myc and c-kit. J Pathol 200: 59–64.
1272. Schaapveld M, Visser O, Louwman WJ, Willemse PH, de Vries EG, van der Graaf WT, Otter R, Coebergh JW, van Leeuwen FE (2008). The impact of adjuvant therapy on contralateral breast cancer risk and the prognostic significance of contralateral breast cancer: a population based study in the Netherlands. Breast Cancer Res Treat 110: 189–197.
1273. Schelfout K, Van Goethem M, Kersschot E, Verslegers I, Biltjes I, Leyman P, Colpaert C, Thienpont L, Van den Haute J, Gillardin JP, Tjalma W, Buytaert P, De Schepper A (2004). Preoperative breast MRI in patients with invasive lobular breast cancer. Eur Radiol 14: 1209–1216.
1274. Schiff R, Osborne CK, Fuqua SAW (2010). Clinical aspects of estrogen and progesterone receptors. In: Diseases of the breast, 4th edition.Harris JR, Lippman ME, Morrow M, Osbourne CK, eds. Wolters Kluwer Lippincott Williams & Wilkins: Philadelphia: pp 408–430.
1275. Schmidt J, Schelling M, Lerf B, Vogt M (2009). Giant lipoma of the breast. Breast J 15: 107–108.
1276. Schmitt FC, Ribeiro CA, Alvarenga S,

Lopes JM (2000). Primary acinic cell-like carcinoma of the breast—a variant with good prognosis? Histopathology 36: 286–289.
1277. Schmitt FC, Soares R, Seruca R (1998). Bilateral apocrine carcinoma of the breast. Molecular and immunocytochemical evidence for two independent primary tumours. Virchows Arch 433: 505–509.
1278. Schmutte C, Marinescu RC, Copeland NG, Jenkins NA, Overhauser J, Fishel R (1998). Refined chromosomal localization of the mismatch repair and hereditary nonpolyposis colorectal cancer genes hMSH2 and hMSH6. Cancer Res 58: 5023–5026.
1279. Schnitt SJ (2003). Benign breast disease and breast cancer risk: morphology and beyond. Am J Surg Pathol 27: 836–841.
1280. Schnitt SJ (2010). Clinging carcinoma: an American perspective. Semin Diagn Pathol 27: 31–36.
1281. Schnitt SJ, Collins LC (2005). Columnar cell lesions and flat epithelial atypia of the breast. Semin Breast Dis 8: 100–111.
1282. Schnitt SJ, Collins LC (2008). Papillary lesions. In: Biopsy interpretation of the breast.Schnitt SJ, Collins LC, eds. Biopsy interpretation series. Wolters Kluwer/Lippincott Williams & Wilkins: Philadelphia: pp 205–235.
1283. Schnitt SJ, Connolly JL, Harris JR, Cohen RB (1984). Radiation-induced changes in the breast. Hum Pathol 15: 545–550.
1284. Schnitt SJ, Connolly JL, Tavassoli FA, Fechner RE, Kempson RL, Gelman R, Page DL (1992). Interobserver reproducibility in the diagnosis of ductal proliferative breast lesions using standardized criteria. Am J Surg Pathol 16: 1133–1143.
1285. Schnitt SJ, Vincent-Salomon A (2003). Columnar cell lesions of the breast. Adv Anat Pathol 10: 113–124.
1285A. Schrader KA, Nelson TN, De LA, Huntsman DG, McGillivray BC (2009). Multiple granular cell tumors are an associated feature of LEOPARD syndrome caused by mutation in PTPN11. Clin Genet 75: 185–189.
1286. Schrager CA, Schneider D, Gruener AC, Tsou HC, Peacocke M (1998). Clinical and pathological features of breast disease in Cowden's syndrome: an underrecognized syndrome with an increased risk of breast cancer. Hum Pathol 29: 47–53.
1287. Schramm N, Pfluger T, Reiser MF, Berger F (2010). Subcutaneous panniculitis-like T-cell lymphoma with breast involvement: functional and morphological imaging findings. Br J Radiol 83: e90–e94.
1288. Schwartz GF, Patchefsky AS, Finklestein SD, Sohn SH, Prestipino A, Feig SA, Singer JS (1989). Nonpalpable in situ ductal carcinoma of the breast. Predictors of multicentricity and microinvasion and implications for treatment. Arch Surg 124: 29–32.
1289. Schwentner L, Kurzeder C, Kreienberg R, Wockel A (2011). Focus on haematogenous dissemination of the malignant cystosarcoma phylloides: institutional experience. Arch Gynecol Obstet 283: 591–596.
1290. Scopsi L, Andreola S, Pilotti S, Bufalino R, Baldini MT, Testori A, Rilke F (1994). Mucinous carcinoma of the breast. A clinicopathologic, histochemical, and immunocytochemical study with special reference to neuroendocrine differentiation. Am J Surg Pathol 18: 702–711.
1291. Scott RJ, McPhillips M, Meldrum CJ, Fitzgerald PE, Adams K, Spigelman AD, du SD, Tucker K, Kirk J (2001). Hereditary nonpolyposis colorectal cancer in 95 families: differences and similarities between mutation-positive and mutation-negative kindreds. Am J Hum Genet 68: 118–127.
1292. Scow JS, Reynolds CA, Degnim AC, Petersen IA, Jakub JW, Boughey JC (2010). Primary and secondary angiosarcoma of the breast: the Mayo Clinic experience. J Surg Oncol 101: 401–407.
1293. Seal S, Thompson D, Renwick A, Elliott A, Kelly P, Barfoot R, Chagtai T, Jayatilake H, Ahmed M, Spanova K, North B, McGuffog L, Evans DG, Eccles D, Easton DF, Stratton MR, Rahman N (2006). Truncating mutations in the Fanconi anemia J gene BRIP1 are low-penetrance breast cancer susceptibility alleles. Nat Genet 38: 1239–1241.
1294. Sek P, Zawrocki A, Biernat W, Piekarski JH (2010). HER2 molecular subtype is a dominant subtype of mammary Paget's cells. An immunohistochemical study. Histopathology 57: 564–571.
1295. Selinko VL, Middleton LP, Dempsey PJ (2004). Role of sonography in diagnosing and staging invasive lobular carcinoma. J Clin Ultrasound 32: 323–332.
1296. Senter L, Clendenning M, Sotamaa K, Hampel H, Green J, Potter JD, Lindblom A, Lagerstedt K, Thibodeau SN, Lindor NM, Young J, Winship I, Dowty JG, White DM, Hopper JL, Baglietto L, Jenkins MA, de la CA (2008). The clinical phenotype of Lynch syndrome due to germ-line PMS2 mutations. Gastroenterology 135: 419–428.
1297. Sgroi DC (2010). Preinvasive breast cancer. Annu Rev Pathol 5: 193–221.
1297A. Shah SP, Morin RD, Khattra J, Prentice L, Pugh T, Burleigh A, Delaney A, Gelmon K, Guliany R, Senz J, Steidl C, Holt RA, Jones S, Sun M, Leung G, Moore R, Severson T, Taylor GA, Teschendorff AE, Tse K et al. (2009). Mutational evolution in a lobular breast tumour profiled at single nucleotide resolution. Nature 461: 809–813.
1298. Shanley S, Fung C, Milliken J, Leary J, Barnetson R, Schnitzler M, Kirk J (2009). Breast cancer immunohistochemistry can be useful in triage of some HNPCC families. Fam Cancer 8: 251–255.
1299. Shehata BM, Fishman I, Collings MH, Wang J, Poulik JM, Ricketts RR, Parker PM, Heiss K, Bhatia AM, Worcester HD, Gow KW (2009). Pseudoangiomatous stromal hyperplasia of the breast in pediatric patients: an underrecognized entity. Pediatr Dev Pathol 12: 450–454.
1300. Shen WH, Balajee AS, Wang J, Wu H, Eng C, Pandolfi PP, Yin Y (2007). Essential role for nuclear PTEN in maintaining chromosomal integrity. Cell 128: 157–170.
1301. Shepherd JJ, Wright DH (1967). Burkitt's tumour presenting as bilateral swelling of the breast in women of child-bearing age. Br J Surg 54: 776–780.
1302. Sheppard DG, Whitman GJ, Huynh PT, Sahin AA, Fornage BD, Stelling CB (2000). Tubular carcinoma of the breast: mammographic and sonographic features. AJR Am J Roentgenol 174: 253–257.
1303. Sheth NA, Saruiya JN, Ranadive KJ, Sheth AR (1974). Ectopic production of human chorionic gonadotrophin by human breast tumours. Br J Cancer 30: 566–570.
1304. Shibata A, Tsai YC, Press MF, Henderson BE, Jones PA, Ross RK (1996). Clonal analysis of bilateral breast cancer. Clin Cancer Res 2: 743–748.
1305. Shien T, Tashiro T, Omatsu M, Masuda T, Furuta K, Sato N, kashi-Tanaka S, Uehara M, Iwamoto E, Kinoshita T, Fukutomi T, Tsuda H, Hasegawa T (2005). Frequent overexpression of epidermal growth factor receptor (EGFR) in mammary high grade ductal carcinomas with myoepithelial differentiation. J Clin Pathol 58: 1299–1304.
1306. Shiloh Y (2003). ATM and related protein kinases: safeguarding genome integrity. Nat Rev Cancer 3: 155–168.
1307. Shin HJ, Kim HH, Kim SM, Kim DB, Lee YR, Kim MJ, Gong G (2007). Pure and mixed tubular carcinoma of the breast: mammographic and sonographic differential features. Korean J Radiol 8: 103–110.
1308. Shin SJ, DeLellis RA, Ying L, Rosen PP (2000). Small cell carcinoma of the breast: a clinicopathologic and immunohistochemical study of nine patients. Am J Surg Pathol 24: 1231–1238.
1309. Shin SJ, Kanomata N, Rosen PP (2000). Mammary carcinoma with prominent cytoplasmic lipofuscin granules mimicking melanocytic differentiation. Histopathology 37: 456–459.
1310. Shin SJ, Rosen PP (2002). Solid variant of mammary adenoid cystic carcinoma with basaloid features: a study of nine cases. Am J Surg Pathol 26: 413–420.
1311. Shin SJ, Simpson PT, Da Silva L, Jayanthan J, Reid L, Lakhani SR, Rosen PP (2009). Molecular evidence for progression of microglandular adenosis (MGA) to invasive carcinoma. Am J Surg Pathol 33: 496–504.
1312. Shirakawa K, Kobayashi H, Heike Y, Kawamoto S, Brechbiel MW, Kasumi F, Iwanaga T, Konishi F, Terada M, Wakasugi H (2002). Hemodynamics in vasculogenic mimicry and angiogenesis of inflammatory breast cancer xenograft. Cancer Res 62: 560–566.
1313. Shirley SE, Duncan ND, Escoffery CT, West AB (2002). Angiomatosis of the breast in a male child. A case report with immunohistochemical analysis. West Indian Med J 51: 254–256.
1314. Shishido-Hara Y, Kurata A, Fujiwara M, Itoh H, Imoto S, Kamma H (2010). Two cases of breast carcinoma with osteoclastic giant cells: are the osteoclastic giant cells pro-tumoural differentiation of macrophages? Diagn Pathol 5: 55
1315. Shousha S (2007). Glandular Paget's disease of the nipple. Histopathology 50: 812–814.
1316. Shousha S, Backhous CM, Alaghband-Zadeh J, Burn I (1986). Alveolar variant of invasive lobular carcinoma of the breast. A tumor rich in estrogen receptors. Am J Clin Pathol 85: 1–5.
1317. Shousha S, Schoenfeld A, Moss J, Shore I, Sinnett HD (1994). Light and electron microscopic study of an invasive cribriform carcinoma with extensive microcalcification developing in a breast with silicone augmentation. Ultrastruct Pathol 18: 519–523.
1318. Shousha S, Tisdall M, Sinnett HD (2004). Paget's disease of the nipple occurring after conservative surgery for ductal carcinoma in situ of the breast. Histopathology 45: 416–418.
1319. Sidwell RU, Rouse P, Owen RA, Green JS (2008). Granular cell tumor of the scrotum in a child with Noonan syndrome. Pediatr Dermatol 25: 341–343.
1320. Silver SA, Tavassoli FA (1998). Primary osteogenic sarcoma of the breast: a clinicopathologic analysis of 50 cases. Am J Surg Pathol 22: 925–933.
1321. Silver SA, Tavassoli FA (2000). Pleomorphic carcinoma of the breast: clinicopathological analysis of 26 cases of an unusual high-grade phenotype of ductal carcinoma. Histopathology 36: 505–514.
1322. Silvera D, Arju R, Darvishian F, Levine PH, Zolfaghari L, Goldberg J, Hochman T, Formenti SC, Schneider RJ (2009). Essential role for eIF4GI overexpression in the pathogenesis of inflammatory breast cancer. Nat Cell Biol 11: 903–908.
1323. Silverman EM, Oberman HA (1974). Metastatic neoplasms in the breast. Surg Gynecol Obstet 138: 26–28.
1324. Silverstein MJ, Lagios MD (2010). Choosing treatment for patients with ductal carcinoma in situ: fine tuning the University of Southern California/Van Nuys Prognostic Index. J Natl Cancer Inst Monogr 2010: 193–196.
1325. Silverstein MJ, Lagios MD, Recht A, Allred DC, Harms SE, Holland R, Holmes DR, Hughes LL, Jackman RJ, Julian TB, Kuerer HM, Mabry HC, McCready DR, McMasters KM, Page DL, Parker SH, Pass HA, Pegram M, Rubin E, Stavros AT et al. (2005). Image-detected breast cancer: state of the art diagnosis and treatment. J Am Coll Surg 201: 586–597.
1326. Silverstein MJ, Lewinsky BS, Waisman JR, Gierson ED, Colburn WJ, Senofsky GM, Gamagami P (1994). Infiltrating lobular carcinoma. Is it different from infiltrating duct carcinoma? Cancer 73: 1673–1677.
1326A. Simpson JF, Sanders ME, Page DL (2011). Diagnostic accuracy of ductal carcinoma in situ: results of Eastern Cooperative Oncology Trial 5194. Lab Invest 91: 64A.
1327. Simpson PT, Gale T, Reis-Filho JS, Jones C, Parry S, Sloane JP, Hanby A, Pinder SE, Lee AH, Humphreys S, Ellis IO, Lakhani SR (2005). Columnar cell lesions of the breast: the missing link in breast cancer progression? A morphological and molecular analysis. Am J Surg Pathol 29: 734–746.
1328. Simpson PT, Gale T, Reis-Filho JS, Jones C, Parry S, Steele D, Cossu A, Budroni M, Palmieri G, Lakhani SR (2004). Distribution and significance of 14-3-3sigma, a novel myoepithelial marker, in normal, benign, and malignant breast tissue. J Pathol 202: 274–285.
1329. Simpson PT, Reis-Filho JS, Lambros MB, Jones C, Steele D, Mackay A, Iravani M, Fenwick K, Dexter T, Jones A, Reid L, Da SL, Shin SJ, Hardisson D, Ashworth A, Schmitt FC, Palacios J, Lakhani SR (2008). Molecular profiling pleomorphic lobular carcinomas of the breast: evidence for a common molecular genetic pathway with classic lobular carcinomas. J Pathol 215: 231–244.
1330. Simpson RH, Cope N, Skalova A, Michal M (1998). Malignant adenomyoepithelioma of the breast with mixed osteogenic, spindle cell, and carcinomatous differentiation. Am J Surg Pathol 22: 631–636.
1331. Singh KA, Lewis MM, Runge RL, Carlson GW (2007). Pseudoangiomatous stromal hyperplasia. A case for bilateral mastectomy in a 12-year-old girl. Breast J 13: 603–606.
1332. Sinha PS, Bendall S, Bates T (2000). Does routine grading of invasive lobular cancer of the breast have the same prognostic significance as for ductal cancers? Eur J Surg Oncol 26: 733–737.
1333. Sinilnikova OM, Egan KM, Quinn JL, Boutrand L, Lenoir GM, Stoppa-Lyonnet D, Desjardins L, Levy C, Goldgar D, Gragoudas ES (1999). Germline brca2 sequence variants in patients with ocular melanoma. Int J Cancer 82: 325–328.
1334. Siponen E, Hukkinen K, Heikkila P,

Joensuu H, Leidenius M (2010). Surgical treatment in Paget's disease of the breast. Am J Surg 200: 241–246.

1335. Siriaunkgul S, Tavassoli FA (1993). Invasive micropapillary carcinoma of the breast. Mod Pathol 6: 660–662.

1336. Skalova A, Vanecek T, Sima R, Laco J, Weinreb I, Perez-Ordonez B, Starek I, Geierova M, Simpson RH, Passador-Santos F, Ryska A, Leivo I, Kinkor Z, Michal M (2010). Mammary analogue secretory carcinoma of salivary glands, containing the ETV6-NTRK3 fusion gene: a hitherto undescribed salivary gland tumor entity. Am J Surg Pathol 34: 599–608.

1337. Sklair-Levy M, Sella T, Alweiss T, Craciun I, Libson E, Mally B (2008). Incidence and management of complex fibroadenomas. AJR Am J Roentgenol 190: 214–218.

1338. Sloane JP, Amendoeira I, Apostolikas N, Bellocq JP, Bianchi S, Boecker W, Bussolati G, Coleman D, Connolly CE, Dervan P, Eusebi V, De MC, Drijkoningen M, Elston CW, Faverley D, Gad A, Jacquemier J, Lacerda M, Martinez-Penuela J, Munt C et al. (1998). Consistency achieved by 23 European pathologists in categorizing ductal carcinoma in situ of the breast using five classifications. European Commission Working Group on Breast Screening Pathology. Hum Pathol 29: 1056–1062.

1339. Sloane JP, Amendoeira I, Apostolikas N, Bellocq JP, Bianchi S, Boecker W, Bussolati G, Coleman D, Connolly CE, Eusebi V, De MC, Dervan P, Drijkoningen R, Elston CW, Faverly D, Gad A, Jacquemier J, Lacerda M, Martinez-Penuela J, Munt C et al. (1999). Consistency achieved by 23 European pathologists from 12 countries in diagnosing breast disease and reporting prognostic features of carcinomas. European Commission Working Group on Breast Screening Pathology. Virchows Arch 434: 3–10.

1340. Sloane JP, Mayers MM (1993). Carcinoma and atypical hyperplasia in radial scars and complex sclerosing lesions: importance of lesion size and patient age. Histopathology 23: 225–231.

1341. Smith BH, Taylor HB (1969). The occurrence of bone and cartilage in mammary tumors. Am J Clin Pathol 51: 610–618.

1342. Smith DN, Denison CM, Lester SC (1996). Spindle cell lipoma of the breast. A case report. Acta Radiol 37: 893–895.

1343. Smith PA, Harlow SP, Krag DN, Weaver DL (1999). Submission of lymph node tissue for ancillary studies decreases the accuracy of conventional breast cancer axillary node staging. Mod Pathol 12: 781–785.

1344. Smith TM, Lee MK, Szabo CI, Jerome N, McEuen M, Taylor M, Hood L, King MC (1996). Complete genomic sequence and analysis of 117 kb of human DNA containing the gene BRCA1. Genome Res 6: 1029–1049.

1345. Smith-Warner SA, Spiegelman D, Yaun SS, van den Brandt PA, Folsom AR, Goldbohm RA, Graham S, Holmberg L, Howe GR, Marshall JR, Miller AB, Potter JD, Speizer FE, Willett WC, Wolk A, Hunter DJ (1998). Alcohol and breast cancer in women: a pooled analysis of cohort studies. JAMA 279: 535–540.

1346. Sneige N, Wang J, Baker BA, Krishnamurthy S, Middleton LP (2002). Clinical, histopathologic, and biologic features of pleomorphic lobular (ductal-lobular) carcinoma in situ of the breast: a report of 24 cases. Mod Pathol 15: 1044–1050.

1347. Sneige N, Yaziji H, Mandavilli SR, Perez ER, Ordonez NG, Gown AM, Ayala A (2001). Low-grade (fibromatosis-like) spindle cell carcinoma of the breast. Am J Surg Pathol 25: 1009–1016.

1348. Sneige N, Zachariah S, Fanning TV, Dekmezian RH, Ordonez NG (1989). Fine-needle aspiration cytology of metastatic neoplasms in the breast. Am J Clin Pathol 92: 27–35.

1349. Soliman AS, Banerjee M, Lo AC, Ismail K, Hablas A, Seifeldin IA, Ramadan M, Omar HG, Fokuda A, Harford JB, Merajver SD (2009). High proportion of inflammatory breast cancer in the population-based cancer registry of Gharbiah, Egypt. Breast J 15: 432–434.

1349A. Solin LJ, Baehner FL, Butler S, Badve S, Yoshizawa C, Shak S, et al. (2011). A quantitative multigene RT-PCR assay for predicting recurrence risk after surgical excision alone without irradiation for ductal carcinoma in situ (DCIS): A prospective validation study of the DCIS Score from ECOG E5194. Cancer Res 71: 108S.

1350. Somerville JE, Clarke LA, Biggart JD (1992). c-erbB-2 overexpression and histological type of in situ and invasive breast carcinoma. J Clin Pathol 45: 16–20.

1351. Somlo G, Frankel P, Chow W, Leong L, Margolin K, Morgan R, Jr, Shibata S, Chu P, Forman S, Lim D, Twardowski P, Weitzel J, Alvarnas J, Kogut N, Schriber J, Fermin E, Yen Y, Damon L, Doroshow JH (2004). Prognostic indicators and survival in patients with stage IIIB inflammatory breast carcinoma after dose-intense chemotherapy. J Clin Oncol 22: 1839–1848.

1352. Soo MS, Dash N, Bentley R, Lee LH, Nathan G (2000). Tubular adenomas of the breast: imaging findings with histologic correlation. AJR Am J Roentgenol 174: 757–761.

1353. Soo MS, Rosen EL, Baker JA, Vo TT, Boyd BA (2001). Negative predictive value of sonography with mammography in patients with palpable breast lesions. AJR Am J Roentgenol 177: 1167–1170.

1354. Soomro S, Shousha S, Taylor P, Shepard HM, Feldmann M (1991). c-erbB-2 expression in different histological types of invasive breast carcinoma. J Clin Pathol 44: 211–214.

1355. Soreide JA, Anda O, Eriksen L, Holter J, Kjellevold KH (1988). Pleomorphic adenoma of the human breast with local recurrence. Cancer 61: 997–1001.

1355A. Sorlie T, Borgan E, Myhre S, Vollan HK, Russnes H, Zhao X et al. (2010). The importance of gene-centring microarray data. Lancet Oncol 11: 719–720.

1356. Sorlie T, Perou CM, Tibshirani R, Aas T, Geisler S, Johnsen H, Hastie T, Eisen MB, van de Rijn M, Jeffrey SS, Thorsen T, Quist H, Matese JC, Brown PO, Botstein D, Eystein LP, Borresen-Dale AL (2001). Gene expression patterns of breast carcinomas distinguish tumor subclasses with clinical implications. Proc Natl Acad Sci U S A 98: 10869–10874.

1357. Sorlie T, Tibshirani R, Parker J, Hastie T, Marron JS, Nobel A, Deng S, Johnsen H, Pesich R, Geisler S, Demeter J, Perou CM, Lonning PE, Brown PO, Borresen-Dale AL, Botstein D (2003). Repeated observation of breast tumor subtypes in independent gene expression data sets. Proc Natl Acad Sci U S A 100: 8418–8423.

1357A. Sotelo-Avila C , Bale PM (1994). Subdermal fibrous hamartoma of infancy: pathology of 40 cases and differential diagnosis. Pediatr Pathol 14: 39–52.

1358. Sotiriou C, Wirapati P, Loi S, Harris A, Fox S, Smeds J, Nordgren H, Farmer P, Praz V, Haibe-Kains B, Desmedt C, Larsimont D, Cardoso F, Peterse H, Nuyten D, Buyse M, Van de Vijver MJ, Bergh J, Piccart M, Delorenzi M (2006). Gene expression profiling in breast cancer: understanding the molecular basis of histologic grade to improve prognosis. J Natl Cancer Inst 98: 262–272.

1359. Sparano JA, Paik S (2008). Development of the 21-gene assay and its application in clinical practice and clinical trials. J Clin Oncol 26: 721–728.

1360. Squillaci S, Tallarigo F, Patarino R, Bisceglia M (2007). Nodular fasciitis of the male breast: a case report. Int J Surg Pathol 15: 69–72.

1361. Srivastava S, Zou ZQ, Pirollo K, Blattner W, Chang EH (1990). Germ-line transmission of a mutated p53 gene in a cancer-prone family with Li-Fraumeni syndrome. Nature 348: 747–749.

1361A. Stacey SN, Manolescu A, Sulem P, Rafnar T, Gudmundsson J, Gudjonsson SA, Masson G, Jakobsdottir M, Thorlacius S, Helgason A, Aben KK, Strobbe LJ, bers-Akkers MT, Swinkels DW, Henderson BE, Kolonel LN, Le ML, Millastre E, Andres R, Godino J et al. (2007). Common variants on chromosomes 2q35 and 16q12 confer susceptibility to estrogen receptor-positive breast cancer. Nat Genet 39: 865–869.

1361B. Stacey SN, Manolescu A, Sulem P, Thorlacius S, Gudjonsson SA, Jonsson GF, Jakobsdottir M, Bergthorsson JT, Gudmundsson J, Aben KK, Strobbe LJ, Swinkels DW, van Engelenburg KC, Henderson BE, Kolonel LN, Le ML, Millastre E, Andres R, Saez B, Lambea J et al. (2008). Common variants on chromosome 5p12 confer susceptibility to estrogen receptor-positive breast cancer. Nat Genet 40: 703–706.

1362. Staff S, Nupponen NN, Borg A, Isola JJ, Tanner MM (2000). Multiple copies of mutant BRCA1 and BRCA2 alleles in breast tumors from germ-line mutation carriers. Genes Chromosomes Cancer 28: 432–442.

1363. Staklenac B, Pauzar B, Pajtler M, Loncar B, Dmitrovic B (2004). An unusual tumour of the breast: cytological findings. Cytopathology 15: 160–162.

1363A. Stalsberg H, Thomas DB (1993). Age distribution of histologic types of breast carcinoma. Int J Cancer 54: 1–7.

1364. Stambolic V, Suzuki A, de la Pompa JL, Brothers GM, Mirtsos C, Sasaki T, Ruland J, Penninger JM, Siderovski DP, Mak TW (1998). Negative regulation of PKB/Akt-dependent cell survival by the tumor suppressor PTEN. Cell 95: 29–39.

1365. Stankovic T, Kidd AM, Sutcliffe A, McGuire GM, Robinson P, Weber P, Bedenham T, Bradwell AR, Easton DF, Lennox GG, Haites N, Byrd PJ, Taylor AM (1998). ATM mutations and phenotypes in ataxia-telangiectasia families in the British Isles: expression of mutant ATM and the risk of leukemia, lymphoma, and breast cancer. Am J Hum Genet 62: 334–345.

1366. Stanley MW, Skoog L, Tani EM, Horwitz CA (1993). Nodular fasciitis: spontaneous resolution following diagnosis by fine-needle aspiration. Diagn Cytopathol 9: 322–324.

1367. Starink TM, van der Veen JP, Arwert F, de Waal LP, de Lange GG, Gille JJ, Eriksson AW (1986). The Cowden syndrome: a clinical and genetic study in 21 patients. Clin Genet 29: 222–233.

1368. Stark M, Hoffmann A, Xiong Z (2011). Mammary myofibrosarcoma: case report and literature review. Breast J 17: 300–304.

1369. Stavros AT, Thickman D, Rapp CL, Dennis MA, Parker SH, Sisney GA (1995). Solid breast nodules: use of sonography to distinguish between benign and malignant lesions. Radiology 196: 123–134.

1370. Steck PA, Pershouse MA, Jasser SA, Yung WK, Lin H, Ligon AH, Langford LA, Baumgard ML, Hattier T, Davis T, Frye C, Hu R, Swedlund B, Teng DH, Tavtigian SV (1997). Identification of a candidate tumour suppressor gene, MMAC1, at chromosome 10q23.3 that is mutated in multiple advanced cancers. Nat Genet 15: 356–362.

1371. Stefanick ML, Anderson GL, Margolis KL, Hendrix SL, Rodabough RJ, Paskett ED, Lane DS, Hubbell FA, Assaf AR, Sarto GE, Schenken RS, Yasmeen S, Lessin L, Chlebowski RT (2006). Effects of conjugated equine estrogens on breast cancer and mammography screening in postmenopausal women with hysterectomy. JAMA 295: 1647–1657.

1372. Stefansson OA, Jonasson JG, Johannsson OT, Olafsdottir K, Steinarsdottir M, Valgeirsdottir S, Eyfjord JE (2009). Genomic profiling of breast tumours in relation to BRCA abnormalities and phenotypes. Breast Cancer Res 11: R47.

1373. Steffen J, Nowakowska D, Niwinska A, Czapczak D, Kluska A, Piatkowska M, Wisniewska A, Paszko Z (2006). Germline mutations 657del5 of the NBS1 gene contribute significantly to the incidence of breast cancer in Central Poland. Int J Cancer 119: 472–475.

1374. Stemke-Hale K, Gonzalez-Angulo AM, Lluch A, Neve RM, Kuo WL, Davies M, Carey M, Hu Z, Guan Y, Sahin A, Symmans WF, Pusztai L, Nolden LK, Horlings H, Berns K, Hung MC, Van de Vijver MJ, Valero V, Gray JW, Bernards R et al. (2008). An integrative genomic and proteomic analysis of PIK3CA, PTEN, and AKT mutations in breast cancer. Cancer Res 68: 6084–6091.

1375A. Stephens P, Edkins S, Davies H, Greenman C, Cox C, Hunter C, Bignell G, Teague J, Smith R, Stevens C, O'Meara S, Parker A, Tarpey P, Avis T, Barthorpe A, Brackenbury L, Buck G, Butler A, Clements J, Cole J et al. (2005). A screen of the complete protein kinase gene family identifies diverse patterns of somatic mutations in human breast cancer. Nat Genet 37: 590–592.

1375. Stephens PJ, McBride DJ, Lin ML, Varela I, Pleasance ED, Simpson JT, Stebbings LA, Leroy C, Edkins S, Mudie LJ, Greenman CD, Jia M, Latimer C, Teague JW, Lau KW, Burton J, Quail MA, Swerdlow H, Churcher C, Natrajan R et al. (2009). Complex landscapes of somatic rearrangement in human breast cancer genomes. Nature 462: 1005–1010.

1376. Sternlicht MD, Kedeshian P, Shao ZM, Safarians S, Barsky SH (1997). The human myoepithelial cell is a natural tumor suppressor. Clin Cancer Res 3: 1949–1958.

1377. Stout AP, Murray MR (1942). Hemangiopericytoma: a vascular tumor featuring Zimmermann's pericytes. Ann Surg 116: 26–33.

1378. Stovall M, Smith SA, Langholz BM, Boice JD, Jr, Shore RE, Andersson M, Buchholz TA, Capanu M, Bernstein L, Lynch CF, Malone KE, Anton-Culver H, Haile RW, Rosenstein BS, Reiner AS, Thomas DC, Bernstein JL (2008). Dose to the contralateral breast from radiotherapy and risk of second primary breast cancer in the WECARE study. Int J Radiat Oncol Biol Phys 72: 1021–1030.

1379. Stutz JA, Evans AJ, Pinder S, Ellis IO, Yeoman LJ, Wilson AR, Sibbering DM (1994). The radiological appearances of invasive cribriform carcinoma of the breast. Nottingham Breast Team. Clin Radiol 49: 693–695.

1380. Su X, Hankinson SE, Clevenger CV, Eliassen AH, Tworoger SS (2009). Energy balance, early life body size, and plasma prolactin levels in postmenopausal women. Cancer Causes Control 20: 253–262.

1381. Su Y, Swift M (2001). Outcomes of adjuvant radiation therapy for breast cancer in women with ataxia-telangiectasia mutations. JAMA 286: 2233–2234.

1382. Sullivan ME, Khan SA, Sullu Y, Schiller C, Susnik B (2010). Lobular carcinoma in situ variants in breast cores: potential for misdiagnosis, upgrade rates at surgical excision, and practical implications. Arch Pathol Lab Med 134: 1024–1028.

1383. Sullivan T, Raad RA, Goldberg S, Assaad SI, Gadd M, Smith BL, Powell SN, Taghian AG (2005). Tubular carcinoma of the breast: a retrospective analysis and review of the literature. Breast Cancer Res Treat 93: 199–205.

1384. Sumpio BE, Jennings TA, Merino MJ, Sullivan PD (1987). Adenoid cystic carcinoma of the breast. Data from the Connecticut Tumor Registry and a review of the literature. Ann Surg 205: 295–301.

1385. Suster S, Wong TY (1994). Polymorphous sweat gland carcinoma. Histopathology 25: 31–39.

1386. Suzuki R, Orsini N, Mignone L, Saji S, Wolk A (2008). Alcohol intake and risk of breast cancer defined by estrogen and progesterone receptor status—a meta-analysis of epidemiological studies. Int J Cancer 122: 1832–1841.

1387. Suzuki T, Miki Y, Takagi K, Hirakawa H, Moriya T, Ohuchi N, Sasano H (2010). Androgens in human breast carcinoma. Med Mol Morphol 43: 75–81.

1388. Swerdlow SH, Campo E, Harris NL, Jaffe ES, Pileri S, Stein H, Thiele J, Vardiman JW, eds (2008). WHO classification of tumours of haematopoietic and lymphoid tissues. WHO classification of tumours, 4th edition. IARC: Lyon.

1389. Swift M, Morrell D, Massey RB, Chase CL (1991). Incidence of cancer in 161 families affected by ataxia-telangiectasia. N Engl J Med 325: 1831–1836.

1390. Symmans WF, Peintinger F, Hatzis C, Rajan R, Kuerer H, Valero V, Assad L, Poniecka A, Hennessy B, Green M, Buzdar AU, Singletary SE, Hortobagyi GN, Pusztai L (2007). Measurement of residual breast cancer burden to predict survival after neoadjuvant chemotherapy. J Clin Oncol 25: 4414–4422.

1391. Taccagni G, Rovere E, Masullo M, Christensen L, Eyden B (1997). Myofibrosarcoma of the breast: review of the literature on myofibroblastic tumors and criteria for defining myofibroblastic differentiation. Am J Surg Pathol 21: 489–496.

1392. Tai YC, Domchek S, Parmigiani G, Chen S (2007). Breast cancer risk among male BRCA1 and BRCA2 mutation carriers. J Natl Cancer Inst 99: 1811–1814.

1393. Tait R, Pinder SE, Ellis IO, Purushotham AD (2005). Adenomyoepithelioma of the breast; a case report and literature review. J BUON 10: 393–395.

1394. Talley C, Kushner HI, Sterk CE (2004). Lung cancer, chronic disease epidemiology, and medicine, 1948-1964. J Hist Med Allied Sci 59: 329–374.

1395. Talman ML, Jensen MB, Rank F (2007). Invasive lobular breast cancer. Prognostic significance of histological malignancy grading. Acta Oncol 46: 803–809.

1396. Talwalkar SS, Miranda RN, Valbuena JR, Routbort MJ, Martin AW, Medeiros LJ (2008). Lymphomas involving the breast: a study of 106 cases comparing localized and disseminated neoplasms. Am J Surg Pathol 32: 1299–1309.

1397. Talwar S, Prasad N, Gandhi S, Prasad P (1999). Haemangiopericytoma of the adult male breast. Int J Clin Pract 53: 485–486.

1398. Tamura G, Monma N, Suzuki Y, Satodate R, Abe H (1993). Adenomyoepithelioma (myoepithelioma) of the breast in a male. Hum Pathol 24: 678–681.

1399. Tamura S, Enjoji M, Toyoshima S, Terasaka R (1988). Adenomyoepithelioma of the breast. A case report with an immunohistochemical study. Acta Pathol Jpn 38: 659–665.

1400. Tan EY, Tan PH, Yong WS, Wong HB, Ho GH, Yeo AW, Wong CY (2006). Recurrent phyllodes tumours of the breast: pathological features and clinical implications. ANZ J Surg 76: 476–480.

1401. Tan H, Zhang S, Liu H, Peng W, Li R, Gu Y, Wang X, Mao J, Shen X (2011). Imaging findings in phyllodes tumors of the breast. Eur J Radiol [Epub ahead of print]

1402. Tan MH, Mester J, Peterson C, Yang Y, Chen JL, Rybicki LA, Milas K, Pederson H, Remzi B, Orloff MS, Eng C (2011). A clinical scoring system for selection of patients for PTEN mutation testing is proposed on the basis of a prospective study of 3042 probands. Am J Hum Genet 88: 42–56.

1403. Tan PH, Aw MY, Yip G, Bay BH, Sii LH, Murugaya S, Tse GM (2005). Cytokeratins in papillary lesions of the breast: is there a role in distinguishing intraductal papilloma from papillary ductal carcinoma in situ? Am J Surg Pathol 29: 625–632.

1403A. Tan PH, Lui GG, Chiang G, Yap WM, Poh WT, Bay BH (2204). Ductal carcinoma in situ with spindle cells; a potential diagnostic pitfall in the evaluation of breas lesions. Histopath 45:343-351.

1404. Tan PH, Jayabaskar T, Chuah KL, Lee HY, Tan Y, Hilmy M, Hung H, Selvarajan S, Bay BH (2005). Phyllodes tumors of the breast: the role of pathologic parameters. Am J Clin Pathol 123: 529–540.

1405. Tan PH, Jayabaskar T, Yip G, Tan Y, Hilmy M, Selvarajan S, Bay BH (2005). p53 and c-kit (CD117) protein expression as prognostic indicators in breast phyllodes tumors: a tissue microarray study. Mod Pathol 18: 1527–1534.

1406. Tan PH, Thike AA, Tan WJ, Thu MM, Busmanis I, Li H, Chay WY, Tan MH, The Phyllodes Tumour Network Singapore (2012). Predicting clinical behavior of breast phyllodes tumors: a nomogram based on histological criteria and surgical margins. J Clin Pathol 65: 69–76.

1407. Tan PH, Tse GM, Bay BH (2008). Mucinous breast lesions: diagnostic challenges. J Clin Pathol 61: 11–19.

1408. Tang F, Wei B, Tian Z, Gilcrease MZ, Huo L, Albarracin CT, Resetkova E, Zhang H, Sahin A, Chen J, Bu H, Abraham S, Wu Y (2011). Invasive mammary carcinoma with neuroendocrine differentiation: histological features and diagnostic challenges. Histopathology 59: 106–115.

1409. Tang G, Shak S, Paik S, Anderson SJ, Costantino JP, Geyer CE, Jr, Mamounas EP, Wickerham DL, Wolmark N (2011). Comparison of the prognostic and predictive utilities of the 21-gene Recurrence Score assay and Adjuvant! for women with node-negative, ER-positive breast cancer: results from NSABP B-14 and NSABP B-20. Breast Cancer Res Treat 127: 133–142.

1410. Tavassoli FA (1991). Myoepithelial lesions of the breast. Myoepitheliosis, adenomyoepithelioma, and myoepithelial carcinoma. Am J Surg Pathol 15: 554–568.

1411. Tavassoli FA (1999). Myoepithelial lesions. In: Pathology of the breast, 2nd edition.Tavassoli FA, ed. Appleton & Lange: New York: pp 763–791.

1412. Tavassoli FA, Bratthauer GL (1993). Immunohistochemical profile and differential diagnosis of microglandular adenosis. Mod Pathol 6: 318–322.

1413. Tavassoli FA, Devilee P, eds (2003). WHO classification of tumours of the breast and female genital organs, 3rd edition. IARC: Lyon, France.

1414. Tavassoli FA, ed. (1999). Pathology of the breast, 2nd edition. 2nd Edition. Appleton & Lange: Stamford, Connecticut.

1415. Tavassoli FA, Eusebi V (2009). Benign soft tissue lesions. In: Tumors of the mammary gland.Tavassoli FA, Eusebi V, eds. AFIP atlas of tumor pathology. Fourth series ; fasc. 10. American Registry of Pathology in collaboration with the Armed Forces Institute of Pathology: Washington, D.C: pp 263–285.

1416. Tavassoli FA, Eusebi V, eds (2009). Tumors of the mammary gland. AFIP atlas of tumor pathology. Fourth series ; fasc. 10. American Registry of Pathology in collaboration with the Armed Forces Institute of Pathology: Washington, D.C.

1417. Tavassoli FA, Norris HJ (1980). Secretory carcinoma of the breast. Cancer 45: 2404–2413.

1418. Tavassoli FA, Norris HJ (1986). Mammary adenoid cystic carcinoma with sebaceous differentiation. A morphologic study of the cell types. Arch Pathol Lab Med 110: 1045–1053.

1419. Tavassoli FA, Norris HJ (1990). A comparison of the results of long-term follow-up for atypical intraductal hyperplasia and intraductal hyperplasia of the breast. Cancer 65: 518–529.

1420. Tavassoli FA, Weiss S (1981). Hemangiopericytoma of the breast. Am J Surg Pathol 5: 745–752.

1421. Tavtigian SV, Oefner PJ, Babikyan D, Hartmann A, Healey S, Le Calvez-Kelm F, Lesueur F, Byrnes GB, Chuang SC, Forey N, Feuchtinger C, Gioia L, Hall J, Hashibe M, Herte B, McKay-Chopin S, Thomas A, Vallee MP, Voegele C, Webb PM et al. (2009). Rare, evolutionarily unlikely missense substitutions in ATM confer increased risk of breast cancer. Am J Hum Genet 85: 427–446.

1422. Tavtigian SV, Oefner PJ, Babikyan D, Hartmann A, Healey S, Le Calvez-Kelm F, Lesueur F, Byrnes GB, Chuang SC, Forey N, Feuchtinger C, Gioia L, Hall J, Hashibe M, Herte B, McKay-Chopin S, Thomas A, Vallee MP, Voegele C, Webb PM et al. (2009). Rare, evolutionarily unlikely missense substitutions in ATM confer increased risk of breast cancer. Am J Hum Genet 85: 427–446.

1423. Tavtigian SV, Simard J, Rommens J, Couch F, Shattuck-Eidens D, Neuhausen S, Merajver S, Thorlacius S, Offit K, Stoppa-Lyonnet D, Belanger C, Bell R, Berry S, Bogden R, Chen Q, Davis T, Dumont M, Frye C, Hattier T, Jammulapati S et al. (1996). The complete BRCA2 gene and mutations in chromosome 13q-linked kindreds. Nat Genet 12: 333–337.

1424. Taylor HB, Robertson AG (1965). Adenomas of the nipple. Cancer 18: 995–1002.

1425. Telesinghe PU, Anthony PP (1985). Primary lymphoma of the breast. Histopathology 9: 297–307.

1426. Teresi RE, Zbuk KM, Pezzolesi MG, Waite KA, Eng C (2007). Cowden syndrome-affected patients with PTEN promoter mutations demonstrate abnormal protein translation. Am J Hum Genet 81: 756–767.

1427. Terrier P, Terrier-Lacombe MJ, Mouriesse H, Friedman S, Spielmann M, Contesso G (1989). Primary breast sarcoma: a review of 33 cases with immunohistochemistry and prognostic factors. Breast Cancer Res Treat 13: 39–48.

1428. Tesluk H, Amott T, Goodnight JE, Jr (1986). Apocrine adenoma of the breast. Arch Pathol Lab Med 110: 351–352.

1429. Thanapaisal C, Koonmee S, Siritunyaporn S (2006). Malignant peripheral nerve sheath tumor of breast in patient without Von Recklinghausen's neurofibromatosis: a case report. J Med Assoc Thai 89: 377–379.

1430. The Breast Cancer Linkage Consortium (1999). Cancer risks in BRCA2 mutation carriers. J Natl Cancer Inst 91: 1310–1316.

1431. The Consensus Conference Committee (1997). Consensus Conference on the classification of ductal carcinoma in situ. Cancer 80: 1798–1802.

1431A.

1431A. Thomas G, Jacobs KB, Kraft P, Yeager M, Wacholder S, Cox DG, Hankinson SE, Hutchinson A, Wang Z, Yu K, Chatterjee N, Garcia-Closas M, Gonzalez-Bosquet J, Prokunina-Olsson L, Orr N, Willett WC, Colditz GA, Ziegler RG, Berg CD, Buys SS et al. (2009). A multistage genome-wide association study in breast cancer identifies two new risk alleles at 1p11.2 and 14q24.1 (RAD51L1). Nat Genet 41: 579–584.

1432. Thomas JS, Julian HS, Green RV, Cameron DA, Dixon MJ (2007). Histopathology of breast carcinoma following neoadjuvant systemic therapy: a common association between letrozole therapy and central scarring. Histopathology 51: 219–226.

1433. Thompson D, Duedal S, Kirner J, McGuffog L, Last J, Reiman A, Byrd P, Taylor M, Easton DF (2005). Cancer risks and mortality in heterozygous ATM mutation carriers. J Natl Cancer Inst 97: 813–822.

1434. Thompson D, Easton D (2001). Variation in cancer risks, by mutation position, in BRCA2 mutation carriers. Am J Hum Genet 68: 410–419.

1435. Thompson D, Easton D (2002). Variation in BRCA1 cancer risks by mutation position. Cancer Epidemiol Biomarkers Prev 11: 329–336.

1436. Thompson D, Easton DF (2002). Cancer incidence in BRCA1 mutation carriers. J Natl Cancer Inst 94: 1358–1365.

1436A. Thompson L, Chang B, Barsky SH (1996). Monoclonal origins of malignant mixed tumors (carcinosarcomas). Evidence for a divergent histogenesis. Am J Surg Pathol 20: 277–285.

1437. Thompson PA, Lade S, Webster H, Ryan G, Prince HM (2010). Effusion-associated anaplastic large cell lymphoma of the breast: time for it to be defined as a distinct clinico-pathological entity. Haematologica 95: 1977–1979.

1438. Thor AD, Eng C, DeVries S, Paterakos M, Watkin WG, Edgerton S, Moore DH, Etzell J, Waldman FM (2002). Invasive micropapillary carcinoma of the breast is associated with chromosome 8 abnormalities detected by comparative genomic hybridization. Hum Pathol 33: 628–631.

1439. Thorlacius S, Struewing JP, Hartge P, Olafsdottir GH, Sigvaldason H, Tryggvadottir L, Wacholder S, Tulinius H, Eyfjord JE (1998). Population-based study of risk of breast cancer in carriers of BRCA2 mutation. Lancet 352: 1337–1339.

1440. Tinat J, Bougeard G, Baert-Desurmont S, Vasseur S, Martin C, Bouvignies E, Caron O, Bressac-de Paillerets B, Berthet P, Dugast C, Bonaiti-Pellie C, Stoppa-Lyonnet D, Frebourg T (2009). 2009 version of the Chompret criteria for Li Fraumeni syndrome. J Clin Oncol 27: e108–e109.

1441. Tischkowitz M, Xia B (2010). PALB2/FANCN: recombining cancer and Fanconi anemia. Cancer Res 70: 7353–7359.

1442. Tognon C, Knezevich SR, Huntsman D, Roskelley CD, Melnyk N, Mathers JA, Becker L, Carneiro F, MacPherson N, Horsman D, Poremba C, Sorensen PH (2002). Expression of the ETV6-NTRK3 gene fusion as a primary event in human secretory breast carcinoma. Cancer Cell 2: 367–376.

1443. Toikkanen S, Kujari H (1989). Pure and mixed mucinous carcinomas of the breast: a clinicopathologic analysis of 61 cases with long-term follow-up. Hum Pathol 20: 758–764.

1444. Toikkanen S, Pylkkanen L, Joensuu H (1997). Invasive lobular carcinoma of the breast has better short- and long-term survival than invasive ductal carcinoma. Br J Cancer 76: 1234–1240.

1445. Toker C (1961). Some observations on Paget's disease of the nipple. Cancer 14: 653–672.

1446. Toker C (1970). Clear cells of the nipple epidermis. Cancer 25: 601–610.

1447. Tommiska J, Bartkova J, Heinonen M, Hautala L, Kilpivaara O, Eerola H, Aittomaki K, Hofstetter B, Lukas J, von Smitten K, Blomqvist C, Ristimaki A, Heikkila P, Bartek J, Nevanlinna H (2008). The DNA damage signalling kinase ATM is aberrantly reduced or lost in BRCA1/BRCA2-deficient and ER/PR/ERBB2-triple-negative breast cancer. Oncogene 27: 2501–2506.

1448. Toombs BD, Kalisher L (1977). Metastatic disease to the breast: clinical, pathologic, and radiographic features. AJR Am J Roentgenol 129: 673–676.

1449. Topalovski M, Crisan D, Mattson JC (1999). Lymphoma of the breast. A clinicopathologic study of primary and secondary cases. Arch Pathol Lab Med 123: 1208–1218.

1450. Tornos C, Soslow R, Chen S, Akram M, Hummer AJ, Abu-Rustum N, Norton L, Tan LK (2005). Expression of WT1, CA 125, and GCDFP-15 as useful markers in the differential diagnosis of primary ovarian carcinomas versus metastatic breast cancer to the ovary. Am J Surg Pathol 29: 1482–1489.

1451. Tot T (2007). Clinical relevance of the distribution of the lesions in 500 consecutive breast cancer cases documented in large-format histologic sections. Cancer 110: 2551–2560.

1452. Toth J (1977). Benign human mammary myoepithelioma. Virchows Arch A Pathol Anat Histol 374: 263–269.

1452A. Toussaint J, Sieuwerts AM, Haibe-Kains B, Desmedt C, Rouas G, Harris AL et al. (2009). Improvement of the clinical applicability of the Genomic Grade Index through a qRT-PCR test performed on frozen and formalin-fixed paraffin-embedded tissues. BMC Genomics 10: 424.

1453. Tresserra F, Grases PJ, Fabregas R, Fernandez-Cid A, Dexeus S (1999). Invasive micropapillary carcinoma. Distinct features of a poorly recognized variant of breast carcinoma. Eur J Gynaecol Oncol 20: 205–208.

1454. Trojani M, de Mascarel I, Coquet M, Coindre JM, De Mascarel A (1989). [Osteoclastic type giant cell carcinoma of the breast]. Ann Pathol 9: 189–194.

1455. Trojani M, Guiu M, Trouette H, de Mascarel I, Cocquet M (1992). Malignant adenomyoepithelioma of the breast. An immunohistochemical, cytophotometric, and ultrastructural study of a case with lung metastases. Am J Clin Pathol 98: 598–602.

1456. Trotman LC, Wang X, Alimonti A, Chen Z, Teruya-Feldstein J, Yang H, Pavletich NP, Carver BS, Cordon-Cardo C, Erdjument-Bromage H, Tempst P, Chi SG, Kim HJ, Misteli T, Jiang X, Pandolfi PP (2007). Ubiquitination regulates PTEN nuclear import and tumor suppression. Cell 128: 141–156.

1457. Troxell ML, Levine J, Beadling C, Warrick A, Dunlap J, Presnell A, Patterson J, Shukla A, Olson NR, Heinrich MC, Corless CL (2010). High prevalence of PIK3CA/AKT pathway mutations in papillary neoplasms of the breast. Mod Pathol 23: 27–37.

1458. Truninger K, Menigatti M, Luz J, Russell A, Haider R, Gebbers JO, Bannwart F, Yurtsever H, Neuweiler J, Riehle HM, Cattaruzza MS, Heinimann K, Schar P, Jiricny J, Marra G (2005). Immunohistochemical analysis reveals high frequency of PMS2 defects in colorectal cancer. Gastroenterology 128: 1160–1171.

1459. Tsang WY, Chan JK (1996). Endocrine ductal carcinoma in situ (E-DCIS) of the breast: a form of low-grade DCIS with distinctive clinicopathologic and biologic characteristics. Am J Surg Pathol 20: 921–943.

1460. Tse GM, Law BK, Ma TK, Chan AB, Pang LM, Chu WC, Cheung HS (2002). Hamartoma of the breast: a clinicopathological review. J Clin Pathol 55: 951–954.

1461. Tse GM, Lui PC, Lee CS, Kung FY, Scolyer RA, Law BK, Lau TS, Karim R, Putti TC (2004). Stromal expression of vascular endothelial growth factor correlates with tumor grade and microvessel density in mammary phyllodes tumors: a multicenter study of 185 cases. Hum Pathol 35: 1053–1057.

1462. Tse GM, Lui PC, Scolyer RA, Putti TC, Kung FY, Law BK, Lau TS, Lee CS (2003). Tumour angiogenesis and p53 protein expression in mammary phyllodes tumors. Mod Pathol 16: 1007–1013.

1462A. Tse GM, Lui PC, Vong JS, Lau KM, Putti TC, Karim R, Scolyer RA, Lee CS, Yu AM, Ng DC, Tse AK, Tan PH (2009). Increased epidermal growth factor receptor (EGFR) expression in malignant mammary phyllodes tumors. Breast Cancer Res Treat 114: 441–448.

1463. Tse GM, Tan PH, Lui PC, Gilks CB, Poon CS, Ma TK, Law BK, Lam WW (2007). The role of immunohistochemistry for smooth-muscle actin, p63, CD10 and cytokeratin 14 in the differential diagnosis of papillary lesions of the breast. J Clin Pathol 60: 315–320.

1464. Tse GM, Tan PH, Moriya T (2009). The role of immunohistochemistry in the differential diagnosis of papillary lesions of the breast. J Clin Pathol 62: 407–413.

1464A. Tse GM, Tan PH, Putti TC, Lui PC, Chaiwun B, Law BK (2006). Metaplastic carcinoma of the breast: a clinicopathological review. J Clin Pathol 59: 1079–1083.

1465. Tsubura A, Hatano T, Murata A, Shoji T, Shikata N, Morii S (1992). Breast carcinoma in patients receiving neuroleptic therapy. Morphologic and clinicopathologic features of thirteen cases. Acta Pathol Jpn 42: 494–499.

1466. Tsuda H, Fukutomi T, Hirohashi S (1995). Pattern of gene alterations in intraductal breast neoplasms associated with histological type and grade. Clin Cancer Res 1: 261–267.

1466A. Tsuda H, Takarabe T, Fukutomi T, Hirohashi S (1999). der(16)t(1;16)/der(1;16) in breast cancer detected by fluorescence in situ hybridization is an indicator of better patient prognosis. Genes Chromosomes Cancer 24: 72–77.

1467. Tung N, Miron A, Schnitt SJ, Gautam S, Fetten K, Kaplan J, Yassin Y, Buraimoh A, Kim JY, Szasz AM, Tian R, Wang ZC, Collins LC, Brock J, Krag K, Legare RD, Sgroi D, Ryan PD, Silver DP, Garber JE et al. (2010). Prevalence and predictors of loss of wild type BRCA1 in estrogen receptor positive and negative BRCA1-associated breast cancers. Breast Cancer Res 12: R95.

1468. Tung N, Wang Y, Collins LC, Kaplan J, Li H, Gelman R, Comander AH, Gallagher B, Fetten K, Krag K, Stoeckert KA, Legare RD, Sgroi D, Ryan PD, Garber JE, Schnitt SJ (2010). Estrogen receptor positive breast cancers in BRCA1 mutation carriers: clinical risk factors and pathologic features. Breast Cancer Res 12: R12.

1469. Turashvili G, Bouchal J, Baumforth K, Wei W, Dziechciarkova M, Ehrmann J, Klein J, Fridman E, Skarda J, Srovnal J, Hajduch M, Murray P, Kolar Z (2007). Novel markers for differentiation of lobular and ductal invasive breast carcinomas by laser microdissection and microarray analysis. BMC Cancer 7: 55.

1469A. Turnbull C, Ahmed S, Morrison J, Pernet D, Renwick A, Maranian M, Seal S, Ghoussaini M, Hines S, Healey CS, Hughes D, Warren-Perry M, Tapper W, Eccles D, Evans DG, Hooning M, Schutte M, van den Ouweland A, Houlston R, Ross G et al. (2010). Genome-wide association study identifies five new breast cancer susceptibility loci. Nat Genet 42: 504–507.

1470. Turner N, Tutt A, Ashworth A (2004). Hallmarks of 'BRCAness' in sporadic cancers. Nat Rev Cancer 4: 814–819.

1471. Turner NC, Reis-Filho JS (2006). Basal-like breast cancer and the BRCA1 phenotype. Oncogene 25: 5846–5853.

1472. Turpin E, Bieche I, Bertheau P, Plassa LF, Lerebours F, de Roquancourt A, Olivi M, Espie M, Marty M, Lidereau R, Vidaud M, de The H (2002). Increased incidence of ERBB2 overexpression and TP53 mutation in inflammatory breast cancer. Oncogene 21: 7593–7597.

1473. Tutt A, Robson M, Garber JE, Domchek SM, Audeh MW, Weitzel JN, Friedlander M, Arun B, Loman N, Schmutzler RK, Wardley A, Mitchell G, Earl H, Wickens M, Carmichael J (2010). Oral poly(ADP-ribose) polymerase inhibitor olaparib in patients with BRCA1 or BRCA2 mutations and advanced breast cancer: a proof-of-concept trial. Lancet 376: 235–244.

1474. Tworoger SS, Hankinson SE (2008). Prolactin and breast cancer etiology: an epidemiologic perspective. J Mammary Gland Biol Neoplasia 13: 41–53.

1475. Uchin JM, Billings SD (2009). Radiotherapy-associated atypical vascular lesions of the breast. J Cutan Pathol 36: 87–88.

1476. Udler MS, Meyer KB, Pooley KA, Karlins E, Struewing JP, Zhang J, Doody DR, MacArthur S, Tyrer J, Pharoah PD, Luben R, Bernstein L, Kolonel LN, Henderson BE, Le ML, Ursin G, Press MF, Brennan P, Sangrajrang S, Gaborieau V et al. (2009). FGFR2 variants and breast cancer risk: fine-scale mapping using African American studies and analysis of chromatin conformation. Hum Mol Genet 18: 1692–1703.

1477. Ueng SH, Mezzetti T, Tavassoli FA (2009). Papillary neoplasms of the breast: a review. Arch Pathol Lab Med 133: 893–907.

1478. Umar A, Boland CR, Terdiman JP, Syngal S, de la Chapelle A, Ruschoff J, Fishel R, Lindor NM, Burgart LJ, Hamelin R, Hamilton SR, Hiatt RA, Jass J, Lindblom A, Lynch HT, Peltomaki P, Ramsey SD, Rodriguez-Bigas MA, Vasen HF, Hawk ET et al. (2004). Revised Bethesda Guidelines for hereditary nonpolyposis colorectal cancer (Lynch syndrome) and microsatellite instability. J Natl Cancer Inst 96: 261–268.

1479. Ursin G, Longnecker MP, Haile RW, Greenland S (1995). A meta-analysis of body mass index and risk of premenopausal breast cancer. Epidemiology 6: 137–141.

1480. Uziel T, Savitsky K, Platzer M, Ziv Y, Helbitz T, Nehls M, Boehm T, Rosenthal A, Shiloh Y, Rotman G (1996). Genomic Organization of the ATM gene. Genomics 33: 317–320.

1481. Vahteristo P, Bartkova J, Eerola H, Syrjakoski K, Ojala S, Kilpivaara O, Tamminen A, Kononen J, Aittomaki K, Heikkila P, Holli K, Blomqvist C, Bartek J, Kallioniemi OP, Nevanlinna H (2002). A CHEK2 genetic variant contributing to a substantial fraction of familial breast cancer. Am J Hum Genet 71: 432–438.

1482. Validire P, Capovilla M, Asselain B, Kirova Y, Goudefroye R, Plancher C, Fourquet A, Zanni M, Gaulard P, Vincent-Salomon A, Decaudin D (2009). Primary breast non-Hodgkin's lymphoma: a large single center study of initial characteristics, natural history, and prognostic factors. Am J Hematol 84: 133–139.

1483. van Asperen CJ, Brohet RM, Meijers-Heijboer EJ, Hoogerbrugge N, Verhoef S, Vasen HF, Ausems MG, Menko FH, Gomez Garcia EB, Klijn JG, Hogervorst FB, van Houwelingen JC, Van't Veer LJ, Rookus MA, van Leeuwen FE (2005). Cancer risks in BRCA2 families: estimates for sites other than breast and ovary. J Med Genet 42: 711–719.

1484. van Beers EH, van Welsem T, Wessels LF, Li Y, Oldenburg RA, Devilee P, Cornelisse CJ, Verhoef S, Hogervorst FB, Van't Veer LJ, Nederlof PM (2005). Comparative genomic hybridization profiles in human BRCA1 and BRCA2 breast tumors highlight differential sets of genomic aberrations. Cancer Res 65: 822–827.

1485. van Bogaert LJ, Maldague P (1977). Histologic variants of lipid-secreting carcinoma of the breast. Virchows Arch A Pathol Anat Histol 375: 345–353.

1486. Van de Vijver MJ, He YD, Van't Veer LJ, Dai H, Hart AA, Voskuil DW, Schreiber GJ, Peterse JL, Roberts C, Marton MJ, Parrish M, Atsma D, Witteveen A, Glas A, Delahaye L, van der Velde T, Bartelink H, Rodenhuis S, Rutgers ET, Friend SH et al. (2002). A gene-expression signature as a predictor of survival in breast cancer. N Engl J Med 347: 1999–2009.

1487. Van den Eynden GG, Van der Auwera I, Van Laere S, Colpaert CG, van Dam P, Merajver S, Kleer CG, Harris AL, Van Marck EA, Dirix LY, Vermeulen PB (2004). Validation of a tissue microarray to study differential protein expression in inflammatory and non-inflammatory breast cancer. Breast Cancer Res Treat 85: 13–22.

1488. Van der Auwera I, Van den Eynden GG, Colpaert CG, Van Laere SJ, van Dam P, Van Marck EA, Dirix LY, Vermeulen PB (2005). Tumor lymphangiogenesis in inflammatory breast carcinoma: a histomorphometric study. Clin Cancer Res 11: 7637–7642.

1489. Van der Auwera I, Van Laere SJ, Van den Eynden GG, Benoy I, van Dam P, Colpaert CG, Fox SB, Turley H, Harris AL, Van Marck EA, Vermeulen PB, Dirix LY (2004). Increased angiogenesis and lymphangiogenesis in inflammatory versus noninflammatory breast cancer by real-time reverse transcriptase-PCR gene expression quantification. Clin Cancer Res 10: 7965–7971.

1490. van Deurzen CH, Cserni G, Bianchi S, Vezzosi V, Arisio R, Wesseling J, Asslaber M, Foschini MP, Sapino A, Castellano I, Callagy G, Faverly D, Martin-Martinez MD, Quinn C, Amendoeira I, Kulka J, Reiner-Concin A, Cordoba A, Seldenrijk CA, van Diest PJ (2010). Nodal-stage classification in invasive lobular breast carcinoma: influence of different interpretations of the pTNM classification. J Clin Oncol 28: 999–1004.

1491. Van Dorpe J, De Pauw A, Moerman P (1998). Adenoid cystic carcinoma arising in an adenomyoepithelioma of the breast. Virchows Arch 432: 119–122.

1492. van Golen KL, Bao LW, Pan Q, Miller FR, Wu ZF, Merajver SD (2002). Mitogen activated protein kinase pathway is involved in RhoC GTPase induced motility, invasion and angiogenesis in inflammatory breast cancer. Clin Exp Metastasis 19: 301–311.

1493. van Golen KL, Wu ZF, Qiao XT, Bao LW, Merajver SD (2000). RhoC GTPase, a novel transforming oncogene for human mammary epithelial cells that partially recapitulates the inflammatory breast cancer phenotype. Cancer Res 60: 5832–5838.

1493A. Van Hoeven KH, Drudis T, Cranor ML, Erlandson RA, Rosen PP (1993). Low-grade adenosquamous carcinoma of the breast. A clinocopathologic study of 32 cases with ultrastructural analysis. Am J Surg Pathol 17: 248–258.

1494. Van Laere S, Van der Auwera I, Van den Eynden GG, Fox SB, Bianchi F, Harris AL, van Dam P, Van Marck EA, Vermeulen PB, Dirix LY (2005). Distinct molecular signature of inflammatory breast cancer by cDNA microarray analysis. Breast Cancer Res Treat 93: 237–246.

1495. van Lier MG, Wagner A, Mathus-Vliegen EM, Kuipers EJ, Steyerberg EW, van Leerdam ME (2010). High cancer risk in Peutz-Jeghers syndrome: a systematic review and surveillance recommendations. Am J Gastroenterol 105: 1258–1264.

1495A. van Wezel T, Lombaerts M, van Roon EH, Philippo K, Baelde HJ, Szuhai K, Cornelisse CJ, Cleton-Jansen AM (2005). Expression analysis of candidate breast tumour suppressor genes on chromosome 16q. Breast Cancer Res 7: R998–1004.

1496. Van't Veer LJ, Dai H, Van de Vijver MJ, He YD, Hart AA, Mao M, Peterse HL, van der Kooy K, Marton MJ, Witteveen AT, Schreiber GJ, Kerkhoven RM, Roberts C, Linsley PS, Bernards R, Friend SH (2002). Gene expression profiling predicts clinical outcome of breast cancer. Nature 415: 530–536.

1497. Varga Z, Kolb SA, Flury R, Burkhard R, Caduff R (2000). Sebaceous carcinoma of the breast. Pathol Int 50: 63–66.

1498. Varga Z, Robl C, Spycher M, Burger D, Caduff R (1998). Metaplastic lipid-rich carcinoma of the breast. Pathol Int 48: 912–916.

1499. Varga Z, Zhao J, Ohlschlegel C, Odermatt B, Heitz PU (2004). Preferential HER-2/neu overexpression and/or amplification in aggressive histological subtypes of invasive breast cancer. Histopathology 44: 332–338.

1500. Vargas AC, Da SL, Lakhani SR (2010). The contribution of breast cancer pathology to statistical models to predict mutation risk in BRCA carriers. Fam Cancer 9: 545–553.

1501. Varghese JS, Easton DF (2010). Genome-wide association studies in common cancers—what have we learnt? Curr Opin Genet Dev 20: 201–209.

1502. Varley JM, McGown G, Thorncroft M, James LA, Margison GP, Forster G, Evans DG, Harris M, Kelsey AM, Birch JM (1999). Are there low-penetrance TP53 alleles? evidence from childhood adrenocortical tumors. Am J Hum Genet 65: 995–1006.

1503. Vasen HF (2005). Clinical description of the Lynch syndrome [hereditary nonpolyposis colorectal cancer (HNPCC)]. Fam Cancer 4: 219–225.

1504. Vasen HF, Morreau H, Nortier JW (2001). Is breast cancer part of the tumor spectrum of hereditary nonpolyposis colorectal cancer? Am J Hum Genet 68: 1533–1535.

1505. Vasen HF, Stormorken A, Menko FH, Nagengast FM, Kleibeuker JH, Griffioen G, Taal BG, Moller P, Wijnen JT (2001). MSH2 mutation carriers are at higher risk of cancer than MLH1 mutation carriers: a study of hereditary nonpolyposis colorectal cancer families. J Clin Oncol 19: 4074–4080.

1506. Vasen HF, Watson P, Mecklin JP, Lynch HT (1999). New clinical criteria for hereditary nonpolyposis colorectal cancer (HNPCC, Lynch syndrome) proposed by the International Collaborative group on HNPCC. Gastroenterology 116: 1453–1456.

1507. Vaz F, Hanenberg H, Schuster B, Barker K, Wiek C, Erven V, Neveling K, Endt D, Kesterton I, Autore F, Fraternali F, Freund M, Hartmann L, Grimwade D, Roberts RG, Schaal H, Mohammed S, Rahman N, Schindler D, Mathew CG (2010). Mutation of the RAD51C gene in a Fanconi anemia-like disorder. Nat Genet 42: 406–409.

1508. Venable JG, Schwartz AM, Silverberg SG (1990). Infiltrating cribriform carcinoma of the breast: a distinctive clinicopathologic entity. Hum Pathol 21: 333–338.

1509. Venkitaraman AR (2009). Linking the cellular functions of BRCA genes to cancer pathogenesis and treatment. Annu Rev Pathol 4: 461–487.

1510. Vera-Sempere F, Llombart-Bosch A (1985). Lipid-rich versus lipid-secreting carcinoma of the mammary gland. Pathol Res Pract 180: 553–558.

1511. Vergier B, Trojani M, de Mascarel I, Coindre JM, Le Treut A (1991). Metastases to the breast: differential diagnosis from primary breast carcinoma. J Surg Oncol 48: 112–116.

1512. Vermeulen PB, van Golen KL, Dirix LY (2010). Angiogenesis, lymphangiogenesis, growth pattern, and tumor emboli in inflammatory breast cancer: a review of the current knowledge. Cancer 116: 2748–2754.

1513. Viacava P, Naccarato AG, Nardini V, Bevilacqua G (1995). Breast carcinoma with osteoclast-like giant cells: immunohistochemical and ultrastructural study of a case and review of the literature. Tumori 81: 135–141.

1514. Viale G, Rotmensz N, Maisonneuve P, Orvieto E, Maiorano E, Galimberti V, Luini A, Colleoni M, Goldhirsch A, Coates AS (2009). Lack of prognostic significance of «classic» lobular breast carcinoma: a matched, single institution series. Breast Cancer Res Treat 117: 211–214.

1515. Vieira CC, Mercado CL, Cangiarella JF, Moy L, Toth HK, Guth AA (2010). Microinvasive ductal carcinoma in situ: clinical presentation, imaging features, pathologic findings, and outcome. Eur J Radiol 73: 102–107.

1516. Vielh P, Validire P, Kheirallah S, Campana F, Fourquet A, Di BL (1993). Paget's disease of the nipple without clinically and radiologically detectable breast tumor. Histochemical and immunohistochemical study of 44 cases. Pathol Res Pract 189: 150–155.

1517. Villa MT, White LE, Petronic-Rosic V, Song DH (2008). The treatment of diffuse dermal angiomatosis of the breast with reduction mammaplasty. Arch Dermatol 144: 693–694.

1518. Villani A, Tabori U, Schiffman J, Shlien A, Beyene J, Druker H, Novokmet A, Finlay J, Malkin D (2011). Biochemical and imaging surveillance in germline TP53 mutation carriers with Li-Fraumeni syndrome: a prospective observational study. Lancet Oncol 12: 559–567.

1519. Vincent-Salomon A, Gruel N, Lucchesi C, MacGrogan G, Dendale R, Sigal-Zafrani B, Longy M, Raynal V, Pierron G, de Mascarel I, Taris C, Stoppa-Lyonnet D, Pierga JY, Salmon R, Sastre-Garau X, Fourquet A, Delattre O, De Cremoux P, Aurias A (2007). Identification of typical medullary breast carcinoma as a genomic sub-group of basal-like carcinomas, a heterogeneous new molecular entity. Breast Cancer Res 9: R24

1520. Vincent-Salomon A, Lucchesi C, Gruel N, Raynal V, Pierron G, Goudefroye R, Reyal F, Radvanyi F, Salmon R, Thiery JP, Sastre-Garau X, Sigal-Zafrani B, Fourquet A, Delattre O (2008). Integrated genomic and transcriptomic analysis of ductal carcinoma in situ of the breast. Clin Cancer Res 14: 1956–1965.

1521. Vinh-Hung V, Burzykowski T, Cserni G, Voordeckers M, Van De Steene J, Storme G (2003). Functional form of the effect of the numbers of axillary nodes on survival in early breast cancer. Int J Oncol 22: 697–704.

1522. Vinh-Hung V, Nguyen NP, Cserni G, Truong P, Woodward W, Verkooijen HM, Promish D, Ueno NT, Tai P, Nieto Y, Joseph S, Janni W, Vicini F, Royce M, Storme G, Wallace AM, Vlastos G, Bouchardy C, Hortobagyi GN (2009). Prognostic value of nodal ratios in node-positive breast cancer: a compiled update. Future Oncol 5: 1585–1603.

1523. Virk RK, Khan A (2010). Pseudoangiomatous stromal hyperplasia: an overview. Arch Pathol Lab Med 134: 1070–1074.

1524. Visscher DW, Pankratz VS, Santisteban M, Reynolds C, Ristimaki A, Vierkant RA, Lingle WL, Frost MH, Hartmann LC (2008). Association between cyclooxygenase-2 expression in atypical hyperplasia and risk of breast cancer. J Natl Cancer Inst 100: 421–427.

1525. Vo T, Xing Y, Meric-Bernstam F, Mirza N, Vlastos G, Symmans WF, Perkins GH, Buchholz TA, Babiera GV, Kuerer HM, Bedrosian I, Akins JS, Hunt KK (2007). Long-term outcomes in patients with mucinous, medullary, tubular, and invasive ductal carcinomas after lumpectomy. Am J Surg 194: 527–531.

1526. Vo TN, Meric-Bernstam F, Yi M, Buchholz TA, Ames FC, Kuerer HM, Bedrosian I, Hunt KK (2006). Outcomes of breast-conservation therapy for invasive lobular carcinoma are equivalent to those for invasive ductal carcinoma. Am J Surg 192: 552–555.

1527. Vollebergh MA, Lips EH, Nederlof PM, Wessels LF, Schmidt MK, van Beers EH, Cornelissen S, Holtkamp M, Froklage FE, de Vries EG, Schrama JG, Wesseling J, Van de Vijver M, van Tinteren H, de Bruin M, Hauptmann M, Rodenhuis S, Linn SC (2011). An aCGH classifier derived from BRCA1-mutated breast cancer and benefit of high-dose platinum-based chemotherapy in HER2-negative breast cancer patients. Ann Oncol 22: 1561–1570.

1528. Vos CB, Cleton-Jansen AM, Berx G, de Leeuw WJ, ter Haar NT, van Roy F, Cornelisse CJ, Peterse JL, Van de Vijver M (1997). E-cadherin inactivation in lobular carcinoma in situ of the breast: an early event in tumorigenesis. Br J Cancer 76: 1131–1133.

1529. Vourtsi A, Zervoudis S, Pafiti A, Athanasiadis S (2006). Male breast hemangioma—a rare entity: a case report and review of the literature. Breast J 12: 260–262.

1530. Vranic S, Bilalovic N, Lee LM, Kruslin B, Lilleberg SL, Gatalica Z (2007). PIK3CA and PTEN mutations in adenoid cystic carcinoma of the breast metastatic to kidney. Hum Pathol 38: 1425–1431.

1531. Vranic S, Frkovic-Grazio S, Lamovec J, Serdarevic F, Gurjeva O, Palazzo J, Bilalovic N, Lee LM, Gatalica Z (2010). Adenoid cystic carcinomas of the breast have low Topo IIalpha expression but frequently overexpress EGFR protein without EGFR gene amplification. Hum Pathol 41: 1617–1623.

1532. Vranic S, Gatalica Z, Deng H, Frkovic-Grazio S, Lee LM, Gurjeva O, Wang ZY (2010). ER-{alpha}36, a novel isoform of ER-{alpha}66, is commonly over-expressed in apocrine and adenoid cystic carcinomas of the breast. J Clin Pathol

1533. Vranic S, Gatalica Z, Deng H, Frkovic-Grazio S, Lee LM, Gurjeva O, Wang ZY (2011). ER-alpha36, a novel isoform of ER-alpha66, is commonly over-expressed in apocrine and adenoid cystic carcinomas of the breast. J Clin Pathol 64: 54–57.

1534. Vu-Nishino H, Tavassoli FA, Ahrens WA, Haffty BG (2005). Clinicopathologic features and long-term outcome of patients with medullary breast carcinoma managed with breast-conserving therapy (BCT). Int J Radiat Oncol Biol Phys 62: 1040–1047.

1535. Vuitch MF, Rosen PP, Erlandson RA (1986). Pseudoangiomatous hyperplasia of mammary stroma. Hum Pathol 17: 185–191.

1536. Waddell N, Arnold J, Cocciardi S, Da Silva L, Marsh A, Riley J, Johnstone CN, Orloff M, Assie G, Eng C, Reid L, Keith P, Yan M, Fox S, Devilee P, Godwin AK, Hogervorst FB, Couch F, Grimmond S, Flanagan JM et al. (2010). Subtypes of familial breast tumours revealed by expression and copy number profiling. Breast Cancer Res Treat 123: 661–677.

1537. Waddell N, Jonnalagadda J, Marsh A, Grist S, Jenkins M, Hobson K, Taylor M, Lindeman GJ, Tavtigian SV, Suthers G, Goldgar D, Oefner PJ, kConFab Investigators, Taylor D, Grimmond S, Khanna KK, Chenevix-

Trench G (2006). Characterization of the breast cancer associated ATM 7271T>G (V2424G) mutation by gene expression profiling. Genes Chromosomes Cancer 45: 1169–1181.

1538. Wahner-Roedler DL, Sebo TJ, Gisvold JJ (2001). Hamartomas of the breast: clinical, radiologic, and pathologic manifestations. Breast J 7: 101–105.

1539. Waite KA, Eng C (2002). Protean PTEN: form and function. Am J Hum Genet 70: 829–844.

1540. Waldman FM, Hwang ES, Etzell J, Eng C, DeVries S, Bennington J, Thor A (2001). Genomic alterations in tubular breast carcinomas. Hum Pathol 32: 222–226.

1541. Walford N, ten Velden J (1989). Histiocytoid breast carcinoma: an apocrine variant of lobular carcinoma. Histopathology 14: 515–522.

1542. Wallis M, Tardivon A, Helbich T, Schreer I (2007). Guidelines from the European Society of Breast Imaging for diagnostic interventional breast procedures. Eur Radiol 17: 581–588.

1543. Walsh MD, Buchanan DD, Cummings MC, Pearson SA, Arnold ST, Clendenning M, Walters R, McKeone DM, Spurdle AB, Hopper JL, Jenkins MA, Phillips KD, Suthers GK, George J, Goldblatt J, Muir A, Tucker K, Pelzer E, Gattas MR, Woodall S et al. (2010). Lynch syndrome-associated breast cancers: clinicopathologic characteristics of a case series from the colon cancer family registry. Clin Cancer Res 16: 2214–2224.

1544. Walsh MM, Bleiweiss IJ (2001). Invasive micropapillary carcinoma of the breast: eighty cases of an underrecognized entity. Hum Pathol 32: 583–589.

1545. Walsh T, Casadei S, Coats KH, Swisher E, Stray SM, Higgins J, Roach KC, Mandell J, Lee MK, Ciernikova S, Foretova L, Soucek P, King MC (2006). Spectrum of mutations in BRCA1, BRCA2, CHEK2, and TP53 in families at high risk of breast cancer. JAMA 295: 1379–1388.

1546. Wang H, Ge J, Chen L, Xie P, Chen F, Chen Y (2009). Melanocytic malignant peripheral nerve sheath tumor of the male breast. Breast Care (Basel) 4: 260–262.

1547. Wang N, Leeming R, Abdul-Karim FW (2004). Fine needle aspiration cytology of breast cylindroma in a woman with familial cylindromatosis: a case report. Acta Cytol 48: 853–858.

1548. Wang W (2007). Emergence of a DNA-damage response network consisting of Fanconi anaemia and BRCA proteins. Nat Rev Genet 8: 735–748.

1549. Wang Y, Klijn JG, Zhang Y, Sieuwerts AM, Look MP, Yang F, Talantov D, Timmermans M, Meijer-van Gelder ME, Yu J, Jatkoe T, Berns EM, Atkins D, Foekens JA (2005). Gene-expression profiles to predict distant metastasis of lymph-node-negative primary breast cancer. Lancet 365: 671–679.

1550. Wapnir IL, Dignam JJ, Fisher B, Mamounas EP, Anderson SJ, Julian TB, Land SR, Margolese RG, Swain SM, Costantino JP, Wolmark N (2011). Long-term outcomes of invasive ipsilateral breast tumor recurrences after lumpectomy in NSABP B-17 and B-24 randomized clinical trials for DCIS. J Natl Cancer Inst 103: 478–488.

1551. Ward BA, McKhann CF, Ravikumar TS (1992). Ten-year follow-up of breast carcinoma in situ in Connecticut. Arch Surg 127: 1392–1395.

1551A. Wargotz ES, Deos PH, Norris HJ (1989). Metaplastic carcinomas of the breast. II. Spindle cell carcinoma. Hum Pathol 20: 732–740.

1551B. Wargotz ES, Norris HJ (1989). Metaplastic carcinomas of the breast. I. Matrix-producing carcinoma. Hum Pathol 20: 628–635.

1551C. Wargotz ES, Norris HJ (1989). Metaplastic carcinomas of the breast. III. Carcinosarcoma. Cancer 64: 1490–1499.

1551D. Wargotz ES, Norris HJ (1990). Metaplastic carcinomas of the breast. IV. Squamous cell carcinoma of ductal origin. Cancer 65: 272–276.

1552. Wargotz ES, Norris HJ (1990). Metaplastic carcinomas of the breast: V. Metaplastic carcinoma with osteoclastic giant cells. Hum Pathol 21: 1142–1150.

1553. Wargotz ES, Norris HJ, Austin RM, Enzinger FM (1987). Fibromatosis of the breast. A clinical and pathological study of 28 cases. Am J Surg Pathol 11: 38–45.

1554. Wargotz ES, Weiss SW, Norris HJ (1987). Myofibroblastoma of the breast. Sixteen cases of a distinctive benign mesenchymal tumor. Am J Surg Pathol 11: 493–502.

1555. Warner NE (1969). Lobular carcinoma of the breast. Cancer 23: 840–846.

1556. Watermann DO, Tempfer C, Hefler LA, Parat C, Stickeler E (2005). Ultrasound morphology of invasive lobular breast cancer is different compared with other types of breast cancer. Ultrasound Med Biol 31: 167–174.

1557. Watson CM, Davison AN, Baker D, O'Neill JK, Turk JL (1991). Suppression of demyelination by mitoxantrone. Int J Immunopharmacol 13: 923–930.

1558. Watson P, Lynch HT (2001). Cancer risk in mismatch repair gene mutation carriers. Fam Cancer 1: 57–60.

1559. Watson P, Vasen HF, Mecklin JP, Bernstein I, Aarnio M, Jarvinen HJ, Myrhoj T, Sunde L, Wijnen JT, Lynch HT (2008). The risk of extra-colonic, extra-endometrial cancer in the Lynch syndrome. Int J Cancer 123: 444–449.

1560. Weaver DL (2010). Pathology evaluation of sentinel lymph nodes in breast cancer: protocol recommendations and rationale. Mod Pathol 23 Suppl 2: S26–S32.

1561. Weaver DL, Ashikaga T, Krag DN, Skelly JM, Anderson SJ, Harlow SP, Julian TB, Mamounas EP, Wolmark N (2011). Effect of occult metastases on survival in node-negative breast cancer. N Engl J Med 364: 412–421.

1562. Weaver DL, Le UP, Dupuis SL, Weaver KA, Harlow SP, Ashikaga T, Krag DN (2009). Metastasis detection in sentinel lymph nodes: comparison of a limited widely spaced (NSABP protocol B-32) and a comprehensive narrowly spaced paraffin block sectioning strategy. Am J Surg Pathol 33: 1583–1589.

1563. Weaver J, Billings SD (2009). Postradiation cutaneous vascular tumors of the breast: a review. Semin Diagn Pathol 26: 141–149.

1564. Weaver MG, Abdul-Karim FW, al-Kaisi N (1993). Mucinous lesions of the breast. A pathological continuum. Pathol Res Pract 189: 873–876.

1565. Weidner N, Semple JP (1992). Pleomorphic variant of invasive lobular carcinoma of the breast. Hum Pathol 23: 1167–1171.

1566. Weigelt B, Baehner FL, Reis-Filho JS (2010). The contribution of gene expression profiling to breast cancer classification, prognostication and prediction: a retrospective of the last decade. J Pathol 220: 263–280.

1567. Weigelt B, Geyer FC, Horlings HM, Kreike B, Halfwerk H, Reis-Filho JS (2009). Mucinous and neuroendocrine breast carcinomas are transcriptionally distinct from invasive ductal carcinomas of no special type. Mod Pathol 22: 1401–1414.

1568. Weigelt B, Geyer FC, Natrajan R, Lopez-Garcia MA, Ahmad AS, Savage K, Kreike B, Reis-Filho JS (2010). The molecular underpinning of lobular histological growth pattern: a genome-wide transcriptomic analysis of invasive lobular carcinomas and grade- and molecular subtype-matched invasive ductal carcinomas of no special type. J Pathol 220: 45–57.

1569. Weigelt B, Horlings HM, Kreike B, Hayes MM, Hauptmann M, Wessels LF, de Jong D, Van de Vijver M, Van't Veer LJ, Peterse JL (2008). Refinement of breast cancer classification by molecular characterization of histological special types. J Pathol 216: 141–150.

1569A. Weigelt B, Mackay A, A'Hern R, Natrajan R, Tan DS, Dowsett M et al. (2010). Breast cancer molecular profiling with single sample predictors: a retrospective analysis. Lancet Oncol 11: 339–349.

1569B. Weigelt B, Kreike B, Reis-Filho JS (2009). Metaplastic breast carcinomas are basal-like breast cancers: a genomic profiling analysis. Breast Cancer Res Treat 117: 273–280.

1569C. Weigelt B, Reis-Filho JS (2009). Histological and molecular types of breast cancer: is there a unifying taxonomy? Nat Rev Clin Oncol 6: 718–730.

1570. Weiss JR, Moysich KB, Swede H (2005). Epidemiology of male breast cancer. Cancer Epidemiol Biomarkers Prev 14: 20–26.

1571. Weiss SW, Nickoloff BJ (1993). CD-34 is expressed by a distinctive cell population in peripheral nerve, nerve sheath tumors, and related lesions. Am J Surg Pathol 17: 1039–1045.

1572. Weitzel JN, Pooler PA, Mohammed R, Levitt MD, Eckfeldt JH (1988). A unique case of breast carcinoma producing pancreatic-type isoamylase. Gastroenterology 94: 519–520.

1573. Wellings SR, Jensen HM, Marcum RG (1975). An atlas of subgross pathology of the human breast with special reference to possible precancerous lesions. J Natl Cancer Inst 55: 231–273.

1574. Wells CA, Ferguson DJ (1988). Ultrastructural and immunocytochemical study of a case of invasive cribriform breast carcinoma. J Clin Pathol 41: 17–20.

1574A. Wells CA, Wells CW, Yeomans P, Vina M, Jordan S, d'Ardenne AJ (1990). Spherical connective tissue inclusions in epithelial hyperplasia of the breast ("collagenous spherulosis"). J Clin Pathol 43: 905–908.

1575. Wessels LF, van Welsem T, Hart AA, Van't Veer LJ, Reinders MJ, Nederlof PM (2002). Molecular classification of breast carcinomas by comparative genomic hybridization: a specific somatic genetic profile for BRCA1 tumors. Cancer Res 62: 7110–7117.

1576. Westenend PJ, Schutte R, Hoogmans MM, Wagner A, Dinjens WN (2005). Breast cancer in an MSH2 gene mutation carrier. Hum Pathol 36: 1322–1326.

1577. Weston VJ, Oldreive CE, Skowronska A, Oscier DG, Pratt G, Dyer MJ, Smith G, Powell JE, Rudzki Z, Kearns P, Moss PA, Taylor AM, Stankovic T (2010). The PARP inhibitor olaparib induces significant killing of ATM-deficient lymphoid tumor cells in vitro and in vivo. Blood 116: 4578–4587.

1577A. Wetterskog D, Lopez-Garcia MA, Lambros MB, A'Hern R, Geyer FC, Milanezi F, Cabral MC, Natrajan R, Gauthier A, Shiu KK, Orr N, Shousha S, Gatalica Z, Mackay A, Palacios J, Reis-Filho JS, Weigelt B (2012). Adenoid cystic carcinomas constitute a genomically distinct subgroup of triple-negative and basal-like breast cancers. J Pathol 226:84–96.

1578. White RR, Halperin TJ, Olson JA, Jr, Soo MS, Bentley RC, Seigler HF (2001). Impact of core-needle breast biopsy on the surgical management of mammographic abnormalities. Ann Surg 233: 769–777.

1579. Whittemore AS, Gong G, John EM, McGuire V, Li FP, Ostrow KL, Dicioccio R, Felberg A, West DW (2004). Prevalence of BRCA1 mutation carriers among U.S. non-Hispanic Whites. Cancer Epidemiol Biomarkers Prev 13: 2078–2083.

1580. Whitten TM, Wallace TW, Bird RE, Turk PS (1997). Image-guided core biopsy has advantages over needle localization biopsy for the diagnosis of nonpalpable breast cancer. Am Surg 63: 1072–1077.

1581. Wiechmann L, Sampson M, Stempel M, Jacks LM, Patil SM, King T, Morrow M (2009). Presenting features of breast cancer differ by molecular subtype. Ann Surg Oncol 16: 2705–2710.

1582. Wijnen J, Khan PM, Vasen H, van der Klift H, Mulder A, van Leeuwen-Cornelisse I, Bakker B, Losekoot M, Moller P, Fodde R (1997). Hereditary nonpolyposis colorectal cancer families not complying with the Amsterdam criteria show extremely low frequency of mismatch-repair-gene mutations. Am J Hum Genet 61: 329–335.

1583. Willemze R, Swerdlow SH, Harris NL, Vergier B (2008). Primary cutaneous follicle centre lymphoma. In: WHO classification of tumours of haematopoietic and lymphoid tissues, 4th edition.Swerdlow SH, Campo E, Harris NL, Jaffe ES, Pileri S, Stein H et al. IARC: Lyon: pp 227–228.

1584. Williams SA, Ehlers RA, Hunt KK, Yi M, Kuerer HM, Singletary SE, Ross MI, Feig BW, Symmans WF, Meric-Bernstam F (2007). Metastases to the breast from nonbreast solid neoplasms: presentation and determinants of survival. Cancer 110: 731–737.

1585. Wilson JR, Bateman AC, Hanson H, An Q, Evans G, Rahman N, Jones JL, Eccles DM (2010). A novel HER2-positive breast cancer phenotype arising from germline TP53 mutations. J Med Genet 47: 771–774.

1586. Wimmer K, Etzler J (2008). Constitutional mismatch repair-deficiency syndrome: have we so far seen only the tip of an iceberg? Hum Genet 124: 105–122.

1587. Winchester DJ, Chang HR, Graves TA, Menck HR, Bland KI, Winchester DP (1998). A comparative analysis of lobular and ductal carcinoma of the breast: presentation, treatment, and outcomes. J Am Coll Surg 186: 416–422.

1588. Winnes M, Molne L, Suurkula M, Andren Y, Persson F, Enlund F, Stenman G (2007). Frequent fusion of the CRTC1 and MAML2 genes in clear cell variants of cutaneous hidradenomas. Genes Chromosomes Cancer 46: 559–563.

1589. Wirapati P, Sotiriou C, Kunkel S, Farmer P, Pradervand S, Haibe-Kains B, Desmedt C, Ignatiadis M, Sengstag T, Schutz F, Goldstein DR, Piccart M, Delorenzi M (2008). Meta-analysis of gene expression profiles in breast cancer: toward a unified understanding of breast cancer subtyping and prognosis signatures. Breast Cancer Res 10: R65.

1590. Wiseman C, Liao KT (1972). Primary lymphoma of the breast. Cancer 29: 1705–1712.

1591. Wolff AC, Hammond ME, Schwartz JN, Hagerty KL, Allred DC, Cote RJ, Dowsett M, Fitzgibbons PL, Hanna WM, Langer A, McShane LM, Paik S, Pegram MD, Perez EA, Press MF, Rhodes A, Sturgeon C, Taube SE, Tubbs R, Vance GH et al. (2007). American Society of Clinical Oncology/College of American Pathologists guideline recommendations for human epidermal growth factor receptor 2 testing in breast cancer. J Clin Oncol 25: 118–145.

1592. Wong AK, Lopategui J, Clancy S, Kulber D, Bose S (2008). Anaplastic large cell lymphoma associated with a breast implant capsule: a case report and review of the literature. Am J Surg Pathol 32: 1265–1268.

1593. Wong AY, Salisbury E, Bilous M (2000). Recent developments in stereotactic breast biopsy methodologies: an update for the surgical pathologist. Adv Anat Pathol 7: 26–35.

1594. Wood B, Sterrett G, Frost F, Swarbrick N (2008). Diagnosis of extramammary malignancy metastatic to the breast by fine needle biopsy. Pathology 40: 345–351.

1594A. Woodard BH, Brinkhous AD, McCarty KS, Sr, McCarty KS, Jr (1980). Adenosquamous differentiation in mammary carcinoma: an ultrastructural and steroid receptor study. Arch Pathol Lab Med 104: 130–133.

1595. Woods MO, Williams P, Careen A, Edwards L, Bartlett S, McLaughlin JR, Younghusband HB (2007). A new variant database for mismatch repair genes associated with Lynch syndrome. Hum Mutat 28: 669–673.

1596. Woodward WA, Vinh-Hung V, Ueno NT, Cheng YC, Royce M, Tai P, Vlastos G, Wallace AM, Hortobagyi GN, Nieto Y (2006). Prognostic value of nodal ratios in node-positive breast cancer. J Clin Oncol 24: 2910–2916.

1597. Wooster R, Bignell G, Lancaster J, Swift S, Seal S, Mangion J, Collins N, Gregory S, Gumbs C, Micklem G (1995). Identification of the breast cancer susceptibility gene BRCA2. Nature 378: 789–792.

1598. Wooster R, Neuhausen SL, Mangion J, Quirk Y, Ford D, Collins N, Nguyen K, Seal S, Tran T, Averill D (1994). Localization of a breast cancer susceptibility gene, BRCA2, to chromosome 13q12-13. Science 265: 2088–2090.

1599. World Cancer Research Fund (2007). Food, nutrition, physical activity, and the prevention of cancer: a global perspective. AICR: Washington, DC.

1599A. World Health Organization (1981). Histological typing of breast tumours: international histological classification of tumours, 2nd edition. WHO, Geneva.

1600. Wrba F, Ellinger A, Reiner G, Spona J, Holzner JH (1988). Ultrastructural and immunohistochemical characteristics of lipid-rich carcinoma of the breast. Virchows Arch A Pathol Anat Histopathol 413: 381–385.

1601. Wu CC, Krahe R, Lozano G, Zhang B, Wilson CD, Jo EJ, Amos CI, Shete S, Strong LC (2011). Joint effects of germ-line TP53 mutation, MDM2 SNP309, and gender on cancer risk in family studies of Li-Fraumeni syndrome. Hum Genet 129: 663–673.

1602. Xiao Y, Ye Y, Zou X, Jones S, Yearsley K, Shetuni B, Tellez J, Barsky SH (2011). The lymphovascular embolus of inflammatory breast cancer exhibits a Notch 3 addiction. Oncogene 30: 287–300.

1603. Yamaguchi R, Tanaka M, Kondo K, Yokoyama T, Kaneko Y, Yamaguchi M, Ogata Y, Nakashima O, Kage M, Yano H (2010). Characteristic morphology of invasive micropapillary carcinoma of the breast: an immunohistochemical analysis. Jpn J Clin Oncol 40: 781–787.

1604. Yang H, Ahmed I, Mathew V, Schroeter AL (2006). Diffuse dermal angiomatosis of the breast. Arch Dermatol 142: 343–347.

1605. Yang H, Jeffrey PD, Miller J, Kinnucan E, Sun Y, Thoma NH, Zheng N, Chen PL, Lee WH, Pavletich NP (2002). BRCA2 function in DNA binding and recombination from a BRCA2-DSS1-ssDNA structure. Science 297: 1837–1848.

1606. Yang M, Moriya T, Oguma M, De La Cruz C, Endoh M, Ishida T, Hirakawa H, Orita Y, Ohuchi N, Sasano H (2003). Microinvasive ductal carcinoma (T1mic) of the breast. The clinicopathological profile and immunohistochemical features of 28 cases. Pathol Int 53: 422–428.

1607. Yap J, Chuba PJ, Thomas R, Aref A, Lucas D, Severson RK, Hamre M (2002). Sarcoma as a second malignancy after treatment for breast cancer. Int J Radiat Oncol Biol Phys 52: 1231–1237.

1608. Yilmaz E, Sal S, Lebe B (2002). Differentiation of phyllodes tumors versus fibroadenomas. Acta Radiol 43: 34–39.

1609. Yoo JL, Woo OH, Kim YK, Cho KR, Yong HS, Seo BK, Kim A, Kang EY (2010). Can MR Imaging contribute in characterizing well-circumscribed breast carcinomas? Radiographics 30: 1689–1702.

1609A. Yorozuya K, Takeuchi T, Yoshida M, Mouri Y, Kousaka J, Fujii K et al. (2010). Evaluation of Oncotype DX Recurrence Score as a prognostic factor in Japanese women with estrogen receptor-positive, node-negative primary Stage I or IIA breast cancer. J Cancer Res Clin Oncol 136: 939–944.

1610. Yoshida S, Nakamura N, Sasaki Y, Yoshida S, Yasuda M, Sagara H, Ohtake T, Takenoshita S, Abe M (2005). Primary breast diffuse large B-cell lymphoma shows a non-germinal center B-cell phenotype. Mod Pathol 18: 398–405.

1611. Young RH, Clement PB (1988). Adenomyoepithelioma of the breast. A report of three cases and review of the literature. Am J Clin Pathol 89: 308–314.

1612. Youngson BJ, Cranor M, Rosen PP (1994). Epithelial displacement in surgical breast specimens following needling procedures. Am J Surg Pathol 18: 896–903.

1613. Yu GH, Fishman SJ, Brooks JS (1993). Cellular angiolipoma of the breast. Mod Pathol 6: 497–499.

1614. Yu JI, Choi DH, Park W, Huh SJ, Cho EY, Lim YH, Ahn JS, Yang JH, Nam SJ (2010). Differences in prognostic factors and patterns of failure between invasive micropapillary carcinoma and invasive ductal carcinoma of the breast: matched case-control study. Breast 19: 231–237.

1615. Yu K, Lee CH, Tan PH, Hong GS, Wee SB, Wong CY, Tan P (2004). A molecular signature of the Nottingham prognostic index in breast cancer. Cancer Res 64: 2962–2968.

1616. Yuan JM, Wang XL, Xiang YB, Gao YT, Ross RK, Yu MC (2000). Non-dietary risk factors for nasopharyngeal carcinoma in Shanghai, China. Int J Cancer 85: 364–369.

1617. Zafrani B, Aubriot MH, Mouret E, De Cremoux P, De Rycke Y, Nicolas A, Boudou E, Vincent-Salomon A, Magdelenat H, Sastre-Garau X (2000). High sensitivity and specificity of immunohistochemistry for the detection of hormone receptors in breast carcinoma: comparison with biochemical determination in a prospective study of 793 cases. Histopathology 37: 536–545.

1618. Zakaria S, Pantvaidya G, Ghosh K, Degnim AC (2007). Paget's disease of the breast: accuracy of preoperative assessment. Breast Cancer Res Treat 102: 137–142.

1619. Zaloudek C, Oertel YC, Orenstein JM (1984). Adenoid cystic carcinoma of the breast. Am J Clin Pathol 81: 297–307.

1620. Zamecnik M, Michal M, Gogora M, Mukensnabl P, Dobias V, Vano M (2002). Gynecomastia with pseudoangiomatous stromal hyperplasia and multinucleated giant cells. Association with neurofibromatosis type 1. Virchows Arch 441: 85–87.

1621. Zandrino F, Calabrese M, Faedda C, Musante F (2006). Tubular carcinoma of the breast: pathological, clinical, and ultrasonographic findings. A review of the literature. Radiol Med 111: 773–782.

1622. Zekioglu O, Erhan Y, Ciris M, Bayramoglu H, Ozdemir N (2004). Invasive micropapillary carcinoma of the breast: high incidence of lymph node metastasis with extranodal extension and its immunohistochemical profile compared with invasive ductal carcinoma. Histopathology 44: 18–23.

1623. Zhang S, Phelan CM, Zhang P, Rousseau F, Ghadirian P, Robidoux A, Foulkes W, Hamel N, McCready D, Trudeau M, Lynch H, Horsman D, De Matsuda ML, Aziz Z, Gomes M, Costa MM, Liede A, Poll A, Sun P, Narod SA (2008). Frequency of the CHEK2 1100delC mutation among women with breast cancer: an international study. Cancer Res 68: 2154–2157.

1624. Zhang SM, Willett WC, Selhub J, Hunter DJ, Giovannucci EL, Holmes MD, Colditz GA, Hankinson SE (2003). Plasma folate, vitamin B6, vitamin B12, homocysteine, and risk of breast cancer. J Natl Cancer Inst 95: 373–380.

1625. Zhao H, Langerod A, Ji Y, Nowels KW, Nesland JM, Tibshirani R, Bukholm IK, Karesen R, Botstein D, Borresen-Dale AL, Jeffrey SS (2004). Different gene expression patterns in invasive lobular and ductal carcinomas of the breast. Mol Biol Cell 15: 2523–2536.

1626. Zhao J, Lang R, Guo X, Chen L, Gu F, Fan Y, Fu L (2010). Clinicopathologic characteristics of pleomorphic carcinoma of the breast. Virchows Arch 456: 31–37.

1626A. Zelek L, Llombart-Cussac A, Terrier P, Pivot X, Guinebretiere JM, Le PC, Tursz T, Rochard F, Spielmann M, Le CA (2003). Prognostic factors in primary breast sarcomas: a series of patients with long-term follow-up. J Clin Oncol 21: 2583–2588.

1626B. Zheng W, Long J, Gao YT, Li C, Zheng Y, Xiang YB, Wen W, Levy S, Deming SL, Haines JL, Gu K, Fair AM, Cai Q, Lu W, Shu XO (2009). Genome-wide association study identifies a new breast cancer susceptibility locus at 6q25.1. Nat Genet 41: 324–328.

1627. Zhou X, Hampel H, Thiele H, Gorlin RJ, Hennekam RC, Parisi M, Winter RM, Eng C (2001). Association of germline mutation in the PTEN tumour suppressor gene and Proteus and Proteus-like syndromes. Lancet 358: 210–211.

1628. Zhou XP, Waite KA, Pilarski R, Hampel H, Fernandez MJ, Bos C, Dasouki M, Feldman GL, Greenberg LA, Ivanovich J, Matloff E, Patterson A, Pierpont ME, Russo D, Nassif NT, Eng C (2003). Germline PTEN promoter mutations and deletions in Cowden/Bannayan-Riley-Ruvalcaba syndrome result in aberrant PTEN protein and dysregulation of the phosphoinositol-3-kinase/Akt pathway. Am J Hum Genet 73: 404–411.

1629. Ziegler RG, Hoover RN, Nomura AM, West DW, Wu AH, Pike MC, Lake AJ, Horn-Ross PL, Kolonel LN, Siiteri PK, Fraumeni JF, Jr (1996). Relative weight, weight change, height, and breast cancer risk in Asian-American women. J Natl Cancer Inst 88: 650–660.

1630. Zou D, Yoon HS, Perez D, Weeks RJ, Guilford P, Humar B (2009). Epigenetic silencing in non-neoplastic epithelia identifies E-cadherin (CDH1) as a target for chemoprevention of lobular neoplasia. J Pathol 218: 265–272.

1631. Zubor P, Kajo K, Dussan CA, Szunyogh N, Danko J (2006). Rapidly growing nodular pseudoangiomatous stromal hyperplasia of the breast in an 18-year-old girl. APMIS 114: 389–392.

Subject index